# HEADACHE AND MIGRAINE IN CHILDHOOD AND ADOLESCENCE

Edited by

**Vincenzo Guidetti** MD PhD
*Department of Neurological and Psychiatric Sciences*
*University 'La Sapienza'*
*Rome*
*Italy*

**George Russell** MB FRCP FRCPE FRCPCH
*Reader (part-time)*
*Department of Child Health*
*University of Aberdeen Medical School*
*Aberdeen*
*UK*
*and*
*Honorary Consultant in Medical Paediatrics*
*Royal Aberdeen Children's Hospital*
*Aberdeen*
*UK*

**Matti Sillanpää** MD PhD
*Professor and Head*
*Department of Child Neurology*
*University of Turku Hospital TYKS*
*Turku*
*Finland*

**Paul Winner** MD
*Clinical Associate Professor of Neurology*
*Premiere Research Institute*
*Palm Beach Headache Center*
*West Palm Beach*
*USA*

MARTIN DUNITZ

© 2002 Martin Dunitz Ltd, a member of the Taylor & Francis group

First published in the United Kingdom in 2002 by Martin Dunitz Ltd, The Livery House, 7–9 Pratt Street, London NW1 0AE

Tel: +44 (0) 20 7482 2202
Fax: +44 (0) 20 7267 0159
E-mail: info@dunitz.co.uk
Webiste: http://www.dunitz.co.uk

A CIP record for this book is available from the British Library.

ISBN 1-85317-810-1

Although every effort has been made to ensure that all owners of copyright material have been acknowledged in this publication, we would be glad to acknowledge in subsequent reprints or editions any omissions brought to our attention.

Distributed in the USA by
Fulfilment Center
Taylor & Francis
7625 Empire Drive
Florence, KY 41042, USA
Toll Free Tel.: +1 800 634 7064
E-mail: cserve@routledge_ny.com

Distributed in Canada by
Taylor & Francis
74 Rolark Drive
Scarborough, Ontario M1R 4G2, Canada
Toll Free Tel.: +1 877 226 2237
E-mail: tal_fran@istar.ca

Distributed in the rest of the world by
ITPS Limited
Cheriton House
North Way
Andover, Hampshire SP10 5BE, UK
Tel.: +44 (0)1264 332424
E-mail: reception@itps.co.uk

Composition by Wearset Ltd, Boldon, Tyne and Wear
Printed in Great Britain by Biddles Ltd, Guildford and King's Lynn

# CONTENTS

# Contributors

**Frank Andrasik** PhD
Senior Research Scientist
Professor of Psychology
Institute for Human and Machine
Cognition
University of West Florida
Pensacola FL 32501
USA

**Maria Bardare** MD
Pediatric Department
University of Milan
20122 Milan
Italy

**Gianfranco Brunelli** MD
Pediatric Department
University of Milan
20122 Milan
Italy

**Oliviero Bruni** MD
Center for Pediatric Sleep Disorders
Department of Developmental Neurology
and Psychiatry
University 'La Sapienza'
00185 Rome
Italy

**Gennaro Bussone** MD
Headache Center
Department of Neurology
National Neurological Institute 'Carlo
Besta'
20133 Milan
Italy

**Sandra Capuccini**
Clinical Psychologist
Department of
Childhood and Adolescent Neurology and
Psychiatry
University 'La Sapienza'
00185 Rome
Italy

**Antonella Cerquiglini** MD
Assistant Professor
Department of Developmental
Neuropsychiatry
University 'La Sapienza'
00185 Rome
Italy

**Alessandra Cherchi** MD
Headache Centre
Department of Neurosciences 'BB Brodie'
University of Cagliari
09124 Cagliari
Italy

**Domenico D'Amico**
Neurologist
Headache Center
Department of Neurology
National Neurological Institute 'Carlo
Besta'
20133 Milan
Italy

**Maria Del Zompo** MD
Headache Centre
Department of Neurosciences 'BB Brodie'
University of Cagliari
09124 Cagliari
Italy

**Deusvenir de Souza Carvalho** MD PhD
Professor of Neurology and Head of
Headache Investigation and Treatment
Sector
Discipline of Neurology and Neurosurgery
Federal University of São Paulo
São Paolo-SP
Brazil

**Fabio Facchinetti** MD
University Centre of Adaptive Disorders
and Headache
Department of Gynaecologic, Obstetric
and Pediatric Sciences
University of Modena and Reggio Emilia
41100 Modena
Italy

**Victor Farkas** MD
University Children's Hospital Budapest
Bokay 53
H-1083 Budapest
Hungary

**Tiziana Franceschini**
Child and Clinical Psychologist
Department of Childhood and Adolescent
Neurology and Psychiatry
University 'La Sapienza'
00185 Rome
Italy

**Federica Galli**
Clinical Psychologist
Department of Childhood and Adolescent
Neurology and Psychiatry
University 'La Sapienza'
00185 Rome
Italy

**Jack Gladstein** MD
Associate Dean for Student Affairs
Associate Professor of Pediatrics
Director, Pediatric Headache Clinic
University of Maryland, School of Medicine
Baltimore MD 20742
USA

**Peter J Goadsby**
Professor of Clinical Neurology
Institute of Neurology
The National Hospital
London WC1N 3BG
UK

**Licia Grazzi** MD
Headache Center
Department of Neurology
National Neurological Institute 'Carlo
Besta'
20133 Milan
Italy

**Vincenzo Guidetti** MD PhD
Department of Neurological and
Psychiatric Sciences
University 'La Sapienza'
00185 Rome
Italy

**Antonio Gullì**
Clinical Psychologist
Department of Childhood and Adolescent
Neurology and Psychiatry
University 'La Sapienza'
00185 Rome
Italy

**Bo Larsson** MD
Associate Professor
Department of Public Healthcare and
Caring Sciences
Uppsala Science Park
S-75183 Uppsala
Sweden

**Antonio La Vitola** MD
Corso Mazzini vico V 1
88100 Catanzaro
Italy

**Massimo Leone** MD
Headache Center
Department of Neurology
National Neurological Institute 'Carlo Besta'
20133 Milan
Italy

**Donald Lewis** MD FAAN FAAP
Associate Professor of Neurology
Children's Hospital of
The King's Daughters
Eastern Virginia Medical School
Norfolk VA 23510
USA

**Vanessa Lilliu** PhD
Child Neurology and Psychiatry Unit
Department of Neurosciences 'BB Brodie'
University of Cagliari
09124 Cagliari
Italy

**Liisa Metsähonkala** MD PhD
Department of Pediatrics
University of Turku Central Hospital
TYKS
20520 Turku
Finland

**Pasquale Montagna** MD
Institute of Neurology
University of Bologna
40123 Bologna
Italy

**Antonio Pascotto** MD
Professor of Childhood and Adolescent
Neurology and Psychiatry
Second University of Naples
80138 Naples
Italy

**J Passchier** PhD
Department of Medical Psychology and
Psychotherapy
Erasmus University Rotterdam
3000 DR Rotterdam
The Netherlands

**Francesco Peltrone** MD
Via Antonio Daniele
88100 Catanzaro
Italy

**Raymund Pothmann**
SPZ- Ev. Krankenhaus
D-46047 Oberhausen
Germany

**Livia N Rossi** MD
Pediatric Department
University of Milan
20122 Milan
Italy

**George Russell** MB FRCP FRCPE FRCPCH
Reader (part-time)
Department of Child Health
University of Aberdeen Medical School
Aberdeen AB9 2ZD
UK
and
Honorary Consultant in Medical
Paediatrics
Royal Aberdeen Children's Hospital
Aberdeen AB25 2ZG
UK

**Stefano Seri** MD
Director, Paediatric Neuroscience
Programme
Department of Clinical Neurophysiology
The Birmingham Children's Hospital
Birmingham B4 6NH
UK
and
Professor of Developmental
Neuropsychiatry
University 'Tor Vergata'
00133 Rome
Italy

**Laura Sgarbi**
University Centre of Adaptive Disorders
and Headache
Department of Gynaecologic, Obstetric
and Pediatric Sciences
University of Modena and Reggio Emilia
41100 Modena
Italy

**Matti Sillanpää** MD PhD
Professor and Head, Department of Child
Neurology
University of Turku Central Hospital
TYKS
20520 Turku
Finland

**David NK Symon** BSc MB ChB FRCP
FRCPCH AIL
Consultant Paediatrician
General Hospital
Hartlepool
TS24 9AH
UK

**Mimma Tafà** PhD
Child and Clinical Psychologist
Family Psychotherapist
University 'La Sapienza'
00185 Rome
Italy

**Francesca Tagliente** MD PhD
Second University of Naples
80138 Naples
Italy

**Susanna Usai** MD
Headache Center
Department of Neurology
National Neurological Institute 'Carlo
Besta'
20133 Milan
Italy

**Paul Winner** DO FANN FAAP
Clinical Associate Professor of Neurology
Premiere Research Institute
Palm Beach Headache Center
5205 Greenwood Avenue
West Palm Beach
Florida
USA

**Çiçek Wöber-Bingöl** MD
Department of Neuropsychiatry of
Childhood and Adolescence
A-1090 Vienna
Austria

**Alessandro Zuddas** MD
Child Neurology and Psychiatry Unit
Department of Neurosciences 'BB Brodie'
University of Cagliari
09124 Cagliari
Italy

# Preface

From Neolithic times to the era of Hippocrates and Plato, history has recorded headache and included it in the mythology of different ages. The foundations of current research into headache in children and adolescents were laid in the 1960s by Bo Bille (Sweden) with his fundamental work 'Migraine in schoolchildren' (1962); during the same period, in Italy Roberto Mayer studied the interplay between organic and psychological development of headache ('La cafalea nell'età evolutiva', 1964). In the 1970s and 1980s, Charles Barlow and Giovanni Lanzi established further keystones in migraine with their books 'Headaches and Migraine' (1984) and the great 'La cefalea essenziale in età evolutiva' (1980) respectively, as did Judith Hockaday and Michael Noronha in the UK in 1988. Without the efforts of all these people, this book would not have been possible.

This book covers the latest treatment and research that has followed the work of those mentioned above. As with many medical specialties, the tendency to treat the child patient as simply a 'miniature adult' does not always work in treating pediatric disease and this distinction is at the forefront of this text. The problems of diagnosis and communication with the very young patient are discussed, and emphasis is placed on the need for understanding and assistance from parents, teachers and other carers. The pathophysiology and the genetics of headache and migraine are substantially covered, as well as the psychological aspects of headache. A variety of treatments is discussed, including psychotherapy, and relaxation and biofeedback treatments. A substantial section is devoted to pediatric and adolescent migraine that has yet to receive its own standardized criteria. A wide range of types of headache are included, thus making this the definitive and most comprehensive book on this subject.

We would like to thank the authors who contributed to this text; their devotion and efforts are much appreciated. Our gratitude also goes to our former and present scholars whose guidance and instruction have been invaluable, in particular to: Dr Randy Peterson, Dr Isabelle Rapin, Dr Alfred Spiro, Dr Niko Moshe, Dr S Schinnar and Dr Seymour Solomon.

*Vincenzo Guidetti, Rome*
*George Russell, Aberdeen*
*Matti Sillanpää, Turku*
*Paul Winner, West Palm Beach*

# I

## Introduction

# 1

# What is hidden behind headache?

*Vincenzo Guidetti, Federica Galli*

It may be surprising to read how many factors are hypothesized to be related to headache (migraine or tension-type) in children and adolescents from both the somatic perspective (allergies, ocular or mandibular problems, constipation, epilepsy, sleep disorders, periodic syndromes) and the psychological one (anxiety, depression, panic, school phobia, lack of concentration, hyperactivity, stress). It is more difficult relating the conditions to headache in a deterministic way (cause–effect), attaining evidence of common predisposing biological substrate or excluding a chance occurrence.

This kind of situation may represent a 'paradigm' of the link between somatic and psychological aspects involved in childhood headache, even though the theme draws issues of wide-ranging interest. Nowadays, increasing attention is dedicated to the importance of getting over the nature/nurture, body/mind or mind/brain dichotomies. The challenge is finding the *rationale* supporting this view, as well as recognizing and accepting weak points of the current status of our knowledge in many fields.

Headache may be seen as a 'distillate' of the strict embedding of variables of nature (genetic), nurture (environment), body–brain (pathophysiology) and mind (emotion, affects). The immediate challenge is finding

reciprocal connections, links between these different dimensions, on the basis of developmental processes. Closure within its own sub-specialty risks limiting the comprehension of and intervention on 'that headache in that patient'. Perhaps, a few pathologies such as headache may need a great deal of expertise in different fields, from diagnosis to treatment.

Neuroscience, neurology, developmental psychology and psychiatry often continue to work in isolation. However, recent study of the human brain by new imaging techniques (computed tomography [CT], magnetic resonance imaging [MRI], functional MRI, MR spectroscopy, positron emission tomography [PET], single photon emission CT [SPECT]) shows that the links between neurology, psychiatry and psychology are not as great as has been thought for a long time, giving a new common foundation and evidence-based language for different areas of research and clinical work.[1] Better communication between different fields of research (from neurology to psychiatry, paediatrics to psychology) could represent an opportunity for a reciprocal enrichment.

Biological functions are influenced, mediated and often elicited by only environmental and social factors. The acquisition of schemata (e.g. reading, writing, language, etc.) during childhood changes the functional neuroanatomy of the brain. Modern neurosciences have soundly supported the fact that the organisms are the product of the interaction of the genes and the environment. 'Anatomical changes in the brain occur throughout the life and are likely to shape the skills and character of an individual'.[2]

This book attempts to synthesize concepts and findings from a wide range of scientific disciplines, obviously focusing on headache, but considering headache as a symptom to be decoded. The primary headache is one of the most diffuse disorders in childhood and adolescence, but many questions about the aetiology, diagnosis and therapy are unsolved. Developmental issues need careful attention. Primary headache (both migraine and tension-type) has a high tendency to change or to remit spontaneously,[3–6] assuming over time age-related features that should be considered in the diagnosis and treatment.[7] Factors predicting the evolution of headache are poorly investigated, even if there is evidence for the negative prognostic value of co-morbid psychiatric disorders,[8] i.e. we are dealing with clinical situations with a natural tendency to change over time.[7] Furthermore, the co-morbid and developmental factors may play a crucial role in influencing headache. It is necessary to stress the wide professional background and the multiplicity of specialties that are needed to handle headache in childhood and adolescence, together with the crucial importance of knowledge about the normal and problematic steps of the developmental ages. This explains the number of chapters that are dedicated to the analysis of co-morbid factors in the headache field and to the psychological framing of patient, by both the normal and the pathological views.

A child is not a 'little adult' and many individual factors can affect the expression of headaches. It is crucial to avoid a restraining and unilateral approach to young patients, beginning by considering the child as a whole in his or her physical and psychological development, and taking into account neurobiological and psychological maturational processes, and familial and social environmental factors. These aspects stress the wide range of competence needed to work in the headache field, some dealing more with the developmental age.

Interpersonal relationships early in life may shape the subsequent patterns of relationships through life, as well as the physiological responses and the ability to cope with future stressful events.[9] The younger the child, the more the body is the main means of communicating discomfort, worries and anxiety. Whether headache may also be a way of communicating these aspects explains the number of chapters of the book dedicated to the psychological factors in developmental, diagnostic and treatment terms. The term 'psychosomatic' is increasingly being replaced by the terms 'biopsychosocial', 'biobehavioural', 'psychophysiological', 'psychoneuroimmunological', etc. These changes denote the multiple causality lying beneath illness, and the importance of genetic, biological, physiological, environmental, social and cultural factors in determining illness.

The problem of the interaction between 'psyche' and 'soma' dates back to the times of Socrates and Hippocrates, currently remaining an intriguing and enigmatic field of interest. The definition of 'psychosomatic disorder' requires, at first, an explanation of the meaning of the term.

Currently, psychosomatic theories outline the complexity and non-linearity of the mind–body relationship. Genetic, physiological, social and psychological variables seem to be differently involved in determining the individual response to diseases. The mind–body relationship raises additional questions when we refer to developmental age. The difficulty of explaining psychological disease verbally can facilitate the 'body way' of communicating it to the environment, to obtain attention or to avoid fearful situations.

We do not know how this primary mode of communication can influence subsequent patterns, with the body as the first choice for expressing diseases. Modern neuroscience supports the inseparability of the mind and brain. The complex interplay between brain structure and social influences represents a point that is now unquestionable, and the consequences need to be taken into account in any field of research and clinical work.

External factors have a critical role to play, starting with the regulation of gene expression. Each gene has a double function: a *template* function that guarantees the fidelity of replication and a *transcriptional* function that is responsive to environmental factors.[10] Exposure to adverse early environments may underlie vulnerability to, and later expression of, physio- and/or psychopathology.[9,11,12] The interaction between the primary caregivers and their offspring is one of the most important early life influences ('attachment system') in shaping the development of personality and psychopathology, along with genetic influences.[9,13,14] Repetitive painful experiences and prolonged exposure to analgesic drugs may alter neuronal and synaptic experiences permanently, even though the plasticity of developing neurons may determine improvement over growth.[15]

Access to pain experiences of infants and analysis of the involved mechanisms may be troublesome and reductive, if we do not take into consideration the complexity of pain experience in a biopsychosocial perspective. 'Pain is always embedded in a complex matrix of biologic, psychological and social interactions', 'clinical pain can never be seen as primarily a biologic phenomenon or as only a psychological event, nor can pain be divorced from the social context'.[16] Factors such as cognitive maturation, language development, self-regulation capabilities, and cultural, familial and individual attributions about pain contribute individually and in combination to the pain experience and to the development of chronic pain.[17] The developmental point of view should always represent the main perspective for analysing pain in general, and head pain specifically. On the basis of an age-related background, pain modulation, transmission and communication involve neurochemical and neurosignalling mechanisms, as well as temperamental, stress-related, cognitive, familial, social and cultural variables. No consideration of the implication of each of these factors may risk weakening our intervention by the use of adult-focused categories of diagnosis and treatment (the child as 'miniature' adult): an approach that is simpler to apply, but limited. However, the sum of the above-mentioned factors is never linear, and the result is always different by the simple total of the single factors.

The complexity of framing head pain is partly related to the difficulties of taking into consideration each of these aspects, in the reciprocal interplay. The mechanism (the relative weight) of each factor is unknown, but it requires consideration in the general framing of head pain, to understand how each element is implicated in 'causing', 'triggering' or 'maintaining' headache over time.

The presence of a genetic liability to headache does not itself exclude the influences of 'external' factors in modulating or triggering headache crises. The joint effect of genetic and specific individual factors on recurrent headaches[18] requires close attention, inasmuch as they should be seen from the perspective of their mutual interplay.

This book represents a great effort to provide a comprehensive framework for the diagnosis and treatment of headache in childhood and adolescence. A cross-section of the contents of each chapter gives an indication of the number of topics related to headache. However, a lot of points need to be cleared up. It is likely that only multidisciplinary work may provide elements for framing 'the headaches' both in a theoretical perspective and in clinical practice. This is the challenge for the immediate future.

The desire for certain and definitive explanations about what happens around us, and putting into definitive categories, is part of the human natural tendency to systematize and organize reality. The natural tendency of clinicians to avoid admissions of ignorance collude with the families' difficulties in not having a clear diagnosis and definite treatments. To date, the current status of scientific knowledge about headache does not allow us to draw clear-cut conclusions about several aspects of headaches. Based on an evidence-based background, it is incumbent upon us to tell, and motivate, our patients and their families that 'to date, we do not know why . . .'.

# References

1. Price BH, Adams RD, Coyle JT, Neurology and psychiatry – closing the great divide. *Neurology* 2000; **54**: 8–14.
2. Kandel ER, Biology and the future of psychoanalysis: A new intellectual framework for psychiatry revisited. *Am J Psychiatry* 1999; **156**: 505–24.
3. Bille B, The prognosis of migraine in schoolchildren. *Acta Paediatr Scand Suppl* 1973; **236**: 38.
4. Bille B, Migraine in childhood and its prognosis. *Cephalalgia* 1981; **1**: 71–5.
5. Dooley J, Bagnell A, The prognosis and treatment of headaches in children—a ten year follow-up. *Can J Neurol Sci* 1995; **22**: 47–9.
6. Guidetti V, Galli F, Evolution of headache in childhood and adolescence: an 8-year follow-up. *Cephalalgia* 1998; **18**: 450–4.
7. Guidetti V, Galli F, Cerutti R, Fortugno S, 'From 0 to 18': what happens to the child and his headache. *Funct Neurol* 2000; **15**(suppl 3): 89–105.
8. Guidetti V, Galli F, Fabrizi P et al, Headache and psychiatric comorbidity: clinical aspects and outcome in an 8-year follow-up study. *Cephalalgia* 1998; **18**: 455–62.
9. Ladd CO, Hout RL, Thrivikraman KV, Nemeroff CB, Meaney MJ, Plotsky PM, Long-term behavioral and neuroendocrine adaptations to adverse early experience. In: Mayer EA, Saper CB, eds, *Progress in Brain Research – The biological basis for mind brain interactions*, Vol 122. Oxford: Elsevier Science BV, 2000: 81–103.
10. Kandel ER, A new intellectual framework for psychiatry. *Am J Psychiatry* 1998; **155**: 457–69.
11. Cui X, Vaillant GE, Antecedents and consequences of negative life events in adulthood: a longitudinal study. *Am J Psychiatry* 1996; **152**: 21–6.
12. Young EA, Abelson JL, Curtis GC, Nesse RM, Childhood and vulnerability to mood and anxiety disorders. *Depression Anxiety* 1997; **5**: 66–72.
13. McGue M, Bouchard TJ, Genetic and environmental influence on human behavioural influences on human behavioural differences. *Annu Rev Neurosci* 1998; **21**: 1–24.
14. Bowlby J, The making and breaking of affectionals. I. Aetiology and psychopathology in

the light of attachment theory. An expanded version of the Fiftieth Maudsley Lecture, delivered before the Royal College of Psychiatrists, 19 November 1976. *Br J Psychiatry* 1977; **130:** 201–10.

15. Anand KJS, Effects of perinatal pain and stress. In: Mayer EA, Saper CB, eds, *Progress in Brain Research – The biological basis for mind brain interactions*, Vol 122. Oxford: Elsevier Science BV, 2000: 17–29.

16. McGrath PJ, Developmental and psychological factors in children's pain. *Pediatr Clin North Am* 1989; **36:** 823–36.

17. Zeltzer L, Bursch B, Walco G, Pain responsiveness and chronic pain: a psychobiological perspective. *Dev Behav Pediatr* 1997; **18:** 413–22.

18. Svensson DA, Larsson B, Lichtenstein P, Genetic and environmental influences on recurrent headaches in eight to nine-year-old twins. *Cephalalgia* 1999, **19:** 866–72.

# II

## Pathophysiology

# 2

# Neurophysiology

*Stefano Seri, Antonella Cerquiglini*

The literature on neurophysiological correlates of migraine is incredibly extensive. In their updated and thorough review, Schoenen and Thomsen[1] selected 143 references, and a far greater number of clinical studies can be found through a Medline search. The difficulty in extracting meaningful information from such a potential wealth of data mainly lies in the variability in study design and methods, and the lack of normative data. This problem is even more striking when we review the sparse literature about children, most of which provides only interesting but anecdotal reports.

In the past decade, in parallel with the increasing sophistication in the techniques of investigating brain morphology and function in vivo, we have witnessed a growth in the understanding of the biological and clinical correlates of the migraine attack. This vast armamentarium has inherent strengths and weaknesses, which need to be understood to exploit their potential as diagnostic and research tools fully. The high spatial resolution of magnetic resonance imaging (MRI) and positron emission tomography (PET) and the millisecond time resolution of such electrophysiological techniques as MEG/EEG (magnetoencephalography/electroencephalography) can potentially provide us with an accurate description of the biological substrates of the migrainous brain in both adults and children. Computer manipulation of biomedical imaging has recently allowed co-registration and fusioning of morphological and functional images to enhance their respective merits. In this chapter we will mainly focus on electrophysiological data and briefly review human models relevant to the pathogenesis of the migraine attack. We also present some original findings on the use of brain electrophysiological imaging in childhood migraine to highlight the possible further mileage inherent in these study techniques.

## Genotype–phenotype relationships

Susceptibility to migraine is thought to be genetically determined, with aggregation in families as a result of a combination of environmental and genetic tendencies. Twin studies have established the multifactorial nature of migraine, with hereditability approaching 50%. In spite of this compelling evidence, familial hemiplegic migraine (FHM) is the only clinical form in which a strong genetic linkage has been isolated. About 50% of families with FHM have a linkage to chromosome 19p13. Mutations have been demonstrated for some families in a brain-expressed calcium channel $\alpha_{1A}$ subunit (CACNA1A). Genetic heterogeneity has also been described.[2] Based on this evidence, the hypothesis that migraine might be a channelopathy has been put forward. However, a purely genetic model of migraine fails to account for the wide variability in the phenotype of migraine sufferers, particularly in children. The occurrence of pure migraine forms in children is a rare occurrence, and symptoms follow an age-related pattern.

A high variability in precipitating factors has also been reported, including foods, stressors and visual stimuli. In a recent Danish study, the problem of genotype–environment interaction was addressed.[3] The best fitting model implied that the liability to migraine without aura resulted from additive genetic effects (61%) and individual-specific environmental effects (39%), indicating that genetic factors play a role in the aetiology of migraine without aura, irrespective of sex. Environmental factors are equally important and these factors are individual to the migraineurs. It is reasonable to believe that the biological substrate (the quantitative differences in excitatory amino acids, opiates, electrolytes, etc.) acts by rendering the central nervous system (CNS) more reactive and vulnerable to changes in the internal and external environments. The relative immaturity of the child's brain could then be responsible for the lack of specificity in the clinical manifestations.

## Cortical spreading depression

The best studied phenomenon and model of the migraine attack is the cortical spreading depression (CSD) of Leao. This disturbance of the cerebral cortical function is associated with metabolic and haemodynamic changes, which have been summarized in recent studies.[4] From the electrophysiological point of view, the main neuronal and glial cell changes include an initial depolarization associated with an increase in extracellular potassium, followed by a short-lasting depression of electrical activity. At the biochemical level, glutamate seems to play a key role, through one of its receptors, the $N$-methyl-D-aspartate (NMDA) receptor.[5] Glutamate increase is caused by a $K^+$-induced removal of the voltage-sensitive $Mg^{2+}$ blockade of NMDA receptors. This, in turn, is responsible for an influx in $Ca^{2+}$, which is accompanied by an increase in nitric oxide (NO) synthesis. The crucial role of extracellular $K^+$ is in agreement with recent findings, suggesting that impairment in glial-cell function (the major scavenger of extracellular $K^+$) can increase the susceptibility of neural tissue to CSD.[6]

The haemodynamic changes associated with CSD are an early and short-lasting vasoconstriction with consequent reduction in regional cerebral blood flow (rCBF),[7] followed by a transient increased cortical flow lasting 1–2 min, and in the later stages by a persistent flow reduction and hypoperfusion lasting up to 1 hour in experimental animals.[8] This phenomenon has been demonstrated in adult patients suffering from migraine using MEG techniques and consists of suppression of spontaneous cortical activity, long duration field changes and large amplitude waves (LAW) of several seconds' duration.[9]

Although changes in rCBF in CSD are strikingly similar to those reported in patients during spontaneous migraine attacks, the mechanisms linking oligaemia to the localized pain is still poorly understood. Some studies have suggested that the pain of migraine is probably mediated via the trigeminal nerve, which releases vasoactive peptides, leading to dilatation of the greater blood vessels.[10]

# Functional imaging data

The concept of idiopathic or primary headache, including migraine, is based on the assumption that this condition is the result of an abnormal brain function with completely normal brain structure. In a retrospective study conducted in an unselected fashion on children referred to a paediatric outpatient clinic for evaluation of headache over a 2-year period, only 3.8% of the patients had an abnormal imaging study.[11] In all of them, CT or MRI findings were not related to the presenting complaint. Recently, some compelling evidence from a study on specific clinical types of headache has, however, challenged this concept of normal structural background. In a quantitative MRI analysis using voxel-based morphometry, May and co-workers[12] were able to identify increased grey matter volume in the inferoposterior hypothalamus, which co-localized with ictal and interictal PET abnormalities. No differences were seen between a subgroup recorded in headache-free state and one recorded during active headache. This new finding, if confirmed, raises the possibility that some of the concepts that we rely upon could merely reflect the technical limitations in the design of some older studies. Longitudinal studies starting early in the course of the disease are needed to address the issue of whether changes are the result of repeated and possibly prolonged attacks.

Functional brain imaging studies have indicated an ictal pattern of hypoperfusion in migraine with aura, which is ipsilateral to the headache pain and contralateral to the symptoms of the aura.[13] There is less agreement about the spreading nature of the hypoperfusion,[14,15] which can easily be detected with nuclear medicine technology. Unambiguous evidence supporting the spreading nature of the phenomenon should take advantage of techniques with a greater time resolution, such as EEG/MEG, as in the study of Welch and co-workers.[16] A better understanding of the complexity and controversy behind these issues and the possible role of CSD and the associated vascular changes are reflected in a recent contribution.[17]

For children, as a result of obvious ethical restrictions, which can skew the investigated sample towards the more severe ends of the spectrum, it is even more difficult to generalize the few experimental data available. In the interictal phase, common migraine sufferers tend to show a normal rCBF profile.[18] In the same study, the authors report, in children for the first time, rCBF changes in 14 of 19 patients suffering from migraine with aura.

# Evoked potential data

Neurophysiological techniques have suggested an abnormal responsiveness of the visual cortex to light stimuli. This concept has been supported by a number of experimental findings. The most consistent were an enhanced photic driving and abnormal steady-state visual evoked response,[19] and enhanced fast rhythms in the β range (20–30 cycles/s) in children after luminance or contrast stimuli.[20] Unfortunately, these last data failed to be confirmed by other investigators.[21] Furthermore, more recent data in adults have revealed the lack of hyperexcitability of the visual cortex of migraine sufferers when exposed to red light.[22] This has been interpreted as the expression of the hypoexcitability of the visual cortex in the interictal phase, and is consistent with data from transcranial magnetic stimulation (TMS) of the motor cortex in the hemisphere responsible for the aura.[23]

Unfortunately, most of the conflicting evidence is intimately related to the diversity of experimental conditions in the studies. The greatest cofounders in the interictal studies are the variability in latency between the recording and the last attack and, more importantly, the duration and severity of the migraine history. It is in fact extremely difficult to unequivocally attribute changes to the pathogenic mechanisms rather than to the effect of more or less prolonged and frequent attacks on the underlying anatomical structures.

## Neurophysiological findings during the migraine attack

The first patients with ictal EEG recording of migraine attacks were described by Navarranne et al.[24] After this report on two adolescents with hemiplegic migraine, 10 further similar cases were described by Degen and coworkers.[25] In a study on ictal and interictal EEG changes, we were the first to use quantitative spectral EEG measures in childhood migraine.[26] No significant differences between migraineurs and age-matched controls were seen in the interictal period. In 10 patients we were able to record a spontaneous attack of migraine with a visual aura. During the early stages of the aura, a unilateral decrease in occipital α power was seen, followed by a bilateral frontal increase in δ power. During the headache phase, we recorded an increased δ activity in posterotemporal and occipital electrode sites. We then set out to investigate the topography and time course of these changes, taking advantage of a newly developed method that enables co-registration and fusion of EEG and MRI data.[27]

The recording of EEG activity was obtained from 32–64 channels. Electrode position and the head geometry were measured using a Polhemus Iso-Track II digitizer, and fiducial points (nasion, inion, left and right preauricular points) were co-registered with the MRI using vitamin gel capsules. This procedure allowed us to translate the coordinates of the three-dimensional EEG localization into the MRI of the individual patient. Data were then acquired and stored on optical media for offline analysis.

The EEG activity was processed offline and artefact-free epochs analysed in the frequency domain. Using the FFT approximation method and a radially weighted minimum norm strategy, the sources of EEG activity in the different EEG bands are reconstructed. Source reconstruction relied on realistic head models computed from the MRI of each patient. The three-dimensional coordinates of the voxel with the highest current density value could be plotted on a MRI-based representation in the Talairach space coordinates. Using a computer-aided image-fusion procedure, the localization could also be superimposed on the MRI of the individual patient, to provide a better understanding of the spatial relationship between anatomical areas and the recorded electrophysiological events. We present data on an illustrative patient recorded ictally, suffering from migraine with unilateral visual aura. In Fig. 2.1 we show the patient during the three-dimensional electrode localization procedure (Fig. 2.1a) and a graphic representation (Fig. 2.1b) of the grid points used for source reconstruction. Using an FFT-approximation technique, we identified the peak frequency in the EEG spectrum during the attack and analysed the three-dimensional topography of its intracranial sources at discrete instants in time. In Fig. 2.2 the time course and the topography of the slow (1 Hz)

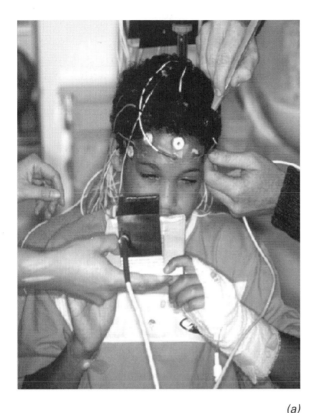

(a)

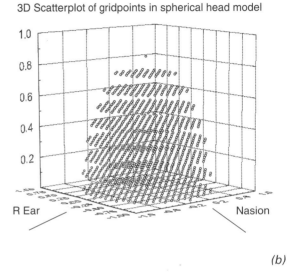

3D Scatterplot of gridpoints in spherical head model

R Ear          Nasion

(b)

**Figure 2.1**
*(a) A child is measured after the recording. Fiducial points (paramagnetic capsules) are seen on the forehead and their three-dimensional position, as well as that of the EEG electrodes, are measured. These coordinates allow co-registration with the patient's MRI. (b) The scattergram of the 1152 discrete gridpoints, at which current density is computed using the inverse solution strategy, forms the basis for the full-head reconstruction.*

frequency activity suggests a posterior onset in the right temporo-occipital leads. Later, there is a progressive spread of slow activity to more anterior locations and 60 min after the onset of the migraine attack, during the pain symptom, bilateral and diffuse abnormal slowing is seen. This last finding might well reflect the associated vascular changes that accompany the attack. These findings were consistent across all the cases that we were able to record during the attack, suggesting that the cascade of activation patterns, and possibly of biochemical–haemodynamic events during the attack, are quite consistent for this specific clinical subtype.

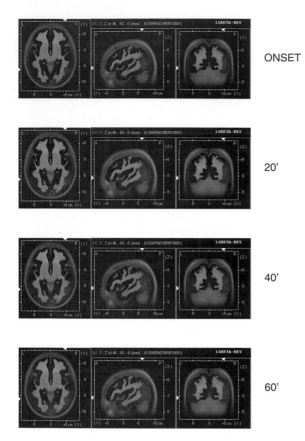

ONSET

20'

40'

60'

**Figure 2.2**
*The four time points at which spectral EEG activity in the δ band is represented correspond to different patterns of cortical activation. The normalized MRI of the subject shows a clear anteroposterior increase in slow-wave activity. At 60 min after the onset of the visual aura, the electrical activity of the whole cortex is characterized by dominant slow-wave frequencies.*

# Conclusion

This short review of current concepts about the neurophysiological aspects of migraine highlights difficulties in reconciling such a vast amount of sometimes contradictory data into a unifying pathogenic model. This may have reflected, at least in part, the fact that we have a remarkable and effective armamentarium for early intervention and treatment of migraine attacks, but little or no preventive treatment. It is, however, encouraging to note the remarkable and parallel technological developments in molecular genetics and modern imaging techniques. The first will improve classification and selection of more robust clinical entities, which in turn will enable basic and clinical scientists to overcome some of the discrepancies and shortfalls of some of the older studies.

# References

1. Schoenen J, Thomsen LL, Neurophysiology and autonomic dysfunction in migraine. In: Olesen J, Tfelft-Hansen P, Welch KMA, eds, *The Headaches*, 2nd edn. Philadelphia: Lippincott Williams & Wilkins, 2000: 301–312.
2. Carrera P, Piatti M, Stenirri S et al, Genetic heterogeneity in Italian families with familial hemiplegic migraine. *Neurology* 1999; **56**: 26–33.
3. Gervil M, Ulrich V, Kaprio J, Olesen J, Russell MB, The relative role of genetic and environmental factors in migraine without aura. *Neurology* 1999; **53**: 995–9.
4. Lauritzen M, Pathophysiology of the migraine aura: the spreading depression theory. *Brain* 1994; **117**: 199–210.
5. Lauritzen M, Hansen AJ, The effect of glutamate receptor blockade on anoxic depolarisation and cortical spreading depression. *J Cereb Blood Flow Metab* 1992; **12**: 223–9.
6. Largo C, Ibarz JM, Herreras O, The effect of gliotoxin fluorocitrate on spreading depression and glial membrane potential in rat brain in situ. *J Neurophysiol* 1997; **78**: 295–307.
7. Duckrow RB, Regional cerebral blood flow during spreading cortical depression in conscious rats. *J Cereb Blood Flow Metab* 1991; **11**: 150–4.

8. Shimazawa M, Hara H, An experimental model of migraine with aura: cortical hypoperfusion following spreading depression in the awake and freely moving rat. *Clin Exp Pharmacol Physiol* 1996; **23**: 890–2.

9. Barkley GL, Tepley N, Simkins R, Moran J, Welch KM, Neuromagnetic fields in migraine: preliminary findings. *Cephalalgia* 1990; **10**: 171–6.

10. Moskowitz MA, Nozaki K, Kraig RP, Neocortical spreading depression provokes the expression of C-fos protein-like immunoiractivity within the trigeminal nucleus caudalis via trigeminovascular mechanisms. *J Neurosci* 1993; **13**: 1167–77.

11. Maytal J, Bienkowski RS, Patel M, Eviatar L, The value of brain imaging in children with headaches. *Pediatrics* 1995; **96**: 413–16.

12. May A, Ashburner J, Buchel C et al, Correlation between structural and functional changes in brain in an idiopathic headache syndrome. *Nature Med* 1999; **5**: 836–8.

13. Olesen J, Friberg L, Skyhoj Olsen T et al, Timing and topography of cerebral blood flow, aura, and headache during migraine attacks. *Ann Neurol* 1990; **28**: 791–8.

14. Olsen TS, Spreading oligemia in the migraine aura – most likely an artifact due to scattered radiation. *Cephalalgia* 1993; **13**: 86–8.

15. Friberg L, Olsen TS, Roland PE, Lassen NA, Focal ischaemia caused by instability of cerebrovascular tone during attacks of hemiplegic migraine: a regional cerebral blood flow study. *Brain* 1987; **110**: 917–34.

16. Welch KM, Barkley GL, Tepley N, Ramadan NM, Central neurogenic mechanisms of migraine. *Neurology* 1993; **43**(suppl 3): S21–5.

17. Vijayan N, O'Brien MD, Blau JN et al, Spreading cerebral hypoperfusion during migraine headache. *N J Engl Med* 1995; **332**: 1516–18.

18. Soriani S, Feggi L, Battistella PA, Arnaldi C, De Carlo L, Stipa S, Interictal and ictal phase study with Tc 99m HMPAO brain SPECT in juvenile migraine with aura. *Headache* 1997; **37**: 31–6.

19. Nyrke T, Kangasniemi P, Lang AH, Difference of steady state visual evoked potential in classic and common migraine. *Electroenceph Clin Neurophysiol* 1989; **72**: 284–94.

20. Good PA, Mortimer MJ, A test for migraine in children: differentiation between migraine with aura and without aura using VER to white, blue or red stimuli. In: Clifford Rose F, ed., *New Advances in Headache Research*, Vol. 2. London: Smith-Gordon, 1991: 93–100.

21. Van Dijk JG, Dorresteijn M, Haan J, Ferrari MD, No confirmation of visual evoked potential diagnostic test for migraine. *Lancet* 1991; **337**: 517–18. (Note: comment in: *Lancet* 1991; **337**: 976–7.

22. Afra J, Ambrosini A, Genicot R, Albert A, Schoenen J, Influence of colors on habituation of visual evoked potentials in patients with migraine with aura and in healthy volunteers. *Headache* 2000; **40**: 36–40.

23. Van der Kamp W, Maassen VanDerBrink A, Ferrari MD, Van Dijk JC, Interictal cortical excitability to magnetic stimulation in familial hemiplegic migraine. *Neurology* 1997; **48**: 1462–4.

24. Navarranne P, Simon-Canton L, Gastaut H, Hemiplegic migraines: 2 cases with EEG recording of the crisis. *Rev Neurol (Paris)* 1967; **117**: 88.

25. Degen R, Degen HE, Palm D, Meiser W, The EEG during the hemiplegic migraine attack of children. *EEG EMG Z Elektroenzephalogr Elektromyogr Verwandte Geb* 1980; **11**: 128–34.

26. Seri S, Cerquiglini A, Guidetti V, Computerized EEG topography in childhood migraine between and during attacks. *Cephalalgia* 1993; **13**: 53–6.

27. Seri S, Cerquiglini A, Pisani F, Michel CM, Pascual Marqui RD, Curatolo P, Frontal lobe epilepsy associated with tuberous sclerosis: electroencephalographic–magnetic resonance image fusioning. *J Child Neurol* 1998; **13**: 33–8.

# 3

# Neurochemistry

*Alessandro Zuddas, Vanessa Lilliu, Maria Del Zompo*

In the last decade, a dramatic increase in the knowledge about molecular and cellular mechanisms in developmental neurobiology has provided impetus for new approaches in the elucidation of the pathophysiology of several disorders of the central nervous system (CNS).

Until recently, mechanisms of diseases investigated in adult patients, or developed using animal models based on adults, had been 'adapted' to disorders of children and adolescents. Molecular genetics indicates how specific alleles of genes, apparently unrelated to the current putative mechanism of a disorder, can be strongly associated with specific diseases with adult onset, and it has been shown that alterations in development can lead to clinically significant changes appearing only in adult life. These findings induced several scientists and clinicians to move from an upside-down approach (i.e. studying adults to understand children) to a downside-up approach: studying children to understand adults or, from a more biological perspective, studying brain development to explain mechanisms of neuropsychiatric disorders in children, adolescents and adults. The aim of this chapter is to describe, from a developmental perspective, the principal neurotransmitters involved in the migraine attack, providing basic information on the differentia-

tion and maturation mechanisms for both serotoninergic and dopaminergic systems. A deeper insight into these developmental mechanisms, together with new information on the genetic predisposition to the disorder, can lead to new, more effective, therapeutic approaches to the disorder, possibly differentiated by the age of onset.

## Pathophysiology of migraine attacks

For many years, two principal hypotheses have been proposed for explaining the pathogenesis of migraine. A vascular hypothesis held that migraine was primarily a disease of cranial blood vessels, the pain occurring as a result of sensory nerve activation by inappropriate vasodilatation in the cranial circulation. On the other hand, a neurogenic hypothesis proposed that neurogenic inflammation (vasodilatation and plasma protein extravasation) in the meninges was responsible for trigeminal sensory nerve activation and the generation of headache.[1] More recently, brain imaging studies during spontaneous migraine have shown the activation of brain-stem regions involved in the central modulation of head pain and craniovascular functions.[2] This observation gave rise to an integrated hypothesis suggesting that migraine has a central neural basis, which leads to dysfunction within various sensory, nociceptive and vascular control pathways.[3] Positron emission tomography (PET) studies further supported the involvement of brain-stem regions in migraine pathogenesis, showing regionally specific increases in cerebral blood flow (an index of neural activity), within the reticular formation, during spontaneous migraine attacks.[2]

The reticular formation is an important neuronal matrix for the integration of many CNS activities. Inputs converge on the reticular formation from almost all somatic and visceral sensory pathways and from the cortex, hypothalamus, corpus striatum, limbic system and spinal cord. The reticular formation provides prominent output via the ascending reticular-activating system to the same structures. The ascending reticular-activating system plays key roles in alertness, behaviour and affects. Neuronal circuits of the reticular formation are also involved in the regulation of cardiovascular function, respiration and other visceral responses by influencing cranial nerve nuclei and by the descending connections to autonomic centres in the spinal cord. Moreover, axons ascending the spinothalamic and trigeminothalamic pain pathways conduct nociceptive information to the lateral columns of the reticular formation and the ascending reticular-activating system; they also activate neurons in the medial column and raphe nuclei in the caudal brain stem. These nuclei have an inhibitory output to spinal dorsal horn and trigeminal nuclei where they can modulate sensory neurotransmission, thereby forming an endogenous pain control system. The nuclei within reticular formation, which are thought to be most significantly activated during migraine attacks, are the raphe and

locus ceruleus, which have high densities of serotoninergic and catecholaminergic (noradrenaline or norepinephrine) neurons, respectively. This brain-stem hyperactivity is not to be considered as a consequence of headache, but rather to be inherent to the attack itself, because it was unaffected by the administration of serotonin (5-hydroxytryptamine or 5HT) agonists that successfully treated the attack and its associated symptoms.

Dysfunction in the reticular formation (raphe nuclei) and neighbouring regions (periaqueductal grey matter and locus ceruleus) could, therefore, potentially interfere with pain perception and pain control mechanisms, and alter neuronal projections governing the autonomic control of the diameter of cranial blood vessels and blood flow.[4] Alteration in integrative functions and output of the brain stem may, therefore, explain many of the neurophysiological symptoms that are specific premonitory signs of migraine and the attack itself. Future anti-migraine strategies will come from studying functional changes within the brain during spontaneous migraine attacks, and studying the effect and the modifications caused by the administration of clinically useful anti-migraine agents.

## Serotonin and migraine

For many years, the principal pharmacological interest in approaching migraine has been directed towards 5HT. This was because circulating levels of 5HT fell during a migraine attack and it was observed that 5HT itself could stop a migraine attack. This gave rise to the theory that the painful vasodilatation occurring in intracranial blood vessels during migraine was a sort of overcompensation in response to the vasoconstrictor effects of 5HT released from platelets. Subsequently, when changes in circulating 5HT levels proved to be pharmacologically small, interest in the humoral role of 5HT in migraine declined. Current theories suggest that parasympathetic projections (containing acetylcholine and vasoactive intestinal peptide – VIP) from brain-stem regions innervate intracranial meningeal blood vessels.[5] The activation of these pathways could trigger headache by releasing nitric oxide (NO), which is a potent vasodilator and activator of perivascular sensory nerves. The existence of other pathways that could cause NO-mediated vasodilatation through 5HT acting at endothelial 5HT receptors has also been proposed (see below). Indeed, anti-migraine prophylactic agents that are 5HT antagonists may act by preventing this initial vasodilator stimulus.[6] These hypotheses provide a potential integrating link between the vascular and the neural theories of migraine.

## Developmental neurobiology of serotoninergic neurons

Serotonin was identified initially as the active substance from brain extracts that produced peripheral vasoconstriction;[7] this substance was later shown to be identical to a contractile substance isolated from the chromaffin cells of the gastrointestinal tract called enteramine.[8] Subsequent studies, using fluorescence histochemistry and immunocytochemical methods,[9,10] demonstrated the localized distribution of 5HT neurons along the midline of the brain stem (dorsal and medial raphe nuclei). From the midbrain, 5HT pericarya send long axons to innervate a wide distribution of receiving areas from the spinal cord to the cortex. Prominent forebrain terminal

regions include the hypothalamus, cortex, hippocampus, amygdala and striatum. These innervation patterns are relatively conserved throughout mammals, including humans.

Serotonin neurons are highly branched, suggesting that they are able simultaneously to modulate the function of several regions of the CNS. 5HT has been shown to be able to influence a broad spectrum of physiological systems, such as cardiovascular regulation, respiration and thermoregulation, as well as a variety of behavioural functions, including circadian rhythms, the sleep–wake cycle, appetite, aggression, sexual behaviour, sensorimotor reactivity and pain sensitivity. Pharmacological modulation of 5HT function is able to influence a wide range of psychiatric and neurological disorders, including depression, schizophrenia, anxiety and eating disorders, degenerative disorders and Alzheimer's disease, as well as a less structured range of impulse-related disorders (gambling, substance abuse, obsessive control and attention deficit disorder).[11]

Neurons producing 5HT are among the earliest to be born in the developing CNS: their differentiation and maturation have been extensively studied in the rat, the gestational period of which is about 20 days. Two clusters of 5HT-expressing neurons can be identified in the embryonic rhomboencephalon at days 12–15 (E12–15): the rostral cluster gives rise to dorsal, median and caudal dorsal–linear raphe; the caudal cluster contributes to the manus, obscurus and pallidus raphe nuclei. Cells with serotoninergic properties are also detectable in the fetal (retro- and suprachiasmatic areas) and adult (dorsomedial) hypothalamus and in the postnatal spinal cord.

The regional restriction of serotoninergic neurons includes the combination of local

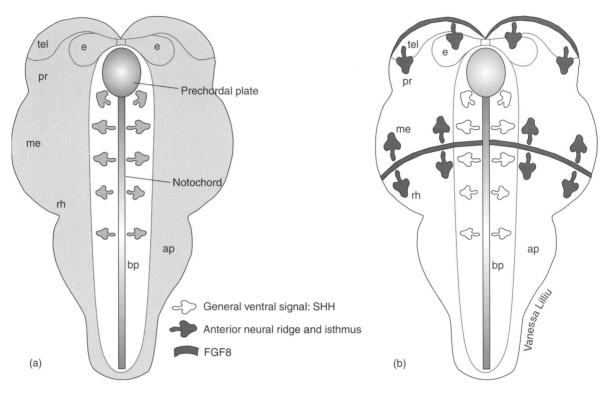

**Figure 3.1**

*(a) Relationship between the neural plate and prechordal plate/notochord (mesendodermal organizers): induction of ventral structures in the neural plate via the sonic hedgehog protein: bp, basal plate; ap, alar plate; tel, telencephalon; e, eyes; pr, prosencephalon; me, mesencephalon; rh, rombencephalon; SHH, sonic hedgehog. (b) Regulation of forebrain, midbrain and hindbrain: patterning of local organizers (anterior neural ridge and isthmus) within the neural plate producing FGF8.*

inductive substances and regional competence to react to these signals.[12] Ventral specification signals (such as the sonic hedgehog protein, SHH) produced by the floor plate (the ventral midline of the developing CNS) and the notocord (a rod-like structure of mesodermal origin that lies just under the floor plate) induce basal plate neurons, including progenitors for 5HT, dopamine and motor neurons. Dorsal signalling centres that produce bone morphogenic proteins (BMPs) repress 5HT neurogenesis in the alar (dorsolateral) plate. Additional signals are produced by the isthmic regions at the midbrain/hindbrain transition (especially fibroblast growth factor 8 – FGF8; Figure 3.1).

Region-specific competence to form serotoninergic neurons is controlled through the regional expression of transcriptional factors. Transcriptional factors are regulatory proteins that recognize short stretches of DNA within the promoter region of a gene: they are defined on the basis of the amino acid sequence of their DNA-binding motifs, which include the homoeodomain helix, loop–helix and a T box ('homoeobox'). The binding of one or more transcriptional factors within a promoter regions determines whether transcription of that gene can proceed. Other regulatory sequences can lie upstream, providing for fine turning of gene transcription. Different classes of homoeobox genes (genes coding for homoeobox transcriptional factors) tend to be expressed in different regions of the brain and are critical to the development of that specific region.[13]

Specific transcriptional factors either repress 5HT phenotype (such as the *Otx* genes in the midbrain and the forebrain) or are permissive for 5HT neurons in the hindbrain (such as *Nkx 2.2* and *Nkx 6.1* homoeobox genes). Finally, brain-derived neurotrophic factor (BDNF) appears to promote the survival of serotoninergic neurons,[14] whereas ciliary neurotrophic factor (CNTF) promotes raphe cells to become cholinergic neurons and reduces the number of 5HT neurons.[15]

Rostral raphe nuclei produce axonal projections that ascend to the midbrain and forebrain; axonal projections from the caudal raphe nuclei descend to the spinal cord.[16] Rostral projections become detectable soon after pericarya, and by E15 they reach the diencephalon via the middle forebrain bundle: medial fibres then project to the frontal pole of the telencephalon (reached at E17), lateral to the hypothalamus, a minority of fibre entering the diencephalon through the ganglionic eminences. 5HT fibres also pass through the diagonal band of Broca and the septum and into the cerebral cortex, where they segregate into two groups: one superficial within the marginal zone, the other deep into the cortical plate. From the anterior regions, 5HT fibres reach the hippocampus through the cingulate cortex. Descending fibres enter the spinal cord at E14 and innervate the intermediolateral column (preganglionic sympathetic neurons) and somatic motor neurons (E17). Later, 5HT fibres innervate the dorsal horn neurons.

After birth, 5HT-immunoreactive fibres can also be detected in the sensory cortex. These fibres are, however, not a raphe projection. They are thalamocortical projections, unable to produce 5HT. They absorb 5HT from the neocortex (and perhaps the reticular nuclei), using a 5HT transporter.[17] In these and other brain regions, 5HT is able to modulate differentiation, cell migration and generation of functional neuronal circuitry (i.e. generation of a so-called vibrissae-related barrel fields in the sensory cortex.[18,19] Several studies have shown that, along the pathways where 5HT fibres grow, the 5HT receptors are expressed early enough to mediate these maturational effects.[20,21]

Moreover, non-neuronal brain tissues express 5HT receptors. The choroid plexus has high level of $5HT_{2C}$ receptors, ependymal cells and radial glia of $5HT_{1A}$ receptors; they have been postulated to regulate the production of neurotrophic factors.[22] 5HT also regulates craniofacial development: ectomesenchymal cells express 5HT transporter and 5HT receptors that are exposed to 5HT derived from maternal circulation; drugs that block 5HT transport or interact with 5HT receptors can be responsible for craniofacial malformations.[23]

## 5HT receptors and the acute attack of migraine

The study and characterization of the 5HT receptors involved in the treatment of the acute attack of migraine have provided a better general understanding of 5HT physiology and pharmacology. At least seven subclasses of 5HT receptors have been pharmacologically and molecularly characterized.[24] The $5HT_1$ subclass consists of the A, B, C, D, E and F subtypes;[25] currently, the more effective and relatively specific anti-migraine compounds are $5HT_{1B/1D}$ receptor agonists. These drugs have three potential distinct mechanisms of action, all of which may well be additive in their anti-migraine action.

The first is a specific direct vasoconstriction which opposes the painful vasodilatation occurring in meningeal blood vessels, thereby decreasing nerve activation; however, evidence for the existence of such a mechanism in human brain is inconclusive, suggesting that other actions may be involved. The second mechanism consists of an inhibitory effect on peripheral trigeminal nerves innervating vascular, pain-producing structures. The inhibition of trigeminal afferents has two possible effects: the inhibition of neurogenic plasma protein extravasation (PPE) and inhibition of neuropeptide release. PPE can be blocked by an array of agents, including aspirin, indometacin, dihydroergotamine, sumatriptan and valproate.[26] This effect appears to be mediated by $5HT_{1B}$ receptors because, in genetically $5HT_{1B}$ knock-out mice, sumatriptan is ineffective in blocking PPE.[27] Sumatriptan and a number of other triptans, (i.e. eletriptan, naratriptan and zolmitriptan) are also agonists at the $5HT_{1F}$ receptors and these receptors can modulate PPE. The role of PPE and peripheral trigeminal 5HT receptors is, however, brought into question by several lines of evidence: other drugs able to block migraine attack and PPE (i.e. almidan) are inactive to $5HT_{1F}$, whereas drugs such as CP

122,288, or the selective $5HT_{1F}$ agonist LY334,370, are able to inhibit PPE, but are ineffective as anti-migraine drugs.[26] The third mechanism of action for $5HT_{1B/D}$ agonists is within the CNS at the trigeminal–cervical complex (TCC) composed of trigeminal nuclei caudalis and cervicalis (superficial laminae of the dorsal horn in C1–C3.[28] Systemic and local administration of $5HT_{1B/D}$ agonists, such as dihydroergotamine, ziratriptan and zolmitriptan, is able to inhibit the firing of TCC neurons and this effect is blocked by specific antagonists such as naratriptan. The inhibition of central neurotransmission from trigeminal sensory nerves interrupts pain processing within the brain, thereby decreasing the central pain transmission.[26]

The fact that sumatriptan does not inhibit the activity of TCC cells unless the blood–brain barrier is disrupted suggests that each of these three mechanisms described above acts, in a complementary manner, to reduce the intense central trigeminal input that occurs during a migraine attack. Altogether they contribute to the relief of headache pain and migraine-associated symptoms such as nausea, vomiting, phonophobia and photophobia.

## Neuropeptides and migraine attack

Trigeminovascular activation (see above) is marked by the release of neuropeptides, derived from three nerve systems: sympathetic, parasympathetic and trigeminal. The vasoconstrictor sympathetic system is marked by neuropeptide Y (NPY), the vasodilator parasympathetic system by vasoactive intestinal peptide (VIP) and trigeminal systems, both sensitive and vasodilator, by substance P (SP), calcitonin gene-related protein (CGRP) and neurokinin A (NKA). The stimulation of the trigeminal ganglion in cats and humans results in a release of both SP and CGRP and this effect is blocked by sumatriptan and zolmitriptan.[29] In humans, CGRP but not SP is released during migraine as well as CGRP and VIP, but not SP, in cluster headache.[30–33] VIP release indicates an activation of the parasympathetic nerves, suggesting the presence of a functional trigeminal–autonomic loop within the brain stem. Such a loop would explain the marked autonomic symptomatology accompanying cluster headache and paroxysmal hemicranias.[34]

## Nitric oxide and magnesium

Several findings demonstrate that monoamine and peptides involved in neural inflammation are not able to cause the nociception responsible for migraine pain. Experimental studies using two different human headache models, based on glyceryl trinitrate administration (an exogenous NO donor) and histamine (which is able to liberate NO from vascular endothelium), have suggested a key role of NO in migraine.[35] NO is a highly reactive, free radical, lipophilic gas. NO is generated from the terminal guanidino nitrogen of L-arginine by a family of enzymes known as NO synthase (NOS). NOS activity has been reported in many tissues (endothelium, brain peripheral nerve, microglia, myocardium, blood cells, etc.). At least three forms of NOS have been identified: two are constitutive, $Ca^{2+}$/calmodulin-dependent forms that release NO from endothelium and neurons (eNOS and nNOS, respectively).[36] The other is inducible and $Ca^{2+}$/calmodulin independent (iNOS) and generates NO for a long period and in large amounts in response to endotoxins and cytokines. NO has a very short half-life (5–30 s): physiological actions of NO are mediated via an activation of soluble guanylyl cyclase and a consequent increase of cyclic guanosine monophosphate (cGMP) and decrease of intracellular $Ca^{2+}$ in target cells.[37] Several physiological effects of NO may be theoretically implicated in the pathophysiology of migraine: several neurotransmitters, in brain tissue, peripheral cerebral nerves and blood, stimulate the formation of NO in brain neurons and arterial endothelium, and possibly interact with NOS-containing nerve terminals. NO is a potent vasodilator for intra- and extracranial arteries: it has been postulated that NO is also able to activate periphery vascular sensory nerve fibres and/or initiate perivascular neurogenic inflammation. NO is considered by Olsen et al[38] to be the earliest neurotransmitter activated in the cascade of biochemical events leading to a migraine attack. This theory has considerable experimental support and drugs are being developed that can block NOS, which might abort migraine.[35]

Magnesium deficiency has also been suspected of playing a role in the pathogenesis of migraine. Magnesium concentration modulates 5HT receptors, NO synthesis and release, N-methyl-D-aspartate (NMDA) receptors and a variety of other migraine-related receptors and neurotransmitters.[39] Available evidence suggests that up to 50% of patients have lowered levels of ionized magnesium during a migraine attack:[40,41] in these patients, infusion of magnesium results in a rapid and sustained relief of the acute attack.[42] Chronic oral magnesium supplementation reduces the frequency of migraine attacks.[43,44]

It is likely that low magnesium levels can be

a strong predisposing factor for many patients. Considering NO as the earliest neurotransmitter activated in the cascade of events leading to a migraine attack, it is now well established that NO production can be modulated by changes in magnesium concentration.[45] Magnesium is also intimately involved in the control of NMDA glutamate receptors, which play an important role in the regulation of cerebral blood flow and in CNS pain transmission.[45] Magnesium ions can be considered as an NMDA receptor antagonist because they modulate the NMDA receptor function; high concentrations of $Mg^{2+}$ block NMDA receptors and do not allow $Ca^{2+}$ to enter the cells. On the contrary, low $Mg^{2+}$ concentrations facilitate NMDA transmission, allowing calcium to exert its effects on both neurons and cerebral vascular muscle.[46,47] $Mg^{2+}$ controls several cellular functions from ionic currents across membranes to mitochondrial respiration and brain intracellular proton concentration. It is likely that many, if not all, $Mg^{2+}$ functions have a role in migraine mechanisms.

# Dopamine and migraine

Together with 5HT, dopamine also appears to play a crucial role in the mechanism of the migraine attack. In the late 1970s, Sicuteri[48] postulated a dopaminergic hypersensitivity in migraine patients and Lance[49] pointed out that, as nausea often precedes headache, changes in the brain-stem dopaminergic neurotransmission must be present in migraine.

In fact, a variety of prodromal symptoms, including yawning, drowsiness, irritability and hyperactivity, is reported by a significant percentage of migraine patients hours or days before the attack onset. Interestingly, in migraine patients yawning can be induced by doses of the dopamine agonist apomorphine (5 µg/kg) that are ineffective in control individuals.[50,51] Higher doses of dopaminergic agonists induce hyperactivity and stereotypes in rodents, mood fluctuations, irritability, hypotension, nausea and vomiting in humans, as well as involuntary movements in predisposed subjects. In migraine patients, all these symptoms can be blocked by dopamine agonists such as haloperidol, chlorpromazine, prochlorperazine, domperidone and metoclopramide. Although the $D_2$-related antiemetic effect of these drugs is well known, in migraine patients they are also able to block the migraine attack.[52] More recently, an increased density of $D_5$-receptors has been reported in peripheral blood lymphocytes of migraineurs[53] and a significant disequilibrium for specific alleles of distinct dopamine $D_2$-receptors has been described.[54,55]

Taken together, all these data indicate that alterations in dopaminergic neurotransmission can modulate clinical susceptibility to migraine and dopamine, at least in a subgroup of migraine patients, and can play an important role in activating the biochemical cascade leading to the migraine attack.

# Developmental neurobiology of dopamine neurons

The catecholamine dopamine plays a key role in the physiology of most vertebrate and invertebrate organisms. Dopamine is an important regulator of many neural functions, including motor integration, neuroendocrine hormone release, cognition, emotional behaviour and reward. In mammals dopamine neurons are relatively few, when compared with the total number of brain neurons. They are mainly located in the ventral midbrain to form the retrorubral nucleus (A8), the substantia nigra (A9) and the ventral tegmental area (A10).[56,57] In rodents, neurons arising from the substantia nigra project into the striatum (corresponding to the caudate putamen in primates) and receive innervation from multiple structures in the diencelphalon and telencephalon. Dopamine midbrain neurons can be distinguished according to the presence of various specific proteins, such as parvalbumin, calbindin, cholecystokinin and calretinin, although no clear functional differences have been attributed to these different subpopulations.[58,59]

The ascending nigrostriatal pathway regulating motor control and its degeneration in humans is associated with Parkinson's disease. Neurons from the ventral tegmental area project to the limbic system and cortex, and are involved in emotional and reward behaviour and in motivation. Disturbances of this system have been associated with schizophrenia, addictive behavioural disorders and attention-deficit hyperactivity disorder (ADHD).[60,61] Dopamine also modulates interactions between the prefrontal cortex and visual association areas, which are important in visual memory.[62] In addition, dopaminergic neurotransmission is involved in learning and memory dysfunction associated with traumatic brain injury.[63] All three dopaminergic mesencephalic nuclei (A8, A9 and A10 regions) project towards the hippocampal formation, although the functional significance of the mesohippocampal dopamine system is largely unknown. In the mammalian forebrain, smaller clusters of dopamine cells lie in the subparafascicular thalamic nucleus (A11 area), the hypothalamic arcuate nucleus (A12 area), the incertohypothalamic nucleus (A13 area), and the olfactory bulb. In all these neurons,

dopamine is synthesized from tyrosine by tyrosine hydroxylase (TH). Upon release from the presynaptic terminals into the synaptic cleft, dopamine acts through $D_{1R}$ ($D_1$ and $D_5$) and $D_{2R}$ ($D_2$, $D_3$, $D_4$) subfamilies of G-protein-coupled receptors.[64] Dopamine neurotransmission is terminated by the uptake of the released messenger into the presynaptic dopamine fibres.

### Dopamine neuron differentiation

The maturation of dopamine neurotransmission follows a complex developmental pattern of activation of various genes, which can be selectively modulated by a specific interaction with the developing target tissues (Figure 3.2). In the mesencephalon, TH, the rate-limiting enzyme in the biosynthetic pathway of catecholamines (i.e. dopamine, noradrenaline and adrenaline), is expressed early during ontogeny and has been used as a marker of catecholaminergic neuroblasts. Dopamine midbrain neuroblasts are generated near the midbrain–hindbrain junction and migrate radially to their final position in the ventral midbrain. In the mouse midbrain, rare and scattered $TH^+$ cells and fibres have been detected by immunocytochemistry starting at embryonic day (E) 9.5 close to the ventricular ependymal layer, suggesting that dopamine differentiation can occur in early postmitotic neural precursors.[65] In humans, $TH^+$ cells appear in the ventral mesencephalon at 6.5 weeks adjacent to the ventricular zone; their ventral migration begins at 6.7 weeks and $TH^+$ neurites are seen initially in the developing putamen at 9.0 weeks.[66] Fibroblast growth factor 2 (FGF2), also known as basic FGF, and epidermal growth factor (EGF) act as mitogens for neuronal precursors in fetal rat mesencephalic cultures and delay their differentiation.

## Transcriptional factors

As for 5HT neurons, dopamine neurons' early development is regulated by two distinct molecules, sonic hedgehog (SHH) and FGF8 that modulate neuronal identities according to the duration, context or concentration of SHH.[67] SHH is necessary and sufficient for induction of the dopamine neurons along the dorsoventral axis; SHH interacts with FGF8, which in turn is responsible for dopamine neuron induction along the antero-posterior axis of the neural tube. SHH and FGF8, as with other inductive secreted molecules, are thought to activate cascades of other signalling molecules and transcription factors which lead to the final differentiation of dopamine neurons. Two transcription factors, *Nurr1* and *Ptx3*, expressed at crucial times in differentiating midbrain dopamine cells, have recently been identified. *Nurr1*, an 'orphan' member of the steroid–thyroid hormone receptor superfamily, is expressed predominantly in the CNS, mainly in limbic areas and the ventral midbrain and, at a lower level, in the diencephalon and olfactory bulbs.[68]

In the mouse, the onset of *Nurr1* expression in the ventral midbrain occurs in dopamine neuroblasts 1 day before the appearance of TH, and its expression continues in mature dopaminergic neurons during adulthood. Lack of *Nurr1* (i.e. *Nurr1* knock-out mice) leads to a genesis of midbrain dopamine neurons in the midbrain, but not in diencephalon (areas A11/A13) or in the olfactory bulb. *Ptx3* is a bicoid-related homoeobox gene, selectively expressed in mesencephalic dopamine neurons shortly after *Nurr1*, in part under FGF8 control. The onset of *Ptx3* expression coincides with that of TH. At later stages, *Ptx3* expression remains restricted to the mesencephalic dopamine system and this association is conserved in the adult brain.[69,70] *Ptx3* is also expressed in the absence of *Nurr1*, but *Nurr1* is essential to commit *Ptx3*-positive ventral mesencephalic precursors towards dopamine differentiation and it is critically involved in maintenance of *Ptx3*-expressing cells.[71] Several lines of evidence indicate that *Ptx3* and *Nurr1*, although regulated independently, may cooperate to regulate terminal differentiation of midbrain dopamine neurons. *Nurr1* is essential for both survival and final differentiation of ventral, mesencephalic, late dopamine precursors into fully functional dopamine neurons, whereas the role of *Ptx3* in dopamine neuron differentiation remains to be clarified.[71]

Soon after the achievement of final commitment, developing midbrain dopamine neurons express the *c-Ret* proto-oncogene and the *GFRa1* gene.[72] These genes encode for components of a multireceptor complex interacting with the glial cell line-derived neurotrophic factor (GDNF), the most potent trophic factor yet described for midbrain dopaminergic neurons and spinal motoneurons.[73] *Ret* belongs to the receptor tyrosine kinase family and is the signalling component of the GDNF receptor complex, where *GFRa1* is anchored to the cell surface via a glycosyl-phosphatidyl-inositol linkage and is the ligand-binding subunit. Their mRNAs are both clearly present in the A9 and A10 DA neurons from E12.5,[74] as well as in other areas that are known targets of GDNF action. Developing dopamine midbrain neurons also express receptors for various neurotrophins which in vitro act as 'dopaminotrophic factors': *trkB*, the high-affinity receptor for BDNF and NT4/5, and *trkC*, the high-affinity receptor for NT3.[75]

Besides the already known molecules, other still unidentified epigenetic factors must be involved in the maturation of the dopamine function. Among these environmental influences, target interactions appear to play an important role in modulating key aspects of midbrain dopamine neurotransmission and target neurons have a pivotal influence on the maturation of midbrain dopamine neurons and modulate dopamine synthesis and uptake.[76,77] The last seems to be dependent on a direct influence of striatal neurons on the regulation of the dopamine transporter (*DAT*) gene expression during development, at least in vitro.

## Dopamine neuron maturation

Once ventral midbrain neurons have acquired a dopaminergic specification, a set of genes involved in the maturation of dopaminergic properties is activated before the establishment of dopamine neurotransmission, which in rodents occurs at around E15–E16 (Figure 3.2).

Among the various specific dopaminergic markers, TH appears early and dopamine neurons also express dopamine receptors (autoreceptors) before the functional onset of dopamine neurotransmission.[78] Autoreceptors belong to the $D_{2R}$ class. In the adult, they are distributed on the dopamine somata, dendrites and nerve terminals. The latter seem to modulate dopamine synthesis and dopamine release, whereas those localized at the cell body or dendrites seem to influence basal firing by modulating the rates of impulse activity. Binding studies and in situ hybridization data show that these autoreceptors appear at E13–E14 in the rat midbrain, 2 days after TH immunoreactivity, and their number increases thereafter.[78] The early prenatal appearance of $D_2$ autoreceptors in the embryonic midbrain suggests that they may have a regulatory role

in the development of dopamine neurons. Indeed, dopamine is accumulated in ventral midbrain neurons shortly after their initial differentiation, when dopamine pathways and functional neurotransmission are not yet established.[79,80] In addition, dopamine is released spontaneously from developing midbrain neurons in cultures.[81,82]

The synaptic vesicle monoamine transporter gene (*VMAT2*) is also expressed early in the rat ventral midbrain (at least E12 in the rat)[80] several days before the establishment of nigrostriatal dopamine neurotransmission. *VMAT2* belongs to the vesicular neurotransmitter transporter family and allows transport and storage of monoamines into dense core vesicles in most aminergic neurons, using the electrochemical gradient generated by a vesicular $H^+$ ATPase.[83] The early appearance of *VMAT2*[80] and dopamine[79] during midbrain ontogeny, and the presence of functional release in the ventral mesencephalon in primary cultures, indicate that vesicular storage also occurs in the embryonic brain. An additional role of VMAT2 could consist of clearing the cytoplasm of free dopamine which readily oxidizes to produce toxic free radicals.

During embryonic development, dopamine synthesis, storage and high-affinity uptake appear to develop asynchronously, in a non-correlated fashion. In cells acutely dissociated from the embryonic rat ventral mesencephalon, measurable dopamine is detected as early as E12.5 and its concentration increases sharply at E16, reaching a plateau before birth. In the striatum, dopamine is first detected at E16, suggesting that dopamine nigral fibres reach their target tissue at this embryonic age,[79] in accordance with morphological data showing the arrival of the first $TH^+$ axons at the striatum at that age.[84] In contrast to the early appearance of endogenous dopamine levels in the mesencephalon, specific high-affinity dopamine uptake in rat mesencephalic cells is found only at E16, and increases sharply between E16 and E18, reaching a plateau before birth. Thus, the onset of dopamine uptake and its subsequent increase seem concomitant with the arrival of the first dopamine fibres to the striatum.

## Development of the dopamine transporter protein

DAT is a member of the multigene family encoding $Na^+/Cl^-$-dependent neurotransmitter transporter, and its gene product mediates high-affinity uptake of the released dopamine into the presynaptic dopamine neuron.[85] Immunohistochemical and in situ hybridization analyses on the adult rodent brain demonstrate that distribution of the transcript and the protein corresponds quite closely with dopamine cell bodies and terminals, respectively.[86] Interestingly, the protein is also localized along nigral dendrites and cell bodies, suggesting that dopamine uptake is involved in the regulation of the extracellular concentration of dopamine in the substantia nigra,[87] where it acts on dopamine autoreceptors to modulate dopamine synthesis and release.

DAT gene inactivation in transgenic mice has confirmed unequivocally the physiological role for DAT as the most critical component in terminating dopamine neurotransmission and its role as an obligatory target for the behavioural and the biochemical action of psychostimulants. Homozygote DAT-null mice show spontaneous hyperlocomotion as a result of protracted persistence of dopamine in the extracellular space, and are insensitive to the action of amphetamine and cocaine.[88] Moreover, the absence of DAT produces extensive

adaptive changes to control dopamine neurotransmission, such as a great decrease in the level of TH and in the content and release of dopamine.[89] Thus DAT not only regulates the duration and intensity of dopamine neurotransmission, but also plays a critical role in regulating presynaptic dopamine homoeostasis, maintaining the delicate balance of dopamine synthesis, release and degradation.

Striatal cells could be involved in the regulation, at a transcriptional level, of a key step in the maturation of dopamine neurotransmission in vivo. The level of DAT gene transcription and the corresponding uptake sites are selectively increased in rat E13 mesencephalic dopamine neurons in vitro, after addition of E16 striatal cells in co-culture.[90] More mature mesencephalic dopamine neuron cultures (E16) are not susceptible to the striatal influences on DAT mRNA and function. These observations suggest that mesencephalic dopamine neurons respond to target influences only within a restricted developmental window. Upregulation of DAT mRNA level by striatal cells in mesencephalic dopamine neurons in culture seems to require direct cell interactions because target cells are ineffective when separated from mesencephalic cells by a barrier, which allows diffusion of soluble molecules. Interestingly, the still unidentified 'signals' derived from target striatal cells appear to be specific because non-target cortical or cerebellar cells fail to stimulate dopamine uptake or DAT gene expression.[90]

Taken together, these data indicate that alteration in dopaminergic neurotransmission can modulate clinical susceptibility to migraine and dopamine, at least in a subgroup of migraine patients, and can play an important role in activating the biochemical cascade leading to the migraine attack.

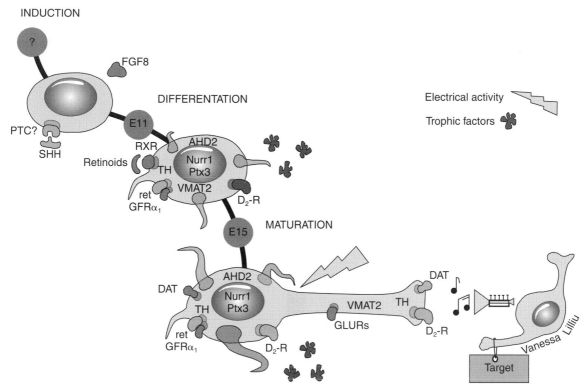

Developmental steps in mesencephalic dopaminergic neurons

**Figure 3.2**
*The diagram resumes the time course and the early events in rodent DA neuronal development. The onset of some key genes is shown, as well as the putative intervention of trophic factors, electrical activity and the influence of striatal target cells: FGF8, fibroblast growth factor; SHH, sonic hedgehog; PTC, 12 transmembrane protein, patched, SHH receptor; RXR, 9-cis-retinoic acid receptor; AHD2, retinoic acid-generating enzyme aldehyde dehydrogenase; TH, tyrosine hydroxylase; VMAT2, synaptic vesicle monoamine transporter, Nurr1 and ptx3, transcription factors; $D_2$-R, $D_2$ type dopamine receptors; ret, receptor tyrosin kinase, Ret, which, together with GFR$\alpha_1$, forms the receptor complex for the glial cell-line-derived neurotrophic factor (GDNF); DAT, dopamine transporter, GLURs, glutamate receptors; E, embtyonic age in days.*

# Future directions

The maturation of dopamine and 5HT transmission follows a complex developmental pattern of activation of various genes, which can be selectively modulated by a specific interaction with the developing target tissue. Timing of maturation is also different among different neurotransmitters: at birth, maturation of serotoninergic function can be considered complete; and dopaminergic function continues developing until early adult life

(8 weeks after birth for rodents, late adolescence for humans). Differences in maturation can explain clinical and neurochemical differences between adults and children/adolescents in several CNS disorders, including migraine. Investigation of the pathophysiology of the migraine attack, which incorporates the developmental perspective described in this chapter, could lead to a new, age-specific therapeutic approach to this disorder.

# References

1. Moskowitz MA, Neurogenic versus vascular mechanisms of sumatriptan and ergot alkaloids in migraine. *Trends Pharmacol Sci* 1992; **13**: 307–11.
2. Weiller C, May A, Limmroth V et al, Brain stem activation in spontaneous human migraine attacks. *Nature Med* 1995; **1**: 658–60.
3. Goadsby PJ, Zagami AS, Lambert GA, Neural processing of craniovascular pain: a synthesis of the central structures involved in migraine. *Headache* 1991; **31**: 365–71.
4. Diener HC, May A, Positron emission tomography studies in acute migraine attacks. In: Sandler M, Ferrari M, Harnett S, eds, *Migraine Pharmacology and Genetics*. London: Chapman & Hall, 1996: 109–16.
5. Goadsby PJ, Uddman R, Edvinsson L, Cerebral vasodilation in the cat involves nitric oxide from parasympathetic nerves. *Brain Res* 1996; **707**: 110–18.
6. Fozard JR, 5-Hydroxytryptamine and nitric oxide: the casual relationship between two endogenous precipitants of migraine. In: Sandler M, Ferrari M, Harnett S, eds, *Migraine Pharmacology and Genetics*. London: Chapman & Hall, 1996: 167–79.
7. Rapport MM, Green AA, Page IH, Crystalline serotonin. *Science* 1948; **108**: 329–30.
8. Ersparmer V, Asero B, Identification of enteramine, specific hormone of enterochromaffin system, as 5-hydroxytryptamine. *Nature* 1952; **169**: 800.
9. Dahlstrom A, Fuxe K, Evidence for the existence of monoamine-containing neurons in the central nervous system. I: Demonstration of monoamines in the cell bodies of brainstem neurons. *Acta Physiol Scand Suppl* 1964; **62**(232): 1–55.
10. Jacobs BL, Azmitia EC, Structure and function of the brain serotonin system. *Physiol Rev* 1992; **72**: 165–229.
11. Lucki I, The spectrum of behaviors influenced by serotonin. *Biol Psychiatry* 1998; **44**: 151–62.
12. Rubenstein JLR, Development of serotonergic neurons and their projections. *Biol Psychiatry* 1998; **44**: 145–50.
13. Rubenstein JLR, Simamura K, Regulation of patterning and differentiation in the embryonic vertebrate forebrain. In: Cowan WV, Jessel TM, Zipursky SL, eds, *Molecular and Cellular Approaches to Neural Development*. Oxford: Oxford University Press, 1997: 356–90.
14. Eaton MJ, Whittemore SR, Autocrine BDNF secretion enhances the survival and serotonergic differentiation of raphe neuronal precursor cells grafted into the adult rat CNS. *Exp Neurol* 1996; **140**: 105–14.
15. Rudge JS, Eaton MJ, Mather P, Lindsay R, Whittemore SR, CTNF induces raphe neuronal precursors to switch from a serotonergic to a cholinergic phenotype in vitro. *Mol Cell Neurol* 1996; **7**: 204–21.
16. Wallace JA, Lauder JM, Development of the serotonergic system in rat and chick embryos. In: Bjorklund A, Hokfelt T, Tohyama M, eds, *Handbook of Chemical Neuroanatomy*, vol 10: *Ontogeny of Transmitters and Peptides in the CNS*. Amsterdam: Elsevier Science, 1992: 619.
17. Lebrand C, Cases O, Adelbrecht C et al, Transient uptake and storage of serotonin in developing thalamic neurons. *Neuron* 1996; **17**: 823–35.
18. Cases O, Vitalis T, Seif I, De Maeyer E, Sotelo C, Gaspar P, Lack of barrels in the somatosensory cortex of monoamine oxidase A deficient mice: a role of serotonin excess during the critical period. *Neuron* 1996; **16**: 297–307.
19. Osterheld-Haas MC, Hornung JP, Laminar development of the mouse barrel cortex: effect

of neurotoxin against monoamines. *Exp Brain Res* 1996; **110**: 183–95.

20. Hellendall RP, Schambra UB, Liu JP et al, Prenatal expression of 5-HT1C and 5-HT-2 receptors in the rat central nervous system. *Exp Neurol* 1993; **120**: 186–201.

21. Tecott L, Shtrom S, Julius D, Expression of a serotonin-gated ion channel in embryonic neural and nonneural tissues. *Mol Cell Neurosci* 1995; **6**: 43–55.

22. Lauder JM, Ontogeny of neurotransmitter systems: substrates for developmental disabilities? *Ment Retard Dev Disabil Res Rev* 1995; **1**: 151–68.

23. Moiseiwitsch JRD, Lauder JM, Serotonin regulates mouse cranial neural crest migration. *Proc Natl Acad Sci USA* 1995; **92**: 7182–6.

24. Hoyer D, Clarke DE, Fozard JR et al, International Union of Pharmacology classification of receptors for 5-hydroxytryptamine (serotonin). *Pharmacol Rev* 1994; **46**: 157–203.

25. Hartig PR, Hoyer D, Humphrey PPA, Martin GR, Alignment of receptor nomenclature with the human genome: classification of 5-HT1B and 5-HT1D receptor subtypes. *Trends Pharmacol Sci* 1996; **17**: 103–5.

26. Goadsby PJ, Serotonin receptors and the acute attack of migraine. *Clin Neurosci* 1998; **5**: 18–23.

27. Yu X-J, Waeber C, Castanon N et al, 5-Carboxamido-tryptamine, CP-122,288 and dihydroergotamine but not sumatriptan, CP-93,129, and serotonin 5-O-carboxymethyl-glycyl-tyrosin-amide block dural plasma protein extravasation in knockout mice that lack 5-hydroxytryptamine 1B receptors. *Mol Pharmacol* 1996; **49**: 761–5.

28. Goadsby PJ, Hoskin KL, The distribution of trigeminovascular afferents in the non-human primate brain macaca nemestrina: a c-fos immunocytochemical study. *J Anat* 1997; **190**: 367–75.

29. Goadsby PJ, Edvinsson L, The trigeminovascular system and migraine: studies characterizing cerebrovascular and neuropeptide changes seen in man and cat. *Ann Neurol* 1993; **33**: 48–56.

30. Goadsby PJ, Edvinsson L, Human in vivo evidence for trigeminovascular activation in cluster headache. *Brain* 1994; **117**: 427–34.

31. Goadsby PJ, Edvinsson L, Ekman R, Vasoactive peptide release in the extracerebral circulation of humans during migraine headache. *Ann Neurol* 1990; **28**: 183–7.

32. Gallai V, Sarchielli P, Floridi A et al, Vasoactive peptides levels in the plasma of young migraine patients with and without aura assessed both interictally and ictally. *Cephalalgia* 1995; **15**: 384–90.

33. Fanciullacci M, Alessandri M, Figini M, Geppetti P, Michelacci S, Increases in plasma calcitonin gene-related peptide from extracerebral circulation during nitroglycerin-induced cluster headache attack. *Pain* 1995; **60**: 119–23.

34. Goadsby PJ, Lipton RB, A review of paroxysmal hemicranias, SUNCT syndrome and other short-lasting headaches with autonomic features, including new cases. *Brain* 1997; **120**: 193–209.

35. Thomsen LL, Olesen J, Nitric oxide theory of migraine. *Clin Neurosci* 1998; **5**: 28–33.

36. Knowles RG, Moncada S, Nitric oxide synthases in mammals. *Biochem J* 1994; **298**: 249–58.

37. Mayer B, Regulation of nitric oxide synthase and soluble guanylyl cyclase. *Cell Biochem Funct* 1994; **12**: 167–77.

38. Olesen J, Thomsen LL, Lassen LH, Jansen-Olesen J, The nitric oxide hypothesis of migraine and other vascular headaches. *Cephalalgia* 1995; **15**: 94–100.

39. Mauskop A, Altura BM, Role of magnesium in the pathogenesis and treatment of migraines. *Clin Neurosci* 1998; **5**: 24–7.

40. Ramadan NM, Halvorson H, Vande-Linde A, Levine SR, Helpern JA, Welch KM, Low brain magnesium in migraine. *Headache* 1989; **29**: 590–3.

41. Soriani S, Arnaldi C, De Carlo L et al, Serum and red blood cell magnesium levels in juvenile migraine patients. *Headache* 1995; **35**: 14–16.

42. Mauskop A, Altura BT, Cracco RQ, Altura BM, Intravenous magnesium sulfate relieves cluster headaches in patients with low serum ionized magnesium levels. *Headache* 1995; **35**: 597–600.

43. Facchinetti F, Sances G, Borella P, Genazzani

AR, Nappi G, Magnesium prophylaxis of menstrual migraine: effects on intracellular magnesium. *Headache* 1991; **31**: 298–301.

44. Peikert A, Wilimizig C, Kohne-Volland R, Prophylaxis of migraine with oral magnesium: results from a prospective, multi-center, placebo-controlled and double-blind randomized study. *Cephalalgia* 1996; **16**: 257–63.

45. Altura BT, Altura BM, Endothelium-dependent relaxation in coronary arteries requires magnesium ions. *Br J Pharmacol* 1987; **91**: 449–51.

46. Foster AC, Fagg GE, Neurobiology. Taking apart NMDA receptors. *Nature* 1987; **329**: 395–6.

47. Huang QF, Gebrewold A, Zhang A, Altura BT, Altura BM, Role of excitatory amino acids in regulation of rat pial microvasculature. *Am J Physiol* 1994; **266**: R158–63.

48. Sicuteri F, Dopamine, the second putative protagonist in headache. *Headache* 1997; **17**: 129–31.

49. Lance JW, Headache. *Ann Neurol* 1981; **10**: 1–10.

50. Blin O, Azulay J, Masson G, Aubrespey G, Serratrice G, Apomorphine-induced yawning in migraine patients: enhanced responsiveness. *Clin Neuropharmacol* 1991; **14**: 91–5.

51. Del Bene E, Poggioni M, Tommasi F, *Video Assessment of Headache*, 1994.

52. Peroutka SJ, Dopamine and migraine. *Neurology* 1997; **49**: 650–6.

53. Barbanti P, Bronzetti E, Ricci A et al, Increased density of dopamine D5 receptor in peripheral blood lymphocytes of migraineurs: a marker for migraine? *Neurosci Lett* 1996; **207**: 73–6.

54. Peroutka SJ, Wilholt T, Jones K, Clinical susceptibility to migraine with aura is modified by dopamine D2 receptor (DRD2) NcoI alleles. *Neurology* 1997; **49**: 201–6.

55. Del Zompo M, Cherchi A, Palmas MA et al, Association between dopamine receptor genes and migraine without aura in a Sardinian sample. *Neurology* 1998; **51**: 781–6.

56. Nelson EL, Liang CL, Sinton CM et al, Midbrain dopaminergic neurons in the mouse: computer-assisted mapping. *J Comp Neurol* 1996; **369**: 361–71.

57. Bjorklund A, Lindvall O, Dopamine containing systems in the CNS. In: Bjorklund A, Hokfelt T, eds, *Handbook of Chemical Neuroanatomy*. Amsterdam: Elsevier, 1984: 55–122.

58. Liang CL, Sinton CM, German DC, Midbrain dopaminergic neurons in the mouse: co-localization with Calbindin-D28K and calretinin. *Neuroscience* 1996; **75**: 523–33.

59. Alfahel-Kakunda A, Silverman WF, Calcium-binding proteins in the substantia nigra and ventral tegmental area during development: correlation with dopaminergic compartmentalization. *Brain Res Dev Brain Res* 1997; **103**: 9–20.

60. Egan MF, Weinberger DR, Neurobiology of schizophrenia. *Curr Opin Neurobiol* 1997; **7**: 701–7.

61. Swanson J, Castellanos FX, Murias M et al, Cognitive neuroscience of attention deficit hyperactivity disorder and hyperkinetic disorder. *Curr Opin Neurobiol* 1998; **8**: 263–71.

62. Williams GV, Goldman-Rakic PS, Modulation of memory fields by dopamine D1 receptors in prefrontal cortex. *Nature* 1995; **376**: 572–5.

63. Tang YP, Noda Y, Nabeshima T, Involvement of activation of dopaminergic neuronal system in learning and memory deficits associated with experimental mild traumatic brain injury. *Eur J Neurosci* 1997; **9**: 1720–7.

64. Gingrich JA, Caron MG, Recent advances in the molecular biology of dopamine receptors. *Annu Rev Neurosci* 1993; **16**: 299–321.

65. Di Porzio U, Zuddas A, Cosenza-Murphy DB et al, Early appearance of tyrosine hydroxylase immunoreactive neurones in the mesencephalon of mouse embryos. *Int J Dev Neurosci* 1990; **8**: 523–32.

66. Freeman TB, Spence MS, Boss BD et al, Development of dopaminergic neurones in the human substantia nigra. *Exp Neurol* 1991; **113**: 344–53.

67. Ericson J, Morton S, Kawakami A et al, Two critical periods of sonic hedgehog signaling required for the specification of motor neuron identity. *Cell* 1996; **87**: 661–73.

68. Zetterstrom RH, Williams R, Perlmann T et al, Cellular expression of the immediate early transcription factors Nurr1 and NGFI-B suggests a gene regulatory role in several brain regions including the nigrostriatal dopamine system.

*Brain Res Mol Brain Res* 1996; **41**: 111–20.

69. Ye W, Shimamura K, Rubenstein JLR et al, FGF and SHH signals control dopaminergic and serotonergic cell fate in the anterior neural plate. *Cell* 1998; **93**: 755–66.

70. Smidt MP, van Schaick HS, Lanctot C et al, A homeodomain gene *Ptx3* has highly restricted brain expression in mesencephalic dopaminergic neurons. *Proc Natl Acad Sci USA* 1997; **94**: 13 305–10.

71. Saucedo-Cardenas O, Quintana-Hau JD, Le WD et al, Nurr1 is essential for the induction of the dopaminergic phenotype and the survival of ventral mesencephalic late dopaminergic precursor neurons. *Proc Natl Acad Sci USA* 1998; **95**: 4013–18.

72. GFR-α Nomenclature Committee, Nomenclature of GPI-linked receptors for the GDNF ligand family. *Neuron* 1997; **19**: 485.

73. Lindsay RM, Yancopoulos GD, GDNF in a bind with known orphan: accessory implicated in new twist. *Neuron* 1996; **17**: 571–4.

74. Nosrat CA, Tomac A, Hoffer BJ et al, Cellular and developmental patterns of expression of Ret and glial cell line-derived neurotrophic factor receptor alpha mRNAs. *Exp Brain Res* 1997; **115**: 410–22.

75. Hyman C, Juhasz M, Jackson C et al, Overlapping and distinct actions of the neurotrophins BDNF, NT-3, and NT-4/5 on cultured dopaminergic and GABAergic neurons of the ventral mesencephalon. *J Neurosci* 1994; **14**: 335–47.

76. Prochiantz A, Di Porzio U, Kato A et al, In vitro maturation of mesencephalic dopaminergic neurons from mouse embryos is enhanced in presence of their striatal target cells. *Proc Natl Acad Sci USA* 1979; **76**: 5387–91.

77. Di Porzio U, Daguet MC, Glowinski J et al, Effect of striatal cells on in vitro maturation of mesencephalic dopaminergic neurons in serum-free conditions. *Nature* 1980; **288**: 370–3.

78. Schambra UB, Duncan GE, Breese GR et al, Ontogeny of D1A and D2 dopamine receptor subtypes in rat brain using in situ hybridization and receptor binding. *Neuroscience* 1994; **62**: 65–85.

79. Fiszman ML, Zuddas A, Masana MI et al, Dopamine synthesis precedes dopamine uptake in embryonic rat mesencephalic neurones. *J Neurochem* 1991; **56**: 392–9.

80. Perrone-Capano C, Tino A, di Porzio U, Target cells modulate dopamine transporter gene expression during brain development. *Neuroreport* 1994; **5**: 1145–8.

81. Daguet MC, Di Porzio U, Prochiantz A et al, Release of dopamine from dissociated mesencephalic dopaminergic neurons in primary cultures in absence or presence of striatal target cells. *Brain Res* 1980; **191**: 564–8.

82. Cragg SJ, Holmes C, Hawkey CR et al, Dopamine is released spontaneously from developing midbrain neurons in organotypic culture. *Neuroscience* 1998; **84**: 325–30.

83. Liu Y, Edwards RH. The role of vesicular transport proteins in synaptic transmission and neural degeneration. *Annu Rev Neurosci* 1997; **20**: 125–56.

84. McCaffery P, Drager UC, High levels of a retinoic acid-generating dehydrogenase in the meso-telecephalic dopamine system. *Proc Natl Acad Sci USA* 1994; **91**: 7772–6.

85. Amara SG, Arriza JL, Neurotransmitter transporters: three distinct gene families. *Curr Opin Neurobiol* 1993; **3**: 337–44.

86. Revay R, Vaughan R, Grant S et al, Dopamine transporter immunohistochemistry in median aminence, amygdala, and other areas of the rat brain. *Synapse* 1996; **22**: 93–9.

87. Hersch SM, Yi H, Heilman CJ, Edwards RH et al, Subcellular localization and molecular topology of the dopamine transporter in the striatum and substantia nigra. *J Comp Neurol* 1997; **388**: 211–27.

88. Giros B, Jaber M, Jones SR et al, Hyperlocomotion and indifference to cocaine and amphetamine in mice lacking the dopamine transporter. *Proc Natl Acad Sci USA* 1996; **379**: 606–12.

89. Jones SR, Gainetdinov RR, Jaber M et al, Profound neuronal plasticity in response to inactivation of the dopamine transporter. *Proc Natl Acad Sci USA* 1998; **95**: 4029–34.

90. Perrone Capano C, Tino A, Amadoro G et al, Dopamine transporter gene expression in rat mesencephalic dopaminergic neurones is increased by direct interaction with target striatal cells in vitro. *Mol Brain Res* 1996; **39**: 160–6.

# 4

# Pharmacology

*Alessandra Cherchi, Maria Del Zompo*

The treatment of migraine in children is not easy to schedule because these subjects cannot easily distinguish pain from migraine and tension-type headache. In addition, there is only a limited number of well-designed studies that demonstrate a clear efficacy of pharmacological agents. Furthermore, the interpretation of the results of therapeutic trials is complicated by a high rate of response to placebo, difficulties in measuring pain and a high variability in the pattern of the attacks. The approach to the treatment of the disease consists mainly in the avoidance of trigger factors, rest and, when required, the use of pharmacological agents. Trigger factors may be identified by teaching children to fill in a 'headache diary' to describe the characteristics of their headache, their food intake, weather changes and associated stress. Initial therapy should prescribe resting in a dark and quiet room because pain is exacerbated by many activities such as watching television or playing board games. Behavioural therapy has also been shown to be effective in managing the frequency and intensity of migraine attacks. The behavioural approach to the disease involves regular sleep and meals, and biofeedback.[1]

The pharmacological treatment of migraine consists of abortive and/or preventive therapy. The former is aimed at relieving or ameliorating the symptoms of an acute attack, whereas preventive therapy, which requires the daily intake of medication for a certain period of time, decreases the frequency of the attacks and the severity of pain.

The aim of this chapter is to describe the mechanism of action of drugs used to treat and prevent the acute attacks of migraine and, when possible, to correlate the mechanism to some of the hypothesized migraine pathogenesis.

## Pharmacology of acute treatment

If attacks are infrequent and mild, simple analgesics could be used, whereas a prophylactic treatment should be considered if the attacks are frequent and highly debilitating.[2,3] Abortive drugs for migraine are simple analgesic drugs, anti-migraine agents and antiemetics.

### Non-steroidal anti-inflammatory drugs

Non-steroidal anti-inflammatory drugs (NSAIDs) represent a heterogeneous group of compounds, often chemically unrelated, which share certain therapeutic actions and side effects. These drugs are able to inhibit cyclooxygenase, one of the enzymes responsible for the biosynthesis of the prostaglandins and some related autacoids. Prostaglandins (PGs) are important mediators of inflammation and are synthesized from arachidonic acid. This acid is not available in a free form, but is obtained from phospholipases A, B and C. The bifunctional enzyme cyclo-oxygenase catalyses the oxygenation of the arachidonic acid to the cyclic endoperoxide $PGG_2$, and, in a peroxidase step, reduces the C-15 hydroperoxide to a hydroxyl $PGH_2$ (Fig. 4.1).[4]

Recently, the existence of two isoforms of cyclo-oxygenase, COX-1 and COX-2, has been demonstrated. Both forms are membrane-associated glycoproteins: COX-1 is the 'constitutive' isoform found in the blood

vessels, stomach and kidney, whereas COX-2 is the 'induced' form synthesized in inflammation sites by cytokines and inflammatory mediators. COX-2 is found in small amounts in human lung, rat kidney and fetal membranes, but most of its activity is the result of an induction; in fact it may increase by more than 20-fold during the inflammatory reaction, with COX-1 being increased two- to threefold. COX-1 activation leads to the production of prostacyclin ($PGI_2$), which is antithrombogenic when released by endothelium and cytoprotective when released by the gastric mucosa. In blood vessels it is essential for the synthesis of thromboxane $A_2$ ($TxA_2$) and its pharmacological inhibition determines a loss of normal platelet aggregation. Inhibition of gastric prostaglandin production is considered to be the cause of the most frequent and dangerous side effects of NSAIDs: gastric ulceration, bleeding and perforation. In the kidney, prostaglandins are synthesized by the renal medulla and influence several functions as total renal blood flow, $Na^+$ and water reabsorption, and renin release. All these functions, with the possible exception of renin secretion, seem to depend on COX-1 activity. Renal side effects of NSAIDs include reduction of glomerular filtration rate and $Na^+$ and water excretion. These effects can lead to acute renal failure and increase of blood pressure. The kinetics of COX-1 inhibition differs from that of COX-2. COX-1 inhibition is competitively reversible because it depends on hydrogen binding, whereas COX-2 inhibition is essentially irreversible, probably as a result of covalent binding. COX-2 inhibitor agents are selective for COX-2 at the range of doses normally used in a clinical regimen. Aspirin is a selective COX-1 inhibitor of platelets at low doses, whereas at high doses the inhibition is

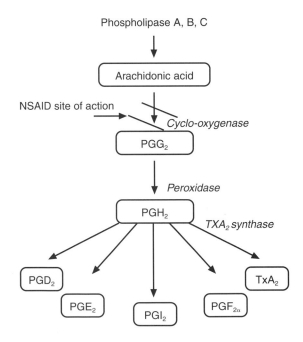

**Figure 4.1**
*Prostaglandin pathway. NSAID, non-steroidal anti-inflammatory drug; PG, prostaglandin; $PGI_2$, prostacyclin; $TxA_2$, thromboxane $A_2$*

generalized. Non-selective COX inhibitors include: indometacin, piroxicam, diclofenac and ibuprofen, and aspirin at high doses. Meloxicam and enolcarboxamide, a compound related to piroxicam, are described as COX-2-selective inhibitors. Celecoxib, a COX-2-selective inhibitor and a 1,5-diarylpyrazole-based compound, was approved by the US Food and Drug Administration (FDA) in 1998 for rheumatoid arthritis but not for analgesia.[4,5]

Chemical classification of analgesic, antipyretic and non-steroidal anti-inflammatory drugs used in migraine therapy includes salicylic acid derivates, *p*-aminophenol derivates, indole and indene acetic acids, heteroarylacetic acids and arylpropionic acids (Table 4.1). Table 4.2 shows the NSAIDs used to treat pain in children.

Although the inhibition of cyclo-oxygenase is thought to be the major mechanism of action of all NSAIDs, numerous differences are observed in their activities, possibly depending on their different action on enzymes.

## Salicylates

Aspirin is a salicylate ester of acetic acid with analgesic, antipyretic and anti-inflammatory effects. Given orally, it is absorbed rapidly, partly from the stomach but mostly from the upper small intestine. The rate of absorption is determined by the pH at the gastric mucosal surface and the presence of food in the stomach. The peak value is reached in about 2 h and then declines, with a half-life of 15 min. The biotransformation of aspirin takes place in the hepatic endoplasmic reticulum and mitochondria; it is excreted in the urine. This drug has not been approved by the FDA for use in babies.[6] Aspirin must be avoided in children under the age of 12 because of its

Salicylates: salicylic acid, aspirin, methyl salicylate
*p*-Aminophenol derivates: acetaminophen
Indole and indene acetic acids: indometacin
Heteroarylacetic acids: diclofenac, ketorolac
Arylpropionic acids: ibuprofen, naproxen, ketoprofen

**Table 4.1**
*Analgesic–antipyretic and non-steroidal anti-inflammatory drugs used in migraine therapy*

| Aspirin | Use: permitted >12 |
|---|---|
| Acetaminophen | Use: permitted >4 |
| Indometacin | Use: not approved in children (FDA) |
| Ketoralac | Use: not approved in children (FDA) |
| Diclofenac | Use: not approved in children (FDA) |
| Ibuprofen | Use: permitted >2 |
| Naproxen | Use: permitted >12 |
| Ketoprofen | Use: not approved in children |

**Table 4.2**
*Analgesic, antipyretic and non-steroidal anti-inflammatory drugs used to treat pain in children*

possible association with Reye's syndrome, although its use is feasible above that age at the adult dosage of 1000 mg/day.[3]

## p-Aminophenol derivates

Acetaminophen, N-acetyl-*p*-aminophenol, is the active metabolite of phenacetin (not available in the U.K.) and has analgesic and antipyretic properties. It is rapidly absorbed from the gastrointestinal tract. Its peak in the plasma is reached in 30–60 min and its half-life is about 2 h. The drug is metabolized in the liver and eliminated mostly with urine. The FDA has authorized the use of the drug in children at a dosage of 240 mg in 4–5 year olds and 480 mg in 11–12 year olds.[6]

### Indole and indene acetic acids

Indometacin is a methylated indole derivative, with analgesic but mainly anti-inflammatory properties. It is rapidly absorbed from the gastrointestinal tract. The peak concentration in the plasma is reached within 2 h, but may be delayed when the drug is taken after meals. The half-life in the plasma is variable but is around 2 h. The agent is metabolized in the liver and eliminated mostly with the urine, but also with the bile and faeces. The FDA has not approved its use in children.[6]

### Heteroarylacetic acids

Ketorolac is a heteroarylacetic acid derivative. It is a potent analgesic and a weak anti-inflammatory agent. Ketorolac is rapidly absorbed when given orally or intramuscularly, achieving the peak plasma concentration in 30–50 min. Its half-life ranges from 4 to 6 h and it is about 90% eliminated in the wine. The FDA has not approved this agent for the treatment of pain in children.[6]

Diclofenac is a phenylacetic acid derivative with anti-inflammatory, analgesic and antipyretic activities. It is rapidly absorbed when given orally and intramuscularly, achieving the peak plasma concentration in 30–50 min. The drug has a half-life of 4–6 h and is eliminated through the kidneys. The FDA has not approved this agent for the treatment of pain in children.[6]

### Arylpropionic acids

Ibuprofen is the main member of the propionic class of NSAIDs. It has anti-inflammatory, antipyretic and analgesic properties. It is rapidly absorbed when given orally. The peak in plasma levels is observed after 1–2 h, with a half-life of about 2 h. The biotransformation occurs in the liver and the excretion is renal. The efficacy of this agent was evaluated compared with acetaminophen in a double-masked, randomized controlled, crossover study performed in a group of 106 children aged 4–16 years who had migraine. The study showed the efficacy of both treatments with respect to placebo. Ibuprofen provided the best relief.[7] The FDA has authorized the use of this agent in children aged over 2 years.[6] The dose of ibuprofen suggested in children aged under 12 is from a quarter to half the adult dose.[1]

Naproxen is fully absorbed when administered orally. The rapidity is influenced by the presence of food in the stomach. Peak plasma concentration occurs in 2–4 h. Naproxen is also absorbed rectally with a half-life in the plasma of about 14 h. The drug is metabolized by the liver and almost entirely excreted in the urine. The FDA has approved the agent for paediatric use at the age of 12 years or over, in the abortive treatment of migraine.[6]

Ketoprofen shares the pharmacological properties of other propionic acid derivatives. It is rapidly absorbed after oral administration, its maximal concentration in the plasma is achieved within 1–2 h and its half-life is about 2 h. The drug is biotransformed in the liver and excreted with urine. This agent is not approved for paediatric use in the treatment of pain.[6]

### Other therapies

Several authors suggest that children should be given a gastrokinetic antiemetic before administration of analgesics, especially if nausea and vomiting are severe. The gastrokinetic antiemetics are domperidone and metoclopramide. Both drugs act as blockers of dopaminergic receptors sited in the chemoreceptor trigger zone (CTZ), but domperidone does not cross the blood–brain barrier. Domperidone is available as a suspension in a concentration of 5 mg/5 ml. It does not cause side effects. Metoclopramide is also prepared as a suspension at the concentration of 5 mg/5 ml. It can determine adverse effects such as restlessness and extrapyramidal effects, as a result of antagonism with dopaminergic receptors in the central nervous system.

## Anti-migraine drugs

Specific acute anti-migraine drugs include sumatriptan, the 'second generation of triptans' and the ergot alkaloids.

### Triptans

Triptans are 5-hydroxytryptamine (5HT or serotonin) derivatives; they are selective agonists for vascular 5HT receptor subtypes such as $5HT_{1D}$, $5HT_{1B}$, $5HT_{1F}$ and $5HT_{1A}$, although they possess low affinity for adrenergic and dopaminergic receptors. The anti-migraine effect seems to occur through different mechanisms:

(1) Inhibition of dural neurogenic inflammation
(2) Direct attenuation of excitability of cells in trigeminal nuclei via stimulation of $5HT_{1B}$ receptors
(3) Vasoconstriction of meningeal, dural, cerebral or pial vessels mediated via stimulation of $5HT_{1B}$ receptors.[8]

Sumatriptan is a $5HT_1$ receptor agonist, with a high affinity for $5HT_{1D}$ and $5-HT_{1B}$

receptors and lower interaction with $5HT_{1A}$ and $5HT_{1E}$ receptors. Sumatriptan is rapidly absorbed after oral administration, with a bioavailability of 14%, as a result of an extensive first-pass metabolism and a half-life of 2.5 h. It is metabolized in the liver and its metabolites are excreted in the urine. Clinical studies in adults have shown that this drug is effective, well tolerated and safe in adults as an anti-migraine agent.[8] Few studies are available about its use in children and adolescents. Some of the studies available are open trials and provide conflicting results about the efficacy and tolerability of the agent. Moreover, its dosage in children has not yet been established.[9] A double-masked, randomized controlled study, carried out on a group of 23 children aged from 8 to 16, failed to demonstrate the efficacy of sumatriptan given orally,[10] whereas another double-masked, randomized controlled trial has shown the efficacy of nasal spray in children migraineurs ($p = 0.01$) without the presence of significant clinical adverse effects.[11] The FDA has approved sumatriptan only for use in adults.[6]

The second generation of triptans include zolmitriptan, naratriptan, rizatriptan, eletriptan and frovatriptan. This new class of agents differs from sumatriptan in their interactions with 5HT receptors and their bioavailability.

Zolmitriptan is a $5HT_{1B/D}$-selective agonist with a bioavailability of 40% and a half-life of 2.5–3.[12] Several open-label studies are reported in the literature, showing the efficacy in pain relief and the safety of this drug in children and adolescents in the treatment of migraine attacks.[12–14] A couple of double-masked, randomized studies performed on groups of patients aged from 12 to 65 suggested the efficacy of this agent, and the absence of clinically serious adverse events associated with zolmitriptan treatment.[15,16] The FDA has approved the drug only for use in adults.[6]

Rizatriptan is a selective $5HT_{1B/D}$ receptor agonist with no or very low activity at other 5HT receptor subtypes, or adrenergic, dopaminergic and histaminergic receptors. This agent is rapidly absorbed after oral administration, with a bioavailability of 40–45% and a plasma half-life of 2–3 h. It is metabolized in the liver by monoamine oxidase A and excreted with its metabolites mostly in the urine. At the present time, several studies are being carried out that evaluate the use of this agent in children and adolescents. The FDA approved the use of this agent only in adults.[6]

Naratriptan is a selective $5HT_{1B}$ and $5HT_{1D}$ agonist. Absorbed when given orally, it presents a bioavailability of 70%. Metabolized in the liver, it is excreted in the urine. The efficacy and safety of this agent in adults have been established in at least four randomized controlled studies, although documentation about use in children is still poor. The FDA approved its use as an anti-migraine agent only in adults.[6]

### Ergotamine

Ergotamine belongs to the class of ergot alkaloids, derivatives of the tetracyclic compound 6-methylergoline. They are non-selective pharmacological agents which interact with various receptors, such as $5HT_1$ and $5HT_2$, adrenergic and dopaminergic receptors. The absorption of the drug when given orally is changable as a result of an extensive first-pass metabolism. The peak plasma concentration is reached in about 70 min. Ergotamine is metabolized in the liver and excreted mostly in the bile. Only traces of unmetabolized drug are found in the urine and faeces. Ergotamine

preparations are available in a variety of preparations and combinations with other agents. Controlled studies in children have been unsuccessful because of high drop-out rates for side effects such as nausea and increase of headache symptoms. Ergotamine is no longer used to treat migraine and is not indicated in children.

## Prophylactic treatment of migraine

Migraine is considered to be a disorder of multifactorial aetiology which can be triggered by external and internal factors. Each attack is characterized by headache combined with autonomic disturbances, mostly nausea, vomiting, photophobia and phonophobia. Migraine prophylaxis is requested in the presence of more than three attacks per month, when attacks do not respond to acute treatment or when the adverse events of acute treatments are severe.

The aim of preventive treatment is to reduce the frequency and severity of attacks while keeping the side effects to a minimum. Many medications studied as preventive treatments of migraine have not been adequately evaluated in children; others were involved in clinical trials carried out before the establishment of the International Headache Society (IHS) migraine classification.

In children, drugs such as β blockers, calcium channel blockers, anti-serotoninergic agents, antidepressant agents and clonidine have been widely studied.[17] The drugs described in this chapter are summarized in Table 4.3.

## β blockers

β-Receptors include $β_1$, $β_2$ and $β_3$, all of which are Gs protein coupled and differ with regard

| | |
|---|---|
| Beta-blockers | Propanolol, Timolol |
| Calcium channel blockers | Flunarizine, Verapamil |
| Antiserotoninergic agents | Methysergide |
| Antidepressants | Tricyclic agents |
| Dopamine agonists | Lisuride |
| Miscellaneous | Valproic acid, Clonidine |

**Table 4.3**
*Prophylactic agents for migraine*

to their location. $\beta_1$-Receptors are located in the heart, kidney and central nervous system (CNS), $\beta_2$-receptors in the smooth muscles and CNS and $\beta_3$-receptors in fat.

β Blockers include propranolol, nadolol, atenolol and timolol; only propranolol and timolol are used clinically in the treatment of migraine. β Blockers are characterized by the relative affinity for $\beta_1$- and $\beta_2$-receptors, intrinsic sympathomimetic activity, blockade of α-adrenergic receptors, differences in lipid solubility and pharmacokinetic properties.

These agents are not indicated for use in patients with asthma, congestive heart failure, atrioventricular conduction defects, diabetes and renal insufficiency. Side effects, including hypotension, exercise intolerance, bradycardia and bradyarrhythmias in patients with atrioventricular conduction defects, are seldom severe and are manifested as a consequence of the β-receptor blockade.

The clinical efficacy of β blockers in the prevention of migraine is still unknown and their pharmacological properties do not provide sufficient explanation for the same.

Propranolol interacts with an equal affinity for $\beta_1$- and $\beta_2$-receptors; it is, however, lacking in intrinsic sympathomimetic activity and does not block α-adrenergic receptors. Propranolol

is highly lipophilic and is almost completely absorbed after oral administration. The drug is mostly metabolized by the liver during the first passage through the portal circulation; only 25% reaches the systemic circulation. The bioavailability of this agent may be increased by the concomitant ingestion of food. The efficacy of propranolol in adult and childhood migraine has been suggested;[18] administration should commence at a low dose (1–2 mg/kg per day) and continue for at least 12 weeks.[19] The FDA has approved the use of propranolol in migraine prophylaxis in adults.[6]

Timolol is a potent, non-subtype-selective, β-adrenergic antagonist, possessing no intrinsic sympathomimetic activity. It is well absorbed in the gastrointestinal tract when given orally and is subject to moderate first-pass metabolism. The FDA has approved the use of this drug only in adults.[6]

## Calcium channel blockers

Voltage-sensitive channels have been divided into various subtypes on the basis of their kinetic and functional properties. According to their kinetic characteristics, they are differentiated into 'low-threshold' and 'high-threshold'

43

channels. The former, also called 'T' channels, can be opened by short depolarizations and play a key role in the control of the excitability and activity of some nervous cells. The latter can be opened by using high depolarizations and include L, N, P and Q channels, which are also represented in the CNS. High-threshold channels are reportedly responsible for the high increases of the cytosolic $Ca^{2+}$ and the release of intracellular calcium necessary for its action as a second messenger. Calcium antagonists (CaCB) inhibit voltage-sensitive calcium by channels blocking the entry of extracellular $Ca^{2+}$ and the release of intracellular $Ca^{2+}$ into vascular smooth muscles, causing vasodilatation. This group of drugs includes compounds such as flunarizine, nimodipine, verapamil and diltiazem.

Flunarizine is considered as a wide-spectrum CaCB: it acts on T- and L-type calcium channels by binding the receptor site at the extracellular surface of the calcium channels of the cardiac muscle, vascular smooth muscles, CNS neurons and chromaffin cells. The mechanism of action of flunarizine in the prevention of migraine is not clear; it is thought to be the result of the blockade of different pathways of intracellular calcium elevation.[20] Several authors have suggested that the anti-migraine effect is related to its ability to interfere with the dopaminergic system blocking $D_2$-receptors. The importance of the role played by the dopaminergic system is based on the evidence that this drug is able to cause extrapyramidal side effects and/or depression.[21] Weizman et al[22] suggested the existence of a pharmacological interaction between flunarizine and the opioid system. They showed that, in mice, the analgesic effect of flunarizine was reversed by naloxonazine, a μ-receptor antagonist.[22] Flunarizine also seems to interfere with

the cholinergic system, which is reportedly involved in the mechanisms of pain regulation, determining a decrease in the release of hippocampal acetylcholine in rats after long-term concomitant administration of pentylenetetrazole.[23] Flunarizine appears to be effective in the prophylaxis of adult and childhood migraine at a dose of 0.1–0.3 mg/kg per day for 12 weeks.[24]

Verapamil, an L-type CaCB, acts on vascular smooth muscle and cardiac cells, inducing a negative inotropic effect on sinoatrial (SA) and atrioventricular (AV) nodes; therefore it should not be used in patients with ventricular or nodal conduction dysfunctions.

When given orally, calcium channel blockers are almost completely absorbed, although their bioavailability is reduced as a result of the first-pass hepatic metabolism; their half-life is widely variable and may range from 1.3 to 64 h. Biotransformation of verapamil results in the production of norverapamil, which is biologically active but less potent. The most common side effects observed with this group of agents are caused by excessive vasodilatation. The FDA has not approved the use of this drug for migraine in children.[6]

## Anti-serotoninergic drugs

The evidence linking 5HT to migraine is circumstantial. During a migraine attack, platelet 5HT decreases, urinary 5HT increases in some patients and 5-hydroxyindole acetic acid (5HIAA), a major metabolite of 5HT, may increase.

This class of agents includes methysergide, a congener of methylergonovine, which blocks $5HT_{2A}$, $5HT_{2B}$ and $5HT_{2C}$ receptors. Methysergide is a $5HT_1$ receptor agonist and its therapeutic effect is dependent on $5HT_2$ blockade and vasoconstriction of the carotid vascular bed.[25,26] Fozard[27] has speculated that the activation of $5HT_{2B}$ and $5HT_{2C}$ receptors by endogenous 5HT could dilate cerebral vessels, resulting in the release of endothelium-derived nitric oxide (NO), which can activate sensory trigeminovascular fibres.[27] Various side effects are manifested with this compound, although they are usually mild and of a transient nature; the most common are diarrhoea, nausea and vomiting. Central disturbances include drowsiness, weakness, nervousness, excitement and psychotic episodes. The onset of inflammatory fibrosis represents a rare but potentially severe complication of prolonged treatment. This condition can develop in different sites, giving rise to retroperitoneal fibrosis, pleuropulmonary fibrosis, and coronary and endocardial fibrosis. Fibrosis usually reverses after drug withdrawal, although persistent damage to cardiac valves has been observed in 1 of 5000 treated patients. Consistently, therapy should be interrupted after 6 months of continuous treatment. In adults, the efficacy of methysergide in the prophylaxis of migraine headache is well documented. The FDA has approved the drug for clinical use in adults although its safety and efficacy in children have not yet been proved.[6]

## Antidepressants

This class of drugs includes tricyclic agents such as amitriptyline, imipramine, nortriptyline, trazodone and selective serotonin reuptake inhibitors.

Amitriptyline is an effective agent for the prophylaxis of migraine in adults. It causes a potent inhibition of 5HT reuptake and antagonizes $5HT_2$ receptors. The prophylactic effect is independent of its antidepressant action and is probably the result of modulation of the serotoninergic system. Side effects are related to the anticholinergic properties of this drug and include dry mouth, dizziness, urinary retention, cardiac arrhythmia and orthostatic hypotension. When given orally, amitriptyline reaches a peak serum level after 4 h, with a half-life of 2–25 h. The hepatic metabolism converts the drug into nortriptyline, an active derivative. The drug is excreted through the kidney. The dose of oral amitriptyline may range from 0.1 to 2 mg/kg per day, as suggested by Hamalainen et al.[19] The FDA has not approved the use of this drug for migraine prophylaxis in children.[6]

To date, the use of other antidepressants such as selective serotonin reuptake inhibitors in the preventive treatment of migraine has not been suggested.

## Dopamine agonists

Lisuride is a semi-synthetic ergot derivative capable of stimulating $D_1$ and $D_2$ dopamine receptor subtypes. Lisuride is characterized by potent antihistaminic, central dopaminergic and anti-serotoninergic activity; data present in the literature report that it may determine a functional response as a full agonist on $5HT_{1B}$ receptors in Chinese hamster ovary cells. Hypotension caused by the stimulation of $5HT_7$ receptors is blocked by lisuride in anaesthetized rats.[26] A hypotensive action has been described at high doses of this drug in adults, as a result of its activity on dopamine receptors.

When given orally, lisuride reaches a peak concentration after 40 min, with a half-life of 2 h. It may cause cardiovascular side effects such as orthostatic hypotension, nausea and vomiting. The use of lisuride as a prophylactic agent is based on the hypothesis of hypersensitivity of the dopaminergic system in migraineurs. Several clinical studies performed in the past with apomorphine, a dopaminergic agonist, showed the presence of a hyperresponsiveness of dopaminergic receptors in migraineurs, compared with controls.[28] Recently, genetic data reinforced the hypothesis of the involvement of the dopaminergic system in the disease.[29,30] The FDA has approved the use of this compound only in adults for the treatment of headache secondary to hypertension and vasculopathy.[6]

## Miscellaneous

Several drugs used in the prevention of migraine have not yet been studied adequately and are therefore not used in the management of the disease. These include trazodone, clonidine, antihistamines and several anticonvulsants, such as valproate.[31]

The action of valproate as an anticonvulsant agent appears to be mediated by a prolonged recovery of voltage-activated $Na^+$ channels from inactivation. The mechanism of action of this compound in the treatment of migraine is still unknown. Welch et al[32] hypothesized that it may inhibit the central neuronal hyperexcitability. Jensen et al[33] focused on the role of valproate as a $\gamma$-aminobutyric acid (GABA)-mimetic agent that acts on GABA receptors located on the dorsal raphe nuclei, resulting in a decreased firing rate of serotoninergic neurons.[33] The FDA has approved use of this compound for the treatment of migraine in subjects aged over 16 years.[6] Hamalainen[19] suggested the administration of 15–30 mg/kg per day divided into two doses.

Clonidine, an imidazoline, is an $\alpha_2$-selective adrenergic agonist acting on the CNS. To date, its efficacy as an anti-migraine drug has been poorly documented. The FDA has not approved the use of this drug in children.[6]

## Conclusions

In children, the approach to migraine treatment should be restricted to that small group in whom frequent and severe attacks occur, and should also take into consideration the age of the child. On prescribing a pharmacological therapy, the proven efficacy of the compound, contraindications and potential side effects of the treatment should all be carefully evaluated.

## References

1. Welborn CA, Pediatric migraine. *Emerg Med Clin North Am* 1997; **15**: 625–36.
2. Welch KMA, Drug therapy of migraine. *N Engl J Med* 1993; **329**: 1476–83.
3. Spierings ELH, *Management of Migraine*. Oxford: Butterworth-Heinemann, 1996.
4. Frolich JC, A classification of NSAIDs according to the relative inhibition of cyclooxygenase isoenzymes. *Trends Pharmacol Sci* 1997; **18**: 30–4.
5. Hawkey CJ, COX-2 inhibitors. *Lancet* 1999; **353**: 307–14.
6. Micromedex: database informatic system for drug and toxicology information. © 1974–1999. Micromedex Inc., vol 101.
7. Hamalainen ML, Hoppu K, Valkeila E, Santavuori P, Ibuprofen or acetaminophen for the acute treatment of migraine in children: a double-blind, randomized, placebo-controlled, crossover study. *Neurology* 1997; **48**: 103–7.
8. Ferrari MD, Migraine. *Lancet* 1998; **351**: 1043–51.
9. McDonald JT, Treatment of juvenile migraine with subcutaneous sumatriptan. *Headache* 1994; **34**: 581–2.
10. Hamalainen ML, Hoppu K, Santavuori P, Sumatriptan for migraine attacks in children: a randomized, placebo-controlled study. *Neurology* 1997; **48**: 1100–3.

11. Ueberall MA, Wenzel D, Intranasal sumatriptan for the acute treatment of migraine in children. *Neurology* 1999; **52**: 1507.

12. Dowson AJ, Fletcher PE, Millson DS, Efficacy and tolerability of 'Zomig' in adolescent migraine. *Cephalalgia* 1998; **18**: 406–7 (abstract).

13. Solomon GD, Cady RK, Klapper JA, Earl NL, Saper JR, Ramadan NM, Clinical efficacy and tolerability of 2.5 mg zolmitriptan for the acute treatment of migraine. *Neurology* 1997; **49**: 1219–25.

14. Goadsby PJ, 311C90, a novel 5-HT1B/1D receptor agonist. The assessment of efficacy and tolerability in the acute treatment of migraine. *Neurology* 1997; **48**(suppl 2): A86 (abstract).

15. Rapoport AM, Ramadan NM, Adelman JU et al, Optimizing the dose of zolmitriptan ('Zomig', 311C90) for the acute treatment of migraine. A multicenter, double-blind, placebo-controlled, dose range-finding study. *Neurology* 1997; **49**: 1210–18.

16. Brown DL, Sweet RM, 311C is effective in patients who respond poorly to existing antimigraine therapies. *Eur J Neurol* 1996; **3**(suppl 5): 152 (abstract).

17. Igarashi M, May WN, Golden GS, Pharmacological treatment of childhood migraine. *J Pediatr* 1992; **120**: 653–7.

18. Forsythe WI, Gillies D, Sills MA, Propranolol ('Inderal') in the treatment of childhood migraine. *Dev Med Child Neurol* 1984; **26**: 737–41.

19. Hamalainen ML, Migraine in children. Guidelines for treatment. *CNS Drugs* 1998; **10**: 105–17.

20. Zapater P, Moreno J, Horga JF, Neuroprotection by the novel calcium antagonist PCA50938, nimodipine and flunarizine, in gerbil global brain ischemia. *Brain Res* 1997; **772**: 57–62.

21. Piccini P, Nuti A, Paoletti AM, Napolitano A, Melis GB, Bonuccelli U, Possible involvement of dopaminergic mechanisms in the antimigraine action of flunarizine. *Cephalalgia* 1990; **10**: 3–8.

22. Weizman R, Getslev V, Pankova IA, Schrieber S, Pick CG, Pharmacological interaction of the calcium channel blockers verapamil and flunarizine with the opioid system. *Brain Res* 1999; **818**: 187–95.

23. Serra M, Dazzi L, Caddeo M, Floris C, Biggio G, Reversal by flunarizine of the decrease in hippocampal acetylcholine release in pentylenetetrazole-kindled rats. *Biochem Pharmacol* 1999; **58**: 145–9.

24. Sorge F, De Simone R, Marano E, Nolano M, Orefice G, Carrieri P, Flunarizine in prophylaxis of childhood migraine. *Cephalalgia* 1988; **8**: 1–6.

25. Silberstein SD, Methysergide. *Cephalalgia* 1998; **18**: 421–35.

26. De Vries P, De Visser PA, Heiligers JPC, Villalon CM, Saxena PR, Changes in systemic and regional haemodynamics during 5-HT7 receptor-mediated depressor responses in rats. *Naunyn-Schmiedeberg's Arch Pharmacol* 1999; **359**: 331–8.

27. Fozard JR, 5HT in migraine: evidence from 5-HT receptor antagonists for a neuronal aetiology. In: Sandler M, Collins GM, eds, *Migraine: A spectrum of ideas*. New York: Oxford University Press, 1990: 128–46.

28. Cerbo R, Barbanti P, Muzzi MG et al, Dopamine hypersensitivity in migraine: role of the apomorphine test. *Clin Neuropharmacol* 1997; **20**: 36–41.

29. Del Zompo M, Cherchi A, Palmas MA et al, Association between dopamine receptor genes and migraine without aura in a Sardinian sample. *Neurology* 1998; **51**: 781–6.

30. Peroutka SJ, Wilhoit T, Jones K, Clinical susceptibility to migraine with aura is modified by dopamine D2 receptor (DRD2) NcoI alleles. *Neurology* 1997; **49**: 201–6.

31. Silberstein SD, Wilmore LJ, Divalproex sodium: migraine treatment and monitoring. *Headache* 1996; **36**: 239–42.

32. Welch KMA, D'Andrea G, Tepley N, Barkly G, Ramadan NM, The concept of migraine as a state of central neuronal hyperexcitability. *Neurol Clin* 1989; **8**: 817–28.

33. Jensen R, Brinck T, Olesen J, Sodium valproate has a prophylactic effect in migraine without aura. *Neurology* 1994; **44**: 647–51.

# III

## Assessment and diagnosis

# 5

# History taking

*Vincenzo Guidetti, Federica Galli*

We investigate a patient with a headache –
headaches do not occur *in vacuo*

Blau (1986)[1]

The diagnosis and treatment of headaches in
children and adolescents cannot leave out of
consideration the crucial importance of considering the patient as a whole: his or her
neurobiological and psychological maturational processes, and familial and social
environmental factors, must be considered in
order to guarantee drug effectiveness and the
compliance of the patients and/or parents.
Taking a detailed and accurate history is the
best starting point for a correct diagnosis.
However, the diagnostic process may be troublesome, because physiological, psychological
and environmental factors are strictly embedded in the occurrence of headaches. The
employment of the International Headache
Society (IHS) Classification[2] represents a
crucial contribution to the systematization of
the classification in both adulthood and childhood. However, the criteria have shown
limitations in their application to childhood
headache and some modifications of diagnostic parameters have been discussed.[3–12]

Headache is always a symptom, but only a
multilevel analysis can ensure a comprehensive framing of the disease. Multilevel analysis
means first to work at integrating the biologi-

cal an psychological perspectives, considering
the specificity of each individual.

The exclusion of symptomatic headache
opens up several additional questions on the
aetiology, pathophysiology and treatment, as
well as on the specificity of handling children
and adolescents. A child is not a 'little adult'
and many individual factors can affect the
expression of headaches. Beginning by considering the child as a result of his or her development, taking into account neurobiological
and psychological maturational processes,
familial and social environmental factors, is
crucial to avoiding a restraining and unilateral
approach to the disease.

The child is often brought for consultation
by the parents, who cannot always give a
complete description of the symptoms, so
introducing bias in the evaluation of the situation. The child can describe the symptoms
only according to his or her intellectual development and experience. Developmental and
psychological factors influence pain perception and response (see Chapter 34).

The entire problem and the reasons for
consultation should be examined minutely,
before a drug is prescribed. Taking a detailed
and accurate history of the patient's development,[12] framing headache in the daily life
context, is the basis for planning a rational
treatment. The moment of history taking is

crucial for building up an alliance with the parents and patient, for addressing the diagnosis and building up a strong basis for compliance. Losing or overlooking the potential of this moment is to risk undermining our work.

The parents and the patient present to the specialist with worries, doubts and sometimes certainties, but always with several ideas. We should always take into account the worries that head pain may evoke in both parents and patients: from the presence of organic disease (e.g. cerebral tumour) to the presence of mental disease (considering also the symbolic meanings related to the head). It is very important to hold and understand these worries, even though they may seem limited and/or incongruous given our knowledge of or mental progressive structuring towards the diagnosis. By encouraging the parents to tell us their explanations of the head pain we give them the confidence of 'holding', and the idea of an open space.

History taking is an art:[1] the personal style takes shape based on a steady and updated background knowledge obtained through clinical experiences. It means asking, observing, building an alliance, holding worries and doubts, collecting objective data, framing and reframing the subjective interpretations, in order to understand 'what it is hidden behind that headache'. It is not easy to consider all these points of observation at the same time. For this reason, we suggest that a physician and psychologist work together from the first step. The subsequent integration of the two perspectives gives the basis for the decision-making process.

## The headache history

We refer mainly to primary headaches, even when exclusion of the occurrence of secondary headache is one of our main diagnostic objectives. In spite of a careful history taking giving us the crucial diagnostic elements, it is not really enough to make the diagnosis. Neurological and general physical examinations also need to be always carried out, and coordination, reflexes, strength, head circumference, optic fundi, eye movements, any sign of trauma, nuchal rigidity and neurocutaneous abnormality should be carefully evaluated and recorded.

The following points relate to a greater likelihood of symptomatic headache and should always be kept in mind and carefully looked at in the process of history taking, when medical examinations are needed to exclude secondary headache:

- Headache attacks become more severe, more lengthy or more frequent
- Headache has acute onset
- Headache lacks alternating lateralization
- Unexplained recurrent syndrome of vomiting or projectile vomiting
- Headache caused by cough, sneezing, straining, exercise, recumbence or sleep
- Headache wakes child in the night and morning headache is current
- Recent head trauma
- Child's personality or behaviour is changed (increased fatiguability, depression, apathy, failure of attention, decreasing school achievement, irritability, lethargy, anorexia, drowsiness)
- Physical or psychical development delay
- Suffering expression
- Pain is not assuaged by mild pain-killing drugs
- Abnormal signs on examination: visual (e.g. diplopia, blurring of vision, visual loss) or neurological (e.g. neck stiffness, papilloedema, incoordination, seizures) symptoms

- Lack of triggering or relieving factors
- The aura is stereotyped or prolonged, or shows a 'march'.[13]

Any abnormality in neurological examination requires further investigation, particularly if it is related to the co-occurrence of one or more of the above points. However, secondary headaches concern a significant number of patients (15–20% in clinical practice), but our main concerns relate to primary headaches.

## How to proceed with history taking

Blau[12] suggested that we should 'treat the patient like a visitor to your home'. We have at least two people in front of us (mother or father and patient), and sometimes three (mother, father and patient) or more. The first step is greeting, shaking everyone's hand, introducing ourselves and the other colleagues (one or two psychologists) in the room, and an invitation to sit down.

It is important to explain our model of working, to avoid confusions and subsequent misunderstandings. The basis of the correct rapport and the starting point for the building of the diagnostic and therapeutic alliance is to be clear and to explain clearly what will happen. It is sometimes sufficient to say: 'We work at many levels, and usually we consider the possible involvement of both medical and psychological causes of headaches . . .'.

During the anamnesis, the questions should be asked by the doctor. The patient and his or her parents bring a medical problem to our attention, so we must therefore answer in medical terms. The patient merits special attention. His or her collaboration is very important. A child or adolescent is usually brought for consultation by one or both parents. At the start of diagnosis, we should take into account the patient's and the parents' viewpoint. A child can describe the symptoms according to his or her intellectual development and experience, even though shyness may be an obstacle to a description of the symptoms. The child should be encouraged to do this, even though children cannot always describe their symptoms as clearly as adults. An adolescent often asks to be treated as an adult, and we have to speak to his or her adult parts. From the beginning of the rapport, it is important to try to build up an alliance with the patient.

The parents are not always able to give a complete description of the symptoms. Anxieties or personal explanations about possible causes of headache may play an important role, introducing a bias in their evaluation of the situation. Their ideas about the causes of head pain give us important areas to think about, and these should be evaluated and then discussed. The parents and the patient should feel directly involved.

During the first examination, it is better to start with 'open questions'. In fact, 'closed questions' result in 'closed answers' ('yes' or 'no'), bringing about defensive attitudes in both parents and patients. The use of structured interviews on headache characteristics is crucial for achieving scientific goals, but this method should not be used during the first examination. It risks freezing the rapport and limiting the analysis to a collection of quantitative data. Qualitative data are better at helping in the general framing of the headache, which is not just a sterile diagnostic label. We have to have 'leading questions' in mind, fitting them to the progress of the communication. Simple questions, in plain words, are preferable.

At the start we ask a general question such as 'What is the reason for coming to see me?'. We know the general reason for the patient's referral, but the content and tone of the answer give us an idea of the urgency of the problem and the possible definitions of the disease, so opening up space for analysis. It is important to note who speaks first, what the mood is and what terms are used in speaking – the details are important. Only a short amount of time is available to get an idea of the characteristics and context of the headache, to go over the history of the patient and his or her family and to reach decisions.

Once these points have been cleared up, we can analyse the characteristics of the headache. It is better to start from the 'history of headache' rather than from 'the patient or family history', because it represents the unequivocal shared field. Our model of consultation promotes our theories on headache, and these might not be shared by the people whom we are dealing with, e.g. if the parents arrive convinced that their son's headaches are related to a visual disturbance, it might be very difficult to explain the reason for clinical interviews with the child. From the start, it is important to catch the perplexities and doubts of our patient and family, to reframe those in our mind, and finally, at the end of the diagnostic period, to give them back for discussion.

We have to analyse at a double level: at the patient's and the parents' viewpoint. Objective and clear data by the parents may not correspond with those of the patient. The patient should always be encouraged to answer, bearing in mind the difference in language and cognition between a child and an adolescent.

An important question should always be addressed to the patient: 'How many types of headaches do you have?' or 'Do you have one type or two types of headache?' If he or she has only one type of headache, he or she will immediately look astonished and say 'only one'. Otherwise, we go on with analysis of the two types. The patient and his or her parents may be worried by the occurrence of migrainous headache, because of its associated vomiting or symptoms of aura, which inhibit activities. Thus, the co-occurrence of episodic tension-type headache may not be reported. In addition, the symptoms of the two types of headache may be confused and overlapped in the report ('sometimes my headache is throbbing, sometimes pulsating'), which does not help the diagnosis.

## The first onset

It is important to know when the headaches first started ('When did your headache start?'), what characteristics they had ('How did your headache start?') and whether the symptoms and frequency have changed over time. Sometimes it may be difficult to describe the onset crises, because the patient was young and has difficulty remembering the onset episodes.

However, it is important to know why he or she has been referred to a specialist now ('Why have you come to see me now?'). The parents may be alarmed by the increasing frequency and/or intensity of the crises, or worried about school performance, or have simply asked for a consultation. It is important to consider the time that has elapsed from the first onset of headache crises to the request for referral. When headache attacks become more severe, more lengthy or more frequent, headache may be a symptom of a structural lesion.

The IHS classification[1] requires at least five attacks for consideration of the diagnosis of migraine. This criterion may be inadequate in developmental ages, because the child could be brought early for examination, before the minimal number of attacks has been reached. It is very important to ask about the occurrence of particular happenings in relation to onset of the crises ('Did something happen in relation to the onset of headaches?' or 'How did the headaches begin?'). The occurrence of 'objective' events (e.g. the birth of a brother or sister, an accident, the death of a relative, etc.) can easily be reported by the parents. Sometimes small daily 'stressors' may play an important role in triggering or exacerbating headaches. Reporting this may be difficult for both parents and patient. Only a psychological examination will give us an idea about the real weight played by life events in modulating head pain, because individual factors are strictly embedded in pain modulation.[14]

It is important to examine the time of onset of single crises ('Do headaches occur at any special time of the day' and 'Do headaches occur at any special time of the week, month or year?'): the time of day (morning, afternoon, evening, night), the week or seasonal periodicity, or the occurrence of an unpredictable or changed trend. All these factors are important for general framing of the headache and to give us ideas about triggering factors ('Do headaches occur under particular conditions?'), e.g. migraine attacks occurring only during school will help in analysis of the weight of school matters on the patient. On the other hand, an unexplained change in the child's personality or behaviour, delay of physical or psychical development associated with a worsening or sudden onset or headache that wakens the child in the night and the presence of morning headache will require exclusion of secondary headache.

## The frequency

Good monitoring of the rate of occurrence of headache attacks has diagnostic and therapeutic implications. Usually, the question 'How often does the headache occur?' is enough to provide information about the latest period (at least 6 months). A sudden worsening in headache frequency should raise an alarm, particularly if it is related to more lengthy and severe head pain. According to the IHS classification,[1] crises occurring more than 15 days per month open up the diagnosis of chronic daily headache (CDH). The prevalence of childhood and adolescence CDH ranges from 0.2% to 0.9%,[15,16] even though the percentage for all the patients referred to headache centres is obviously much higher (15–20%).

The choice of prophylactic therapy depends on the frequency of crises.

## The length

Evaluation of the length of headache crises ('How long has the headache been present?') may be difficult without the aid of a diary card. Frequently the patient seeks sleep as a relieving factor and the effectiveness of analgesic drugs may make it difficult to quantify exactly the length of the headache. However, headache attacks in children may be briefer and more frequent than in adolescents. For migraine crises, the IHS parameters[1] do not provide for attacks lasting less than 2 h, even though the duration in children may be below this. The item 'length' of the crisis might be modified and reduced, at least to 1 hour, to be adequate for classifying migraine crises with early onset.

## The intensity

The IHS classification[1] requires the presence of 'moderate or severe intensity (inhibits or prohibits daily activities)' to diagnose migraine with or without aura and 'mild or moderate intensity (may inhibit, but not prohibit activities)' for episodic or chronic tension-type headache. The younger the child, the more difficult it is to obtain objective and personal evaluation of the pain's intensity, because individual parameters play the most relevant part in the evaluation of the child's pain. The amount of school absence may be taken into account as another index of frequency and severity of headache. However, school attendance may be regular, with only occasional absences related to headache crises.[17]

Asking the child to evaluate the pain's intensity on a subjective scale from 1 to 10, may be useful for comparing different crises in the same child; alternatively, it can give a general idea, even if it gives weak information about the absolute level of pain, because this is too closely related to the developmental level, memory and cognition categories, the familial context, and present and past environmental answers.

In most cases, behavioural information gives the most important data for evaluation of the pain's intensity. The changes in behaviour can in children fulfil the item 'aggravation by routine physical activity', increasing the accuracy of the diagnosis. During migraine attacks, the child usually stops playing and goes to bed in the dark. Often the child asks to lie down on the sofa and may fall asleep. In tension-type headache, the parent usually becomes aware of headache only if informed by the child.

Pain that is not assuaged by mild pain-killing drugs or reduced by rest becomes more severe and/or is caused by cough, sneezing, straining, recumbence or sleep may alert the physician to a probable occurrence of secondary headache.

## Localization

The child is usually able to locate the side and the point of the head pain; sometimes this is not possible, and the child is able to report the exact localization and the trend of head pain only at the next visit.

The unilateral location of pain is not a specific feature of juvenile migraine, and several authors[3,18] agreed on the predominance of bifrontal location in over 55% of patients. However, unilaterality seems to be more frequent in adolescents than in children, in whom the pain is frequently bilateral and becomes unilateral with increasing age.[3,4,18]

Unilateral headache does not exclude episodic tension-type headache. Migraine and tension-type headache can occur in the same child, and attention to the differential analysis of symptoms for each type may avoid the overlap in symptoms and the generic labels of 'unclassifiable' or 'mixed' headache.

The younger the patient, the more other diagnoses should be taken into account when head pain is always unilateral, with no change in the side:[19] in children, rare primary forms (chronic paroxysmal hemicrania, cluster headache or hemicrania continua) or secondary headache (mainly arteriovenus malformations or malignant or benign tumours) may present a unilateral and unchanging location of pain.

## Quality

The pulsating quality of pain is not a specific feature of childhood migraine, even if its presence is helpful in excluding tension-type headache. It may not be easy to establish the quality of pain, and well-tailored questions are crucial ('What is the quality of pain?' 'Is it pressing, heavy, pulsating, excruciating?').

It has been emphasized[5] that about 15% of migrainous children, especially the youngest, refer to the 'burdening' or 'heavy' quality of the pain. The child should be helped in describing the headache quality by asking for examples or metaphors. Soliciting the description by questions such as 'When you have a headache, do you feel the pain as a throbbing hammer or something that is heavy or pressing?' may be very helpful. Distinguishing between the pressing or tightening quality of pain may be difficult for a child, requiring particular questions.

## Accompanying symptoms

The presence of many and distressing symptoms may frequently account for the request for specialist intervention. The parents' worries may originate from awareness of the symptoms accompanying the head pain.

An in-depth and complete analysis of accompanying symptoms is the starting point for addressing elements in order to obtain a correct differential diagnosis. Non-headache symptoms are not necessarily present in each attack and in each patient. Such symptoms consist of changes in vasomotor control, pallor or flushing, tachycardia, alterations of mood (e.g. irritability or grouchiness) and/or appetite (e.g. anorexia), sleep (e.g. lethargy), fluid balance (e.g. thirsty) and temperature (e.g. shivering or feeling cold). Lacrimation, rings under the eyes and glassy eyes may be reported, mainly by the parents.

Gastrointestinal symptoms (mostly nausea and vomiting) seem to be the most distinctive symptoms of childhood migraine. The absence of both is not typical of migraine in children.

The occurrence of nausea or abdominal symptoms related to headache is not easily recognized. In the youngest patients, clear-cut elements are more difficult to obtain, mainly because of the difficulty in defining a temporal association between head pain and abdominal disorders. The experience of recurrent abdominal pain is common in the developmental ages, and it frequently co-occurs in headache patients, so much so that the term 'abdominal migraine' has been used.[20] By avoidance of the speculative analysis about the effective relationship between abdominal and head pain, it is important to bear in mind that in some patients the co-occurrence of headache and abdominal disorders and/or other 'functional pains' may open up the diagnosis of anxiety disorders.[21] The choice and effectiveness of the drug depend on the correct framing of 'that headache in that patient', and the evaluation of psychological functioning, after the exclusion of structural lesions, should address the best choice.

Photophobia and phonophobia do not seem to present age-related features. The presence of both leads more clearly to the diagnosis of migraine. The presence of vertigo should also be considered carefully by specific questions. Benign paroxismal vertigo is recognized by the IHS classification[1] as a precursor syndrome (also called a variant or equivalent) of migraine, even though objective or subjective vertigo may represent the most prominent feature of migraine both in children and in adults.[22]

In children, the presence of muscle contraction headache is less frequent than in adolescents or adults, but, if it is present, it may be helpful for excluding migraine. Headache with acute onset and associated with neck stiffness, lethargy and vomiting may alert the doctor to exclude structural lesions, particularly if linked to abnormal signs on examination, or visual or neurological symptoms.

## Triggering factors

'What makes the headache begin or become worse?' or 'Are headache attacks related to specific circumstances – foods or other factors?'. Usually, the parents are able to identify triggering factors and have several (often fanciful and unscientific) explanations. For the youngest patient, it may be more difficult to identify triggering factors, but sometimes an explanation in plain words and a little persistence may help to get information, mainly when the difficulties are related to the patient's shyness. It is relevant to recognize triggering factors for two main reasons. On the one hand, the intervention on 'real' triggering factors gives us an additional possibility of reducing the frequency or intensity of the headache crises. On the other, bearing in mind the 'rationalization', even unrealistic, of the headache as presented by parents or patient, this could give a basis for starting a discussion at the time of the presentation of findings. The weight given, respectively, to organic and psychological elements, tell us a great deal about the probable difficulties with the following diagnostic steps, and make strategic suggestions for better implementation of the diagnostic and therapeutic alliance.

## Relieving factors

The question 'What makes headache better?' will give us relevant information on the attitude about drugs, the efficacy of both analgesic drugs and self-help attempts (and results) to relieve headache.

The absolute absence of relieving (and triggering factors) may represent an alarming symptom of symptomatic headache.

## The aura

Any element that suggests the presence of aura symptoms should be obtained and analysed in detail, bearing in mind the cognitive level of the child. In fact, it is usual for the child to report visual phenomena not related to headache, because he or she is unable to recall the temporal sequence of the symptoms' presentation. In this case, it is important to ask for an accurate description and explanations of the context in which and occasions when aura occurs.

Psychic symptoms, such as hallucinations and perceptual distortion, are, however, difficult for children to describe, and require persistent questioning.[23] It may be useful to invite the patients to describe their visual aura by freehand drawings or by showing them some sketches. The symptoms of aura are most typically visual disturbances (flashing lights, patchy scotomata, fortification spectra, blurring of vision, diplopia, spots, coloured circles), but also sensory or motor (paraesthesias, limb weakness, disorders of body image and of size, stiffness in a hand) and speech (aphasia or dysarthria) disorders. As in adults, the aura may precede or accompany head pain, which may be absent all together.

A detailed analysis of the co-occurring

symptoms is crucial for the differential diagnosis, management and therapy. Variants of migraine such as hemiplegic migraine, basilar artery migraine, ophthalmoplegic migraine, retinal migraine, chronic paroxysmal migraine and other variants ('Alice in Wonderland syndrome', confusional migraine, migraine stupor and transient global amnesia) are considered to be unusual forms of migraine, with typical onset during developmental age; noticeable and persistent specific neurological symptoms are associated with the usual diagnostic criteria for migraine. The relationship between migraine and epilepsy is controversial.[23]

To end with 'Do you have anything to ask about?' or 'Do you have anything to add?' may be very useful in order to increase the background for general framing of headache, developing the basis on which to build up the diagnostic and therapeutic alliance.

## The history of the patient

A detailed reconstruction of the developmental steps of child growth (see Chapter 34) is absolutely indispensable in history taking, but the exhaustive treatment of the topic is beyond the aims of this chapter. Briefly we consider some key factors that are indispensable to complete framing of the headache and to address the differential diagnosis (at the start between primary and secondary headache).

A few prospective studies have been carried out to detect factors predicting the onset of headache in children. Factors such as hyperreactivity in the first month of life,[24] nocturnal confusion seizures and enuresis, sleeping difficulties, long-term diseases, concentration difficulties and travel sickness have, however, been recognized as probably predicting the onset of headache at school entry.[25]

The occurrence of recurrent co-morbid somatic complaints (e.g. recurrent abdominal pain, unexplained fatigue, asthma, etc.) and periodic syndromes (cyclic vomiting, benign paroxysmal torticollis of infancy, kinetosis, dizziness, sleep disorders, growth pains, hyperactivity syndrome) in our patients' past (or present) should be carefully detected for both diagnostic and therapeutic aims. Some of these disorders have usually been recognized as 'equivalents of migraine', even though the subject is still far from clear systematization (the IHS classification[2] codes only benign paroxysmal vertigo and alternating hemiplegia of infancy as 'precursors of migraine'). For instance, the occurrence of recurrent abdominal pain and migraine-like headache may be related to both secondary (such as temporal lobe epilepsy or metabolic disorders, namely abdominal coeliac disease, urea cycle disorder, mitochondrial cytopathy)[23] and primary headache (as probable symptoms of the tendency to express psychological distress through somatic symptoms in somatization or anxiety disorders).[20,21]

Allergies and diet-triggering factors should be asked about, even though the exact implication in affecting headache has not been found.

Cerebral contusion and minor and non-concussive head injury may provoke migraine-like attacks, which may occur after a latent interval. Focused questioning should always be done on timing, ways, probable loss of consciousness, etc.

School matters should be carefully evaluated, from the start. Reactions to first separations from caregivers, change in school achievement and relationships with schoolfriends and teachers give us important information about the social world of the child or adolescent, and the probable weight of current school matters in influencing headache, leading more clearly to the psychological assessment.

The past occurrence of psychopathological disorders should be asked for, even during the first steps of history taking, as anamnestic data; the negative prognostic value related to the presence of co-morbid psychiatric disorders and headache should also be considered.[26] However, only the following psychological assessment provides sound diagnostic elements about the current situation.

## The history of the family

In spite of a high positive family history for migraine (about 50–70%, mostly on the maternal side),[27,28] at the present time this is not considered to be a diagnostic parameter, because there is no strong empirical support for the clear-cut implication of genetic determinants in causing migraine. Genetics has frequently been called into question to explain the high familial recurrence of migraine, even though only a rare subtype of migraine (familial hemiplegic migraine) has been established to have clear-cut genetic linkages.[29–31]

To the best of our knowledge, few studies have been published on the familial occurrence of headache other than migraine, even though in chronic tension-type headache the involvement of genetic factors has been suggested.[32,33]

Both environmental and genetic factors seem, however, to play a significant role in determining migraine (mainly without aura),[34] even though the subject is as yet far from any definitive explanations.[35]

Careful analysis of the presence of headache (onset, type, drug or non-drug therapy, behaviour patterns related to the attacks, etc.) in both parents and relatives may give us information about the weight of such disorders in supporting the request for medical intervention, and about the ordinary life demands and family quality of life. The role of the family in modelling and reinforcement of illness, family health problems and parental concerns about illness, and certain family characteristics have been emphasized as having a role in influencing the occurrence of some disease for which there is a role for psychological determinants.[36]

Family history taking should consider the occurrence of specific diseases that run in the family (such as hypertension, diabetes, epilepsy, thyroid problems, gastrointestinal diseases or surgical interventions) through the use of explicit questions. Knowledge about these 'familial' disorders (onset, length, therapeutic interventions, etc.) is important to evaluate the individual's (genetic?) susceptibility to certain diseases and the probable links to the occurrence of headache, but it is also important to call attention to the weight of related (present or past) worries and the current influences on coping with illnesses.

The presence (past or current) of psychiatric disorders should be carefully analysed, together with related drug and/or psychological treatments. The analysis of family relationship patterns by the planning of psychological assessment is relevant to display their probable influences on child development (see Chapter 34).

## Final comment

Paying special attention to history taking is crucial to achieve elements for the global framing of headache. It addresses the diagnosis and further assessment on both the neurological and the psychological fronts. Genuine listening to our patient and his or her parents is the basis for any step thereafter.

# References

1. Blau JN, Headache: history, examination, differential diagnosis and special investigations. In: *Handbook of Clinical Neurology*, vol. 4. Amsterdam: Elsevier, 1986: 43–58.
2. Headache Classification Committee of the International Headache Society, Classification and diagnostic criteria of headache disorders, cranial neuralgias and facial pain. *Cephalalgia* 1988; 8(suppl 7).
3. Rothner AD, Headache in children: A review. *Headache* 1979; **19**: 156–62.
4. Prensky AL, Sommer D, Diagnosis and treatment of migraine in children. *Neurology* 1979; **29**: 506–10.
5. Silberstein SD, Twenty questions about headaches in children and adolescents. *Headache* 1990; **30**: 716–24.
6. Guidetti V, Bruni O, Cerutti R et al, How and why childhood headache and migraine differ from that of the adults. In: Galli V, Guidetti V, eds, *Juvenile Headache*. Amsterdam: Excerpta Medica, 1991: 27.
7. Metsähonkala L, Sillanpää M, Migraine in children – an evaluation of the IHS criteria. *Cephalalgia* 1994; **14**: 285–90.
8. Hamalainen ML, Hoppu K, Santavouri PR, Effect of age on the fulfillment of the IHS criteria for migraine in children at a headache clinic. *Cephalalgia* 1995; **15**: 404–9.
9. Winner P, Martinez W, Mate L, Bello L, Classification of pediatric migraine: proposed revision to the IHS criteria. *Headache* 1995; **35**: 407–10.
10. Seshia SS, Specificity of IHS criteria in childhood headache. *Headache* 1996; **36**: 295–9.
11. Wöber-Bingöl Ç, Wöber C, Karwautz A et al, IHS criteria for migraine and tension-type headache in children and adolescents. *Headache* 1996; **36**: 231–8.
12. Raieli V, Raimondo D, Gangitano M, D'Amelio M, Cammalleri R, Camarda R, The IHS classification criteria for migraine headaches in adolescents need minor modifications. *Headache* 1996; **36**: 362–6.
13. Hockaday JM, Definitions, clinical features, and diagnosis of childhood migraine. In: Hockaday JM, ed., *Migraine in Childhood*. London: Butterworths, 1988: 12–13, 16–24.
14. McGrath PJ, Developmental and psychological factors in children's pain. *Pediatr Clin North Am* 1989; **36**: 823–36.
15. Sillanpää M, Piekkala P, Kero P, Prevalence of headache at preschool age in unselected child population. *Cephalalgia* 1991; **11**: 239–42.
16. Abu-Arefeh I, Russell G, Prevalence of headache and migraine in schoolchildren. *BMJ* 1994; **309**: 765–9.
17. Passchier J, Orlebeke JF, Headache and stress in schoolchildren: an epidemiological study. *Cephalalgia* 1985; **5**: 167–76.
18. Bille B, Migraine in schoolchildren. *Acta Paediatr* 1962; **51**(suppl 136): 1–151.
19. Guidetti V, Fabrizi P, Galli F, De Cesare C, Unilateral headache in early and late childhood. *Int J Neurol Sci* 1999; **20**: S56–9.
20. Arav-Boger R, Spirer Z, Periodic syndromes of childhood. In: *Advances in Pediatrics*. Chicago: Mosby Year Book, 1997.
21. Garralda ME, Somatisation in children. *J Child Psychol Psychiatry* 1996; **1**: 13–33.
22. Deonna TW, Paroxysmal disorders which may be migraine or may be confused with it. In: Hockaday JM, ed., *Migraine in Childhood*. London: Butterworths, 1988: 78–80.
23. Hocakday JM, Newton RW, Migraine and epilepsy. In: Hockaday JM, ed., *Migraine in Childhood*. London: Butterworths, 1988: 60–2, 88–104.
24. Guidetti V, Ottaviano S, Pagliarini M, Childhood headache risk: warning signs and symptoms present during the first months of life. *Cephalalgia* 1984; **4**: 237–42.
25. Aromaa M, Rautava P, Helenius H, Sillanpää M, Factors of early life as predictors of headache in children at school entry. *Headache* 1998; **36**: 409–15.
26. Guidetti V, Galli F, Fabrizi P, Giannantoni AS, Napoli L, Bruni O, Trillo S, Headache and psychiatric comorbidity: clinical aspects and

outcome in an 8-year follow-up study. *Cephalalgia* 1998; **18**: 455–62.

27. Chu ML, Shinnar S, Headaches in children younger than 7 years of age. *Arch Neurol.* 1992; **49**: 79–82.

28. Messinger HB, Spierings EL, Vincent AJ, Lebbink J, Headache and family history. *Cephalalgia* 1991; **11**: 13–18.

29. Ophoff RA, van Eijk R, Sandkuijl LA et al, Genetic heterogeneity of familial hemiplegic migraine. *Genomics* 1994; **22**: 21–6.

30. Gardner K, Barmada MM, Ptacek LJ and Hoffman EP, A new locus for hemiplegic migraine maps to chromosome 1q31. *Neurology* 1997; **49**: 1231–8.

31. Silberstein SD, Lipton RB, Goadsby PJ, eds, *Headache in Clinical Practice*. Oxford: Isis Medical Media, 1998: 26–7.

32. Østergaard S, Russell MB, Bendsten L, Olesen J, Comparison of first-degree relatives and spouses of people with chronic tension-type headache. *BMJ* 1997; **314**: 1092–3.

33. Russell MB, Østergaard S, Bendsten L, Olesen J, Familial occurrence of chronic tension-type headache. *Cephalalgia* 1999; **19**: 207–10.

34. Russell MB, Genetic epidemiology of migraine and cluster headache. *Cephalalgia* 1997; **17**: 683–701.

35. Ophoff RA, *The Molecular Basis of Familial Hemiplegic Migraine*. Enschede, The Netherlands: PrintPratners Ipskamp, 1997.

36. Garralda ME, Somatisation in children. *J Child Psychol Psychiatry* 1996; **1**: 13–33.

# 6

# Psychological assessment

*Federica Galli, Mimma Tafà, Sandra Capuccini, Antonio Gullì and Vincenzo Guidetti*

A correct and complete assessment of headaches with onset in childhood requires a multilevel framing, taking into consideration the number of organic and psychological factors that influence headache crises. This chapter addresses the basic elements for a psychological assessment for all who deal with childhood headache; it considers the multiplicity of psychological factors that need attention in the assessment process.

In childhood diseases, the involvement of somatic and psychological factors seems to be more the rule than the exception, in terms of a reciprocal modulation of the two dimensions, even if not considering the issue of a cause–effect relationship.

A study[1] on the kind of patients seen in a paediatric outpatient clinic showed that only 12% presented physical diseases, 36% had purely psychological problems and 52% had a mixture of physical and psychological problems.

Studies carried out in paediatric settings showed that a minority of paediatric clinic patients had only physical diseases, whereas the majority had a mixture of physical and psychological problems.[1–6] Psychological problems seen in consultation by paediatricians seem to exceed the number of those seen jointly by psychologists and psychiatrists.[3] However, less than 1% of children are referred for either psychological or psychiatric services by paediatricians.[7] On the other hand, research in childhood and adolescence psychopathology refers to 'somatic complaints' (most commonly 'abdominal pain or headaches') such as co-occurring symptoms in young psychiatric patients. Other studies on adults[8–10] showed that individuals with psychological problems are more likely to come to a primary medical setting than to traditional mental health settings.

Livingston et al[11] found that between 25% and 30% of children admitted to a psychiatric hospital had physical symptoms, including headache, food intolerance, abdominal pain, nausea and dizziness. Between 2% and 10% of children present the so-called 'functional' pains, for which a 'cause' is not found.[12] However, the lack of evidence for an organic cause does not mean in itself that the problem is exclusively 'psychological'. A biological substrate always exists, even if we do not consider or know its origin. Psychological factors interact with this biological basis, even though we do not yet know how (triggers, shared background, or both?).

This view opens up the need for close collaboration between physicians and psychologists in general paediatric settings. The presence of clinical psychologists in paediatric medical settings may take on a preventive value. Psychological or psychiatric problems may be brought to attention by means other than 'psychological channels'; this happens more than ever in children, when parents may more easily accept a physical complaint, and children more often 'choose' the 'body's way' of expressing psychological disease.

For headache, the role of psychological factors in influencing the occurrence of crises is highlighted by clinical and research remarks (see Chapters 14 and 24).

Daily clinical practice with children or adolescents who have headaches shows a high number of signs and symptoms affecting patients at any moment or reported through the clinical history. Experimental data have suggested the occurrence of neurological signs,[13] sleep disturbances,[14] allergy,[15] problems with school achievement,[16] unhappy family environment,[17] lack of concentration,[16] school phobia,[16] hyperactivity,[18] periodic syndromes,[19] anxiety,[20] depression,[20] panic attacks,[21] etc. (for a review of psychosocial factors related to headache crises see Karwantz et al[22]). Moreover, the involvement of psychological factors in childhood and adolescence headache displayed a negative prognostic value.[23]

This kind of situation represents a 'paradigm' of the involvement of somatic and psychological aspects of headaches in childhood and adolescence, even though the role and reciprocal modulation of organic and psychological factors in influencing headache are unclear. The strict embedding is stressed equally by psychiatric research, even if the subsequent interpretations sometimes appear weak. The American Academy of Child and Adolescent Psychiatry[24] classifies migraine as a disease to consider for a differential diagnosis with anxiety, because it is 'a physical condition that may mimic anxiety disorders'. A community study on somatization[25] reported headaches in 10–30% of children and adolescents. Headache is always a symptom, but only a multilevel analysis can ensure comprehensive framing of the disease.

The above studies represent the rationale behind the need for clinical and paediatric psychologists in childhood and adolescence headache centres. In clinical practice, not giving consideration to the psychological factors that influence headache risks rendering the diagnostic and therapeutic process unsuccessful, or at least partially successful.

Historically the relationship of medicine and psychology has been oscillating between cooperative and antagonistic, and is traditionally linked more to psychiatry. Until the mid-1960s, clinical psychologists were primarily employed in assessment roles in mental health hospitals. In 1959, 44% of clinical psychologists were employed in testing activities. In 1976, assessment were the main activities for only 24% of clinical psychologists.[26] Since the early 1980s,[6] an increasing number of psychologists have been employed in medical settings. Consultation, direct intervention, research, and training medical students and interns, in addition to assessment activities, represent the main areas of work.[27] Currently, the practice of psychologists in clinical and scientific roles, and in areas of medical specialty other than psychiatric services, represents an important challenge for the psychological professions.[27]

The contribution of clinical psychologists to medical settings may not be straightforward.[28] The timing and methods of diagnostic and therapeutic work differ considerably, needing to discuss and integrate strategies. Psychologists may risk mimicking the medical role, overly characterizing the use of the medical system by overidentification. Physicians may risk applying only medical–organic categories when analysing diseases.

The duration of the psychological assessment is much longer than the medical one. Establishing a rapport with the parent(s) and patient is fundamental, and uses different methods from those of doctors. The patient's medical problem in a medical setting may have a clear-cut need for psychological work. It may be very difficult to make progress on both the medical and psychological sides, matching two different time periods and methods of work. Much depends on the specific rules of the different organization within which the headache centre is located, on the number of the patients being referred and the members of staff; however, from our own experience, we suggest giving the psychological work some autonomy, e.g. by fixing the appointments at shorter intervals than the medical visits.

Medical settings for children represent areas in which the involvement of clinical and child psychologists is necessary, because of the predilection for children to use the 'body's way' of communicating and the possible psychological consequences of illnesses in the development of a child's personality. In line with this viewpoint, the role of clinical psychologists is crucial in a childhood and adolescence headache centre.

Several issues must, however, be addressed to pursue real interdisciplinary work. Medical systems have different rules and language from psychological ones. Reciprocal misconceptions may make the working relationship difficult.[6] A specific period of training for psychologists (at least 6 months) is totally necessary to achieve the basic tools of knowledge in the headache field. The scientific basis of working with children and adolescents who have headaches should be well known to avoid mis-

understanding and to build a common work plan, for the two professionals. We believe that collaborative work using a combination of medical and psychological expertise may improve the general framing of headache.

There are many models of consultation. It is important that psychologists have a wide theoretical and experiential background to work in this field. Assessment represents the initial step in all clinical work for determining clinical diagnoses and establishing treatment plans and recommendations. The full diagnostic assessment requires data gathering from the patients, families and, when possible, the school, as well as from the primary physician and any other source.

A complete and detailed anamnesis represents the starting point to address the following assessment plan, tailoring it for the specific situation. The initial encounter represents a unique opportunity for observing verbal and non-verbal interactions between parent(s) and patient, in order to analyse how arguments are dealt with and how communication is modulated between the two (who is the first to speak; how are problems formulated and discussed, etc.). A shift in the direction of a psychological assessment may not be expected and needs a careful explanation to avoid doubts and assumptions, which if not discussed could have a negative influence on the psychological evaluation process. A focus on the headache may be more comfortable than discussing other problems, when bringing the patient and parent(s) to consider the child's inner world. This is even more important and tactful when dealing with parents and patient who has 'chosen' the somatic way to manifest his or her distress.[29,30] For these reasons the shift from the presenting problem ('headache') to the psychological view may not be easy (see

Chapter 1). Parents come with their own ideas about the causes of the headache crises: sometimes they present defensive attitudes (often not explicitly verbalized) when we propose psychological assessment. The headache is simply reported from an organically based view. Sometimes, the patient simply does not return, once reassurance has been given about the primary nature of the headache. The clinician must be able to determine and then transmit to the parents the subtle boundaries between the fear of being blamed and the ability to embrace new perspectives for framing their child's headache. General psychology teaches us about our basic tendency to reduce knowledge about reality to clear-cut categories of classification, which are undoubtedly useful in our daily lives, but possibly insufficiently flexible to embrace the subtle differences in aspects of our experience. It is very difficult to make the parent(s) or patient aware that the absence of physical illness does not indicate the absence of biophysiological mechanisms. The reality of head pain should be stressed, as well as the importance of the psychological assessment, in order to decode the role of psychological factors in the aetiology, triggering and/or maintenance of headache crises. However, the point of looking at psychological aspects should be clarified, and it is important to give clear explanations. The implication of headache may account for the ideas related to the fear of 'mental illness'. An awareness of these worries and subsequent discussion with the parent(s) and patient may improve rapport.

In the evaluation process, it is crucial to focus on, and decode, the presence of questions about issues other than the 'headache'. Once it is clear that we are dealing with a primary headache, our aim is to understand 'what is behind headache'. The range of problems which are brought to the clinician's attention during the diagnostic process reflects a wide variety; this supports the need for an eclectic background of knowledge and an extensive training in different fields of clinical and developmental psychology.

The implication of involvement of psychological factors in headache crises may be suggested by the following:

- The presence of a time relationship between the onset of headache and the occurrence of any stressor, such as important changes in daily life (e.g. transferring to secondary school)
- Present or past concurrent psychiatric disorder(s)
- Disabilities following headache crises which would not be expected based on the severity and frequency of the attacks
- The nature of parental concerns (familial illnesses, bereavements or change in school achievement, etc.)
- Personality characteristics, such as extreme conscientiousness, adult-like behaviour and even insecurity, obsessiveness and anxiety.

Headache may be an indirect way of asking for support for a wide range of difficulties with which the parents and/or patients are coping. Times of conflict, hurt, parental separation, bereavement, school or peer relationship problems, sexual or psychological abuse may be brought to the clinician's attention (to consider just a few of the possibilities).

In the following sections we provide the basic tools of reference for proceeding with the psychological evaluation of children or adolescents and their families. However, we stress the importance of tailoring methods and timing assessments in line with the characteristics of each case, and avoiding a rigid approach. The history of the patient and family and the initial interactions should be the main domain of analysis, in order to address timing and methods for any subsequent psychological evaluation.

In general, there should be direct and separate interviews with the patient and parent(s). Sometimes, it may be helpful to see the whole family. It has been stressed that the headache symptom would be supported by relationship difficulties within a family, which inhibit the child's disengagement and autonomy.[31] The weight of the family relationship and the dynamics of the psychological development of the child or adolescent account for a large section of the clinical work with the families of our patients. However, there is a lack of controlled studies on this issue, in spite of the strong support given by clinical experience to the importance of a familial framing of the patient – sometimes leading to indications for 'family therapy'. Considering the above diagnostic steps, the chapter gives the basic tools for assessment of the patient and family, but with no pretense of being exhaustive.

# The patient assessment

The psychological evaluation depends on the age of the patient. The various difficulties presented by our patients require multidisciplinary work and the use of several *qualitative* and *quantitative* instruments of assessment, according to age, cognitive level and specificities of the clinical case.

Psychometric tests and clinical interviews are the main tools of our work, even if this integration of the two sources gives us only global knowledge about the patient and his or her environment. The integration of results from different sources is usually enough to formulate a diagnosis based on the DSM-IV [32] criteria, or to give elements for reaching good framing of the patient's psychological status.

Working with a child or an adolescent in itself requires different techniques of evaluation. The child is brought by his or her parents to the clinic (he or she does not make the demand), and the motivation to collaborate may need to be strengthened. Shyness, inhibition and worries may weaken the psychological evaluation. However, much will depend on the way that the parent(s) prepare, explain and comprehend the meaning of the psychological evaluation. On the other hand, the adolescent may have better comprehension of the assessment process and feel that the involvement of the parents is harmful to his or her autonomy. Adolescence may represent a time of conflict, hurt, separation and loss. Taking on a more adult identity implies the modification of previous balances, and it often needs painful renunciation – entailing renunciation of the childhood self-image in favour of a sexually defined body, with all the emotional upset and psychological adjustment involved; it also entails renunciation of the satisfaction with being a child, together with the risks involved in the first move towards autonomy.[33] It appears as the typical ambivalence of adolescence, which may be totally reproduced during the assessment process.

# The clinical interview

The clinical interview may be considered as the main instrument for exploring the child's or adolescent's perceptions of the presenting problem, as well as for assessing the overall developmental, mental and relationship status, providing information that may not be available from other sources.[34] The aim of this session is to give some theoretical and practical suggestions for conducting clinical interviews with children and adolescents, even though space does not allow exhaustive treatment. Most of the following suggestions are applicable for both children and adolescents, with adjustments for age and particular characteristics of the case.

The child's age and cognitive level of development must be taken into account at the start of the clinical interview. Once a rapport has been established, it is necessary to maintain the cooperation of the child. Maintenance of the rapport is the essence of information gathering. Information taking in clinical interviews is an *art*, and there is no unique technique; theoretical and personal experiences and techniques should lead the way, according to the case.[35–40]

A child as young as 5 years can give useful information in the clinical interview, if age-related strategies are employed. Several areas need to be explored, to become acquainted with the patient's perspective (at all times, even when we have just collected information by an anamnesis) on school, interpersonal relations (family, peers, other adults), future plans, self-concept, feeling states (general, anxiety, depression, anger), reality testing, fantasy, sex concepts, etc.[39] Clearly, the method of information gathering changes with age. Playing (e.g. with puppets, small figures) and drawing may be very useful with children, providing inferential material about the child's inner world, concerns, worries, regulation of affects and impulses. Playing and drawing may also be very useful in providing information

about the cognitive status, leading to probable ad hoc investigations when we note inadequate responses.

There is no fixed way of conducting the interview: much depends on the nature of the main problem, the mutual interplay of the patient and clinician, the context, and the kind and amount of previous information. The key areas should be on our minds and tactful attention should guide questioning, particularly when certain information does not emerge spontaneously or the patient deviates defensively away from key points. This simple observation is an important diagnostic element.

It may be very useful to ask the patient for adjectives (at least three) to describe the self, followed by a description of his or her mother and father; this should be done at the initial encounter, because it is not demanding, and could give important data about the perception of self and others. The observation of delays in response and the capacity to report specific examples for each adjective will give us an idea about the defence strategy of the child, without being too invasive or too similar to school testing. The older the child, the more realistic the information obtained. Asking the child to describe a dream, a movie or a cartoon may provide information about the child's interests, preoccupations and distortions.[34]

Interviewing adolescents needs a particular approach that takes into consideration age-related psychological characteristics. It is uncommon for an adolescent to be referred for headache on his or her volition and even more uncommon for an adolescent to ask for a psychological consultation. This aspect entails the delicate link between autonomy from and dependency on the main caretakers. With adolescents it is essential to assure the confidentiality of the information given during the course of the assessment. It is critical to have the patient's perspective on what is discussed during the history taking, in order to achieve a good diagnostic alliance.

An important aim relates to the involvement and motivation of the adolescent in the interviews. The adolescent should have motivation and our role is crucial in achieving this. The clinician tends to be seen by the adolescent as a parent or friend figure. Modulation of the right distance for strengthening the diagnostic alliance and perceiving the diagnostic elements depends on the clinician's role and experience. Sincere interest and sensible openings represent a good approach towards understanding the adolescent's inner and interpersonal world. It is useful to plan, with the patient, a limited number of interviews (from three to five), specifying the assessment value of the encounters and proposing a final setting for the 'restitution of findings'. The information obtained and involvement of the parents should be discussed according to each case, even though consideration of the adolescent as our main interlocutor may support his or her adult parts. There may, however, be insistent and often worried questioning from the parents who want to know 'what is happening' to their son or daughter, 'what is the diagnosis', etc. It is important to give the parents explanations about the 'object' and 'time' of the psychological assessment, telling them that there will be a dedicated time for discussion of the findings and related indications for therapy. This is a very delicate point that needs to be dealt with tactfully. We must not risk failing to recognize and support the parents, but, at the same time, we must not

exclude the adolescent from the whole diagnostic process. Fantasies of collusion between parents and clinicians should be reduced to a minimum and always discussed with the patient, at an opportune moment. At the same time, the diffidence and defensive attitudes of the parents may be counterproductive to the diagnostic process. Parents should be seen and persuaded to become our allies, supporting the value of the psychological assessment for headache patients. On the other hand, it is necessary to explain to the patient that the course of the psychological evaluation will depend on his or her motivation outline and to recognize his or her capacity for autonomous choice, avoiding reducing the patient to an infantile position, and allowing the adolescent to be an active participant in the whole process. The clinician must also guarantee the confidentiality of what comes up in the clinical interviews.

The clinical interview needs to be articulated, taking into consideration any age-related characteristics. Knowledge about the developmental tasks and relationship dynamics is the best starting point for work with adolescents, e.g. the typical ambivalence between autonomy and dependence may be exactly mirrored by the verbal and non-verbal behaviours shown by the adolescent during the clinical interviews. Any conflict may emerge in the form of worries, anxiety, hesitancy, indecision or open resistance to collaborative attitudes. 'Many adolescents who consciously want help approach a clinical evaluation with anxiety about revealing problems that they may regard as shameful weakness and with concerns about being criticized, controlled, or overwhelmed or becoming regressively dependent. These apprehensions may take the form of bland denials of any difficulties or insistence that either 'everything is ok' or 'I can handle it by myself'.[41]

Several points should lead the clinical interview. We should have a sort of grid in our mind, with key points to consider and explore progressively, but without rigid adherence to a planned scheme or list of questions that may risk mimicking an examination rather than a clinical interview. An interactive model should be pursued, even taking into account the psychological characteristics of headache patients. Questions should arise fluently, giving the adolescent space to proceed by free association. However, a defensive attitude and attempts to omit crucial issues should be dealt with tactfully. Requests for clarification may guide the adolescence in acknowledging ambivalent emotions, giving cues for further reflections, or dealing with new and more complex issues.

To obtain a full picture, it is important not to limit the interview to areas of difficulty. The adolescents should know that the interviewer is interested in learning about him or her as a whole person, including areas of strength, enjoyment, and accomplishment. Adolescents may become defensive or blandly deny difficulties in the face of a too-exclusive focus on pathology. The experienced and empathic diagnostician conveys a genuine interest in learning about the nature, quality, and depth of the young person's interests, hobbies, and recreations. Rather than demonstrating or feigning one's familiarity with the latest rock group, sports cars, or athletic team, it is preferable to let the adolescent teach one about his or her particular interests. In so doing, the adolescent is able to enjoy a sense of mastery and control and some sense of parity with the adult examiner. At the same time, the clinician is able to learn what blend of interests, identifications, sublimations, and direct instinctual and narcissistic gratifications animate the adolescent.[41]

Several areas need to be explored absolutely, because of the adolescents' particular interests, such as school functioning (e.g. satisfaction, motivation, achievement, etc.), quality of current relationships (family, peer, friends), emotional experiences (e.g. emotional closeness or investment, probable discrepancy between what to say and emotion), reflective functions (e.g. use of abstract thought, self–other awareness), mood, usual state, anxiety reasons, hobbies and interests, and expectations for the future.

The area of relationships with friends plays a crucial role in the adolescent's life and requires tactful investigation: 'with whom does the patient hang out? what do they do for fun? how do they get along? Friends may be chosen on many grounds, including shared interests, admired virtues, or repudiated aspects of adolescent's self. Friends may function as sources of support or admiration, as partners for sexual or aggressive exploitation, as collusive companions in regression or delinquency, as targets for projections, and so on'.[41]

Others areas to be evaluated are the adolescent's values and models for emulation. These values may be congruent or in conflict with those of the patient's family, subculture or wider society, and they should be analysed as such.

It is important also to have the adolescent's view of the future, e.g. what is the adolescent's sense of the future, which aspirations, realistic or not, does the adolescent have for it, are such aspirations in agreement with his or her familial or cultural world? A way of preparing the patient for leaving is to close any interview with 'Anything else to be added before we say goodbye?' Often, the most significant things are communicated during the final part of the encounter: leave a brief space to discuss them or delay everything to the next time, depending on the specific case.

## Psychometric tests

The problem of objectivity and subjectivity affects psychological assessments, and the standardization of psychological diagnostic instruments has been an attempt to limit the involvement of subjectivity in the diagnosis. However, the issue of limiting the involvement of subjectivity in diagnostic work is not simple; there are as many solutions as there are variables influencing the psychological sphere.

The choice of psychometric test should be tailored to the case's characteristics and predilection, but always on the basis of sound basic criteria, such as adequate standardization, reliability (regardless of who is administering the test, it produces the same result) and validity (the test is valid if it measures what it is supposed to measure).[42] The use of rating scales and questionnaires that measure particular characteristics requires evaluation of the sensitivity (the proportion of true cases that the test selects) and specificity (the portion of true cases among a group that the test identifies as cases).[43]

Test scores alone do not have an absolute value if they are not compared with data from clinical interviews with patients, and in conjunction with elements drawn from the parents' view (or other sources, such as those of school teachers or previous psychological evaluation).

Several guidelines should be always taken into account,[44] in the choice and administration of any psychometric test:

- Tests are samples of behaviour.
- Tests do not directly reveal traits or capacities, but may allow inferences to be made about the child.
- Tests should have adequate reliability and validity.
- Test scores and other test performance may be adversely affected by: temporary states of fatigue, anxiety or stress; disturbances in temperament and personality; or brain damage.
- Test results should be interpreted in the light of the child's cultural background, primary language and any handicapping conditions.
- Test results are dependent on the child's cooperation and motivation.

Rating scales and a checklist may be part of the clinical assessment,[45] and the choice of the best depends on the specificity of the case (e.g. cognitive level, learning and attentional ability). The objectivity of these scales does not permit by itself to allow formulation of a diagnosis, but only the addition of diagnostic elements.

Data gathering from different sources is useful for a whole evaluation of the patient. Comparing by crosschecking data from the highest number of informants should represent the best way for complete framing of the patient's situation. Parents are considered to be the best informants of behavioural problems[46] and teachers of the child's social functioning,[47] whereas children themselves are the best sources of information for depression, anxiety or other internalizing problems.[45,48,49]

Psychometric properties of rating scales and the checklist may vary widely, and careful attention should be paid to the evaluation of the clinical and statistical adequacy. The use of these interviews may raise problems related to clinical applicability, even more so during the developmental age. If the use of structured interviews helps the objectivity of data collection, the possibility that the introduction of an instrument based on questions and answers may 'freeze' the rapport with the patient should be taken into account. A patient may be inhibited by the interview, because of shyness or because a list of questions may evoke a school situation for the patient, provoking a defensive attitude, which is counterproductive to the diagnostic and therapeutic alliance.

Many attempts have been made to detect psychopathology or psychiatric symptoms in children through the use of structured or semistructured interviews. The structured interviews are more directive than any clinical interview, because the area of investigation, the questions and the sequence are predetermined. The semistructured interviews uses a preset sequence of topics, with sections providing for a structured sequence of questions, and others with exclusion or inclusion criteria to be used to proceed with open questions on the basis of the clinician's advice.

The choice of structured or semistructured interview should be based on the focus and purposes characterizing it, deciding on a wide range of possibilities and considering the specificity of the clinical case (e.g. age, diagnostic reasons). We suggest limiting the use to research situations or when we need to test diagnostic hypotheses that are not otherwise clearly verifiable. The introduction of a structured interview should be explained to the patient, taking into account the eventuality of being administered by a different clinician.

The Child Behavior Checklist (CBCL)[50] is currently one of the checklists used most for statistical and practical properties: it has the best performance data available, takes only 20 min to administer, does not require high literacy, and has extensive coverage and adequate length.[43] Other standardized diagnostic interviews are the Diagnostic Interview for Children and Adolescents (DICA)[51,52] and the Diagnostic Interview Schedule for Children (DISC).[53] Both permit diagnoses according to DSM criteria and have undergone extensive revisions.

Study of the personality of headache sufferers is an important line of research. The Minnesota Multiphasic Personality Inventory (MMPI)[54] is the most widely used and exhaustively standardized personality inventory. MMPI and MMPI-2 have been largely used in research on adult headache sufferers.[55–64] A revision of the MMPI – MMPI-Adolescent[65,66] – has been designed specifically for adolescents (14–18 years inclusive). For children (3–16 years), the Personality Inventory for Children (PIC)[67] is comparable to the MMPI in construction and theoretical basis. It consists of a 600-item true–false questionnaire that is answered by mothers. The PIC has been used with young migraine sufferers,[68,69] showing clinical utility in the diagnostic process.

A revised version of PIC[70] and a self-report version of it – the Personality Inventory for Youth (PIY),[70,71] – have been designed more recently to give a measure of child and adolescent psychopathology, providing standard scores based on contemporary national samples.

An assessment of the patient's intelligence may be useful, when headache is associated with learning disabilities or poor achievement in schooling. The most widely used[72,73] tests for the assessment of intelligence and cognitive functioning are the three Wechsler scales,[74–76] all of which are derived by the Wechsler–Bellevue Intelligence Scale.

## Projective techniques

The concept of a 'projective test' derives from the projective hypothesis that ambiguous stimuli may evoke contents of the examinee's 'inner world', otherwise not so evident. The patient's difficulties in verbalizing affects, emotions and fears may be a sound component of the personality's structure (very typical of patients prone to somatization), or defensively related to the psychological evaluation (is the diagnostic alliance wanting?). Projective techniques may be an indirect technique for the investigation of personality structure, private concerns, needs, interests, coping styles, perception, interpretation, and reaction in response to environmental and interpersonal stimuli. However, the results from projective tests assume a sound helpfulness for framing the patient's psychology only if they are examined together with the findings from clinical interviews with the patient and parents.

In general, for the patient's assessment we suggest use of a projective test, together with at least two clinical interviews. The clinical interview may also start by discussing relevant points that are brought up by the testing.

With children, one of the most common techniques is the invitation to draw a picture. The content may be free, or indications can be given ('Draw yourself . . . a person . . . a family . . . a tree . . .') according to the areas that we need to investigate. Emotional, relational and/or cognitive aspects may be evaluated according to the assessment models.[77–79]

Common and useful questions are asking the child with whom he or she would like to go to a desert island, which wishes he or she would make real, or what animal he or she would most like or least like to be.

The choice of projective test depends on the professional background, personal experience and preference, the patient's age, and clinical impressions during the first encounter. On the basis of our experience, for children between the ages of 3 and 10, the Children's Apperception Test (CAT)[80,81] is adequate to obtain sufficient information to address the successive steps of assessment. The CAT constitutes 10 cards depicting animals, following the principle that children tend to identify more easily with animals than with people. The CAT was specifically developed for children on the basis of the Thematic Apperception Test (TAT).[82] It is applicable at or after 10 years of age. It consists of 30 black and white pictures and one black card. The subject has to tell a story for each card. Eleven cards have to be used with all patients, the others selected according to age, sex or themes represented in the pictures, presupposing that they evoke conflicts and worries on the part of the examinee.

The Rorschach test is historically the first of the projective techniques, and emblematic of the concept of 'projective'. It consists of 10 bilaterally symmetrical inkblots (five achromatic, five coloured), with amorphous, nonspecific stimuli. The theoretical premise is that unconscious processes (e.g. needs, conflicts, etc.) may be revealed by unstructured stimuli. The administration and interpretation of Rorschach require extensive formal training and experience.

The validity and reliability of the Rorschach

for children and adolescents have not been completely studied,[72] even if the numbers of studies are increasing and the methodology is improving.[83] Specific methods and norms have been fixed.[84,85]

The most relevant difference between children and adults is a smaller number of responses in children.[72] In spite of the long tradition of research, the conclusions about the validity of Rorschach are not definitive, even though the contradictory findings are often ascribed to the different methods of administration and scoring.[72]

In spite of the support for clinical utility of Rorschach with children and adolescents who have headache by a control study,[86,87] its use with children should be cautiously tailored according to each case's specificity, because it is more distressing than CAT or other projective techniques and there are fewer normative data than for adolescents or adults.

## Evaluation of the family within the systemic approach

Opinion is now widespread about the definition of the problem of the individual throughout the evaluation of the wider family system. Authors who use different approaches hold that it is no longer possible to overlook the fact that patients live 'within' the family, with whom they have relationships that are meaningful for their development.

Although the framework of interpersonal development is the focus of the analysis of individual difficulties, evaluation of the single patient involves the relationship context to which he or she belongs. In this sense, the relational systemic approach, on the one hand, allows understanding of the symptom within the meaningful context of the family and, on the other, identifies a mutual influence of the patient and the interactive context. The usefulness of the theoretical reference provided by the systemic approach relies on the possibility of connecting the different levels of the patient's clinical situation: the individual, his or her family and, if necessary, the broader social network, all of which aim to find the basic patterns as well as the mutual and circular interactions. Thus, the systemic epistemology allows the integration of the different aspects of the individual, his or her biology, emotions, thoughts, and relationships with the external environment and reality. Pathology becomes a complex plot involving both the patient's emotional experience, thoughts, fears and expectations, and the way the basic membership group respond and organize around pathology itself.

Communication within the family and the extended ecosystem can provide the individual with the competence necessary for development and maintenance of the symptom. Moving away from a linear approach, which risks a reduction in the symptom to a specific behaviour or a chain of behaviours, it is believed that every pathological manifestation is determined by a complex interaction, of different levels, including the communication among the family members, their history and myths, and the phase of the life cycle that the individual and the whole family are undergoing.[88–90] (Systemic psychotherapy has long been dealing with the genesis and identification of family myths. Family myths are a series of shared and integrated beliefs that look at all family members, their roles and positions within the family organization. These beliefs are not questioned by any of the people concerned, although they imply clear distortion of reality. The powerfulness of family myths in the evaluation of the family cannot be over-looked. The myth is a representation of reality, although it cannot be reduced to it. But the myth is also an interpretation of the reality to which all family members adhere.)

## *Evaluation is intervention*

An *evaluation* of a family system should allow improvement of knowledge about the points of strength and vulnerability of the patient and his or her family. Consequently, the phase of evaluation is generally considered as the basic step of any intervention: evaluating a system is already intervening in it.[91,92] Data collection in the phase of evaluation entails a choice on the part of the therapist, which already encompasses the start of the intervention. Thus, the evaluation becomes a fundamental part of the therapy; and, besides coming from what actually emerges within the relationship between the observer and the observed, it is the product of the options made by the clinician.

Unlike the medical perspective, the systemic diagnosis is linked to the feedback that derives from meeting the family. The evaluation, the intervention and the diagnosis do not appear to be different and neatly distinguished phases, but they are all embedded within the same framework represented by the meeting with the family. Therefore, it is not possible to conceive of a static evaluation, separate from the very moment of intervention. The task of the therapist is not so much to discriminate the authenticity of the symptoms and the difficulties shown by the patient, as to start focusing on the shared and explicit explanation in order to 'deconstruct' the symptom and to widen the maps through which the family interpret reality.

The first matter with which the therapist has to deal during the evaluation is who to summon? All the members or only some of them? The solution to this problem is already a first therapeutic intervention. The *ideal* unit of evaluation includes all the family members who are part of the problem and without whom it is difficult to gain complete understanding of the dynamics underlying the symptom and, thus, to promote the change. However, the intervention in the family is not connected so much to the number of people taking part in the treatment, as to the way the therapist conceives of the difficulties that the system is going through. In this perspective, a determinant is to consider the relational family process and the way in which it is connected to the psychological organization of each member. It must be stressed that the therapist, by summoning all the family in order to work with them, conveys to the family themselves messages that are profoundly different from those of the therapist who works with the single patient. In the latter option, the therapeutic contract as well as the privileged focus of the relationship change, although this does not limit the number of people to be summoned in subsequent meetings. However, consideration *who has come* and *who has not* is, for the therapist, an important feedback to be included in the evaluation of the context. Therefore, it has to be stressed that the therapist's choices become part of the evaluation from the very beginning and this results in a unique and peculiar construction of reality. In this sense, the process of evaluation can be seen as a means of amplification of the power of therapy, whether or not it is followed by a clinical intervention.

The encounter with the family begins with what Haley[93] defines as the *social phase*: the family members are involved in the action from the beginning, in order to avoid exclusively drawing the attention to the *designated patient* and to start placing the symptom within the context of relationships to which it belongs. This phase is meant to make the family feel at their ease and to begin the process of recognition. The therapist's attention will therefore be focused on the self-definitions provided by the members and their co-location within the organization of the family. Sometimes a first piece of useful information about the family organization can be drawn by simply observing the spatial disposition assumed by the family within the room. For instance, if the patient sat between the two parents the therapist could make a provisional hypothesis, to be verified, about the function of the symptom in the parents' union. It is useful for the therapist to respect the hierarchy of the family in order to gain their collaboration. This should be done with reference to the problem presented by the family and not on the basis of the therapist's stereotypes.

The evaluation should take into account two levels of investigation: the history of the symptomatic behaviour and the history of the nuclear and origin family.

An adequate evaluation of necessity includes the reconstruction of the history of the symptoms: their emergence, presentation, the relational context in which they appeared, and their pragmatic effects.[94] Meaningful family events can thus be singled out that are close in time to the emergence of the symptomatic behaviour. It is not superfluous to remember that such links do not deterministically establish cause–effect relations (past–present), rather they represent suggestions for connections between events, what Bateson calls the 'patterns which connect'.[95]

The phase after the social exchange is the definition of the problem. Here, the first level of investigation is represented by narration about the symptom and description of the person or relation having difficulties. In this phase of listening, it is important to create room that is suitable for understanding the way in which each family member, and not just the patient, sees the problem. It will also prove useful to know *who* decided to ask for help and the deep reasons, both individual and relational, behind this request and why it takes place at that particular moment of family life. In this phase, the therapist has to encourage the members to express their points of view, helping them to build an open, plain and cooperative context. It is as well to take into account the feedback from the family with respect to evaluation with the therapist.

In this phase the therapist is supposed to draw attention to the communicative style, as well as to the ways in which the family face their problems and their developmental tasks, to the distribution of roles and functions, to the ways of dealing with conflicts, the beliefs and the attitude towards the stranger.[96] It is also useful to consider the units of reciprocal influence emerging from the complex plot of family relationships: the individual, the generational subsystems (parents and children), the triads formed by the components of the different subsystems, the family system and the extended system.

Moreover, it is necessary to verify whether or not opinions about the symptom are shared by the family. For instance, given a certain adolescent difficulty, the position of the parents may be. 'We've come to know how to help our son with *his* problem' or 'My son has a problem, but we think he is reacting to something happening in our family'. To understand the dynamics and family interplay in which the adolescent takes part, the therapist should also understand whether parents assume a common or a different point of view. The circulation of unrecognized messages and emotions has, in brief, to be regarded as the foundation of the symptom.

Thus, the therapist investigates the organization of the system to find out why the family has not been successful in solving their difficulty, instead solving it inadequately through use of the symptom. The phase of analysing the request presented by the family is such a shared and explicit moment that it is impossible not to consider it as a starting context for change. Even though the objectives and necessities of the system have not yet been defined, sharing of the points of view of the expectations towards and the resources for the problem may become a highly therapeutic moment. It has to be stressed that the request for help does not exist as such, but it is organized and defined, as is any other human behaviour, within a relationship.[97]

In this investigation, it will also prove useful to understand whether there have been previous attempts to ask for help and what the characteristics of such attempts were: who made them and why, the period of the family life in which they were made and what they produced; all should be regarded as indications of the way the system dealt with the previous efforts for change.

Thus, evaluation of the family revolves around the opinions of the family members, which are the product of what each one thinks about the difficulties with which the system is dealing. It is important to consider that intervention with the family depends greatly on the emergence of these hypotheses and to consider the possibility of examining them with the

family. Moreover, the evaluation cannot neglect the importance of observing the relationships between family members. To allow such observation, it is useful for the therapist to facilitate the interactions between the members. Although the phase of definition of the problem requires direct involvement on the part of the therapist, in the following phase of interaction it is more opportune for him or her to stay in the background, encouraging the members to talk to each other. The members could even be moved from their seats in order to facilitate or not hinder their interactions. Besides the content of the communication, the therapist has to pay attention to the type of relationships characterizing the interactions between the family members, as well as the emotions that emerge during the meeting, both between family members and between the members and the therapist.

Working with the family means taking into account two different and mutually interactive levels. A *synchronic* level of interactive and communicative models is interwoven with a *diachronic* level of individual and collective histories, shared meanings and values, individual and family myths, which cross the past and live in the present to influence the future.

A further level of investigation is represented by the history of the nuclear family, starting from the first meeting of the parents, and the relational events that have characterized the phases of the couple and family life cycle. The motives that lead to the choice of partner and the intergenerational influences may represent a useful indication for understanding the disengagement phase from the family of origin carried out by each partner, and their attachment styles.[98,99] Investigation into the couple's first years underlines the emotional mechanism that is the basis of the marriage.

Such a mechanism can be obscured later in time by the symptoms manifested by the child. Furthermore, throughout this enquiry, the important change that happened in the nuclear family from its start can emerge. The system of relationships that *organizes* itself around the symptom also becomes clear, as well as the prevailing emotional mechanisms of that system and its possibilities for change.

An evaluation context should also take into account the phase of the *life cycle* that the family is going through (see also Chapter 34). Each stage is actually characterized by specific developmental issues and tasks to which the system has to be ready to respond to.[100] It is obviously different when the children are in the adolescent phase and when they are younger.

In this sense, it will definitely be useful to know how the system has dealt with the normative and incidental paranormative events, and how it has adjusted to the changes and tackled the difficulties. All these responses of the system represent its history, which influences current perceptions and sets constraints for the future. For instance, with respect to the paranormative events, it has emerged that a trauma in the parents' generation can influence the somatic and psychological manifestation of the psychosomatic disorders in childhood, by reducing the parental capacity to face the children's illnesses adequately.[101]

The therapist may be able to understand whether the family difficulties can be attributed to an overload of life events or to a low degree of family resiliency.[102] In any case, throughout this broad enquiry, the attention has shifted from the symptom and the individual, to the network of relationships.

The relational complexity increases further with the investigation into the *extended family*. The multigenerational context can represent the informative and diagnostic tool, attributing a wider meaning to the psychopathological manifestations, by referring them to elements that transcend the present relationships and are rooted in the families of origin of each partner of the couple.[98,99] Therefore, the symptom becomes the product of the intergenerational history, continuing its existence and changing as time goes by as a result of intergenerational debts and credits.[103]

To accomplish this task, *family genograms* can be employed. These are a tool that is peculiar to the systemic methodology; it is able to show the relational plot, the members' affective dimensions and the degree of self-differentiation in a temporal perspective. The family genogram is based on a kind of representation of the genealogical tree, collecting information about the family members and their relationships within the span of at least three generations, and presenting the complex family patterns.[104] This tool, therefore, adds the dimension of time to the description of the system, allowing schemes to be drawn and to stress both positive and negative family events in a chronological manner.

Once the phase of evaluation has been terminated, it is useful to build a new definition of what has emerged, for and with the family. An overall reading of the information collected, the individual perceptions of the problem and the deep emotional difficulties expressed by each member allow the proposal of a view of the symptom, within the context of the network of relationships that generated and maintained it over time. In the phase of evaluation of the family, the definition of the relational context of the problem is fundamental.[105] The relational context also includes the therapist's position, and grids and categories specifically employed with *each* family. The use of key words drawn from the family lexicon, the elaboration of narrative crucial situations and their reformulation in developmental terms become the prerequisite for joint work between the therapist and the family. The co-construction ensuing from this work creates a framework of meanings and connections, aimed at pointing out the resources of each member and the whole family; at the same time, this lays down the lines of future therapeutic work. The evaluation, therefore, not only stresses the vulnerability of the system, but also takes into consideration its resources[91,92,106] so that the most suitable intervention can be organized with respect to the specific family's competence. In this way, an attempt is made to make sense of behaviour that otherwise appears inexplicable and is labelled as 'mad'. The specific symptom is placed and defined within the specific family relationships and the specific multigenerational history.

Thus, evaluation of the path so far followed by the family, the possible alternatives and the important themes to deal with, is not done merely by the therapist, but is carried out by the whole family, *co-constructed* with them, in order to broaden all the family members' comprehension of the situation, to render the family expectations more coherent with the therapeutic project, to empower the experience of the system by overcoming the attitude of delegation, and to reformulate the homeostatic request initially presented by the family.[107]

There are many levels to take into account in the evaluation of the family organization: the process, the relationship, the evolution of the system and its life cycle are all components contemporarily playing a role in the meeting with the family, not to mention the grids and modalities employed by the therapist in the evaluation. If there is to be an evaluation, then it has to be of a *shared* quality. On the one hand, we certainly need the patient to know and to understand; on the other, the categories of the evaluation are built jointly throughout a constant procedure of self-correction by the therapist, which comes out of the meeting with the family.

# The specific case of adolescence

So far it has been pointed out that it is very important to pay attention to the family life cycle. In this sense, adolescence represents a basic moment for the growth of the system. We now move to the individuation of its specificity, which may be useful for the work of evaluation.

Adolescence entails a great deal of change for the family, who have to transform the previous organization of role, functions and relationships, and adopt a new and more functional one. The family have to accomplish a developmental and transitional process similar and parallel to the one in which the adolescent is involved. The physical growth of the adolescent and the growth of the family 'body' are regarded as interdependent by various systemic authors; they cannot take place separately. Adolescence, thus, becomes a double-faced reality, a process of co-evolution concerning *both* the boy or girl *and* the family.

From this perspective, the families with symptomatic children and adolescents are explained by a broader family crisis, attributable to an uneasiness that presents as a result of various aspects: the difficulty of the couple to accept and support the children's separation, resulting from the anguish of loss of parental functions, which are felt to be irreplaceable; the difficulty, often associated with the acceptance of putting under the microscope a conjugal relationship that is fraught with a high degree of latent tension and unresolved conflicts, which cannot be dealt with to preserve the stability of the affective bond; the necessity to compensate for a marriage that is not expressed positively because it is experienced as threatening, with the consequent persistence of a parental attitude that becomes indispensable and needs the presence of a child to survive.[33] It is in these family situations, in which the boundaries between the generational subsystems are weak and confused,[108] that the child becomes involved in the parental subsystem, which is thus transformed into a triad by the stable presence of a third element. In this triangular configuration, the adolescent, whether he or she is equidistant from the parents or is involved with one of the parents in a privileged way, becomes the indispensable mediator, the bridge for the emotional communication between the partners. The concurrence of adolescence and parental separation renders the situation even more complex. In this case, the adolescent assumes the role of 'spokesperson' or 'spy' for one of the two parents. It seems that it is not as much the separation itself and the loss of the parent who has not been entrusted, as the feeling of being caught between the parents that affects the psychological well-being.[109,110]

The suffering involved with this situation, which slows and severely hinders the adolescent's developmental process, may result in symptomatic manifestations. Such manifestations, while expressing the adolescent's difficulties and developmental need for change, stabilize the pathological balance of the family system, placing the adolescent in a situation of childhood dependence and guaranteeing the parents the persistence of their functions.

According to Haley,[111] the adolescent's symptom – expression of a difficulty of disengagement from the family – allows the parents to continue to communicate 'across' and 'on' him or her, while the family organization stays the same and, with time, there is also a block in the family life cycle. Behind these interactive and structural aspects of the family system, a deep emotional stream flows, which specifically concerns the adolescent. The boy or girl may experience the conflict between the opposite tendencies, which appear to be incompatible. The opposition is between the individual needs for growth and autonomy and the feelings of solidarity towards the parents or the family member perceived as weaker, and between reactions of opposition, often disguised by the symptom, and bonds of loyalty towards the family cohesion, which is sometimes represented as a shared myth. We are referring to the 'invisible loyalties'[103] which can induce feelings of guilt for every move towards autonomy, experienced as a betrayal.

In such situations, separations and detachments are not perceived as developmental transformations, but as the breakage of affective bonds. The binomial identity/membership, pivotal in the dynamics of adolescence, runs the risk of breaking, because the identity is perceived as a betrayal of membership. But, taking on a more adult identity also implies the necessity of modifying former balances and often requires painful renunciations: the renunciations of the childhood self-image in favour of a sexually defined body, with all the emotional upset and psychological adjustments that this entails; plus the renunciations of the safe environment of childhood, together with the risks involved in the first move towards autonomy.[33]

Thus appears the typical ambivalence of adolescence. The oscillation between autonomy and request for support, and between the necessity to loosen the bonds and, at the same time, to verify their maintenance, is characteristic of this age of transition. The adolescent feels the necessity to become independent from the parents, but at the same time he or she needs to count on them; the boy or the girl realizes the necessity of reassurance that the parents are strong and independent and that he or she is allowed to move away or differentiate him- or herself from them without feeling guilty. The adolescent's 'symptomatic' attitudes may be seen as the proposal of an autonomous identity, or that the bond with the parents has not been broken by this difference. The adolescent's expectation is that the bond should be enriched and transformed by the difference itself,[95] without undergoing traumatic and irreversible disruptions.

The problems of adolescence may be related to the integration of different levels of reality, in which individual, familiar and social aspects have to be connected and contemporaneously taken into consideration. For this reason, family therapy may be a likely solution in adolescence, because it does not label the patient as 'the problem', and it may help all the family to cope with the changing exigencies of the life cycle. Moreover, successful family treatment can often be followed by individual treatment with another therapist. An integrated individual and familiar approach is the most suitable indication for adolescent disorders, both in diagnostic and in therapeutic terms.

Adolescence may represent a time of conflict, hurt, separation and loss. These peculiarities compel an approach considering the age-related characteristics, the understanding of what is 'normal' though 'conflictual' and 'critical' and of what is 'pathological'.

## Acknowledgement

Dr Mimma Tafà, Family Psychotherapist, University of Rome 'La Sapienza' edited the section on 'Evaluation of the family within the systemic approach'. Special thanks to Riccardo Williams for his contribution to the translation of this chapter.

## References

1. Duff RS, Rowe DS, Anderson FP, Patient care and student learning in pediatric clinic. *Pediatrics* 1973; **50**: 839–46.
2. Stewart W, Breslau N, Kech PE, Comorbidity of migraine and panic disorders. *Neurology* 1994; **44**(suppl 7): S23–7.
3. Kempe CH, *Report of the American Academy of Pediatrics 1978.* Prepared by the Task Force on Pediatric Education. Evanston IL.
4. McClelland CQ, Staples WP, Weisberg I, Begen ME, The practioner's role in behavioral pediatrics. *J Pediatr* 1978; **82**: 325–31.
5. Wright L, A comprehensive program of mental health and behavioral medicine in a large children hospital. *Profess Psychol* 1979; **10**: 458–66.
6. Huszti HC, Walker CE, Critical issues in consultation and liaison. In: Sweet JJ, Rozensky RH, Tovian SM, eds, *Handbook of Clinical Psychology in Medical Settings.* New York: Plenum Press, 1991: 603–14.
7. Pruitt SD, Elliott CH, Pediatric psychology: current issues and developments. In: Walker CE, Roberts MC, eds, *Handbook of Clinical Child Psychology*, 2nd edn. New York: John Wiley & Sons, 1992: 868.
8. Shapiro S, Skinner EA, Kessler LG et al, Utilization of health and mental health services. *Arch Gen Psychiatry* 1984; **41**: 971–8.

9. Rosen BM, Locke BZ, Goldberg ID, Babigian HM, Identification of emotional disturbance in patients seen in general medical clinics. *Hosp Commun Psychiatry* 1972; **23**: 364–70.

10. Rosen JC, Wiens AN, Changes in medical problems and use of medical services following psychological intervention. *Am Psychol* 1979; **34**: 420–31.

11. Livingston R, Taylor JL, Crawford SL, A study of somatic complaints and psychiatric diagnosis in children. *J Am Acad Child Adolesc Psychiatry* 1988; **27**: 185–7.

12. Goodaman JE, McGrath PJ, The epidemiology of pain in children and adolescents: A review. *Pain* 1991; **46**: 247–64.

13. Ottaviano S, Guidetti V, Temperament and migraine. In: Gallai V, Guidetti V, eds, *Juvenile Headache*. Amsterdam: Excerpta Medica, 1991: 125–8.

14. Guidetti V, Bruni O, Fabrizi P, Ottaviano S, Cortesi F, Giannotti F, Prevalence of sleep disorders in childhood and adolescence. *Cephalalgia* 1997; **17**(4): 17–22.

15. Hurrelmann K, Engel U, Holler B, Nordlohne E, Failure in school, family conflicts, and psychosomatic disorders in adolescence. *J Adolesc* 1988; **1**: 237–49.

16. Abu-Arefeh I, Russell G, Prevalence of headache and migraine in school children. *BMJ* 1994; **309**: 765–8.

17. Anttila P, Metsähonkala L, Helenius H, Sillanpää M, Predisposing and provoking factors in childhood headache. *Headache* 2000; **40**: 351–6.

18. Guidetti V, Ottaviano S, Pagliarini M et al, Psychological peculiarities in children with recurrent primary headache. *Cephalalgia* 1983; **41**(suppl 1): 215–17.

19. Lanzi G, Balottin U, Ottolini A et al, Cyclic vomiting and recurrent abdominal pains as migraine and epileptic equivalents. *Cephalalgia* 1983; **3**: 115–18.

20. Merikangas KM, Fenton B, Ramadan NM, Comorbidity and migraine. *Semin Headache Manage* 1996; **1**: 4.

21. Stewart W, Breslau N, Kech PE, Comorbidity of migraine and panic disorders. *Neurology* 1994; **44**(suppl 7): S23–7.

22. Karwautz A, Wöber C, Lang T et al, Psychosocial factors in children and adolescents with migraine and tension-type headache: a controlled study and review of the literature. *Cephalalgia* 1999; **19**: 32–43.

23. Guidetti V, Galli F, Fabrizi P et al, Headache and psychiatric comorbidity: clinical aspects and outcome in an 8-year follow-up study. *Cephalalgia* 1998; **18**: 455–62.

24. Bernstein GA, Shaw K, Practice parameters for the assessment and treatment of children and adolescents with anxiety disorders. *J Am Acad Child Adolesc Psychiatry* 1997; **36**(suppl 10): 69S–84S.

25. Campo JV, Fritsch SL, Somatization in children and adolescents. *J Am Acad Child Adolesc Psychiatry* 1994; **33**: 1223–35.

26. Reisman JM, *A History of Clinical Psychology*. Hemisphere Publishing Corporation, New York 1991.

27. Wright L, Friedman AG, Challenge of the future. Psychologists in medical settings. In: Sweet JJ, Rozensky RH, Tovian SM, eds, *Handbook of Clinical Psychology in Medical Settings*. New York: Plenum Press, 1991: 603–14.

28. Belar CD, Professionalism in medical settings. In: Sweet JJ, Rozensky RH, Tovian SM, eds, *Handbook of Clinical Psychology in Medical Settings*. New York: Plenum Press, 1991: 81–92.

29. Garralda ME, Somatisation in children. *J Child Psychol Psychiatry* 1996; **1**: 13–33.

30. Garralda ME, Practitioner review: Assessment and management of somatization in childhood and adolescence: A practical perspective. *J Child Psychol Psychiatry* 1999; **40**: 1159–67.

31. Fornara R, Cerutti R, Marioni P, Moschetta A, Guidetti V, The child with migraine and his family: A systemic approach. *Cephalalgia* 1989; **9**(suppl 10): 234–6.

32. American Psychiatric Association, *Diagnostic and Statistical Manual of Mental Disorders*, 4th edn (DSM-IV). International Version with ICD-10 codes. Washington: American Psychiatric Association, 1994.

33. Onnis L, Adolescenza e devianza tra indi-

viduo e sistema: il dilemma di una doppia crisi. *Psicobiettivo* 1994; **XIV**(1): 57–67.

34. AACAP Official Action, Practice parameters for the psychiatric assessment of children and adolescents. *J Am Acad Child Adolesc Psychiatry* 1997; **36**(suppl 10): 4S–20S.

35. Simmons JE, *Psychiatric Examination of Children*, 4th edn. Philadelphia: Lea & Febiger, 1987.

36. Greenspan SI, Greenspan NT, *The Clinical Interview of the Child*, 2nd edn. Washington DC: American Psychiatric Press, 1991.

37. Lewis M, Psychiatric assessment of infants, children and adolescents. In: Lewis M, ed., *Child and Adolescent Psychiatry: A Comprehensive Textbook*. Baltimore: Williams & Wilkins, 1991: 447–63.

38. King RA, Noshpitz JD, *Pathways of Growth: essentials of child psychiatry*, Vol II, *Psychopathology*. New York: Wiley, 1991.

39. Kestenbaum CJ, The clinical interview of the child. In: Wiener JM, ed., *Textbook of Child and Adolescent Psychiatry*. Washington: American Psychiatric Press, 1991: 79–88.

40. Diamond CB, General issues in the clinical assessment of children and adolescents. In: Kestenbaum CJ, Williams DT, eds, *Handbook of Clinical Assessment of Children and Adolescents*, Vol. 1. New York: University Press, 1988: 43–55.

41. King RA, Schowalter JE, The clinical interview of the adolescent. In: Wiener JM, ed., *Textbook of Child and Adolescent Psychiatry*. Washington: American Psychiatric Press, 1991: 89–93.

42. Rodrigue JR, Goldman J, Psychological testing. In: Noshpitz JD, ed., *Handbook of Child and Adolescent Psychiatry*, Vol 5. New York: John Wiley & Sons, 1998: 643–63.

43. Costello AJ, Use of rating scales and questionnaires. In: Wiener JM, ed., *Textbook of Child and Adolescent Psychiatry*. Washington: American Psychiatric Press, 1997.

44. Sattler JM, Assessment of children's intelligence. In: Walker CE, Roberts MC, eds, *Handbook of Clinical Child Psychology*, 2nd edn. New York: John Wiley & Sons, 1992: 868.

45. Goldman J, Rodrigue JR, Rating scales. In: Noshpitz JD, ed., *Handbook of Child and Adolescent Psychiatry*, Vol 5. New York: John Wiley & Sons, 1998: 633–43.

46. Chamberlain P, Reid J, Parent observation and report of child symptoms. *Behavioral Assessment* 1987; **9**: 97–109.

47. Hughes J, Assessment of social skills: Sociometric and behavioural approaches. In: Reynolds C, Kamphaus R, eds, *Handbook of Psychological and Educational Assessment of Children: Personality, Behaviour, and Context*. New York: Guilford Press, 1990: 423–44.

48. Hughes HM, Measures of self-concept and self-esteem for children ages 3–12 years: A review and recommendations. *Clin Psychol Rev* 1984; **4**: 657–92.

49. Kendall P, Ahead to basics: Assessments with children and families. *Behavioral Assessment* 1987; **9**: 321–32.

50. Achenbach TM, Edelbrock C, *Manual for the Child Behavior Checklist and Revised Child Behavior Profile*. Burlington: University of Vermont, Department of Psychiatry, 1983.

51. Herjanic B, Campbell W, Differentiating psychiatrically disturbed children on the basis of a structured interview. *J Abnorm Child Psychol* 1977; **5**: 127–34.

52. Herjanic B, Reich W, Development of a structured psychiatric interview for children: agreement between children and parent on individual symptoms. *J Abnorm Psychol* 1982; **10**: 307–24.

53. Costello EJ, Edelbrock CS, Dulcan MK, Kalas R, Klaric SH, *Report on the NIMH Diagnostic Interview Schedule for Children (DIS-C)*. Washington, DC: National Institute of Mental Health, 1984.

54. Butcher JN, Dahlstrom WG, Graham JR et al, *Manual for Restandardized Minnesota Multiphasic Personality Inventory, MMPI-2: An administrative and interpretative guide*. Minneapolis: University of Minnesota Press, 1989.

55. Andrasik F, Blanchard EB, Arena JG, Teders SJ, Teevan RC, Rodichok LD, Psychological functioning in headache sufferers. *Psychosom*

*Med* 1982; **44**: 171–82.

56. Naliboff BD, Cohen MJ, Yellen AN, Does the MMPI differentiate chronic illness from chronic pain? *Pain* 1982; **13**: 333–41.
57. Weeks R, Baskin S, Rapoport A, Sheftell F, Arrowsmith F, A comparison of MMPI personality data and frontalis electromyographic readings in migraine and combination headache patients. *Headache* 1983; **23**: 75–82.
58. Ellertsen B, Klove H, MMPI patterns in chronic muscle pain, tension headache, and migraine. *Cephalalgia* 1987; **7**: 65–71.
59. Invernizzi G, Gala C, Buono M, Cittone L, Tavola T, Conte G, Neurotic traits and disease duration in headache patients. *Cephalalgia* 1989; **9**: 173–8.
60. Mongini F, Ferla E, Maccagnani C, MMPI profiles in patients with headache or craniofacial pain: a comparative study. *Cephalalgia* 1992; **12**: 91–8.
61. De Benedittis G, Lorenzetti A, Minor stressful life events (daily hassles) in chronic primary headache: relationship with MMPI personality patterns. *Headache* 1992; **32**: 330–4.
62. Williams DE, Raczynski JM, Domino J, Davig JP, Psychophysiological and MMPI personality assessment of headaches: an integrative approach. *Headache* 1993; **33**: 149–54.
63. Mongini F, Ibertis F, Ferla E, Personality characteristics before and after treatment of different head pain syndromes. *Cephalalgia* 1994; **14**: 368–73.
64. Mongini F, Ibertis F, Barbalonga E, Raviola F, MMPI-2 profiles in chronic daily headache and their relationship to anxiety levels and accompanying symptoms. *Headache* 2000; **40**: 466–72.
65. Butcher JN, Williams CL, Graham JR et al, *Minnesota Multiphasic Personality Inventory – Adolescent: Manual for Administration, Scoring, Interpretation*. Minneapolis: University of Minnesota Press, 1992.
66. Archer RP, Overview of the Minnesota Multiphasic Personality Inventory – Adolescent (MMPI-A). In: Maruish ME, ed., *The Use of Psychological Testing for Treatment Planning*

*and Outcomes Assessment*, 2nd edn. Mahwah, NJ: Lawrence Erlbaum Associates, 1999: 341–80.
67. Lachar D, *Personality Inventory for Children (PIC), Revised Format Manual Supplement.* Los Angeles: Western Psychological Services, 1982.
68. Guidetti V, Fornara R, Cortesi F, Petrilli A, Ottaviano S, Seri S, Personality Inventory for Children and Childhood Migraine. *Cephalalgia* 1987; **7**: 225–30.
69. Bruni O, Romoli M, Diamanti R, Fornara R, Guidetti, Personality Inventory for Children and Adolescents with Headache and Migraine: a case control study. *Cephalalgia* 1991; **11**(suppl 11): 127–8.
70. Lachar D, Inventory for Children, 2nd edn (PIC-2), Personality Inventory for Youth (PIY), and Student Behavior Survey (SBS). In: Maruish ME, ed., *The Use of Psychological Testing for Treatment Planning and Outcomes Assessment*, 2nd edn. Mahwah, NJ: Lawrence Erlbaum Associates, 1999: 399–427.
71. Lachar D, Kline RB, Personality Inventory for Children and Personality Inventory for Youth. In: Maruish ME, ed., *The Use of Psychological Testing for Treatment Planning and Outcomes Assessment*. Illsdale, NJ: Lawrence Erlbaum Associates, 1994: 479–516.
72. Rodrigue JR, Goldman J, Psychological testing. In: Noshpitz JD, ed., *Handbook of Child and Adolescent Psychiatry*, Vol 5. New York: John Wiley & Sons, 1998: 643–63.
73. Rieger RE, Baron IS, Psychological and neuropsychological testing. In: Wiener JM, ed., *Textbook of Child and Adolescent Psychiatry*. Washington: American Psychiatric Press, 1997: 133–52.
74. Wechsler D, *Wechsler Adult Intelligence Scale – Revised*. San Antonio, TX: Psychological Corporation, 1981.
75. Wechsler D, *Wechsler Pre-school and Primary Scale of Intelligence-Revised*. San Antonio, TX: Psychological Corporation, 1989.
76. Wechsler D, *Wechsler Intelligence Scale for*

*Children*, 3rd edn. San Antonio, TX: Psychological Corporation, 1989.

77. Harris DB, *Children's Drawings as Measures of Intellectual Maturity: A revision and extension of the Goodenough Draw-A-Man Test*. New York: Harcourt Brace and World, 1963.

78. Koppitz EM, *Psychological Evaluation of Children's Human Figure Drawing*. New York: Grune & Stratton, 1968.

79. DiLeo JH, *Children's Drawings as Diagnostic Aids*. New York: Brunner/Mazel, 1970.

80. Bellak L, Bellak SS, *Children's Apperception Test Manual*. New York: CPS, 1952.

81. Bellak L, Adelman C, The children's apperception test (CAT). In: Rabin AI, Haworth MR, eds, *Projective Techniques with Children*. New York: Grune & Stratton, 1960: 62–94.

82. Murray HA, *Thematic Apperception Test Manual*. Cambridge: Harvard University Press, 1943.

83. Levitt EE, French J, Projective testing of children. In: Walker CE, Roberts MC, eds, *Handbook of Clinical Child Psychology*, 2nd edn. New York: John Wiley & Sons, 1992: 149–63.

84. Levitt EE, Truumaa A, *The Rorschach Technique with Children and Adolescents: Application and Norms*. New York: Grune & Stratton, 1972.

85. Exner JE, Weiner IB, *The Rorschach: A comprehensive system*, Vol 3. *Assessment of children and adolescents*. New York: Wiley, 1982.

86. Guidetti V, Ottaviano S, Pagliarini M, Seri S, Rorschach test and childhood migraine. *Cephalalgia* 1985; 5(suppl 3): 160–1.

87. Guidetti V, Mazzei G, Ottaviano S, Pagliarini M, Paolella A, Seri S, Rorschach test and childhood migraine. *Cephalalgia* 1986; 6: 87–93.

88. Haley J, *Uncommon Therapy*. New York: WW Norton & Co., 1973.

89. Bowen M, *Dalla famiglia all'individuo*. Rome: Astrolabio, 1979.

90. Walsh F, ed., *Normal Family Processes*, 1st edn. New York: The Guilford Press, 1982.

91. Colapinto J, Terapia familiare strutturale. In: Gurman AS, Kniskern DP, eds, *Manuale di Terapia della Famiglia*. Turin: Bollati Boringhieri, 1995: 451–75.

92. Lankton SR, Lankton CH, Matthews WJ, Terapia familiare ericksoniana. In: Gurman AS, Kniskern DP, eds, *Manuale di Terapia della Famiglia*. Turin: Bollati Boringhieri, 1995: 241–84.

93. Haley J, *La terapia del problem solving*. Rome: La Nuova Italia Scientifica, 1985.

94. Watzlawitck P, Beavin JH, Jackson DD, *Pragmatica della Comunicazione Umana*. Rome: Astrolabio, 1971.

95. Bateson G, *Steps to an Ecology of Mind*. Chandler Publishing Co., San Francisco, 1972.

96. Kerr ME, Bowen M, *Family Evaluation*. New York: WW Norton & Co., 1988.

97. Onnis L, *Famiglia e malattia psicosomatica*. Rome: La Nuova Italia Scientifica, 1988: 43–59.

98. Tafà M, Malagoli Togliatti M, La coppia: dal vincolo allo scioglimento del legame. *Interazioni* 1996; **2**: 73–96.

99. Tafà M, Malagoli Togliatti M, L'attaccamento oltre l'infanzia: continuità intergenerazionale e potenzialità evolutive del legame di coppia. *Rassegna di Psicologia* 1998; **XV**(3): 31–57.

100. McGoldrick M, Carter E, The family life cycle. In: Walsh F, ed., *Normal Family Processes*, 1st edn. New York: The Guilford Press, 1982.

101. Wanboldt MZ, Weinstraub P, Krafchick D, Berce N, Wanboldt FS, Links between past parental trauma and the medical and psychological outcome of asthmatic children: a theoretical model. *Family Systems Medicine* 1995; **13**(2).

102. Olson D, Family stress and coping: A multisystem perspective. In: Cusinato M, ed., *Research on Family Resources and Need across the World*. Milan: Edizioni Universitarie di Lettere Economia Diritto, LED, 1996: 73–105.

103. Boszormenyi-Nagy I, Spark G, *Invisible Loyalties: Reciprocity in Intergenerational Family*

*Therapy.* New York: Harper & Row, 1973.

104. McGoldrick M, Greson FG, *Genogram in Family Assessment.* New York: WW Norton & Co., 1985.

105. Wynne LC, McDaniel SH, Weber TT, Consulenza familiare e consulenza sistemica. *Terapia Familiare* 1988; **27**: 43–56.

106. Boszormenyi-Nagy I, Grunebaum J, Ulrich D, Terapia Contestuale. In: Gurman AS, Kniskern DP, eds, *Manuale di Terapia della Famiglia.* Turin: Bollati Boringhieri, 1995: 201–39.

107. Telfener U, La valutazione del processo clinico: l'ottica sistemica. *Psicobiettivo* 1996; **XVI**(1): 37–48.

108. Minuchin S, *Families and Family Therapy.* Cambridge: Harvard University Press, 1976.

109. Buchanan CM, Maccoby EE, Dornbusch SM, Caught between parents: Adolescents' experience in divorced homes. *Child Dev* 1991; **62**: 1008–29.

110. Tafà M, Il concetto di Sé nei figli dei separati: difficoltà relazionali e percezione di autoefficacia durante l'adolescenza. *Psicologia Clinica dello Sviluppo*, 2001: in press.

111. Haley J, *Leaving Home. The therapy of disturbed young people.* New York: McGraw Hill, 1980.

# 7

# Neurophysiological methods
*Viktor Farkas*

Various neurophysiological methods have been applied to explore central nervous system (CNS) dysfunctions between attacks in primary headache patients, particularly in migraine, and healthy controls. Most of these studies have produced results of dysfunction in cortical activity; the observations reported in migraineurs are interpreted as a modified cortical excitability (mostly hyperexcitability), which is thought to be implicated in the pathogenesis of migraine disease.[1] By using dynamic neurophysiological methods, recent evidence in the literature suggests that the time interval to the next migraine attack has a considerable influence on this CNS dysfunction.

The main purposes of clinical neurophysiological studies in children with headaches have been the differential diagnosis between primary and secondary headaches, the diagnosis of subtypes of primary headache, and the contribution of data to the pathophysiology of primary headaches in children. Electrophysiological studies on childhood and adolescent headache, particularly in young children, are interesting in view of both the need for an exact, non-invasive clinical diagnosis and the efficacy of neurophysiological studies at an early age attributable to the recent outcome of the illness, with less clinical modification by environmental factors or drug use. Furthermore, by identifying parameters that discrimi-

nate between, for example, patients with migraine and controls in the interval, it would be possible to assess interictal effects of migraine treatment, and whether the effects of pharmacological intervention are the result of a re-normalization of underlying migraine pathophysiology.[2] For the most part, electrophysiological studies in childhood headache concern migraine and electroencephalographic (EEG) evaluations, but also evoked potentials, event-related potentials and, less often, electromyographic (EMG) studies have been performed.[3]

## Visual evoked potentials and the habituation process in migraine

The increased sensitivity to environmental stimuli in migraine and the occurrence of prodromal visual disturbances motivated the use of evoked potentials, particularly visual evoked potentials (VEPs), in the study of primary headaches. VEPs reflect the sensory visual pathways but not the cognitive processing of visual stimuli. A number of studies have been carried out to detect interictal abnormalities in VEPs to transient stimuli or continuous flicker (steady state VEPs, SVEPs) in adults. Few studies are reported in childhood migraine. An earlier quantitative analysis of VEPs to continuous flicker, using two posterior electrodes in children and adults with migraine, demonstrated that the response of photic driving was dependent on age and a history of migraine. Children, independent of whether or not they have migraine, had poor photic driving at lower frequencies of photic stimulation.[4] However, by using topographic methods in juvenile migraine, an increased amplitude of the F1 component of SVEPs was reported with a tendency for visual reactivity in migraine with and without aura to spread.[5] In a follow-up study on the correlation between electrophysiological abnormalities and clinical migraine parameters, the pattern of SVEPs appeared independently of age, age of onset of migraine, duration of illness and type of migraine; visual responsiveness was significantly increased in patients with a family history of migraine.[6] These results in childhood migraine may indicate that there is a genetic predisposition to the illness, based on a primary neural dysfunction on the subcortical–cortical modulation, underlying the observed abnormal visual response.[3]

Amplitudes of averaged VEPs with flash or pattern-reversal stimulation were higher in migraineurs than in healthy controls in a number of studies, but not in all.[7–10] Different stimulus parameters have been used previously and this may explain the inconsistent results. Several studies found increased midline VEP amplitudes,[11–15] whereas others found negative ones.[8–10,16–18] The increased amplitudes of pattern-reversal VEPs in children with migraine correspond to findings of sensitivity and specificity for the amplitude and latency of the P300 component (see later). A reduced amplitude of the lateral VEP has been observed.[14,19] Variable results were reported by studying the latency of the P100 component in children with migraine.[11,13,20–23] Reduction of the P100 amplitude after treatment with β blockers has been observed.[12] An inverse correlation with magnesium levels was found in children suffering from migraine with and without aura in the interval period.[3,11]

Changes of amplitudes during repeated visual stimulation differ between migraine patients in the headache-free phase and controls. During uninterrupted pattern-reversal stimulation with constant intensity, the sequentially measured VEP amplitudes are decreased (habituation) in healthy participants, but remained stable (loss of habituation) or even increased (potentiation) in migraine patients.[24,25] This habituation process is found to occur in many evoked and event-related cortical potentials in normal individuals, but not in migraine patients (see later). On the other hand, a recent study failed to find reduced habituation in migraineurs.[26]

The habituation of neurophysiological parameters in migraine underlies periodic changes during the pain-free interval and is maximally reduced before an attack. Habituation is thought to protect the organism against sensory overload, i.e. against excessive cortical lactate accumulation during sustained stimulation. Migraine patients are characterized by impaired oxidative energy metabolism and elevated lactate in the brain during pain-free intervals.[27,28] The exact cause of the deficient habituation is not known. It may be inversely related to dysfunction of brain centres that modulate the state of cerebral cortex excitability.[29] Periodically occurring changes in cortical excitability may also be responsible for both reduced habituation and metabolic deficit in the migrainous brain. The lack of habituation in migraine patients represents a probably fundamental dysfunctioning of cortical information processing, which might result from the high level of cortical arousal and alertness.[30] These findings are consistent with different biobehavioural and psychological studies in migraineurs, because the highly aroused participants are introverted and low sensation seekers.[31–33] The lack of habituation in migraine patients may be a result of an action of several neurotransmitter systems, the cholinergic, dopaminergic, GABAergic (γ-aminobutyric acid) and serotoninergic neuronal functions or nitric oxide action in the brain.[34] Similarly, the cortical arousal level also depends on the actions of different neurotransmitter systems from the brain stem projecting to the cortex, e.g. the activity of noradrenaline.[35] Nevertheless, among these systems, serotonin (5HT) has a 'gain control' function between unspecific facilitating (noradrenergic) and specific inhibitory (cholinergic) systems,[36,37] particularly those that originate in the raphe nuclei and project to the sensory cortices.[38] Indeed, when facing repetitive stimuli, the 5HT neuron does not habituate for a long period; instead it inhibits activities of noradrenergic neurons.[39] Thus, 5HT may mediate behavioural inhibition and regulation of emotion.[40]

## Cortical auditory evoked potentials

Significant differences have been found between migraine sufferers and healthy controls in the intensity dependence of cortical auditory evoked potentials (AEPs). The intensity–amplitude function of the cortical long-latency AEP was found to be increased in migraineurs.[41] In migraine, the amplitude of the potential is strongly dependent on the intensity of the auditory stimulus, resulting in a step amplitude/stimulus function slope. The strong intensity dependence of cortical AEPs was observed in patients with migraine both with (MA) and without (MO) aura, and it might be a consequence of the reduced central serotoninergic transmission which is responsible for decreased cortical preactivation levels.[42,43] On the other hand, the AEP amplitudes evoked by low-intensity stimuli seemed to be low in migraine patients, which also suggested that cortical preactivation level is decreased in the headache-free period in migraineurs;[44,45] this is thought to be inversely related to the level of CNS serotoninergic neurotransmission. The AEP amplitude–intensity function (ASF) slope has been suggested to reflect cortical 5HT activity.[43] Increased AEP intensity–amplitude steepness can be found even in children and adolescents who have MO.[46]

## Brain-stem auditory evoked potentials

Brain-stem AEPs (BAEPs) are a sensitive measure of CNS dysfunction[47] and amplitudes of the late (pontomesencephalic) waves are suppressed by 5HT in rats.[48,49] The hypothesis has been proposed that BAEP amplitudes may reflect serotoninergic activity in the brain stem, and further studies may possibly shed more light on the hypothesized brainstem hyperexcitability, which is related to phonophobia in migraine.[48] Brain-stem nuclei have been found to be activated during migraine attacks and 5HT-depleting drugs may alter BAEPs in migraineurs.[50] BAEP latencies seem to be normal in the headache-free period;

however, some asymmetry has been observed.[50,51] Latency abnormalities were observed in basilar migraine.[53] There are no convincing results on BAEPs in migraine, but wave IV–V amplitude increases almost linearly with increasing stimulus intensity.[54]

# Contingent negative variation and event-related potentials

Contingent negative variation (CNV) is a slow negative potential appearing during a reaction-time task with a warning and an imperative stimulus, and it could be recorded primarily from association areas of the brain. In various cognitive event-related potentials (ERPs), such as CNV, particularly the day before the attack, increased amplitude was found in both adult and childhood migraines compared with healthy controls and patients with tension-type headache (TTH); this suggested that CNV could be used successfully as a diagnostic instrument for distinguishing between migraine and TTH.[3,55,56] The CNV appears to have a value in the prediction of the clinical efficacy of some prophylactic agents[57,58] in migraine. The CNV of healthy children did not differ from that of their siblings suffering from migraine, so a family-related cortical hypersensitivity is suggested, which does not necessarily lead to the development of migraine.[59]

Trigeminal/neuronal hyperexcitability and activation of the trigeminovascular system by spreading depression is proposed in migraine pathophysiology. Some data suggest that cutaneous and mucosal trigeminal nerve fibres may be involved,[60,61] although the degree of involvement of peripheral and central parts of the trigeminonociceptive system in migraine is

unclear.[2] In migraineurs, the symptoms of olfactory dysfunction could be observed in both the interictal and the ictal periods. Odours can provoke migraine attacks. There are reports dealing with olfactory aura, mostly olfactory hallucinations. Sensory hyper-excitability is frequently manifested by osmophobia.[62,63] On the other hand, a deficit in olfactory thresholds was also observed because higher prevalence of anosmia or hyposmia has been reported in the headache-free interval in migraineurs.[64] These findings may be related to the severity and frequency of migraine attacks. By studying trigeminal and olfactory ERPs in migraineurs, trigeminal hyperexcitability is suggested. However, the general increased nasal chemosensitivity is not supported because smaller ERP amplitudes were observed in migraineurs. Most recently, it has been noted that, in general, olfactory ERPs discriminate better than trigeminal interictal ERPs between migraineurs and controls, emphasizing the role of the olfactory system in migraine. A higher amplitude of trigeminal ERPs might reflect an increased trigeminal nociceptive excitability in migraine; however, the smaller amplitudes of olfactory ERPs could indicate decreased olfactory sensitivity. These observations could be interpreted by the involvement of the serotoninergic system in migraine pathophysiology, because the serotoninergic neurons in the brainstem have a modulatory role in cortical information processing.[65] Low activity in this system leads to high cortical reactivation[39,66] and may also diminish habituation. However, from studies on animals, low activity of the serotoninergic system could have caused glomerular atrophy in the olfactory bulb.[67] In addition to 5HT, the dopaminergic system could contribute, because dopamine is a major neurotransmitter in the first relay station of the olfactory system.[62,64]

There are few studies of ERPs in children with headache. The P300 potential is linked to the processes of perception and cognition, but also to the processes involving memory, which was found to be impaired in short- and long-term components in juvenile migraine.[3,68] The P300 latency is related to the cholinergic mediator, whereas the N2–P3 amplitude depends on the aminergic one: a decrease in acetylcholine leads to a prolongation of the information processing time, whereas an increase in the aminergic mediator during the information processing analysis, enhancing cortical arousal, increases the N2–P3 amplitude.[69] The changes in N2–P3 amplitude observed during a spontaneous attack confirm a previous study on P300 in adolescent migraine, during an attack induced by intravenous administration of histamine, and in juvenile headache patients during spontaneous attacks.[70,71]

The interictal lack of habituation in cortical processing of visual and auditory information is reported in migraine. Most studies on habituation in migraine were performed based on analyses of cognitive ERPs as the P300 component of AEPs and VEPs and the CNV. The periodic changes of amplitude and habituation of CNV are related especially to early and total CNV, but not to the late component. The early CNV component is often discussed as being associated with activity of the frontal cortex.[72] Furthermore, the variability of CNV habituation is accompanied by abnormal extinction of central components of the orienting response.[73] Loss of visual and auditory P300 (an ERP elicited by an oddball paradigm: the active 'oddball' VERP P3b and the passive 'oddball' AERP P3a) latency habituation (i.e. potentiation) during successive stimulation has been reported in migraine children, adolescents and adults.[57,74–76] However, the loss of habituation is age dependent, with a significant positive correlation between age and acceleration of P300 latency. It is suggested that specific cognitive migraine processing depends on brain development and evolves before puberty only in a few cases.[74] Evaluation of cortical habituation, as measured by the amplitude and latency of the P300 component, provides a diagnostic tool with high specificity, but low sensitivity to differentiate between migraine and TTH in childhood and adolescence.[74]

A recent study, however, failed to find VEP amplitude habituation differences (reduced habituation) in migraineurs,[26] and cognitive-processing abnormalities were not observed.[77] Cognitive evoked potentials have more complex generators than the sensory evoked potentials and it is far from clear how P300 latency relates to CNV and VEP amplitudes.

# Migraine attack–interval cycle

Clinical observations of the premonitory symptoms of migraine and several electrophysiological studies suggest that dynamic changes of cortical information processing have a close temporal relationship to the migraine attack cycle. It has been concluded that the time interval to the next attack influences the EEG background activity, VEP amplitude, CNV amplitude and cognitive P300 latency habituation.[48] Latency habituation (shortening) of the visual event-related component P3 also normalizes during the attack.[78] The dynamic changes of neurophysiological abnormalities, if replicable, possibly describe an important mechanism of migraine attack and are related to changes in cortical hyperexcitability, but the underlying mechanism remains unknown. The BAEP ASF slope presumably reflects hyperexcitation or loss of inhibition in the pre-attack period.[48] It may be speculated that brain-stem activation coexists with (and possibly causes) visual cortex inhibition in the pre-attack period. Dynamic changes in the activity of 5HT, dopamine, noradrenaline and cortical arousal between attacks have been observed,[78–80] but these do not sufficiently explain the mechanisms of periodic neurophysiological abnormalities.

Recent studies report that the habituation/potentiation state of VEP amplitudes and the brain-stem activation state are related to the migraine attack–interval cycle. Lack of habituation in the interval period of migraineurs and increased amplitudes, particularly on the day before the attack, are also present using ERPs. Periodic CNV changes are described in migraineurs: loss of habituation continuously increases during migraine interval, with a maximum of a few days before an attack, and is followed by an abrupt normalization during the attack.[57,75,78,80–82] The increased CNV amplitude found on the day before the attack was interpreted as a sign of changed cortical excitability, possibly an adaptive process to control brain-stem intrinsic hyperactivity.[81]

It was proposed that the higher the CNV amplitude, the greater the susceptibility of the brain to a migraine attack. The strong negative correlation between initial potential amplitudes and amplitude potentiation confirms that the latter is probably the result of a reduced cortical preactivation level and it may be a consequence of low serotoninergic brain-stem 'state setting'.[44] It has been demonstrated

that children and adolescents with migraine are also characterized by increased amplitudes and reduced habituation, which occur with a similar periodicity to that during the headache-free interval in adults.[82] It is suggested that the migraine attack occurs when the high negative amplitude of the early CNV component and the greatest failure of habituation coincide with other precipitating factors. These abnormalities return to normal during the attack. Although loss of normal P300 latency habituation was found up to 1 day before a migraine attack, normal habituation seemed to reappear on the attack day.[78] Studies reporting ERP deviations related to the migraine cycle may shed considerable light on the pathogenesis of migraine. It is speculated that response dishabituation to external stimuli overloads a metabolic strain on the brains of migraineurs, which increases the energy demands, triggers activation of the trigeminovascular system and leads to a migraine attack. The persistent dishabituation and higher level of cortical arousal can be normalized during the migraine attack.[34] A similar normalization process just before and during the attack was reported by using pattern-reversal VEPs (PR-VEPs) and strong intensity dependence of cortical AEPs.[83] Concordantly, the normalization around the attack seems to hold true for various evoked/event-related potentials (presumably reflecting a normalization of the inhibitory process).[48] The normalization process is initiated the day before the attack, probably at a time point when prodromes/premonitory symptoms may appear. It is thus likely that the variability of evoked potential (EP) findings in migraine results partly from the fact that in most previous studies the delay between recordings and the next attack (time interval to the next attack) was not taken into consideration, e.g. normalization of VEP habituation in the periattack period might partly explain previous contradictory results on VEP amplitudes in migraineurs. Other studies that use transcranial magnetic stimulation of the visual and/or motor cortex in migraine are also inconclusive; hypoexcitability,[84] hyperexcitability[85] or no differences were reported.[86]

# Transcranial magnetic stimulation

The pathogenesis of cerebral dysfunction in migraine is the subject of controversial discussion. Neurological symptoms such as visual auras might be the result of (1) mechanisms similar to spreading depression, (2) ictal hypoperfusion or (3) generalized hyperexcitability followed by an inhibition of the cortex.[86] There are only a few techniques that allow the investigation of inhibitory and excitatory mechanisms of the cortex in vivo in humans. At low intensities transcranial magnetic stimulation (TMS) activates the corticospinal system trans-synaptically through activation of excitatory or inhibitory interneurons, leading to excitation or inhibition as judged by the amplitude of the EMG activity elicited by a test shock to the ipsilateral sensorimotor cortex.[87,88] Studies investigating motor cortical excitability in MA or MO in the interval period do not support the concept of persistent general cortical hyperexcitability as a major mechanism of cortical dysfunction in migraine secondary to genetic predisposition, or a structural alteration of inhibitory interneurons in the cortex caused by repeated parenchymal insults during attacks, although excitability might undergo dynamic changes.[84,86,89] An increased excitability of the

visual system was suggested by a study which showed that the threshold for phosphenes evoked by TMS in patients with migraine is decreased.[90] However, others could not confirm this result.[84]

# Conclusions

Studies of cortical sensory EPs in primary headache patients have yielded variable results. Consistent changes in conventional VEPs and AEPs have not been observed.[48] EPs and ERPs have been extensively studied in migraineurs during the interictal period, compared with healthy volunteers, and the results are interpreted as functional abnormalities of cortical information processing. However, so far the EPs and ERPs are of little use in the routine clinical diagnosis of headache/ migraine, because these neurophysiological parameters have considerable inter- and intraindividual variability (e.g. variation within study participants over different recordings). On the other hand, these findings can be used for pathophysiological differentiation of groups, as has been done previously for migraineurs versus non-migraineurs and MA versus MO. The hypothesis of neuronal hyperexcitability in migraine was generated based on observations in a number of studies of higher amplitudes of VEPs and somatosensory EPs,[14,15,91] deficient habituation,[44,92,94] increased CNV,[57] alterations of the trigeminovascular system[93] and migraine as a cerebral channelopathy.[2,94,95] It has been suggested that the specific cognitive migraine processing is age dependent and evolves before puberty only in a few cases. Furthermore, recent dynamic studies of neurophysiological methods, particularly ERPs, provided interesting information in relation to the migraine cycle, which may shed considerable light on migraine pathogenesis.[48]

# Conventional EEG

Earlier EEG was traditionally considered a useful adjunct to the clinical evaluation of headache in children. A large number of studies have reported EEG abnormalities in migraine during headache-free periods, whereas there are only a few EEG studies in other primary headaches. In a group of children with TTH, no significant EEG changes were observed.[96] Visual analysis of the EEG background activity in migraine patients has revealed no obviously abnormal EEG rhythm.[97]

The literature concerning EEG abnormalities in migraine patients is confusing because, in earlier reports, there was no clear consensus on diagnostic criteria for childhood migraine, so there was enormous variability in the definition of migraine and diagnostic approaches of paediatric neurologists to this problem. However, there were no strict criteria to determine what constituted an EEG abnormality. Further most studies have serious methodological flaws, e.g. there are only few published controlled studies with masked EEG evaluation in headache patients, particularly in children. These earlier studies suggest that the EEG by conventional evaluation in headache-free migraine patients may differ from EEGs in healthy children and from EEGs in patients with TTH. Although EEG abnormalities have been reported in 44–70% of migraine patients, the specificity of these findings is doubtful because they are nearly as prevalent in controls as in migraineurs:[98] i.e. the interictal focal slow-wave activity, sharp waves and spikes reported in migraineurs are probably not greater than those in healthy controls.[79,99–101] However, the prevalence of EEG abnormalities further reduced as the new uniform criteria for defining migraine came into widespread use. Epileptiform EEG abnormalities were observed in 4% of both healthy and migraine children.[18] Despite these controversial reports on the prevalence and type of EEG abnormalities found in the headache-free periods of migraine children, as a result of the lack of objectivity in earlier retrospective studies, it is clear that migrainous children could be characterized by paroxysmal discharges typical of specific childhood epileptic syndromes.[97,101]

The only consistently reported EEG abnormality in both adult and childhood migraine patients during asymptomatic periods is a prominent photic driving response at flash rates beyond 20 Hz – the 'H-response'. This phenomenon is equivalent to the steady-state VEPs. Recent EEG mapping studies in children and adolescents confirmed photic driving in migraine; the increased amplitude of the steady-state VEP F1 component, with the tendency for spread of visual reactivity, seems to be a consistent electrophysiological pattern in the interval period of migraine attacks, independent of age and type of migraine.[102] However, in a previous report using only two posterior electrodes, children had poor photic driving at lower frequencies of photic stimulation independent of whether or not they had migraine.[4] The 'H-response' can be found in up 90% of migraineurs and 78% of normal study participants.[79,103] In the routine clinical evaluation of the headache patient, the usefulness of photic driving is rather limited because of its low specificity. Thus, the presence of a prominent photic driving response may have interesting implications for the underlying pathogenesis of migraine. Since the seminal observation by Golla and Winter of an increased photic drive of the EEG in migraineurs, cortical hyperreactivity to visual stimuli – a dysfunction of visual processing – has been demonstrated with various methods, e.g. epidemiological surveys, functional tests, and steady-state, flash or pattern-reversal VEPs. It is not clear whether the cortical excitability is the result of lack of inhibition by intrinsic GABAergic neurons[104] or of an abnormal modulation of the cortex by subcortical (monoaminergic) pathways.[24] It was hypothesized that the former, which postulates a loss of cortical interneurons, might be an acquired consequence of the repeated insults of migraine attacks (hypoxia, spreading depression), whereas the latter could be a genetic abnormality. A positive correlation is reported between visual reactivity and family history of migraine or autonomic symptoms during the attack, which favours the hypothesis of an inherited subcortical dysfunction.[3]

We may conclude that, in children with recurrent, chronic headache, the use of standard EEG as a diagnostic tool is not routinely indicated. Despite the EEG's high specificity for epilepsy, the great majority of children presenting epileptiform abnormalities only on the EEG (without any clinical seizure) will not have epilepsy.[105] According to the recommendation of the Quality Standard Subcommittee of the American Academy of Neurology, the EEG is not indicated in routine evaluation of adult patients presenting with headache, but may be useful in patients presenting with symptoms suggestive of a seizure disorder or with atypical migraine aura symptoms.[29,106] A similar recommendation is yet not available for children and adolescents with chronic recurrent headache (migraine). This conclusion does not, however, exclude the use of EEG to evaluate headache sufferers with associated symptoms that suggest a seizure disorder, particularly in children, where the distinctive features of migraine have been found in childhood epilepsy syndromes, including benign occipital epilepsies of childhood, benign rolandic epilepsy with migraine, mitochondrial encephalomyopathy with lactic acidosis and stroke (MELAS), basilar migraine with seizure and migraine with absence seizures.

During migraine attacks with typical visual aura, EEG abnormalities have been reported with somewhat inconsistent results.[97] During migraine aura, bursts of spike activity may have a superficial resemblance to the ictal EEG of an epileptic seizure; however, the usual progressive decline in frequency of rhythmic epileptiform activity of ictal EEGs in epilepsy will not be present in migraine.[107] A normal EEG or non-specific slowing is the usual finding in patients who have MA or MO.[108] Taken together, the results suggest that during the headache phase a normal EEG may be found in some patients (possibly when neural dysfunction is limited to the interhemispheric visual cortex); depression of the amplitude of the α activities may be present (possibly when the cortical dysfunction is mild) or occipital δ activity may occur (a possible combined cortical/subcortical dysfunction). During migraine attacks with complex and/or prolonged neurological aura symptoms, contralateral (unilateral) focal slowing in the form of polymorphic δ or θ activity that lasts for several hours or days has been observed, in addition to the decrease in α power often reactive to eye opening. During basilar migraine attacks, prolonged bursts of repetitive posterior rhythmic sharp waves, alternating with normal background activity, were reported.[109] It remains to be determined whether the focal or diffuse slowing reported between attacks in MA could be related to the persistence of the acute changes and to an insufficient delay between the attack and the EEG recording.[110] Periodic unilateral sharp-slow waves and/or paroxysmal lateralizing epileptiform discharges (PLEDs) or PLED-like activity were reported during and several days after the onset of hemiplegic migraine, prolonged migraine aura or incipient migrainous infarction, but were followed by complete recovery.[97] These patients with PLED-like activity did not have any of the usual entities associated with PLEDs, such as stroke, brain abscess, glioblastoma or herpes encephalitis, and their PLEDs usually resolved within 24 hours.[107]

## Quantitative EEG

By using recent methods of EEG quantitative analysis, it has been possible to perform statistical evaluation and to reduce subjectivity. Studies performed using quantitative EEG are reported in childhood migraine with conflicting results. During the headache-free periods, three major abnormalities have been observed in migraine patients: (1) interhemispheric asymmetry of α rhythm, (2) diffuse or focal slowing and (3) increase of fast activities.[110] These EEG patterns appeared to be variable in relation to the type of migraine and age.[111] The EEG abnormalities in the interval periods of migraine patients, similiar to other electrophysiological parameters, could be subtended by a fluctuating disorder which culminates during the migraine attack.[79]

By using spectral analysis and topographic EEG mapping in children, it was concluded that the spontaneous brain electrical activity in migraine could vary with age, duration of illness and interval from the last or to the next attack. In children the presence of interhemi-

spheric α asymmetry discriminated between MA and MO, but only in adults,[112] although even attacks of MO in children were associated with a diffuse increase of θ activity compared with normal controls.[113] In children with TTH, no significant EEG modification was detectable during the headache phase, in contrast to the migraine attack.[114] The failure to detect a spontaneous characteristic EEG feature that is useful for clinical diagnostic purposes could exclude the clinical use of quantified EEG in the diagnosis of childhood headache. However, the evidence of modifications in EEG background activity in migraine children during the attack and persisting in the interval period might suggest the use of the quantitative EEG techniques in monitoring the pathophysiological alterations of migraine.[3]

## Epilepsy and migraine

The relationship between migraine and epilepsy has intrigued neurologists for over a century. Headaches have been associated with seizures as ictal or postictal phenomena, particularly on occipital lobe seizure; however, migraine aura may trigger seizures. Gowers wrote that 'some surprise may be felt that migraine is given a place in the borderland of epilepsy, but the position is justified by many relations amongst them and by the fact that the two maladies are sometimes mistaken and more often their distinction is difficult'.[115] However, the relationship between epilepsy and migraine has been postulated for over 100 years, although the nature of this interaction is still unresolved. In addition, the diagnosis of atypical migraine symptoms can be difficult, and a number of epileptic and non-epileptic syndromes may mimic migraine.[116,117] The relationship of migraine and epilepsy is often considered to be coincidental in adults, because of the high prevalence of each disorder. Most people with migraine and epilepsy have headaches without apparent temporal association. The term 'migralepsy' for 'a seizure that may be a composite of symptoms encountered in epilepsy and migraine' has been reintroduced.[118] In a more recent review, the term 'migraine-induced epilepsy' was suggested, when seizures occurred during or immediately after a migraine aura.[119] This is similar to the earlier term of 'intercalated seizure' which was used to denote epileptic seizures occurring between the aura phase and the headache phase of migraine.[120] The EEG can be misleading in the differential diagnosis. Despite the EEG's high specificity for epilepsy, in a setting where the pre-test probability of epilepsy is low, the vast majority of patients with epileptiform EEG activity will not have epilepsy.[105] For this reason, the routine use of EEG as a screen for epilepsy in headache patients should be avoided. In patients presenting with headache, in whom atypical associated symptomatology makes seizure disorder reasonably probable, however, epileptiform activity on an EEG could significantly raise the probability of epilepsy.[98] Some migraine patients have paroxysmal discharges on EEG, and even sharp waves with an epileptiform appearance could be presence in migraineur children. It is important to remember that the differential diagnosis is not the only issue; when migraine and epilepsy occur together, both conditions must be diagnosed.[107]

There are mostly anecdotal reports of patients with 'coexisting epilepsy and migraine', e.g. with both photosensitive occipital seizure induced by intermittent photic stimulation and migraine with visual aura remote in time from the epileptic manifestation.[121,122]

Patients with migraine and later development of temporal seizures during the course of migraine disease have also been observed, when episodes were no longer triggered by the migraine aura, and a secondary epileptogenesis was suggested.[118] The frequency of epilepsy in patients with migraine, and migraine in those with epilepsy, seems to be higher than one would expect, suggesting that there may be a co-morbidity for both conditions. Earlier epidemiological findings in this area are difficult to interpret, because of variation in the definitions of migraine used in different studies and the absence of controls. A definite association between migraine and epilepsy was found in about 3% of adult patients with seizures, in every subgroup of epilepsy defined by seizure type, age at onset, aetiology of epilepsy or family history of epilepsy.[118,123–125] The causes of the co-morbidity of migraine and epilepsy are unknown. It cannot be fully explained by a shared genetic susceptibility to both disorders, or by a head injury that is a known risk factor for both disorders.

The co-morbidity of migraine and epilepsy has implications for diagnosis and treatment. Clinicians treating patients with either epilepsy or migraine should be sensitive to the symptoms and familiar with the diagnostic and treatment principles of both disorders.[124] The differential diagnosis between migraine and epilepsy can sometimes be difficult on a purely clinical basis. Some of the symptoms used for classification of migraine are similar to those reported by subjects with partial-onset seizures (e.g. nausea or visual symptoms such as flashing lights).[121] Presumably, the most helpful clinical features are duration of aura, with more than 5 min favouring migraine aura and less than 5 min favouring epileptic aura and aura symptom profile. Alteration of consciousness, automatisms and positive motor features favour epileptic aura, and a mix of positive and negative features, such as a scintillating scotoma, favours migraine. During migraine aura, paroxysmal spike activity could be present. In most of the reported cases, however, these EEGs do not show the usual progressive decline in frequency of rhythmic, repetitive, epileptiform activity typical of ictal EEGs in epilepsy. Another striking EEG pattern – PLEDs or PLED-like activity – has been associated with hemiplegic migraine, prolonged aura or incipient migrainous infarction.[107]

In migraine, as in epilepsy, there is a tendency to excessive response to intermittent photic stimulation, but the pattern of the response is different in the two conditions. It is speculated that a common genetic dysfunction of the occipital lobes could lead to both migraine and epilepsy.[122] Moreover, visual evoked responses are enhanced both in patients with photosensitive epilepsy and in those with migraine.[126] The biochemical abnormalities and pathophysiological mechanisms responsible for the migraine–epilepsy relationship are speculative. An intriguing hypothesis is that occipital brain hyperexcitability in migraine and photosensitive epilepsies could be the result of a defect in the dopaminergic system. In photosensitive patients, dopaminergic agonists block the photoparoxysmal response and migraine patients are hypersensitive to dopamine agonists.[127,128] The metabolic changes that occur during a migrainous aura accompanied by a period of decreased regional cerebral blood flow (focal ischaemia) reduce seizure thresholds in animals.[129] Seizure threshold is also reduced in animals during spreading depression, an effect thought to result from increased extracellular glutamate and potassium.[130] Spreading depression is believed to be associated with migrainous aura. Although spreading depression itself has not been documented on EEGs in humans, this may be secondary to technical difficulties in recording slow shifts of direct current. It consists of pronounced depolarization of neurons and glia, which propagate across the cortex,[131] and it may be associated with seizures. The evidence for the spreading depression of Leao, underlying the migrainous march, is not universally accepted, although the clinical findings strongly suggest it. However, the exact mechanism of the transition from MA to an epileptic seizure has not been proved.[122] Presumably, a common disturbance of cellular excitability could trigger both diseases. It is known that spreading depression does not cross the major sulci. Should it, however, exceptionally cross the central sulcus, as may happen in some patients, it would account for motor epileptic manifestations.[132]

## Epilepsy and migraine in children: special aspects

Although a greater overlap has been suggested between epilepsy and migraine in children and adolescents, compared with adults, it is not clear why migraine should have a stronger influence in children with epilepsy. The explanation may be linked to the greater frequency of occipital or parietal lobe, high-voltage, epileptogenic abnormalities in children compared with adults.[133] The posterior epileptogenic abnormalities may be triggered by the migrainous changes because the metabolic and blood flow changes of the migraine attacks involve the posterior cerebral regions. There may be a confusing overlap of clinical and electrographic features between these two entities. Positive visual symptoms (visual hallucinations and scintillating scotoma) and negative visual symptoms (amaurosis and scotoma) are frequent prodromal manifestations of migraine but are also common ictal characteristics in patients with occipital lobe or parietal lobe epilepsy. However, one must bear in mind that it is very difficult, sometimes impossible to detect sensory phenomena in small children. Photoparoxysmal response in idiopathic, photosensitive, occipital lobe epilepsy could be accompanied by headache and vomiting.[134] Adolescents who had migraine, particularly basilar migraine, developed occasional seizures.

Children and adolescents often have very striking ongoing seizure activity on their EEGs, mostly sharp- and slow-wave discharges. The very impressive seizure activity is usually lateralized and involves posterior temporal and occipital regions. Characteristically, the activity blocks with opening of the eyes, to return only with eye closure.[135] Older individuals often have normal interictal EEGs.[136] One of the most intriguing associations between migraine and epilepsy concerns the high incidence of migrainous headache in children with benign partial epilepsies of childhood and their first-degree relatives.[137] Benign centrotemporal (rolandic) epilepsy of childhood, as with other seizure disorders, has been associated with a higher than expected incidence of migraine. In children with epilepsy, the incidence of migraine was 62% of the patients with centrotemporal epilepsy, 35% of those with absence epilepsy and 8% of those with partial epilepsy.[137,138]

Gastaut, reviewing his experiences with occipital epilepsies in childhood, described the concept of the benign occipital epilepsies.[133,139] A symposium on the migraine–epilepsy relationship was organized by Professor Lugaresi and a monograph was published by Butterworths in 1987. In recent years the term 'childhood seizure susceptibility syndrome' has been suggested in relation to the idiopathic benign childhood partial seizures.[135,140] This may be because of a common, genetically determined, mild or reversible, functional derangement of the maturational process of the brain cortices.[141,142] Recently, it has been proposed to subdivide the idiopathic childhood occipital epilepsies into two groups: early onset benign childhood occipital seizures (EBOS) or Panayiotopoulos-type childhood occipital seizures and late-onset idiopathic childhood occipital epilepsy (LIOE) of Gastaut type.[143] EBOS has a prevalence of 26.3%, the second most common, benign childhood partial epilepsy syndrome after rolandic epilepsy, whereas LIOE had a prevalence of 8.4% in a large-scale study of benign childhood partial seizures.[144] EBOS seizures are prolonged, usually over 5–30 min in duration, often nocturnal, infrequent (mainly one to three in an entire lifetime and usually within 1 year), with a peak of age of 4–5 years at onset and excellent prognosis. In EBOS, even in diurnal seizures, visual hallucination has not been described. Conversely, LIOE seizures are short, usually seconds to less than 1–3 min, mainly diurnal, frequent and often daily, with a protracted period of 5 years, consistently associated with visual hallucinations and with an uncertain prognosis with respect to seizure control.[135] However, with regard to the pathophysiology of occipital seizure activities, it is important to realize that childhood epileptic disorders, with occipital discharges that are suppressed or strikingly reduced by eye opening, can be either idiopathic or symptomatic, even with a normal EEG background activity. These EEG abnormalities may be in both types of idiopathic occipital seizures – bilateral and synchronous – not only because of subcortical, thalamocortical mechanisms, but also because occipital cortical hyperexcitability is bilaterally activated by fixation of sensitivity.[140,145,146] However, high-amplitude spike/sharp waves in the occipital and posterotemporal regions, which may be unilateral or bilateral and are usually asymmetrical, occur in 0.5–1% of normal children with a peak onset at 4–5 years; they are 2.5 times less frequent than centrotemporal spikes and share with them a similar morphology and course of attrition, often appearing together in the same or subsequent EEG.[143]

Occipital epilepsies of childhood, particularly the LIOE of Gastaut type, are associated with migrainous headache as well as visual hallucinations in the form of frequent, diurnal, simple, partial seizures accompanied by elementary visual hallucinations, blindness, or both, which last mainly for seconds and often less than 3 min.[140] However, it may be rather difficult to objectively evaluate visual symptoms in children. It is noteworthy that even ictal EEGs may be normal in one-third of occipital epilepsies, indicating the significance of establishing firm clinical criteria for the diagnosis of visual seizures.[147] It is suggested that misdiagnosis of occipital visual seizures, mostly LIOE, as migraine with visual aura is common, with a detrimental effect on these children. Usually these patients are not examined in a wider context, and later they will not get adequate treatment, e.g. starting to discontinue antiepileptic treatment. The pathogenesis of idiopathic occipital (visual) seizures with ictal blindness and ictal headache is not well understood. Ictal blindness may be related to spreading of bioccipital seizure.

Ictal headache is much more difficult to explain. The ictal elementary visual hallucinations are characterized in LIOE by rapid development and brief duration,[148] and are dominated by multicoloured and small circular or spherical patterns/spots flashing or multiplying in a temporal hemifield,[143] in contrast to the predominantly achromatic or black-and-white linear patterns of migrainous aura. By studying the visual aura symptoms of 163 migraine patients, it was reported that 'it started as a flickering, uncoloured, zigzag line in the centre of the visual field and affected the central vision. It gradually progressed over >4 min usually lasting <30 min towards the periphery of one hemifield and often left a scotoma. The total duration of visual auras was 60 min. Only four patients had exclusively acute onset visual aura'.[149] Drawbacks to this interpretation are that these migraine aura symptoms were observed mostly in adults, not in age-matched children with migraine with visual aura; it is also known that the duration of migrainous aura in children is shorter than in adults. Taken together, it is suggested that the clinical diagnosis of epilepsy with visual seizures in children is not complicated if individual elements of duration, colour, shape, size, location, movement, speed of development and progress are identified, and it is suggested that visual aura of migraine is different from visual seizures when all their components are considered. Although duration is the main differentiating factor, this is not always a safe criterion to use.[135] Nonvisual ictal occipital symptoms, such as eye and head deviation and repetitive eyelid closures, do not occur during a migraine attack. This clustering of symptoms would secure an accurate clinical diagnosis of occipital seizures.

In addition, other conditions, e.g. reversible posterior leukoencephalopathy syndrome (RPLS), an increasingly recognized brain disorder of various aetiologies, may include occipital lobe dysfunction and seizure, preceded by auras of visual dysfunction and hallucinations with severe headache, nausea, altered mental function and seizure. In childhood, RPLS may be associated with a variety of conditions such as malignant hypertension, immunosuppressive drug toxicity, fluid overload and chronic uraemia.[151,152]

## Postictal headache

Postictal headache, often severe and indistinguishable from migraine, occurred in two-thirds of patients with occipital seizures, even after brief visual seizures without convulsions.[135] This postictal headache is frequently associated with vomiting, phonophobia and photophobia. The mechanism of postictal headache, common even after idiopathic or symptomatic visual seizures, is unknown. It is likely that the occipital seizure discharge could trigger a migraine attack/disease, probably by activating trigeminovascular or brain-stem mechanisms.[143] Postictal headache of occipital seizures may be related to serotoninergic mechanisms and may thus respond to oral sumatriptan.[141] There are data for the distinction between migraine and LIOE, in contrast to a 'causative relation between migraine and occipital seizures'.[153] The seizure–migraine sequence is the opposite to migraine–seizure propositions. The possibility of seizures directly following migraine aura has been reported, more commonly in young people, particularly adolescents, but occasionally also in older individuals. The early clinical manifestations are entirely in keeping with migraine, but then motor manifestations supervene which are clearly of an epileptic nature. The aura symptoms may point to one hemisphere or suggest basilar involvement with blindness or symptoms attributable to the brain stem. After the seizure, a migraine-like headache is usually present.[132] The mechanism of the transition from a migraine with aura attack to an epileptic seizure has not been proved. Recently, it has been reasonable to propose that occipital seizures often generate migraine. This 'occipital seizure–migraine' sequence appears to be much more common than the previously prevailing view of migraine with visual aura triggering epileptic seizures.[135]

## References

1. Schoenen J, Cortical electrophysiology in migraine and possible pathogenetic implications. *Clin Neurosci* 1998; **5**: 10–17.
2. Grosser K, Oelkers R, Hummel T et al, Olfactory and trigeminal event-related potentials in migraine. *Cephalalgia* 2000; **20**: 621–31.
3. Puca FM, de Tomasso M, Clinical neurophysiology in childhood headache *Cephalalgia* 1999; **19**: 137–46.
4. Simon RH, Zimmerman AW, Sanderson P, Tasman AW, EEG markers of migraine in children and adults. *Headache* 1983; **23**: 201–5.
5. Genco S, de Tomasso M, Prudenzano AMP et al, EEG features in juvenile migraine: topographic analysis of spontaneous and visual evoked brain electrical activity: a comparison with adult migraine. *Cephalalgia* 1994; **14**: 41–6.
6. Puca FM, de Tomasso M, Tota P, Sciruicchio V, The photic driving in migraine: correlation with clinical features. *Cephalalgia* 1996; **16**: 246–50.
7. Benna P, Bianco C, Costa P et al, Visual evoked potentials and brainstem auditory evoked potentials in migraine and transient

ischemic attacks. *Cephalalgia* 1985; **2**(suppl 2): 53–8.

8. Mariani E, Moschini V, Pastorino G et al, Pattern-reversal visual evoked potentials and EEG correlations in common migraine patients. *Headache* 1988; **28**: 269–71.

9. Drake ME, Pakalnis A, Hietter SA, Padaman H, Visual and auditory evoked potentials in migraine. *Electromyogr Clin Neurophysiol* 1990; **30**: 77–81.

10. Tagliati M, Sabbadini M, Bernardi G, Silvestrini M, Multichannel visual evoked potentials in migraine. *Electroencephalogr Clin Neurophysiol* 1995; **96**: 1–5.

11. Aloisi P, Marrelli A, Porto C et al, Visual evoked potentials and serum magnesium levels in juvenile migraine patients. *Headache* 1997; **37**: 383–5.

12. Diener H-C, Scholz E, Dichgans J et al, Central effects of drugs used in migraine prophylaxis evaluated by visual evoked potentials. *Ann Neurol* 1989; **25**: 125–30.

13. Lahat E, Nadir E, Barr J et al, Visual evoked potentials: a diagnostic test for migraine headache in children. *Dev Med Child Neurol* 1997; **39**: 85–7.

14. Shibata K, Osawa M, Iwata M, Simultaneous recording of pattern reversal electroretinograms and visual evoked potentials in migraine. *Cephalalgia* 1997; **17**: 42–7.

15. Shibata K, Osawa M, Iwata M, pattern reversal visual evoked potentials in migraine with aura and migraine aura without headache. *Cephalalgia* 1998; **18**: 319–23.

16. Kennard C, de Gawel MM, Rudolph N, Rose FC, Visual evoked potentials in migraine subjects. *Res Clin Stud Headache* 1978; **6**: 73–80.

17. Ozden Sener H, Haktanir I, Demirci S, Pattern-reversal visual evoked potentials in migraineurs with or without visual aura. *Headache* 1997; **37**: 449–51.

18. Polich J, Ehlers CL, Dalessio DJ, Pattern-shift visual evoked potentials and EEG in migraine. *Headache* 1986; **26**: 451–6.

19. Tagliatti M, Sabbadini M, Bernardi G, Silvestrini M, Multichannel visual evoked potentials in migraine. *Clin Neurophysiol* 1995; **96**: 1–5.

20. Wenzel D, Brandl U, Harms D, Visual evoked potentials in juvenile complicated migraine. *Electroencephalogr Clin Neurophysiol* 1982; **53**: 59P.

21. Brinciotti M, Guidetti V, Matricardi M, Cortesi F, Responsiveness of the visual system in childhood migraine studied by means of VEPs. *Cephalalgia* 1986; **6**: 1.

22. Rossi LN, Pastorino GC, Bellettini G et al, Pattern reversal visual evoked potentials in children with migraine or tension-type headache. *Cephalalgia* 1996; **16**: 104–9.

23. Tsounis S, Milonas J, Gilliam F, Hemicrania continua-field pattern reversal visual evoked potentials in migraine. *Cephalalgia* 1993; **13**: 267–71.

24. Schoenen J, Wang W, Albert A, Delwaide PJ, Potentiation instead of habituation characterizes visual evoked potentials in migraine patients between attacks. *Eur J Neurol* 1995; **2**: 115–22.

25. Áfra J, Proietti Cecchini A, De Pasqua V et al, Visual evoked potentials during long periods of pattern reversal stimulation in migraine. *Brain* 1998; **121**: 233–41.

26. Oelkers R, Grosser K, Lang E et al, Visual evoked potentials depend on pattern spatial frequency. *Brain* 1999; **122**: 1147–55.

27. Watanabe H, Kuwabara T, Ohkubo M et al, Evaluation of central lactate detected by localised 1H-magnetic resonance spectroscopy in migraine during the interictal period. *Neurology* 1996; **47**: 1093–5.

28. Montagna P, Cortelli P, Monari L et al, 31P-magnetic resonance spectroscopy in migraine without aura. *Neurology* 1994; **44**: 666–9.

29. Lozza A, Proietti Cecchini A, Áfra J, Schoenen J, Neurophysiological approach to primary haeadache pathophysiology. *Cephalalgia* 1998; **18**(suppl 21): 12–16.

30. Schoenen J, Clinical neurophysiology of headache. *Neurol Clin* 1997; **15**: 85–105.

31. Eysenck HJ, Eysenck MH, *Personality and Individual Differences: A Natural Science Approach*. New York: Plenum Press, 1985.

32. Ellis L, Relationships of criminality and psychopathy with eight other apparent

behavioral manifestations of sub-optimal arousal. *Person Individ Diff* 1987; **8**: 905–25.

33. Cloninger CR, A systematic method for clinical description and classification of personality variants – a proposal. *Arch Gen Psychiatry* 1987; **44**: 573–88.

34. Wang W, Wang G-P, Ding X-L, Wang Y-H, Personality and response to repeated visual stimulation in migraine and tension-type headache. *Cephalalgia* 1999; **19**: 718–24.

35. Gray JA, *The Neuropsychology of Anxiety: An Inquiry into the Functions of the Septo-hippocampal System.* New York: Oxford University Press, 1982.

36. Swonger AK, Rech RH, Serotonergic and cholinergic involvement in habituation activity and spontaneous alteration of rats in a Y maze. *J Comp Physiol Psychol* 1972; **81**: 509–22.

37. Hughes RN, Cholinergic and monoaminergic substrates of startle habituation. *Life Sci* 1984; **34**: 2101–5.

38. Steriade M, McCormick DA, Sejnowski TJ, Thalamocortical oscillations in the sleeping and aroused brain. *Science* 1993; **262**: 679–85.

39. Jacobs BL, Azmitia EC, Structure and function of the brain serotonin system. *Physiol Rev* 1992; **72**: 165–229.

40. Spoont MR, Modulatory role of serotonin in neural information processing: implications for human psychopathology. *Psychol Bull* 1992; **112**: 330–50.

41. Wang W, Timsit-Berthier M, Schoenen J, Intensity dependence of auditory evoked potentials is pronounced in migraine. *Neurology* 1996; **46**: 404–9.

42. Wang W, Timsit-Berthier M, Schoenen J, Intensity dependence of auditory evoked potentials in migraine: an indication of cortical potentiation and low serotonergic neurotransmission? *Neurology* 1996; **46**: 1404–9.

43. Hegerl U, Juckel G, Intensity dependence of auditory evoked potentials as an indicator of central serotoninergic neurotransmission: a new hypothesis. *Biol Psychiatr* 1993; **33**: 173–87.

44. Schoenen J, Deficient habituation of evoked cortical potentials in migraine: a link between brain biology, behavior and trigeminovascular activation? *Biomed Pharmacother* 1996; **50**: 71–8.

45. Áfra J, Proietti Cecchini A, Sandor PS, Schoenen J, Comparison of visual and auditory evoked cortical potentials in migraine patients between attacks. *Clin Neurophysiol* 2000; **111**: 1124–9.

46. Siniatchkin M, Kropp P, Neumann M et al, Intensity dependence of auditory evoked cortical potentials in migraine families. *Pain* 2000; **85**: 247–54.

47. Sand T, Clinical correlates of brainstem auditory evoked potential variables in multiple sclerosis. Relation to click polarity. *Electroencephalogr Clin Neurophysiol* 1991; **80**: 292–7.

48. Sand T, Vanagaite Vingen J, Visual, long-latency auditory and brainstem auditory evoked potentials in migraine: relation to pattern size, stimulus intensity, sound and light discomfort thresholds and pre-attack state. *Cephalalgia* 2000; **20**: 804–20.

49. Bhargava VK, McKean CM, Role of 5-hydroxytryptamine in the modulation of acoustic brainstem (farfield) potentials. *Neuropharmacology* 1977; **16**: 447–9.

50. Weiller C, May A, Limmroth V et al, Brain stem activation in spontaneous human migraine attacks. *Nature Med* 1995; **1**: 658–60.

51. Podoshin L, Ben-David J, Pratt H et al, Auditory brainstem and visual evoked potentials in patients with migraine. *Headache* 1987; **27**: 27–9.

52. Schlake HP, Grotemeyer KH, Hofferberth B et al, Brainstem auditory evoked potentials in migraine: evidence of increased side differences during pain-free interval. *Headache* 1990; **30**: 129–32.

53. Yamada T, Stokes Dickens Q, Arensdorf K et al, Basilar migraine: polarity-dependent alteration of brainstem auditory evoked potential. *Neurology* 1986; **36**: 1256–60.

54. Zöllner C, Karnahl T, Stange G, Input-output function and adaptation behaviour of the five early potentials registered with the earlobe

vertex pickup. *Arch Oto Rhino Laryngol* 1976; **212**: 23–33.

55. Schoenen J, Timsit-Berthier M, Contingent negative variation: methods and potential interest in headache. *Cephalalgia* 1993; **13**: 28–32.

56. Besken E, Pothmann R, Sartory G, Contingent negative variation in childhood migraine. *Cephalalgia* 1993; **13**: 42–3.

57. Kropp P, Gerber W-D, Is increased amplitude of contingent negative variation in migraine due to cortical hyperactivity or to reduced habituation? *Cephalalgia* 1993; **13**: 37–41.

58. Maertens de Noordhout A, Timsit-Berthier M, Timsit M, Schoenen J, Effects of beta blockade on contingent negative variation in migraine. *Ann Neurol* 1987; **21**: 111–12.

59. Kropp P, Kirbach U, Detlefsen JO et al, Slow cortical potentials in migraine: a comparison of adults and children. *Cephalalgia* 1999; **19**(suppl 25): 60–4.

60. Bonuso S, Marano E, Di Stasio E et al, The frontotemporal region plays a role in the genesis of migraine without aura. *Headache* 1995; **35**: 154–7.

61. O'Connor TP, van der Kooy D, Pattern of intracranial and extracranial projections of trigeminal ganglion cells. *J Neurosci* 1986; **6**: 2200–7.

62. Blau JN, Solomon F, Smell and other sensory disturbances in migraine. *J Neurol* 1985; **232**: 275–6.

63. Silberstein SD, Migraine symptoms: results of a survey of self-reported migraineurs. *Headache* 1995; **35**: 387–96.

64. Hirsch AR, Olfaction in migraineurs. *Headache* 1992; **32**: 233–6.

65. Hegerl U, Gallinat J, Mrowinski D, Intensity dependence of auditory evoked dipole source activity. *Int J Psychophysiol* 1994; **17**: 1–13.

66. Grossberg S, Gutowski WE, Neural dynamics of decision making under risk: affective balance and cognitive-emotional interactions. *Psychol Rev* 1987; **94**: 300–18.

67. Moriizumi T, Tsukatani T, Sakashita H, Miwa T, Olfactory disturbance induced by deafferentation of serotonergic fibers in the olfactory bulb. *Neuroscience* 1994; **61**: 733–8.

68. Puca FM, Genco S, Savarese MA et al, Juvenile migraine and memory. In: Gallai V, Guidetti V, eds, *Juvenile Headache*. Amsterdam: Elsevier, 1991: 145–8.

69. Callaway E, The pharmacology of human information processing. *Psychophysiology* 1983; **20**: 359–70.

70. Gallai V, Firenze C, Mazzotta G, Del Gatto F, P300 and memory in adolescents with common migraine. *Acta Neurol* 1987; **5**: 87–91.

71. Mazzotta G, Gallai V, The event-related potential (P300) through brain mapping in juvenile headache. In: Gallai V, Guidetti V, eds, *Juvenile Headache*. Amsterdam: Elsevier, 1991: 341–4.

72. Rohrbaugh WJ, Gaillard AG, Sensory and motor aspects of the contingent negative variation. In: Gaillard AG, Ritter W, eds, *Tutorials in Event-related Potentials Research: Endogenous Components*. Amsterdam: Elsevier, 1983: 269–310.

73. Siniatchkin M, Gerber W-D, Kropp P et al, Are the periodic changes of neurophysiological parameters during pain-free interval in migraine related to abnormal orienting activity? *Cephalalgia* 2000; **20**: 20–9.

74. Evers S, Bauer B, Grotemeyer KH et al, Event-related potentials (P300) in primary headache in childhood and adolescence. *J Child Neurol* 1998; **13**: 322–6.

75. Evers S, Bauer B, Suhr MD et al, Cognitive processing in primary headache: a study on event related potentials. *Neurology* 1997; **48**: 108–13.

76. Wang W, Schoenen J, Interictal potentiation of passive 'oddball' auditory event-related potentials in migraine. *Cephalalgia* 1998; **18**: 261–5.

77. Palmer JE, Chronicle EP, Cognitive processing in migraine: a failure to find facilitation in patients with aura. *Cephalalgia* 1998; **18**: 125–32.

78. Evers S, Quibeldey F, Grotemeyer KH et al, Dynamic changes of cognitive habituation and serotonin metabolism during the migraine interval. *Cephalalgia* 1999; **19**: 485–91.

79. Nyrke T, Kangasniemi P, Lang H, Alpha rhythm in classical migraine (migraine with aura): abnormalities in the headache-free interval. *Cephalalgia* 1990; **10**: 177–81.

80. Siniatchkin M, Gerber W-D, Kropp P, Vein A, How the brain anticipates an attack – a study of neurophysiological periodicity in migraine. *Funct Neurol* 1999; **24**: 69–78.

81. Kropp P, Gerber W-D, Prediction of migraine attacks using a slow cortical potential, the contingent negative variation. *Neurosci Lett* 1998; **257**: 73–6.

82. Siniatchkin M, Kropp P, Gerber W-B, Stephani U, Migraine in childhood – are periodically occurring migraine attacks related to dynamic changes of cortical information processing? *Neurosci Lett* 2000; **279**: 1–4.

83. Áfra J, Sándor S, Schoenen J, Habituation of visual and intensity dependence of auditory evoked cortical potentials tend to normalize just before and during the migraine attack. *Cephalalgia* 2000; **20**: 714–19.

84. Áfra J, Mascia A, Gerard P et al, Interictal cortical excitability in migraine: a study using transcranial magnetic stimulation of motor and visual cortices. *Ann Neurol* 1998; **44**: 209–15.

85. Aurora SK, Welch KMA, Brain excitability in migraine: evidence from transcranial magnetic stimulation studies. *Curr Opin Neurol* 1998; **11**: 205–9.

86. Werhahn KJ, Wiseman K, Herzog J et al, Motor cortex excitability in patients with migraine with aura and hemiplegic migraine. *Cephalalgia* 2000; **20**: 45–50.

87. Day BL, Dressler D, de Noordhut AM et al, Electric and magnetic stimulation of human motor cortex: surface EMG and single motor unit responses. *J Physiol* 1989; **412**: 449–73.

88. Rothwell JC, Thompson PD, Day BL et al, Stimulation of the human motor cortex through the scalp. *Exp Physiol* 1991; **76**: 159–200.

89. Van der Kamp W, Maassen VA, Ferrari MD, Van Dijk JG, Interictal cortical hyperexcitability in migraine patients demonstrated with transcranial magnetic stimulation. *J Neurol Sci* 1996; **139**: 106–10.

90. Aurora SK, Ahmad BK, Welch KM et al, Transcranial magnetic stimulation confirms hyperexcitability of occipital cortex in migraine. *Neurology* 1998; **50**: 111–14.

91. Firenze C, Del Gatto F, Mazzotta G, Gallai V, Somatosensory-evoked potential study in headache patients. *Cephalalgia* 1988; **8**: 157–62.

92. Kropp P, Gerber W-D, Contingent negative variation during migraine attack and interval: evidence for normalization of slow cortical potentials during the attack. *Cephalalgia* 1995; **15**: 123–8.

93. Moskowitz MA, The neurobiology of vascular head pain. *Ann Neurol* 1984; **16**: 157–68.

94. Kors EE, Haan J, Ferrari MD, Genetics of primary headaches. *Curr Opin Neurol* 1999; **12**: 249–54.

95. Gardner K, The genetic basis of migraine: how much do we know? *Can J Neurol Sci* 1999; **26**(suppl 3): 37–43.

96. Nevo Y, Kramer U, Rieder-Grosswasser I, Harel S, Clinical categorization of 312 children with chronic headache. *Brain Dev* 1994; **16**: 441–4.

97. Sand T, EEG in migraine. *Funct Neurol* 1991; **6**: 7–22.

98. Gronseth GS, Greenberg MK, The utility of the electroencephalogram in the evaluation of patients presenting with headache: a review of the literature. *Neurology* 1995; **45**: 1263–7.

99. Kellaway P, An orderly approach to visual analysis: parameters of the normal EEG in adults and children. In: Klaas DW, Daly DD, eds, *Current Practice of Clinical Electroencephalography*. New York: Raven Press, 1979: 69–147.

100. Jonkman EJ, Lelieveld MHJ, EEG computer analysis in patients with migraine. *Electroencephalogr Clin Neurophysiol* 1981; **52**: 652–5.

101. Guidetti V, Fornara R, Marchini R et al, Headache and epilepsy in childhood: analysis of a series of 620 children. *Funct Neurol* 1987; **11**: 323–41.

102. Genco S, de Tommaso M, Prudenzano AMP et al, EEG features in juvenile migraine: topo-

graphic analysis of spontaneous and visual evoked brain electrical activity: A comparison with adult migraine. *Cephalalgia* 1994; **14**: 41–6.

103. Nyrke T, Lang AH, Spectral analysis of visual potentials evoked by sin wave modulated light in migraine. *Electroencephalogr Clin Neurophysiol* 1982; **53**: 436–42.

104. Chronicle EP, Wilkins AJ, Coleston DM, Threshold for detection of a target against a background grating suggest visual dysfunction in migraine with aura but not in migraine without aura. *Cephalalgia* 1995; **15**: 117–22.

105. Goodin DS, Aminoff MJ, Does the interictal EEG have a role in the diagnosis of epilepsy? *Lancet* 1984; **1**: 837–9.

106. Quality Standards Subcommittee of the American Academy of Neurology. Practice parameter: the electroencephalogram in the evaluation of headache. *Neurology* 1995; **45**: 1411–13.

107. Lipton RB, Ottman R, Ehrenberg BL, Hauser WA, Comorbidity of migraine: The connection between migraine and epilepsy. *Neurology* 1994; **44**(suppl 7): 28–32.

108. Hockaday JM, Whitty CWM, Factors determining the electroencephalogram in migraine: a study of 500 patients according to clinical type of migraine. *Brain* 1969; **92**: 769–88.

109. Mark DA, Ehrenberg BL, Migraine-related seizures in adults with epilepsy, with EEG correlation. *Neurology* 1993; **43**: 2476–83.

110. Schoenen J, Clinical neurophysiology studies in headache: a review of data and pathophysiological hints. *Funct Neurol* 1992; **7**: 191–204.

111. de Tommaso M, Sciruicchio V, Guido M et al, EEG sepctral analysis in migraine without aura attacks. *Cephalalgia* 1998; **18**: 324–8.

112. Seri S, Cerquilini A, Guidetti V, Computerized EEG topography in childhood migraine between and during attacks. *Cephalalgia* 1993; **13**: 53–6.

113. Guidetti V, Seri S, Cerquilini A, Brinciotti M, Computerized EEG topography in childhood migraine. *Cephalalgia* 1989; **9**(suppl 10): 191–2.

114. Pothmann R, Topographic EEG mapping in childhood headaches. *Cephalalgia* 1993; **13**: 57–8.

115. Gowers WR, *The Borderland of Epilepsy: Faints, Vagal Attacks, Vertigo, Migraine, Sleep Symptoms, and their Treatment.* London: Churchill, 1907.

116. Andermann E, Andermann FA, Migraine-epilepsy relationships: epidemiological and genetic aspects. In: Andermann FA, Lugaresi E, eds, *Migraine and Epilepsy*. Boston: Butterworths, 1987: 281–91.

117. Ehrenberg BL, Unusual clinical manifestations of migraine, and 'the borderland of epilepsy' reexplored. *Semin Neurol* 1991; **11**: 118–27.

118. Marks DA, Ehrenberg BL, Migraine-related seizures in adults with epilepsy, with EEG correlation. *Neurology* 1993; **43**: 2476–83.

119. Welch KMA, Lewis D, Migraine and epilepsy. *Neurol Clin* 1997; **15**: 107–14.

120. Terzano MG, Parrino L, Pietrini V, Galli L, Migraine-epilepsy syndrome: intercalated seizures in benign occipital epilepsy. In: Andermann F, Beaumanoir A, Mira L, Roger J, Tassinari CA, eds, *Occipital Seizures and Epilepsies in Children*. London: John Libbey & Company Ltd, 1993: 93–9.

121. Velioglu SK, Özmenoglu M, Migraine-related seizures in an epileptic population. *Cephalalgia* 1999; **19**: 797–801.

122. Donnet A, Bartolomei F, Migraine with visual aura and photosensitive epileptic seizures. *Epilepsia* 1997; **38**: 1032–4.

123. Ottman R, Susser M, Strategies for data collection in genetic epidemiology: The Epilepsy Family Study of Columbia University. *J Clin Epidemiol* 1992; **45**: 721–7.

124. Ottman R, Lipton RB, Comorbidity of migraine and epilepsy. *Neurology* 1994; **44**: 2105–10.

125. Flanagan D, Ghose K, Co-morbidity of migraine and epilepsy: a review of clinical features. *J Headache Pain* 2000; **1**: 137–44.

126. Gawel M, Connolly JF, Rose FC, Migraine patients exhibit abnormalities in the visual evoked potentials. *Headache* 1993; **23**: 49–52.

127. De Carolis P, Tinuper P, Sacquegna T, Migraine with aura and photosensitive epileptic seizures: a case report. *Cephalalgia* 1991; **11**: 151–3.

128. Quesney LF, Andermann FA, Dopaminergic mechanism in photosensitive epilepsy and its possible relevance to migraine. In: Andermann FA, Lugaresi E, eds, *Migraine and Epilepsy*. Boston: Butterworths, 1987: 391–404.

129. Kogure K, Schwartzman RJ, Seizure propagation and ATP depletion in the rat stroke model. *Epilepsia* 1980; **21**: 63–72.

130. Van Gelder NM, Calcium mobility and glutamic acid release associated with EEG abnormalities, migraine and epilepsy. In: Andermann FA, Lugaresi E, eds, *Migraine and Epilepsy*. Boston: Butterworths, 1987: 367–78.

131. Somjen CG, Aitken PG, Czeh GL et al, mechanisms of spreading depression: a review of recent findings and a hypothesis. *Can J Physiol Pharmacol* 1992; **70**: 248–54.

132. Andermann FA, Andermann E, Migraine and epilepsy, with special reference to the benign epilepsies of childhood. *Epilepsy Res* 1992; **6**(suppl 6): 207–14.

133. Gastaut H, A new type of epilepsy: Benign partial epilepsy of childhood with occipital spike-waves. *Clin Electroencephalogr* 1982; **13**: 13–22.

134. Guerrini R, Dravet C, Genton P et al, Idiopathic photosensitive occipital lobe epilepsy. *Epilepsia* 1995; **36**: 883–91.

135. Panayiotopoulos CP, Visual phenomena and headache in occipital epilepsy: a review, a systematic study and differentiation from migraine. *Epileptic Disorders* 1999; **1**: 205–16.

136. Andermann F, Clinical features of migraine-epilepsy syndromes. In: Andermann FA, Lugaresi E, eds, *Migraine and Epilepsy*. Boston: Butterworths, 1987: 3–30.

137. Giroud M, Couillault G, Arnould S et al, Centro-temporal epilepsy and migraine, A controlled study. Evidence for a non-fortuitous association. *Pediatrie* 1989; **44**: 659–64.

138. Holmes GL, Rolandic epilepsy: clinical and electroencephalographic features. *Epilepsy Res* 1992; **??**(suppl 6): 29–43.

139. Gastaut H, Die benigne Epilepsie des Kindesalters mit okzipitalen Spike-wave. *Z EEG EMG* 1982; **13**: 3–8.

140. Panayiotopoulos CP, Letters to the Editor. *Epilepsia* 1999; **40**: 1320–4.

141. Ogunyemi A, Adams D, Migraine-like symptoms triggered by occipital lobe seizures: response to sumatriptan. *Can J Neurol Sci* 1998; **25**: 151–3.

142. Kuzniecky R, Gilliam F, Morawetz R et al, Occipital lobe developmental malformations and epilepsy: clinical spectrum, treatment, and outcome. *Epilepsia* 1997; **38**: 175–81.

143. Panayiotopoulos CP (ed), *Benign Childhood Partial Seizures and Related Epileptic Syndromes*. London: John Libbey & Company Ltd, 1999.

144. Fejerman N, Atypical evolutions of benign partial epilepsies in children. *Int Pediatrics* 1996; **11**: 351–6.

145. Salanova V, Andermann F, Olivier A et al, Occipital lobe epilepsy: electroclinical manifestations, electrocorticography, cortical stimulation and outcome in 42 patients treated between 1930 and 1991. Surgery of occipital lobe epilepsy. *Brain* 1992; **115**: 1655–80.

146. Panayiotopoulos CP, Basilar migraine? Seizures, and severe epileptic EEG abnormalities. *Neurology* 1980; **30**: 1122–5.

147. Guerrini R, Battaglia A, Dravet C et al, Outcome of idiopathic childhood epilepsy with occipital paroxysms. In: Andermann F, Beaumanoir A, Mira L, Roger J, Tassinari CA, eds, *Occipital Seizures and Epilepsies in Children*. London: John Libbey & Company Ltd, 1993: 165–71.

148. Panayiotopoulos CP, Elementary visual hallucinations, blindness and headache in idiopathic occipital epilepsy, differentiation from migraine. *J Neurol Neurosurg Psychiatr* 1999; **66**: 536–40.

149. Russel MB, Olesen J, A nosographic analysis of the migraine aura in general population. *Brain* 1996; **119**: 355–61.

150. Muranaka H, Fujita H, Goto A et al, Viusal symptoms in epilepsy and migraine: Localiza-

tion and patterns. *Epilepsia* 2001; **42**: 62–6.

151. Bakshi R, Bates VE, Mechter LL et al, Occipital lobe seizures as the major clinical manifestation of reversible posterior leukoencephalopathy syndrome: Magnetic resonance imaging findings. *Epilepsia* 1998; **39**: 295–9.

152. Hinchey J, Chaves C, Appignani B et al, A reversible posterior leukoencephalopathy syndrome. *N Engl J Med* 1996; **334**: 494–500.

153. Rossi GP, Santucci M, Gobbi GD et al, Epidemiological study of migraine in epileptic patients. In: Andermann FA, Lugaresi E, eds, *Migraine and Epilepsy*. Boston: Butterworths, 1987: 313–22.

# 8

# Diagnosis: neuroradiology

*Viktor Farkas*

Diagnosis of headache disorders in children is complex for specialists and even more so for general paediatricians. Although recurrent headache remains one of the most common medical complaints, it is rarely caused by an organic lesion of the central nervous system (CNS) in children. The first step in the diagnostic algorithm for headaches is to distinguish primary and secondary headache disorders, and then to make a further diagnosis within the primary or secondary headache group in the simplest way. The scheme of dividing headaches into primary and secondary disorders is useful in primary care because similar distinctions are made in other diseases, such as epilepsy, hypertension, etc. However, general paediatricians in Hungary are very concerned, and rightly so, about secondary headache, so paediatricians should be encouraged to recognize that primary headache disorders are much more common than secondary headache disorders, even in children. Headache disorders can also exist with no obvious structural or metabolic cause at younger ages, so it is important to emphasize that recurrent episodic headaches are rarely the result of structural lesions, and can in most cases be excluded by a simple physical and paediatric neurological examination, together with taking a good history. The availability of high-tech modalities should

never be an indication for further investigation in the absence of clinical signs. The detection rate of tumours, arteriovenous malformations (AVMs) or aneurysms by using cranial computed tomography (CT) in patients with chronic headache is similar to that expected in the general population, provided that the neurological findings are normal.[1] The cost of detecting intracranial lesions in this patient population is high.

Primary headache disorders, inclusive of migraine, are a so-called clinical diagnosis with a wide variety of neurological and non-neurological manifestations. Until now, in clinical practice there are no confirmatory tests for the diagnosis of migraine in children, so the diagnosis is often based solely on an extended history and physical examination. Recently, the information for diagnosis has been rather subjective, and basically derives from interpretations made by the child and parents. Another problem is that, currently, we know very little about headaches in children other than migraine. However, the diagnosis of primary headache, particularly migraine, is not obtained solely by exclusion of other disorders; a positive diagnosis is also possible in children. This positive diagnosis should be based on information about the attack profile, identification of probable triggers and understanding of the clinical spectrum, variability and natural history of the migraine.[2] It is essential that the paediatrician should record a comprehensive history from the patient who complains of headache and also from the parents to achieve a reliable diagnosis. The history is taken to allow the child to participate, because even very young children can give an account of their symptoms, including accompanying symptoms and any triggers, although with an infrequent and episodic problem it can be difficult for the child to recall symptoms, e.g. 1 month previously, and to identify different types of headaches.

The aim of the physical and neurological examinations is to support the tentative diagnosis – first and foremost to rule out serious underlying diseases, but also to reassure the child and the family. As a rule, the physician will already at this point recognize the type of headache, but the course of events may occasionally demonstrate the need to revise the diagnosis. Information about the child's headache should be as precise as possible, and for this purpose follow-up consultations and the use of a 'diagnostic headache diary for children' are important. During this period of observation, it can usually be established that the child will remain otherwise well, and that growth and development continues normally.[3]

Only very rarely is hospitalization needed for correct clinical diagnosis with a child who has recurrent headaches, e.g. suspicion of serious underlying illness of the CNS which cannot be evaluated quickly enough on an outpatient basis, or rarer types of headache where the diagnosis depends on observation of headache episodes.

There are no standard examinations and diagnostic guidelines for recurrent headache in children and adolescents. The detailed paediatric neurological investigation done by a specialist should also include an assessment of the teeth/mouth/jaw and the spine. If the headache is monosymptomatic, with pericranial muscle tenderness as the only clinical finding, then a serious underlying illness is unlikely and further tests can often be omitted. Currently, a skull radiograph is considered obsolete in the evaluation of headache. Radiological examination of the cervical column will seldom contribute to diagnosis and specific steps for treatment. Radiological examination of the sinuses should be carried out only if there is a definite suspicion of sinusitis.[4] Developmental differences in headache characteristics, which change and evolve as children age, may limit the use of recent International Headache Society (IHS) criteria, which were created and adapted primarily for adults. There is clearly a need to improve the diagnosis of primary headache disorders in children, so it is more often necessary for children aged under 6 years to be referred for brain imaging to rule out potential serious disease of the CNS.[5] However, CT and magnetic resonance imaging (MRI) are not routinely warranted in children with recurrent headache; with a proliferation of imaging facilities, increasing parents' demand for thorough and 'high-tech' evaluation and the increasing practice of 'defensive medicine', neuroimaging is too widely used in the evaluation of recurrent headaches.[6] The realities of our medico-legal climate are such that many physicians feel compelled to conduct neuroimaging studies on patients with headache even though the likelihood of finding pathology is about the same as in the general population. The same may apply to children; however, suspicion of intracranial pathology should be stronger among children with headache than in adults with headache.[7]

Indeed there is only a very limited number of children who have chronic, recurrent headache, with an absolute indication for cerebral neuroimaging. Evaluation of the role of neuroimaging and clinical predictors of surgical space-occupying lesions in children with chronic headache identified two criteria as the strongest predictors: sleep-related headache and no family history of migraines.[8]

The introduction of CT in the 1970s was an important development in the diagnostic evaluation of patients with symptomatic headache. It rendered obsolete the routine use in headache patients of other radiological studies of the CNS. The potential limitations of CT in symptomatic headache included low diagnostic yield for some surgical pathologies, i.e. tumours and vascular anomalies, inability to perform multiplanar imaging, radiation exposure, and difficulty in differentiating grey and white matter structures and bony artefacts.[9,10] Investigators at Nottingham University first applied MRI to the study of the brain in 1980.[11] MRI is a non-invasive technique that has no known biological toxicity and does not involve ionizing radiation. Recently, MRI and CT have been the structural neuroimaging procedures of choice in evaluating patients with a tentative diagnosis of secondary headache.[12,13] CT has been replaced by MRI, which has a higher yield (superior sensitivity and specificity to CT in several aspects). MRI without use of gadolinium paramagnetic contrast media will detect almost all lesions seen with contrasted CT, with the possible exception of small meningiomas. MRI is more sensitive than CT for gliomas, pituitary tumours, white matter lesions, developmental venous anomalies and AVMs.[6] The greater resolution and discrimination of MRI, however, appears to be of little clinical impor-

tance in the evaluation of children with non-acute headache.

There are two particular diagnostic problems in the evaluation of patients with headache disorders: (1) organic conditions that mimic primary headache and (2) organic conditions that coexist, e.g. with migraine, because migraine is such a common disorder in childhood. For example, a patient may have a brain tumour or an aneurysm, as well as migraine; later, the patient may in the same period have several different types of headache. The common vascular anomalies associated with migraine-like headache are AVMs, haemangiomas and aneurysms. Recurrent headache and seizures may in fact be the only clinical manifestation associated with AVM and haemangioma. Other vascular anomalies, such as developmental venous anomalies, venous angiomas and capillary telangiectasias, are usually incidental findings and are rarely associated with headache. MRI is essential for the recognition and diagnosis of haemangiomas and occult AVMs (angiographically negative vascular lesions).[14,15]

Although clinicians have frequently reported symptoms mimicking migraine in patients with cerebral AVM, the IHS classification indicates that 'the relation of migraine and other headaches to this condition is poorly substantiated'.[16] The relationship between migraine and AVM is a subject of controversy, with arguments being based mainly on case reports and retrospective data.[17] A past history of migraine was present in up to 58% of women with AVM in some series, but, in others, occurrence of positive history was no different from that of the general population.[18] There are well-documented cases of migraine attacks eliminated by surgical removal of the AVM, but there are equally well-documented cases of migraine attacks persisting unchanged after neurosurgery.[18] In a recent report, a proportion of occipital AVMs did cause headache that satisfied the current IHS criteria for migraine, and radiosurgery headaches in most of the treated patients.[19] Taken together, although there are strong suggestions (but not conclusions) that the association between migraine and AVM is not coincidental, large prospective studies are recommended to define the clinical characteristics of migraine headaches, which would help to identify those patients at higher risk for an AVM. Anecdotal literature abounds with the specifics of the headache history that increase suspicion for vascular malformation.[6,18] These include change in headache pattern, unilateral headaches that never change sides ('side-locked' headache), and whether the aura is stereotyped or prolonged, or shows a 'march' of neurological symptoms during the headache. Vascular malformations should be taken into account if there is a cranial bruit, or any seizures either with headache or at other times.[20]

The major positive outcome derived from neuroimaging in headache is identification of a treatable lesion. Treatment modality, e.g. for AVMs, includes surgery, endovascular therapy or radiotherapy. With the advent of radiosurgical and interventional endovascular techniques, the risk–benefit ratio is changing and may favour earlier intervention.[6]

Particular warning signs that a paediatrician should be aware of and investigate are listed in Table 8.1. So-called 'sudden onset "first" headache' and the 'worst headache ever' should both be investigated with neuroimaging. There are case reports of negative CT scan and lumbar punctures in patients with aneurysms, so it is recommended that at least magnetic resonance angiography (MRA) is used to explore subarachnoid haemorrhage and aneurysm (see later). Headache with fever, rash and neck stiffness might arise from meningitis or other conditions. Headache with papilloedema must be investigated for signs of

---

Headache with focal neurological findings
Headache accompanied by focal neurological symptoms
Headache in patient with a history of seizures
In patient with atypical headache pattern (ophthalmoplegic migraine, thunderclap headache)
Sudden onset 'first' headache
Hyperacute severe headache ('worst headache ever')
Progressively increasing headache (change in pattern, rapidly increasing headache frequency)
Headache with mental changes (changes in personality and/or cognition)
Headache with papilloedema
New onset headache in a patient with HIV or cancer
History of headache causing awakening from sleep
Headache worsened by Valsalva maneuver
No family history of recurrent headache (migraine)

**Table 8.1**
*Factors indicating cerebral neuroimaging in childhood headache disease.*

intracranial pressure involving a tumour, and new onset headache in a child with cancer or HIV must also be investigated.[2]

According to the Quality Standard Subcommittee of the American Academy of Neurology, in adult patients with recurrent headaches that have been defined as migraine – including those with visual aura – with no recent change in pattern, no history of seizure and no other focal neurological signs or symptoms, the routine use of neuroimaging is not warranted.[21] Neuroimaging is indicated first of all for patients clinically considered to have secondary headache and in patients with atypical headache patterns, a history of seizures or focal neurological signs or symptoms.[22] Similar summary statements are not available for children. A retrospective study assessing the utility of neuroimaging in the evaluation in children with uncomplicated migraine and chronic daily headache, whose physical and neurological examinations were normal, discovered exclusively abnormalities that did not influence the diagnosis, management or outcome of the patients. The neuroimaging findings included arachnoid cysts, Arnold–Chiari I malformation, sinus disease, occult vascular malformations, developmental venous anomalies and 'dilated Virchow–Robin spaces'.[23] None of the abnormalities necessitated surgical intervention or was associated with the headache presentation.

Taken together, these results indicate that neuroimaging studies have very limited value in the clinical evaluation of children with defined clinical headache syndromes whose physical and neurological examinations are normal, so the routine use of neuroimaging is not warranted in such cases. Neuroimaging should be reserved for those patients with clinical evidence suggestive of an underlying structural lesion. Generally, in children with chronic headache, cerebral neuroimaging may be necessary only in exceptional cases, if there is suspicion of serious underlying illness, in the presence of atypical/rare cases of migraine or other unusual type of headache (thunderclap headache, ophthalmoplegic migraine), therapy resistance, different types of headache and facial paint, or children with focal neurological signs as well as a history of seizures. However, it is not infrequently the case that parents may request neuroimaging of the CNS, even though there are no medical indications for this. It is therefore important that the paediatrician explains why such a scan is generally not considered necessary; many parents are, however, anxious that their child with recurrent headache may be suffering from something serious, e.g. a brain tumour. Unfortunately, doctors normally do not have as much time as the patients and parents usually need; they do not have enough time for a constructive interview and neurological examination. Regional traditions and resources will be decisive in determining whether there will be referral and, if so, to whom. It could be important for physicians to make quite clear to the child and parents the purpose of the referral.

However, neuroimaging does have very limited value in the clinical evaluation of children and adolescents with defined headache syndrome diagnoses, whose neurological examination is normal; there are some rare, unique, primary headache syndromes that remain a diagnosis only by exclusion of potentially serious underlying pathology. One of them is the non-aneurysmal thunderclap headache (TCH). TCH is a hyperacute, fiercely intense headache associated with nausea, vomiting, photophobia and normal neurological examination. It can signify a subarachnoid haemorrhage, thrombosis of an intracranial dural venous sinus or pituitary apoplexy.[24-26] However, it may also occur spontaneously without provocation or during sustained physical exertion (during light activities, intense exertion or a Valsalva manoeuvre), but in the absence of a serious underlying intracranial pathology. The extent to which these patients are evaluated and the exact sequence of investigations continue to be debated. All patients require a careful and thorough evaluation, even when the CT and cerebrospinal fluid (CSF) do not demonstrate blood. MRI is unrevealing, but reversible, diffuse, segmental and multifocal cerebral vasospasm may occur in patients with idiopathic TCH. This phenomenon may be illustrated with MRA, which in the appropriate clinical setting obviates the need for conventional catheter angiography. The exposure of vasospastic cerebral blood vessels to contrast dye may further exacerbate the vasospasm. There is no convincing evidence that unruptured intracranial aneurysms present with TCH in the absence of blood on CT or in the CSF and in the presence of diffuse cerebral vasospasm.[27-30] Recently, investigations such as MRI with MRA are recommended and MR venography in TCH patients with bloodless CT and CSF.[27]

Ophthalmoplegic migraine is an uncommon disorder, usually starting in childhood. Until recently, its diagnosis relied on clinical grounds and the exclusion of other disorders. Neuroimaging techniques are required to exclude causes such as the Tolosa–Hunt syndrome, tumours, or vascular or infectious diseases, especially in patients with a first episode. Recently, through use of MRI, occasionally long-lasting abnormalities of the cis-

ternal portion of the oculomotor nerve have been observed (enhancement and enlargement of the cisternal portion of the oculomotor nerve with a spontaneous resolution) in patients with ophthalmoplegic migraine.[31-33] Thickening of the nerve in the interpeduncular cistern can be encountered on a CT scan.[34] However, not all patients with ophthalmoplegic migraine show such a radiological abnormality on MRI; its presence can be considered a useful diagnostic tool (similar to a neuroradiological marker) for this peculiar headache disorder.

# References

1. Dumas MD, Pexman JH, Kreeft JH, Computed tomography evaluation of patients with chronic headache. *Can Med Assoc J* 1994; **151**: 1447–52.
2. Matthew NT, Differential diagnosis in headache – identifying migraine in primary care. *Cephalalgia* 1998; **18**(suppl 22): 32–9.
3. Hockaday JM, Definitions, clinical feature, and diagnosis of childhood migraine. In: Hockaday JM, ed., *Migraine in Childhood*. Cambridge: Butterworth, 1988: 5–24.
4. Danish Neurological Society and the Danish Headache Society, Guidelines for the management of headache. *Cephalalgia* 1998; **18**: 9–22.
5. Massiou H, What is lacking in the treatment of pediatric and adolescent migraine? *Cephalalgia* 1997; **17**(suppl 17): 21–4.
6. Frishberg BM, The utility of neuroimaging in the evaluation of headache patients with normal neurologic examination. *Neurology* 1994; **44**: 1191–7.
7. Hämäläinen ML, Autti L, Salonen O, Santavuori P, Brain MRI in children with migraine: a controlled morphometric study. *Cephalalgia* 1996; **16**: 541–4.
8. Medina LS, Pinter JD, Zurakowski D, Davis RG, Kuban K, Barnes P, Children with headache: clinical predictors of surgical space-occupying lesions and the role of neuroimag-

ing. *Radiology* 1997; **202**: 819–24.

9. Shorvon S, Magnetic resonance imaging in epilepsy: The central clinical research question. In: Shorvon S, Fish DR, Andermann F, Bydder GM, Stefan H, eds, *Magnetic Resonance Scanning and Epilepsy*. New York: Plenum Press, 1994.

10. Cascino G, Advances in neuroimaging: Surgical localization. *Epilepsia* 2001; **42**: 3–12.

11. Holland RC, Hawkes GN, Moore WS, Nuclear magnetic resonance (NMR) tomography of the brain: Coronal and sagittal sections. *J Comput Assist Tomogr* 1980; **4**: 429–33.

12. Aysun S, Yetuk M, Clinical experience on headache in children: analysis of 92 cases. *J Child Neurol* 1998; **13**: 202–10.

13. Deda G, Caksen H, Ocal A, Headache etiology in children: a retrospective study of 125 cases. *Pediatr Int* 2000; **42**: 668–73.

14. Friedland RJ, Bronen RA, Magnetic resonance imaging of neoplastic, vascular, and indeterminate substrates. In: Cascino GD, Jack CR Jr, eds, *Neuroimaging in Epilepsy: Principles and Practice*. Boston: Butterworth-Heinemann, 1996: 29–50.

15. Hofmeister C, Stapf C, Hartman A et al, Demographic, morphological, and clinical characteristics of 1289 patients with brain arteriovenous malformation. *Stroke* 2000; **31**: 1307–10.

16. Massiou H, Bousser MG, Headache related to vascular disorders in the International Headache Society classification. Strengths and weaknesses. In: Olesen J, ed., *Headache Classification and Epidemiology*. New York: Raven Press, 1994: 167–78.

17. Monteiro JM, Rosas MJ, Correia AP, Vaz AR, Migraine and intracranial vascular malformation. *Headache* 1993; **33**: 563–5.

18. Haas DC, Arteriovenous malformation and migraine. Case reports and an analysis of the relationship. *Headache* 1991; **31**: 509–13.

19. Kurita H, Ueki K, Shin M et al, Headaches in patients with radiosurgically treated occipital arteriovenous malformations. *J Neurosurg* 2000; **93**: 224–8.

20. Guidetti V, Migraine in children. *EHF News* 1998; **11**: 1–3.

21. Report of the quality subcommittee of the American Academy of Neurology, Practice parameter: The utility of neuroimaging in the evaluation of headache in patients with normal neurologic examination (Summary statement). *Neurology* 1994; **44**: 1353–4.

22. Maytal J, Bienkowski RS, Patel M, Eviatar L, The value of brain imaging in children with headaches. *Pediatrics* 1995; **96**: 413–16.

23. Lewis DW, Dorbad D, The utility of neuroimaging in the evaluation of children with migraine or chronic daily headache who have normal neurological examinations. *Headache* 2000; **40**: 629–32.

24. Sturm JW, Macdonell R, Recurrent thunderclap headache associated with reversible intracerebral vasospasm causing stroke. *Cephalalgia* 2000; **20**: 132–5.

25. De Bruijn SF, Stam J, Kapelle LJ, Thunderclap headache as first symptom of cerebral venous sinus thrombosis. *Lancet* 1996; **348**: 1623–5.

26. Dodick DW, Wijdicks EFM, Pituitary apoplexy presenting as a thunderclap headache. *Neurology* 1998; **50**: 1510–11.

27. Dodick DW, Brown RD, Britton JW, Huston J III, Nonaneurysmal thunderclap headache with diffuse, multifocal, segmental, and reversible vasospasm. *Cephalalgia* 1999; **19**: 118–23.

28. Harling DW, Peatfield RC, Van Hille PT, Abbott RJ, Thunderclap headache: is it migraine? *Cephalalgia* 1989; **9**: 87–90.

29. Wijdicks EF, Kerkhoff H, van Gijn J, Long-term follow-up of 71 patients with thunderclap headache mimicking subarachnoid haemorrhage. *Lancet* 1988; **ii**: 68–70.

30. Markus HS, A prospective follow-up of thunderclap headache mimicking subarachnoid haemorrhage (letter). *J Neurol Neurosurg Psychiatry* 1991; **54**: 1117–18.

31. Mark AS, Casselman J, Brown D et al, Ophthalmoplegic migraine: Reversible enhancement and thickening of the cisternal segment of the oculomotor nerve on contrast-enhanced MR images. *AJNR* 1998; **19**: 1887–91.

32. Wong V, Wong WC, Enhancement of oculomotor nerve: A diagnostic criterion for ophthalmoplegic migraine? *Pediatr Neurol* 1997; **17**: 70–3.

33. Ostergaard JR, Moller HU, Christensen T, Recurrent ophthalmoplegia in childhood: diagnostic and etiologic considerations. *Cephalalgia* 1996; **16**: 276–9.

34. Prats JM, Mateos B, Garaizar C, Resolution of MRI abnormalities of the oculomotor nerve in childhood ophthalmoplegic migraine. *Cephalalgia* 1999; **19**: 655–9.

# 9

# Compliance and presentation of findings

*Vincenzo Guidetti, Federica Galli*

## Compliance: problems of definition in a multilevel perspective

There is no systematic definition of 'compliance' and the term 'adherence' has been used interchangeably in the literature.[1] However, the term 'compliance' seems to suggest a more passive role on the part of the patient to the instructions and prescriptions than adherence, which implies a more active, voluntary, collaborative involvement of the patient in a mutually acceptable behaviour to achieve preventive or therapeutic results.[2]

The assessment of correct treatment adherence is important for both clinical and research purposes. Non-compliance with therapy is an important obstacle in clinical practice and medical research and, despite its role, it is not commonly assessed.

Compliance rates are of 7–89% for short-term therapy and of 11–83% for long-term therapy.[3] The large span of these percentages outlines the weight of the problem, raising several questions about 'what' should be considered 'non-compliance' and 'which' methods should be used for assessment.

A uniform assessment of compliance does not exist and could refer to dose omissions, incorrect dosage, failure to fill prescriptions, premature ending of the drug and active avoidance of ingestion of medications. It is important to establish the minimum standard required to achieve the therapeutic results, considering the weight shown by placebo in the studies on drug treatment of headaches.

In a similar way, we have several methods for measuring adherence: treatment outcome, drug assays, self and/or parents' reported and pill counts.

In general terms, non-compliance during the developmental ages is comparable to that in adults, even if the analysis of children's compliance is more delicate, inasmuch as it must take into account the compliance of both the parent and the child.

However, compliance is not related exclusively to drug consumption. We might say that compliance concerns 'that headache' in 'that patient' within 'that family'.

Family variables such as adaptability, cohesion, satisfaction and coping have been found to be related to the rates of drug compliance.[4] The parents often come to the specialist with opinions about headache and drugs. It is important to know which are the general and which the specific personal attitudes on drug intake, and the results of previous pharmacological attempts to face headache crises. During history taking, it is important to catch these points in order to implement the therapy that is most appropriate to each patient, and to designate elements for evaluation of the adherence to the resultant treatment.

The problem of 'drug compliance' represents only a part of the general concept of 'adherence to medical regimens'. We arrive at a drug prescription after a complex diagnostic process, on both the medical and the psychological perspectives. A good diagnostic alliance is a better starting point for building a therapeutic alliance. To achieve good therapeutic results, all the factors of the diagnostic process have to be taken into account in the implementation of therapy.

The recognition of triggering factors by parents, patient and clinicians should be considered an essential part of the therapeutic framing. In most cases, we have two points for attacking head pain: through drug interventions on the pathophysiological side, and acting on triggering factors, reducing their effect to a minimum. It is clear that working simultaneously on the two levels gives us additional possibilities for reaching headache relief. This approach sometimes implies debate with parents and the patient about their personal viewpoints and explanations. The tendency to delegate a cure to a drug may be strong, for both the clinician and the parents. By not considering the avoidance of trigger factors in therapeutic terms could risk trapping the framing of headaches in a scotomic view. These factors are an integral part of the medical therapeutic regimen, and the evaluation of compliance should understand this.

It is clear that, in the field of headaches, several factors should be taken into account in the assessment of compliance. Whether the headache crises are monthly or daily and whether in a child or an adolescent are some of these different factors. The implementation of prophylactic treatment brings about a series of different problems into the evaluation of compliance, compared with symptomatic therapy.

## Factors affecting youngsters' compliance

Biological, psychological, cognitive, familial and social factors may interfere with or modulate the adherence to treatment on a developmental basis. All these factors are strictly embedded in determining the nature of the headache, and have relevant consequences on headache compliance. Drug therapy should always be part of a more comprehensive treatment regimen. A treatment plan should be developed together with the parents and should include participation by the child or adolescent, as appropriate to his or her understanding, to provide a tailor made approach to case. In the same way, treatment should be individualized and several additional measures (before and after drug prescription) should be taken into account to guarantee correct drug management and to evaluate the real effectiveness of the drugs.

To prepare a correct drug dose, it is important to evaluate the patient's previous experience with efficacy and side effects of drugs. Side effects must be carefully explained to the parents and/or patient and closely monitored, taking consideration of the adverse consequences on daily life (sleep disturbances, weight gain, sedation, etc.).

Advice about avoiding trigger factors, such as stress, dietary (cheese, chocolate, citrus fruits) or visual stimuli, and about supplementary intervention measures (avoid noise, have a rest, etc.) should always be given.

## Developmental issues

The treatment of headache and migraine in children and adolescents requires a specific approach, taking account of the particular nature on a neurobiological level (pharmacokinetics, pharmacodynamics and pharmacogenetics) and with regard to psychological or environmental factors that are implicated in the pathogenesis (such as triggering factors) and outcome (e.g. drug compliance) of primary headache.

The stage of development markedly influences the absorption, distribution, metabolism and excretion of drugs. A rational drug therapy in children and adolescents requires individual treatment, recognizing individual (co-morbidity, concurrent medications), developmental (pharmacodynamics, pharmacokinetics) and environmental (diet, daily life) factors, which could influence drug disposition and response.

The pharmacokinetics is concerned with how the human body handles a drug, the degree of absorption into the plasma (bioavailability), the time taken to achieve a peak plasma concentration, the drug distribution (from plasma to site of action), the metabolism and the excretion.

The pharmacodynamics concerns the effects and the mechanisms of action once the drug has reached specific receptors.

The pharmacogenetics concerns the genetically related variations in drug response. Developmental and environmental factors can influence genetic determinants in drug metabolism (e.g. drug-metabolizing enzyme activity).

Lack of information on reciprocal modulation between pharmacogenetic, developmental changes in physiology and pharmacokinetics in children can produce either toxicity or a lack of efficacy.[5] The application to childhood psychopharmacology of animal research data is still unclear and insufficient systematic clinical data are available.[6] Moreover, data are not simply transposable, e.g. in rats and mice most cells of the cerebral cortex are generated during the second half of gestation to birth, whereas in humans and monkeys it occurs at the end of the second trimester, before birth.[7] Furthermore, we know very little about the interplay between developing organism characteristics and drug action. An outline of these points is crucial. Psychological and environmental factors play a crucial role in determining compliance.

## Compliance at developmental ages: practical issues for headache treatment

Cognitive, social and emotional factors are related to the perception and modulation of the illness, e.g. cognitions and emotions influence headache sufferers in the process of taking drugs.[8]

The problem of analysing compliance in headache sufferers is probably related to the characteristics of the headache, and the implementation of symptomatic or prophylactic treatment. Compliance in acute disease seems to be better than in asymptomatic or chronic diseases or to prevent them.[3] In addition, compliance decreases enormously as soon as the child sees an improvement in symptoms.[3]

It is clear that, in the headache field, compliance with symptomatic therapy is better than with prophylactic therapy. However, there are few specific studies in adults,[9–11] and our best knowledge is not with children and adolescents.

It is very important to give the parents and patients clear explanations about the disease, even if their knowledge of the disease and its treatment does not seem to be sufficient for achieving good compliance; the beliefs of the patient and parents seem to be related to this.[3] It stresses the importance of closer examinations of the viewpoints of the parents and patient and of discussion about antecedents, and related and triggering factors. Understanding of parents' troubles and expectations is crucial to achieve compliance.[3]

Educational strategies (verbal and written) are generally effective in improving compliance.[3] Explicit instructions should be provided, also taking into consideration the daily routine of life. The collaboration of the child or adolescent is important, and the self-monitoring of crises by diary cards should be encouraged. The constant and complete monitoring of the situation requires evaluation of the following points for at least 2 months:

- Frequency, intensity and length of the attacks
- Assessment of therapeutic effects with respect to the reduction of disability
- Assessment of adequate drug compliance (correct dosage, correct dosing intervals, continuous drug taking).

The use of a diary card improves diagnosis, giving more detailed data about the headache characteristics (duration and characteristics of pain and aura) than face-to-face interviews.[12] Moreover, the patient is directly involved, even though, sometimes, it might be better to avoid paying too much attention to the headache.

Educational strategies should be addressed to prevent drug abuse, stimulating patients' self-monitoring of the crises and finding solutions other than drug use (e.g. acting on triggering factors or non-drug therapies).

Self-care attempts through use of over-the-counter drugs should be studied more in adolescent headache sufferers. In adult migraineurs, the use of over-the-counter drugs ranges from 60% to 90%.[13,14]

Overuse of drugs may predispose to chronic daily headache, with symptomatic drug dependence and refractoriness to prophylactic medication.[15] In adults, the role of analgesic overuse in the exacerbation and maintenance of headaches over time was stressed some time ago.[16–19] Adult patients with chronic daily headache frequently refer the onset of headache to their infancy or adolescence.[15–20] The adolescent patients seem to be more resistant to achieving good compliance with prescriptions.[21,22] Non-compliance can not only compromise the efficacy of medication regimens, but can also lead to inadequate changes in treatment doses, with risks for toxicity.[3] The risk of 'rebound headache' from childhood has been outlined.[23]

During childhood, the culture of a correct drug intake assumes preventive significance. As the youngster ages, the prevention of drug overuse should be pursued as part of the general management, making the parents and, when possible, the patients aware of this. Self-care attempts should be analysed. With adolescent patients, it may be convenient to discuss drug planning with them, explaining, if possible, the nature and characteristics of the headache and the treatment choices. This involves addressing their future as adults, which is important to consider in the work with adolescents.

Non-compliance or refusal to take drugs should be analysed and seen in the diagnostic framing of 'that patient': 'secondary gains' and the possible 'role' of headache in the relationship with caregivers, or within the family, represent possible obstacles to achieving compliance.

Other factors should be taken into account to improve compliance.[3] Drug compliance is easier to achieve when fewer drugs are prescribed, and when the drug is taken a maximum of once or twice daily, especially when children attend school and parents work. Compliance decreases enormously as soon as the patient begins to show an improvement in symptoms. Taking a drug for asymptomatic conditions or for the prevention of disease is related to non-compliance. Seeing the same doctor seems to be related to better compliance.

## Presentation of findings

This represents the last, but not the least important, step of the diagnostic process. A well-built diagnostic alliance represents the presupposition of achieving a sound therapeutic alliance. The compliance of patient and parents is strongly related to the provision of relevant medical findings.[24]

Now, we have the complete history from the patient, the physical and laboratory findings, and the interviews with the patient and family. One or two months have passed since the first examination. In addition, there has also been brief monitoring of the trend of headaches. During the diagnostic process, we may sometimes note an unexplained diminution in headache crises. We do not know the reason but, undoubtedly, it gives us details and matters for discussion.

The presentation of findings must be preceded by 'dedicated time' for all the staff members to discuss the medical and psychological results. Some of the findings are almost always given during the diagnostic process. However, it is convenient to reframe all the elements, presenting them in an integrated way. It is better to present the findings with all family members present.

The method of presentation should be tailored to the psychosocial characteristics of the family. The use of technical terms does not have to be absolutely avoided, but they should be clarified through the use of explanations, examples and metaphors to both the parents and the patient. Even in families of a high sociocultural level clarifications in plain words should be given, inasmuch as technical terms may not have the same meaning as in the professional setting. Any abnormal results should be clarified. It is important to avoid the most commonplace ways of thinking about headache, discussing them in line with scientific data. However, we will not have a solution for each question and a tendency to explain every issue with a sort of 'rage for explanations' should be avoided. Many aspects of headaches do not have scientific explanations and should be explained with the proviso that everything is being done to try to help the patient – to reassure the parents.

It is important to try to discuss doubts, perplexities and beliefs with the parents and patient, to avoid any brooding. The explanations given by the parents or patient during the history taking should be discussed in the light of the general findings.

The solution to the findings may vary from psycho-educational suggestions to indications for psychotherapy. Often, a shift from organic to psychological explanations may be difficult, when the conviction (or the request) has been to investigate (or exclude) organic causes of headache. However, when secondary headache has been excluded, parents may be more reassured by an explanation that the headache is genetic, in terms of allergies or ocular diseases. Once the review of the medical investigations has been done, it is important to stress that lack of physical illness does not mean that there is a lack of underlying physiological mechanisms to explain the headache. However, the actuality and true nature of the symptoms should be emphasized. It is very important for families to feel that their concerns about physical symptoms are heard.[25] An explanation of the diagnosis as a complex interaction of physical, social and emotional factors may be the best way to describe the clinical situation. Encouraging parents to explore emotional aspects, or secondary gains related to headache, may be helpful in modifying negative factors in the child's environment, such as reducing the pressure by parents for excessive academic performance or analysing the concerns about peer relationships.

Garralda[25] suggested drawing attention to the fact that 'lack of confidence by the child in his or her ability to meet the demands of ordinary life, fear that this will lead to a deterioration of the condition and to psychological distress, sadness about the loss of the positive aspects of ordinary life, and despondency about future recovery can contribute to the maintenance of somatization disorders. It is important to underline the role of psychological factors in maintaining or exacerbating a headache.

Sometimes, parents may feel a sense of guilt and responsibility, which could result in parents becoming defensive and not responding. This could result in a failure to follow therapeutic indications or a clear-cut drop-out. The engagement of families is crucial for therapeutic success.

A diagnostic alliance should be built on the basis of the strengths and the resources of the children and their families, emphasizing the importance of a partnership between the patient, doctor and family. It is also important to stress the importance of learning to live with the headaches and waiting for the benefits of treatment.

Reorganization of patterns of family relationships or better modulation of the patient's emotional responses to daily challenges requires time and specific interventions other than analgesic intervention.

# References

1. La Greca AM, Schuman WB, Adherence to prescribed medical regimens. In: Roberts MC, ed., *Handbook of Pediatric Psychology*, 2nd edn. New York: Guilford Press, 1995: 55–83.
2. Turk DC, Meichenbaum D, Adherence to self-care regimens. The patient's perspective. In: Sweet JJ, Rozensky RH, Tovian SH (eds). Handbook of Clinical Psychology in medical settings. Plenum Press New York, 1991; 249–66.
3. Matsui DM, Drug compliance in pediatrics. *Ped Clin North Am* 1997; **44**: 1–14.
4. Chaney JM, Peterson L, Family variables and disease management in juvenile rheumatoid arthritis. *J Pediatr Psychol* 1989; **14**: 489–503.
5. Leeder JS, Kearnes GL, Pharmacogenetics in paediatrics. *Pediatr Clin North Am* 1997; **44**: 55–77.
6. Vitiello B, Pediatric psychopharmacology and interaction between drugs and developing brain. *Can J Psychiatry* 1998; **48**: 582–4.
7. Nowakowski RS, Hayes NL, CNS development: An overview. *Dev Psychopathol* 1999; **11**: 395–417.
8. Passchier J, Mourik J, Brienen JA, Hunfeld JAM, Cognitions, emotions, and behavior of patients with migraine when taking medication during an attack. *Headache* 1998; **38**: 458–64.
9. Mulleners WM, Whitmarsh TE, Steiner TJ, Non-compliance may render migraine prophylaxis useless, but once-daily regimens are better. *Cephalalgia* 1998; **18**: 52–6.
10. MacGregor EA, The doctor and the migraine

patient: improving compliance. *Neurology* 1997; **48**(suppl 3): S16–20.

11. Packard RC, O'Connell P, Medication compliance among headache patients. In: Adler CS, Morrisey Adler S, Packard RC, eds, *Psychiatric Aspects of Headache*. Baltimore: Williams & Wilkins, 1987: 280–8.

12. Metsähonkala L, Sillanpää M, Tuominen J, Headache diary in the diagnosis of childhood migraine. *Headache* 1997; **37**: 240–4.

13. Celentano DD, Stewart WF, Lipton RB, Reed ML, Medication use and disability among migraineurs: a national probability sample survey. *Headache* 1992; **32**: 223–8.

14. Edmeads J, Findlay H, Tugwell P, Pryse-Phillips W, Nelson RF, Murray TJ, Impact of migraine and tension-type headache on life-style, consulting behaviour, and medication use: a Canadian population survey. *Can J Neurol Sci* 1993; **20**: 131–7.

15. Solomon S, Lipton RB, Newman LC, Clinical features of chronic daily headache. *Headache* 1992; **32**: 325–9.

16. Mathew NT, Stubits E, Nigam MR, Transformation of episodic migraine into daily headache: analysis of factors. *Headache* 1982; **22**: 66–8.

17. Mathew NT, Kurman R, Perez F, Drug induced refractory headache-clinical features and management. *Headache* 1990; **30**: 634–8.

18. Mathew NT, Chronic daily headache: clinical features and natural history. In: Nappi G, Bono G, Sandrini G, Martignoni E, Miceli G, eds, *Headache and Depression*. New York: Raven Press, 1991: 49–58.

19. Silberstein SD, Appropriate use of abortive medication in headache treatment. *Pain Management* 1991; **4**: 22–8.

20. Silberstein SD, Tension-type and chronic daily headache. *Neurology* 1993; **43**: 1644–9.

21. La Greca AM, Social consequences of pediatric conditions: Fertile area for furniture investigation and intervention? *J Pediatr Psychol* 1990; **15**: 285–308.

22. Kovacs M, Goldston D, Obrosky DS, Iyengar S, Prevalence and predictors of pervasive non-compliance with medical treatment among youths with insulin-dependent diabetes mellitus. *J Am Acad Child Adol Psychol* 1992; **31**: 1112–19.

23. Vasconcellos E, Piña-Garza JE, Millan EJ, Warner JS, Analgesic rebound headache in children and adolescents. *J Child Neurol* 1998; **13**: 443–7.

24. Bird HR, Presentation of findings and recommendations. In: Wiener JM, ed., *Textbook of Child and Adolescent Psychiatry*, 2nd edn. Washington: American Psychiatric Press, 1997: 180.

25. Garralda ME, Practitioner review: assessment and management of somatization in childhood and adolescence: a practical perspective. *J Child Psychol Psychiatry* 1999; **40**: 1159–67.

# IV

## Migraine

# 10

# Classification of migraine
*Matti Sillanpää*

## Classification

### Pre-IHS classifications

Despite a history of thousands of years, migraine still awaits the detection of basic mechanisms and classification based on aetiologies. Therefore, in the absence of knowledge about the pathogenesis, the diagnostic criteria must be established through observed clinical features. After various definitions of migraine had been used, the first serious attempt was made to develop a common international definition of migraine when the criteria of the Ad Hoc Committee on Classification of Headache[1] were introduced in 1962. Although widely applied in epidemiological studies, the Ad Hoc criteria did not satisfy the need for more standardized criteria of migraine and other headaches to enable internationally comparable studies. The next step was the introduction of the set of criteria by the Headache Classification Committee of the International Headache Society (IHS) in 1988.[2] The IHS criteria are primarily for the purpose of adult migraine and are now widely used.[3] Although far from optimal,[4] they provide researchers with a tool that can be used while waiting for a better one. Several validation studies of the IHS criteria have shown that the IHS set can classify 85%[5] of adult headaches. The method's specificity is excellent (93%) but its sensitivity is poor (44%).[6] The criterion variance ensures that the Ad Hoc criteria yield cases of migraine 1.7 times most often than the IHS criteria.[5]

In children, too, several definitions have been employed. The most widely used definition, before the introduction of the IHS criteria, was that of Vahlquist.[7] His criteria include recurrent paroxysmal headaches separated by symptom-free intervals and two or more of the following individual criteria: scotomata or related phenomena, nausea and/or vomiting, unilaterality and a positive family history.

Table 10.1 shows that there is a great deal of commonality with the definitions introduced before the IHS criteria. The most common individual criteria include visual or other prodromal symptoms, nausea and/or vomiting, recurrent or periodic nature of headache, and a positive family history of migraine. Unilaterality is not invariably included in the criteria. Furthermore, there are some additional qualitative and quantitative conditions in some definitions. Qualitative conditions include symptom-free interval,[7,8] relief by a brief period of rest or sleep,[8,9] and nausea or anorexia as an indispensable symptom.[10] Congdon and Forsythe[11] consider nausea and vomiting as different and equal

| Author | Criterion | | | | |
|---|---|---|---|---|---|
| | Recurrent/ periodic | Prodromal | Nausea/ vomiting | Unilateral | Family history |
| Vahlquist[7] | + | + | + | + | + |
| Holguin and Fenichel[8] | | + | + | + | + |
| Deubner[9] | + | + | + | | |
| Sparks[10] | | + | + | + | + |
| Congdon and Forsythe[11] | + | + | + | | + |
| Prensky and Sommer[12] | + | + | + | + | + |
| Kurtz et al[13] | + | + | + | | |

**Table 10.1**
*Diagnostic criteria of migraine employed in children and adolescents before the International Headache Society criteria (1988)[2]*

criteria. One definition also included throbbing or pulsatile quality of pain and abdominal pain in the symptomatology.[7,10,12,13] The minimum number of different symptoms is either two, three,[8,11] or none.[9]

## Classification of the International Headache Society

The IHS operational diagnostic criteria for migraine are shown in Table 10.2. Not unexpectedly, the IHS classification has evoked discussion and its validity has been questioned.[4,14] As to its application to children, agreement between the IHS-based diagnosis and expert clinical diagnosis of migraine has been poor, with the full agreement being only 47–66%.[15–18] Subsequently, the IHS criteria are probably too restrictive for daily clinical paediatric practice.

One of the debatable issues is the duration of migraine attacks. For adult patients, it is 4–72 hours and for children aged under 15 years 2–48 h. In prior adult studies, the interpolated median duration of attacks[19] is less than 4 h.[20,21] Among children and adolescents, the same median is from 1.5 to 2.7 hours.[9,22,23] The duration of attacks defined by the IHS criteria was less than 4 h in 50% of 11–14 year olds,[24] and 2 h or less in 11–81%.[15,17,25–27] Indeed, the duration of 1 h or less, instead of 2 h, as the shortest duration of migraine attack, has been suggested in children.[15,16,28,29]

In adults, the five most important individual symptoms associated with migraine were, in rank order of relative importance: nausea/vomiting, throbbing pain, unilateral pain, positive family history and photophobia.[30] In children, the order appears to be different. Golferini et al[31] used linear discriminant analysis for new child patients, visiting an ambulatory clinic for chronic and recurrent headaches to evaluate the importance of individual symptoms in migraine. They used a precodified form with 23 items to standardize in advance the data-collecting pro-

1. Migraine without aura
A. At least five attacks fulfilling B–D
B. Headache attacks lasting 2–48 hours (untreated or unsuccessfully treated)
C. Headache has at least two of the following characteristics:
   1. Unilateral location
   2. Pulsating quality
   3. Moderate-to-severe intensity (inhibits or prohibits daily activities)
   4. Aggravated by walking up stairs or similar routine activity
D. During headache of at least one of the following:
   1. Nausea and/or vomiting
   2. Photophobia and phonophobia
E. At least one of the following:
   1. History, physical and neurological examinations do not suggest one of the disorders listed in groups 5–11 (including headache associated with head trauma, vascular and non-vascular disorders, substances or their withdrawal, non-cephalic infection, metabolic disorder, and disorders of the cranium, neck, eyes, ears, nose, sinuses, teeth, mouth, or other facial or cranial structures)
   2. History and/or physical and/or neurological examination do suggest such disorder, but it is ruled out by appropriate investigations
   3. Such disorder is present, but migraine attacks do not occur for the first time in close temporal relationship to the disorder

2. Migraine with aura
A. At least two attacks fulfilling B
B. At least three of the following four characteristics:
   1. One or more fully reversible aura symptoms indicating focal cerebral cortical and/or brain-stem dysfunction
   2. At least one aura symptom develops gradually over more than 4 min or two or more occur in succession
   3. No aura symptoms last more than 60 min. If more than one aura symptom is present, accepted duration is proportionally increased
   4. Headache follows aura with a free interval of less than 60 min (it may also begin before or simultaneously with the aura)
C. At least one of the following:
   1. History, physical and neurological examinations do not suggest one of the disorders listed in groups 5–11 (including headache associated with head trauma, vascular and non-vascular disorders, substances or their withdrawal, non-cephalic infection, metabolic disorder, and disorders of the cranium, neck, eyes, ears, nose, sinuses, teeth, mouth, or other facial or cranial structures)
   2. History and/or physical and/or neurological examination do suggest such disorder, but it is ruled out by appropriate investigations
   3. Such disorder is present, but migraine attacks do not occur for the first time in close temporal relationship to the disorder

**Table 10.2**
*Operational diagnostic criteria for childhood migraine by IHS (1988)[2]*

cedures. On analysis, five variables of importance emerged: frequency of attacks, type of pain, neurological deficits, nausea and vomiting. For migraine, these variables yielded 95% sensitivity and 100% specificity. The presence of vomiting and neurological deficits was found to be a strong indicator of migraine.

Family history has previously often been included in the set of criteria for migraine diagnosis. However, its value has been questioned.[13,32] There may be inaccuracies and underreporting in family history.[33] A direct interview of family members might improve the validity. Family history was not a differentiating factor between migraine and psychogenic migraine.[31] Family history is not included in the set of the IHS migraine criteria.[2]

Unilaterality of pain is one important characteristic of adult migraine.[31] In children, it is often but not always unilateral, especially during the first years of onset of migraine.[15,16,18,26,27,32] However, because unilaterality has a high specificity (86%) and positive predictive value (85%),[18] its inclusion in the criteria of migraine is warranted.

The combination of photophobia and phonophobia as a parameter of childhood migraine has evoked criticism. Preferably, photophobia and phonophobia should be independent characteristics.[17,18]

Although nausea and vomiting are easily reported by children, many other headache features, as subjective experiences, are often difficult to ascertain, especially in younger children. They may have difficulties in describing, for instance, an intensity or throbbing nature of headache, and there may be either reporter or interviewer bias or both. The sensitivity for a pulsating quality of headache varies from 36% to 86%[15,18,24,27] and that of

moderate-to-severe intensity from 57% to 97%.[18,24,27] However, these features are useful for an experienced clinician when carefully examined and ascertained.

# Socioeconomic factors

## Headache

There are many studies about the socioeconomic factors related to the occurrence of childhood overall headache, but there are only a few about the socioeconomic background of children with migraine. Passchier and Orlebeke[34] investigated the association of headache and stress in an epidemiological study of schoolchildren. No significant difference in the occurrence of stress was found between children with any headache and their matched controls. Zuckermann et al[35] examined the effect of the child's sex, presence of siblings at the time of birth, mother's age, place of birth, level of education and socioeconomic status between children with and those without headache or stomachache, but no significant difference was shown. No difference by socioeconomic group or living with two or one parent was reported in another study,[36] but number of siblings (three or more) significantly increased the prevalence of migraine compared with one-sibling families. Borge and Nordhagen[37] studied risk factors of the occurrence of headache and stomachache, and found a significant association between stomachache only and symptom-free controls, but a non-significant association between headache and controls.

Sillanpää et al,[38] however, found associations between some aspects of social background and the occurrence of headache. In their unselected, population-based study of

4405 5-year-old children, 19.5% had disturbing headache, but only 0.2% were 'frequent' and 0.5% 'fairly frequent' headaches. Pairwise comparisons showed that the prevalence of headache was significantly higher in children with headache, in cases of lower housing standards, poorer present living conditions, and more than median number of inhabitants per room. The self-reported economic status of the family was significantly poorer in families of children with headache than in controls (3.9% vs 1.7%). In multivariate analysis, the only independent predictor of headache was a lower housing standard, with the average risk 1.5 (odds ratio 1.3, 1.8) times that of families with symptom-free children. Low social status was associated more often with the main breadwinner than in controls. A higher prevalence of headache was associated with children who had leisure activities than with those who did not (2.3% vs 19.7%; $p = 0.0001$). The effect of social factors on the occurrence of headache could later only partly be reconfirmed in the same patient series at the age of 8–9 years;[39] the authors found a significant relationship between headache of girls and mother's educational level, but a non-significant relationship between conjugal parenting and socioeconomic status. Nor was the number of children of significance from the viewpoint of headache, although headache occurred highly significantly more often if the study subject was the eldest child.

## Migraine

Bille,[40] referring to previous work on a higher prevalence of migraine in upper social class people, studied the social class of 2554 children aged 7–13 years with migraine and their matched controls in his population-based study. The father's occupation, or in the case of the single working mother, her occupation, was used as the marker of the social class, divided into upper class, middle class and working class. No demonstrable difference was found in the migraine distribution among the families by social class. As an exception to the previous literature, one study showed that the prevalence of migraine was lower in adult upper class people.[41] This last group probably consults a doctor more readily than others. Subsequently, clinic-based studies may have had a selection bias and led to incorrect conclusions.[42]

Later studies yielded results in children that were similar to Bille's results. Deubner[13] reported a non-significant difference in the prevalence of migraine by social class, but headache was more severe, frequent and of long duration in lower social class children. The social background, defined by parents' occupations or divorce or separation of the parents, did not differentiate children with migraine from their matched controls.[43] Social class did not distinguish between the presence or absence of migraine in children.[44]

In a Nigerian community-based study,[45] a significantly greater proportion of 298 children with migraine belonged to the uppermost social class than of their matched controls. They also had a higher incidence of neurotic disorders than controls, but there was no difference in behaviour or intelligence level.

# Epidemiology of migraine
## Prevalence

Migraine occurs at all ages from newborns to late adulthood. The incidence varies only by age and other variables. The youngest

| Author(s) | Age (years) | n | Headache at large | | Migraine definition | Migraine | |
|---|---|---|---|---|---|---|---|
| | | | Male | Female | | Male | Female |
| Sillanpää et al[49] | 4–15 | 1683 | | | 'Ascertained by doctor' | 5.5 | |
| Sillanpää et al[50] | 4–15 | 629 | | | 'Ascertained by doctor' | 10.0 | |
| Abu-Arefeh and Russell[43] | 5–15 | 1754 | | | IHS | 9.7 | 11.5 |
| Bille[40] | 7 | 8993 | 58 | 59 | Vahlquist | 1.1 | 1.7 |
| | 7–15 | | | | Vahlquist | 3.3 | 4.4 |
| Sillanpää[48] | 7 | 4825 | 38 | | Vahlquist | 3.2 | |
| Sillanpää and Peltonen[51] | 7 | 314 | 41 | 35 | Vahlquist | 1.2 | |
| | 7–15 | 314 | 46 | 64 | Vahlquist | 3.8 | |
| Pothmann et al[36] | 8–9 | 1189 | 83 | | IHS; MO | 3.4 | |
| | | | | | IHS; MA | 8.6 | |
| | 12–13 | 1005 | 90 | | IHS; MO | 4.8 | |
| | | | | | IHS; MA | 5.5 | |
| | 15–16 | 984 | 93 | | IHS; MO | 4.9 | |
| | | | | | IHS; MA | 5.6 | |
| Raieli et al[24] | 11 | 252 | 17 | 17 | IHS; MO | 3.6 | 0.5 |
| | | | | | IHS; MA | 0.6 | 0.5 |
| | 12 | 421 | 22 | 28 | IHS; MO | 2.8 | 3.3 |
| | | | | | IHS; MA | 0.4 | 1.4 |
| | 13 | 374 | 26 | 35 | IHS; MO | 1.6 | 3.2 |
| | | | | | IHS; MA | 0.5 | 0.5 |
| | 14 | 204 | 18 | 56 | IHS; MO | 1.6 | 3.9 |
| | | | | | IHS; MA | 0 | 1.3 |
| | 11–14 | 1445 | 20 | 28 | IHS; MO | 2.3 | 0.4 |
| | | | | | IHS; MA | 0.4 | 0.9 |
| Sillanpää et al[52] | 13 | 3784 | 80 | 84 | Vahlquist; MO | 6.2 | 8.0 |
| | | | | | Vahlquist; MA | 1.9 | 6.5 |
| Sillanpää and Piekkala[53] | 14 | 3863 | 65 | 71 | Vahlquist; MO | 2.1 | 4.6 |
| | | | | | Vahlquist; MA | 5.9 | 8.9 |

IHS, International Headache Society; MO, migraine without aura; MA, migraine with aura; Vahlquist, Vahlquist's criteria of migraine.

**Table 10.3**
*Epidemiology of childhood and adolescence migraine (%)*

reported case of migraine is a child who, at the age of 2 weeks, began to have cyclical vomiting and later developed migraine, in a family with several members who had migraine.[46]

Several cases of patients with migraine in infancy have been published.[47]

Table 10.3 shows studies on the epidemiology of migraine in childhood and adolescence.

Sillanpää et al[49,50] studied simultaneously two unselected child populations at the ages of 4–15 years in south-western Finland. One study included only Finnish-speaking children and another study only Swedish-speaking children. If headache had been ascertained by a doctor to be migraine, the diagnosis was approved for the study. The prevalence of migraine among Swedish-speaking children proved to be double that of Finnish-speaking children (10% vs 5.5%). Applying the IHS criteria for the same age groups, Abu-Arefeh and Russell[43] achieved similar prevalence rates.

At age 7, the age for starting school in Nordic countries, the prevalence of migraine by the Vahlquist criteria varies from 1.2% to 3.2%.[40,48,51] During compulsory schooling, the average rate is from 3.8% to 3.9%.[40,51]

## Temporal changes in prevalence

Several cross-sectional studies show a marked increase in the prevalence from 7 to 15 years of age (Tables 10.3 and 10.4). Studies employing the Vahlquist criteria[40] yield figures from 1.4% to 5.3%, those based on a medical ascertainment[49,53] from 2.8% to 10.3%, and those using the application of the IHS criteria from 3.5% to 13.8%. The prevalences appear to have doubled in the 1980s and 1990s, compared with the 1950s and 1960s.

Few longitudinal follow-up data are avail-

| Age (years) | Bille[40] (n = 8993) | | | Sillanpää et al[49] (n = 1683) | Sillanpää et al[50] (n = 629) | Abu-Arefeh and Russell[43] (n = 2165) | | |
|---|---|---|---|---|---|---|---|---|
| | Male | Female | Total | Total | Total | Male | Female | Total |
| 4 | | | | 0.9 | 2.7 | | | |
| 5 | | | | 0 | 0 | 3.7 | 3.0 | 3.4 |
| 6 | | | | 0 | 5.3 | 6.8 | 8.1 | 7.4 |
| 7 | 1.1 | 1.7 | 1.4 | 2.8 | 6.9 | 2.8 | 4.1 | 3.5 |
| 8 | 2.7 | 2.7 | 2.7 | 3.5 | 21.2 | 8.5 | 5.9 | 7.3 |
| 9 | 3.5 | 2.9 | 3.2 | 7.2 | 3.5 | 6.6 | 5.9 | 6.3 |
| 10 | 4.0 | 3.3 | 3.6 | 7.1 | 10.6 | 11.4 | 11.6 | 11.5 |
| 11 | 3.7 | 5.7 | 4.7 | 2.8 | 11.8 | 15.3 | 11.4 | 13.2 |
| 12 | 3.5 | 6.9 | 5.2 | 8.5 | 10.5 | 20.2 | 18.0 | 19.1 |
| 13 | 4.0 | 5.9 | 5.0 | 7.4 | 9.0 | 14.8 | 23.7 | 19.0 |
| 14 | 5.4 | 4.8 | 5.1 | 9.7 | 20.4 | 4.0 | 27.0 | 16.2 |
| 15 | 1.5 | 8.2 | 5.3 | 7.6 | 10.3 | 14.0 | 13.6 | 13.8 |
| 4–15 | | | | 5.5 | 10.0 | | | |
| 5–15 | | | | | | 9.7 | 11.5 | 10.6 |
| 7–15 | 3.3 | 4.4 | 3.9 | | | | | |

IHS, International Headache Society; MO, migraine without aura; MA, migraine with aura; Vahlquist, Vahlquist's criteria of migraine.

**Table 10.4**
Prevalence of migraine in children aged under 16 years (%)

able on children. Sillanpää[54] undertook a prospective, population-based study of 4235 children aged 7 years, 2921 of whom could be re-studied 7 years later at the age of 14 years. The Vahlquist set of criteria was used. During follow-up, the prevalence rate had increased from 37% to 69% in the study population. The rise was found in all frequency categories of more than once a month. A similar increase was shown in migraine: from 2.7% to 10.6%. The prevalence rate rose more significantly in girls than in boys: from 2.5% to 14.8% vs from 2.9% to 6.4%. Migraine with aura was reported by 0.7% of 7-year-old and 4.1% of 14-year-old girls. The corresponding figures for boys were 0.2% and 1.0%. Migraine disappeared during follow-up totally in 25% (in 23% of boys and 26% of girls). The discontinuation of migraine attacks was more probable if the onset had been before the age of 7 years. A subgroup of the 1205 patients could be followed for 15 years, from 7 to 22 years of age.[55] At the final follow-up, 7.1% suffered from migraine. Of children who had migraine at age 7, 11.6% persisted with attacks, but of children who had had no attacks at age 7, 5.0% had migraine at age 22.

Bille[56] followed a subgroup of 73 children with 'pronounced migraine' from his patient cohort for 40 years. Using the Vahlquist criteria, he showed that about one-third had persistent migraine through the years of follow-up and approximately a quarter had migraine with symptom-free years. The proportion of subjects with persistent migraine gradually decreased from puberty and young adulthood to the age of 47–53 years (from 38% to 29%). Considering subjects with recurring periods of migraine, the proportion of people who were migraine free during the entire follow-up period was 62% at puberty and young adulthood, and thereafter 40–46%. From puberty or young adulthood (up to age 25) to the last contact, a permanent freedom from migraine attacks had been experienced by 23% (34% of boys and 15% of girls). The significant sex difference found in the prevalence of migraine attacks during follow-up, could not be seen in the frequency or intensity.

The follow-up study of Bille[56] also clearly revealed a memory bias about the occurrence of aura symptoms. At the 40-year follow-up, 48% stated that they had a visual aura, but 70% of them had reported the same at the previous examinations. Similarly, 52% denied any migraine attacks with aura but, based on previous documents, no more than 21% belonged to this category.

## Secular trends

An increasing trend in time has been found in the prevalence of adult headache (US Department on Health and Human Services 1991,[57] Stang et al 1992).[58] Similar secular trend appear clearcut in children. Sillanpää and Anttila (1996)[59] undertook a population-based cross-sectional study in Finnish 7-year-old children with a virtually identical study design applied previously[48] for a subpopulation of the same age in the same city of Turku. The data collection took place using the same methodology and the same (Vahlquist) criteria of migraine. The overall current (6 preceding months) prevalence of headache had increased from 14% in 1974 to 52% in 1992. Similarly, the increase in the prevalence of migraine was from 1.9% in 1974 to 5.7% in 1992. In 1974, the migraine prevalence was 1.9% in both boys and girls, but the rate was higher in boys than in girls in 1992 (6.3% vs 5.0%).

The results of the Finnish study are supported by the Rochester Epidemiology Project,[60] which made use of the records-linkage method. They included a recorded headache database for the 3-year period 1979–1981 and the 2-year period 1989–1990, reanalysed the data for incidence cases and assigned the diagnosis using the IHS classification. The incidence of medically recognized migraine had increased for all ages between the two periods of observation, but particularly in the age group 10–49 years. The relative increase in the peak incidence rate at age 20–29 years was 56%. In females, the increase was in all types of migraine but particularly in the type 'migrainous disorder not fulfilling above criteria'. In males, the migraine had increased in the age group 10–19 years, with a relative increase of 89%.

## Triggering and avoiding factors

Triggering factors are not uncommon in childhood migraine. In a community-based study of 1083 children aged 3–11 years,[44] 4.7% of boys and 5.0% of girls had migraine, defined by the Ad Hoc Committee.[1] Any trigger was reported by the child and family in 18% of 3 to 7 year olds and in 44% of 8 to 11 year olds.

Triggering factors can be divided into three categories: organic, dysfunctional and psychogenic (Table 10.5). There are reports on migraine concurring with other diseases, but there are few data on the prevalence of concurrent diseases in patients with migraine. In a population-based study of 1205 people, girls with any allergic disease at the age of 7–22 had migraine significantly more often than those who had no allergy (24% vs 15%). The difference was not as great in boys (11% vs 7%). On the other hand, in boys with bronchial asthma, migraine was significantly more common than in those without asthma (30% vs 7%) (M Sillanpää, unpublished data). In patients with any epilepsy, the prevalence of migraine is from 8% to 15%.[61,62] The prevalence is substantially higher in patients with centrotemporal epilepsy in childhood (63%), absence epilepsy (33%), and partial epilepsy (7%).[63] Another paroxysmal cerebral disorder, Tourette's syndrome, also provokes migraine attacks more often than expected (in 33%).[64]

Dysfunctional triggers include well-known stroboscopic effects, which appear to be by far the most common ones in this category.[40] Hormonal factors play a marked role in the form of catamenial migraine.[10,40] Ice-cream headache is an unexpectedly common trigger, too. Physical stress has been associated with migraine,[11,40] but its role is controversial. Boys who participated in large amounts of leisure physical activity had significantly more headache than than those who were not so active.[74] One-third to one-half of the patients who have autonomic nervous system dysfunction, including, for example, motion sickness and stomachaches, also evolve migraine.[40,69,70] Cold or hot weather or weather changes give rise to migraine in some patients.

Foods and food additives have often been suggested as triggers of migraine attacks. According to Bille,[40] 2% of children with migraine get attacks from food. However, the prevalence rate of food additive intolerance in the Danish general population aged 5–16 years is around the same (1–2%).[75] In the series of Mortimer et al,[44] dietary factors were accountable in 12% of 3 to 7 year olds and in 8% of children aged 8–11 years. Recently,

| Trigger | % | Author(s) |
|---|---|---|
| *Organic* | | |
| Allergic diseases, girls | 24 | Sillanpää, unpublished data |
| Bronchial asthma, boys | 30 | Sillanpää, unpublished data |
| Epilepsy, overall | 8–15 | Paskind,[61] Ely[62] |
| – centrotemporal | 63 | Septien et al[63] |
| – absence | 33 | Septien et al[63] |
| – partial | 7 | Septien et al[63] |
| Tourette's syndrome | 27 | Barabas et al[64] |
| Trauma | 9–32 | Passchier and Orlebeke,[34] Septien et al,[63] Barlow[65] |
| *Dysfunctional* | | |
| Stroboscopic effects | 84 | Bille[40] |
| Menstruation | 21–45 | Bille,[40] Sparks[10] |
| Ice-cream | 33 | Aromaa et al[66] |
| Physical stress | 4–25 | Bille,[40] Congdon and Forsythe[67] |
| Hunger | 19–35 | Bille,[40] Maratos and Wilkinson[68] |
| Noise | 7–19 | Bille,[40] Passchier and Orlebeke[34] |
| Motion sickness | 15–45 | Bille,[40] Barabas et al,[69] Aromaa et al[70] |
| Heat | 11 | Passchier and Orlebeke[34] |
| Windy or cold weather | 8–14 | Bille,[40] Congdon and Forsythe[11] |
| Television | 3 | Bille[40] |
| Special foods, smells | 2–12 | Bille,[40] Mortimer et al,[44] Bruni et al[71] |
| *Psychogenic* | | |
| Emotional factors | 86 | Maratos and Wilkinson[68] |
| School work | 59 | Bille[40] |
| Sleep disturbances | 29–47 | Bille,[40] Bruni et al[71] |
| Lack of sleep | 17 | Passchier and Orlebeke[34] |
| Stress, conflicts | 20–40 | Cooper et al,[72] Egermark-Eriksson,[73] Passchier and Orlebeke[34] |
| Fear | 36 | Aromaa et al[66] |
| Anxiety | 28 | Aromaa et al[66] |
| Fatigue, uneasiness | 11 | Bille[40] |
| Suffocating atmosphere | 8 | Passchier and Orlebeke[34] |

**Table 10.5**
*Triggering factors in childhood and adolescence migraine*

Bruni et al[71] compared the prevalence of food allergy in children and adolescents in a clinic-based case–control setting, and found it to be 10% for migraine, 7% for tension-type headache subjects and 5% for controls. Cows' milk allergy was also significantly higher in subjects with migraine than in controls (13% vs 7%).

Tyramine has been generally suggested as a trigger in the adult population, but it does not appear to be a precipitant in childhood migraine.[67,76] Foods suggested as responsible for migraine attacks in an Italian study were cocoa, banana, egg and hazelnuts.[77] Furthermore, glutamate, nitrites and red wine are included in this category.[65]

Psychogenic factors are undoubtedly the most important triggers (see Table 10.5). Harmful stress is often a background mechanism that appears from many sources, including school work, conflict situations, sleep disturbances, fatigue, and an uneasiness and suffocating atmosphere, and is accompanied by migraine attacks. In addition, children and adolescents with psychiatric problems suffer significantly more often from migraine than those who have no psychiatric morbidity (17% vs 10%) (M Sillanpää, unpublished data).

Avoidance of migraine attacks is naturally easier if the triggers are known. Avoidable factors include ice-cream and other foods, flickering lights and clearly stressful situations. In patients with frequent and severe attacks of migraine, an oligoantigenic or few food diet prevented attacks in 87%.[78] In the study of Aromaa et al,[66] a pain-relieving drug was taken by 90% compared with 74% of patients with tension-type headaches. A darkened room was also preferred significantly more often in association with migraine compared with tension-type headache (74% vs 34%). A quarter (26%) of migraine patients, but none of the controls, provoked vomiting to achieve relief.

The coping studies reported by Pothmann et al[36] included continuation of the current activity in case of headache in 27%, stopping of the activity in 8%, having a short rest by 31%, with the remaining 34% retiring to bed. 'Lying down' (40%) and 'relaxing' were the most frequently helpful measures used.

*Other headaches*
Tension-type headache
Muscle contraction headache
Secondary headache

*Epilepsy*
Late-onset idiopathic occipital epilepsy
Idiopathic photosensitive occipital epilepsy
Other occipital epilepsies
Other photosensitive epilepsies
Complex partial epilepsy
Centrotemporal epilepsy
Absence epilepsy

*Vertigo*
Tumours of brain stem and auditory nerve
Benign paroxysmal vertigo of childhood
Dizzy spells

*Abdominal disorders*
Stomachache
Vomiting

*Cardiovascular disorders*
Arteriovenous malformation
Arterial hypertension
Vascular stroke
Alternating hemiplegia
Recurrent ophthalmoplegia

*Other*
Syncope
Raised intracranial pressure
Hartnup's disease
Leigh's disease

**Table 10.6**
*Differential diagnosis of migraine*

# Differential diagnosis

Some differential diagnostic aspects of migraine are presented in Table 10.6. It is not always easy to draw a line between migraine and tension-type headache, particularly because they may concur. The IHS criteria of migraine and tension-type headache also overlap in more than half the cases.[79] Secondary headache includes, for example, neoplasma masses, intracranial infections, congenital malformations and other structural changes.

Epilepsies may give rise to differential diagnostic problems. Migraine often concurs with certain types of epilepsy, such as late-onset idiopathic occipital epilepsy,[80] idiopathic photosensitive occipital epilepsy[81] and other photosensitive epilepsies. Complex partial seizures may be mixed up with confusional migraine.[82]

Vertigo and dizziness may be caused by migraine but many other mechanisms, both central and peripheral, can be involved.[83,84] Brain-stem, cerebellopontine angle and auditory nerve tumours may cause intermittent symptoms. Benign paroxysmal vertigo of childhood is considered as a precedent of migraine. Abdominal and gastrointestinal disturbance are very common, but abdominal migraine and cyclic vomiting are infrequently identified and ascertained as migraine. Vascular collapse may be caused by migraine[85] and should be considered among other mechanisms of syncope.

# References

1. Ad Hoc Committee on Classification of Headache, *JAMA* 1962; **179**: 717–18.
2. Headache Classification Committee of the International Headache Society, Classification and diagnostic criteria for headache disorders, cranial neuralgia, and facial pain. *Cephalalgia* 1988; **8**(suppl 7): 1–96.
3. Olesen J, Lipton RB, Migraine classification and diagnosis. International Headache Society criteria. *Neurology* 1994; **44**(suppl 4): 6–10.
4. Bruyn GW, Headache classification: status praesens. *Cephalalgia* 1993; **13**(suppl 12): 12–17.
5. Merikangas KR, Whitaker AE, Angst J, Validation of diagnostic criteria for migraine in the Zürich longitudinal cohort study. *Cephalalgia* 1993; **13**(suppl 12): 47–53.
6. Michel P, Henry P, Letenneur L et al, Diagnostic screen for assessment of the IHS criteria for migraine by general practitioners. *Cephalalgia* 1993; **13**(suppl 12): 54–9.
7. Vahlquist B, Migraine in children. *Int Arch Allergy* 1955; **7**: 348–55.
8. Prensky AL, Sommer D, Diagnosis and treatment of migraine in children. *Neurology* 1979; **29**: 506–10.
9. Sparks J, The incidence of migraine in schoolchildren. *Practitioner* 1978; **221**: 407–11.
10. Kurtz Z, Dilling D, Blau JN, Peckham C, Migraine in children: findings from the National Child Development Study. In: Rose FC, ed., *Progress in Migraine Research*. London: Pitman Books, 1984: 9–17.
11. Congdon PJ, Forsythe WI, Migraine in childhood: a study of 300 children. *Dev Med Child Neurol* 1979; **21**: 209–16.
12. Holguin J, Fenichel G, Migraine. *J Pediatr* 1967; **70**: 290–7.
13. Deubner DC, An epidemiologic study of migraine and headache in 10–20 year olds. *Headache* 1977; **17**: 173–80.
14. Blau JN, Diagnosing criteria: are the criteria valid or invalid? *Cephalalgia* 1993; **13**(suppl 12): 21–4.
15. Wöber-Bingöl C, Wöber C, Karvautz A et al, Diagnosis of headache in childhood and adolescence: a study of 437 patients. *Cephalalgia* 1995; **15**: 13–21.
16. Winner P, Martinez W, Mante L, Bello L, Classification of pediatric migraine: proposed revisions to the IHS criteria. *Headache* 1995; **35**: 407–10.
17. Winner P, Gladstein J, Hamel R et al, Multicenter prospective evaluation of proposed pediatric migraine revisions to the IHS criteria. Presented at the American Association for the study of Headache Scientific Meeting, San Diego, CA, May 1996.
18. Maytal J, Young M, Schechter A, Lipton RB,

Pediatric migraine and the International Headache Society (IHS) criteria. *Neurology* 1997; **48:** 602–7.

19. Stewart WF, Shechter A, Lipton RB, Migraine heterogeneity. Disability, pain intensity, and attack frequency and duration. *Neurology* 1994; **44**(suppl 4): 24–39.

20. Clarke GJR, Waters WE, Headache and migraine in a London general practice: In: Waters WE, ed., *The Epidemiology of Migraine.* London: Bracknell-Berkshire, 1974: 14–22.

21. Mills CH, Waters WE, Headache and migraine of the Isles of Scilly: In: Waters WE, ed., *The Epidemiology of Migraine.* London: Bracknell-Berkshire, 1974: 49–58.

22. Small P, Waters WE, In: Waters WE, ed., *The Epidemiology of Migraine.* London: Bracknell-Berkshire, 1974: 59–67.

23. Andrasik F, Holroyd KA, Abell T, Prevalence of headache within a college student population: a preliminary analysis. *Headache* 1979; **19:** 384–7.

24. Raieli V, Raimondo D, Cammalleri R, Camarda R, Migraine headache in adolescents: a student population-based study in Monreale. *Cephalalgia* 1995; **15:** 5–12.

25. Gladstein J, Holden EW, Perotta L, Raven M, Diagnosis and symptom patterns in children presenting to a pediatric headache. *Headache* 1993; **33:** 497–500.

26. Metsähonkala L, Sillanpää M, Migraine in children – an evaluation of the IHS criteria. *Cephalalgia* 1994; **14:** 285–90.

27. Gallai V, Sarchielli P, Carboni F, Benedetti P, Mastropaolo C, Puca F, on behalf of the Juvenile Headache Collaborative Study Group, Applicability of the 1988 IHS criteria to headache patients under the age of 18 years attending 21 Italian headache clinics. *Headache* 1995; **35:** 146–53.

28. Shinnar S, An approach to the child with headaches. *Ital Pediatr* 1991; **6:** 140–8.

29. Seshia SS, Wolstein JR, Adams C, Booth FA, Reggin JD, International Headache Society criteria and childhood headache. *Dev Med Child Neurol* 1994; **36:** 419–28.

30. Marcus DA, Nash JM, Turk DC, Diagnosing recurring headaches: IHS criteria and beyond. *Headache* 1994; **34:** 329–36.

31. Golferini F, Facchin P, Cavinato M, Lovison L, Pitassi I, Battistella PA, Diagnostic factors in pediatric primary headache. *J Clin Epidemiol* 1988; **41:** 27–33.

32. Hockaday JM, Definitions, clinical features and diagnosis of childhood migraine. In: Hockday JM, ed., *Childhood Migraine.* London: Butterworth, 1988: 5–9.

33. Ottman R, Hong S, Litpn RB, Validity of family history data on severe headache and migraine. *Neurology* 1993; **43:** 1954–60.

34. Passchier J, Orlebeke JF, Headaches and stress in schoolchildren: an epidemiological study. *Cephalalgia* 1985; **5:** 167–76.

35. Zuckermann B, Stevenson J, Bailey V, Stomachaches and headaches in a community sample of preschool children. *Pediatrics* 1987; **79:** 677–82.

36. Pothmann R, v. Frankenberg SV, Mueller B, Sartory G, Hellmeier W, Epidemiology of headache in children and adolescents: evidence of high prevalence of migraine among girls under 10. *Int J Behav Med* 1994; **1:** 76–89.

37. Borge AIH, Nordhagen R, Development of stomach-ache and headache during middle childhood: co-occurrence and psychosocial risk factors. *Acta Paediatr* 1994; **84:** 795–802.

38. Sillanpää M, Piekkala P, Kero P, Prevalence of headache at preschool age in an unselected child population. *Cephalalgia* 1991; **11:** 239–42.

39. Metsähonkala L, Sillanpää M, Tuominen J, Social environment and headache in 8- to 9-year-old children: a follow-up study. *Headache* 1998; **38:** 222–8.

40. Bille B, Migraine in school children. A study of the incidence and short-term prognosis, and a clinical, psychological and encephalographic comparison between children with migraine and matched controls. *Acta Paediatr* 1962; **51**(suppl 136): 1–151.

41. Stewart WF, Lipton RB, Celentano DD, Reed ML, Prevalence of migraine headache in the United States. *JAMA* 1992; **267:** 64–9.

42. Waters WE, Migraine: intelligence, social class, and familial prevalence. *BMJ* 1971; **ii:** 77–81.

43. Abu-Arefeh I, Russell G, Prevalence of headache and migraine in schoolchildren. *BMJ* 1994; **309**: 765–9.
44. Mortimer MJ, Kay J, Jaron A, Childhood migraine in general practice: clinical features and characteristics. *Cephalalgia* 1992; **12**: 238–43.
45. Iloeje SO, Orji GI, Childhood migraine in Nigeria II: psychosocial aspects. *West Afr Med J* 1997; **16**: 237–41.
46. Russell JW, Case of migraine with ophthalmoplegia. *BMJ* 1903; **i**: 1020.
47. Vahlquist B, Hackzell G, Migraine of early onset: a study of thirty-one cases in which the disease first appeared between one and four years of age. *Acta Paediatr* 1949; **38**: 622–36.
48. Sillanpää M, Prevalence of migraine and other headache in Finnish children starting school. *Headache* 1976; **15**: 288–90. (Swedish, with English summary.)
49. Sillanpää M, Urponen H, Pitkäaikaissairaat ja vammaiset lapset Turun ja Porin läänissä. Yleisyys, sosiaalinen tausta ja kuntoutuspalvelut. (Children with long-term illnesses, disabilities and handicaps in the Province of Turku and Pori. Prevalence, social background and habilitation services.) *Lääkintöhall Tutk 30* 1984 (Helsinki: Lääkintöhall) 1–127. (In Finnish, with English summary.)
50. Sillanpää M, Westerén l, Urponen H, Kroniska sjuka och handikappade barn i Åboland. Prevalens, social bakgrund och habiliteringstjänster. (Children with long-term illnesses, disabilities and handicaps in Åboland. Prevalence, social background and habilitation services.) *Kansanterveystiet Julk* M 77, 1984 (Turku: Gillot OY); 1–84.
51. Sillanpää M, Peltonen T, Occurrence of headache amongst schoolchildren in a Northern Finnish community. In: Sicuteri F, ed., *Headache: New vistas.* Florence: Biomedical Press, 1977: 5–8.
52. Sillanpää M, Prevalence of headache in prepuberty. *Headache* 1983; **23**: 10–14.
53. Sillanpää M, Piekkala P, Prevalence of migraine and other headaches in early puberty. *Scand J Prim Health Care* 1984; **2**: 27–32.
54. Sillanpää M, Changes in the prevalence of migraine and other headaches during the first seven school years. *Headache* 1983; **23**: 15–19.
55. Aromaa M, Sillanpää M, Aro H, A population-based follow-up study of headache from age 7 to 22. Submitted.
56. Bille B, A 40-year follow-up of school children with migraine. *Cephalalgia* 1997; **17**: 488–91.
57. US Department of Health and Human Services/Public Health Services. Prevalence of chronic migraine headaches in the United States 1980–1985. *MMWR Morbid Wkly Rep* 1991; **40**: 337–8.
58. Stang PE, Yanagihara T, Swanzon JW et al, Incidence of migraine headache: A population-based study in Olmsted County Minnesota *Neurology* 1992; **42**: 1657–62.
59. Sillanpää M, Anttila P. Increasing prevalence of headache in 7-year-old school children. *Headache* 1996; **36**: 466–70.
60. Rozen TD, Swanzon JW, Stang PE, McDonnell SK, Rocca WA, Increasing incidence of medically recognized migraine headache in a United States population. *Neurology* 1999; **53**: 1468–73.
61. Paskind HA, The relationship of migraine and epilepsy and some other neuropsychiatric disorders. *Arch Neurol Psychiatry* 1934; **32**: 45–50.
62. Ely FA, Migraine-epilepsy syndrome: statistical study of heredity. *Arch Neurol Psychiatry* 1930; **24**: 943–9.
63. Septien L, Pelletier JL, Brunotte F, Giroud M, Dumas R, Migraine in patients with centro-temporal epilepsy in childhood. *Cephalalgia* 1991; **11**: 281–4.
64. Barabas G, Matthews WS, Ferrari M, Tourette's syndrome and migraine. *Arch Neurol* 1984; **41**: 871–2.
65. Barlow CF, Precipitating factors of the migraine attack. In: Barlow CF, ed., *Headaches and Migraine in Childhood.* Oxford: Blackwell Scientific, 1984: 30–45.
66. Aromaa M, Sillanpää M, Rautava P, Helenius H, Childhood headache at school entry. A controlled clinical study. *Neurology* 1998; **50**: 1729–36.
67. Congdon PJ, Forsythe WI, Migraine in childhood. *Dev Med Child Neurol* 1974; **21**: 209–16.

68. Maratos J, Wilkinson M, Migraine in children: a medical and psychiatric study. *Cephalalgia* 1982; **2**: 179–87.

69. Barabas G, Matthews WS, Ferrari M, Childhood migraine and motion sickness. *Pediatrics* 1983; **72**: 188–90.

70. Aromaa M, Rautava P, Helenius H, Sillanpää M, Factors of early life as predictors of headache at school entry. *Headache* 1998; **38**: 23–30.

71. Bruni O, Fabrizi P, Ottaviano S, Cortesi F, Giannotti F, Guidetti V, Prevalence of sleep disorders in childhood and adolescence with headache: a case-control study. *Cephalalgia* 1997; **17**: 492–8.

72. Cooper PJ, Bawden HN, Camfield PR, Camfield CS, Anxiety and life-events in childhood migraine. *Pediatrics* 1987; **79**: 999–1004.

73. Egermark-Eriksson I, Prevalence of headache in Swedish schoolchildren. A questionnaire survey. *Acta Paediatr Scand* 1982; **71**: 135–40.

74. Kujala UM, Taimela S, Viljanen T, Leisure physical activity and various pain symptoms among adolescents. *Br J Sports Med* 1999; **33**: 325–8.

75. Madsen C, Prevalence of food additive intolerance. *Human Exp Toxicol* 1994; **13**: 393–9.

76. Kohlenberg RJ, Tyramine sensitivity in dietary migraine: a critical review. *Headache* 1982; **22**: 30–4.

77. Guariso G, Bertoli S, Cernetti R, Battistella PA, Setari M, Zacchello F, Migraine and food intolerance: a controlled study in pediatric patients. *Pediatr Med Chir* 1993; **15**: 57–61. (In Italian.)

78. Soothill JF, Finch HE, Wilson J, Migraine can be cured by the few food diet. In: Gallai V, Guidetti V, eds, *Juvenile Headache.* Amsterdam: Elsevier Science Publishers BV, 1991: 257–60.

79. Messinger HB, Spierings ELH, Vincent AJP, Overlap of migraine and tension-type headache in the International Headache Society classification. *Cephalalgia* 1991; **11**: 233–7.

80. Panayiotopoulos CP, To the Editor. *Epilepsia* 1999; **40**: 1320–4.

81. Guerrini R, Dravet C, Bureau M, Bonanni P, Ferrari AR, Roger J, Idiopathic photosensitive occipital lobe epilepsy. *Epilepsia* 1995; **36**: 883–91.

82. Shaabat A, Confusional migraine in childhood. *Pediatr Neurol* 1996; **15**: 23–5.

83. Fried MP, The evaluation of dizziness in children. *Laryngoscope* 1980; **90**: 1548–60.

84. Abu-Arafeh I, Russell G, Paroxysmal vertigo as a migraine equivalent in children in a population-based study. *Cephalalgia* 1995; **15**: 22–5.

85. McHarg ML, Shinnar S, Rascoff H, Walsh CA, Syncope in childhood. *Pediatr Cardiol* 1997; **18**: 367–71.

# 11

# The genetics of migraine headaches

*Pasquale Montagna*

That migraine runs in families is a fact well known since antiquity, and it is only too natural to consider that migraine may have a genetic basis when different generations in a family are affected one after another with the same disease.[1,2] Migraine is, however, a disease so prevalent in the general population, affecting up to 33% of females and 13% of males (lifetime prevalence[3]), that the concourse of several cases in the same family may be the result of chance or environmental influences rather than a genetic predisposition. The high prevalence among the general population is just one of the problems encountered in the quest for the genetic basis of this enigmatic disease. Not only does migraine show prevalence rates that vary according to sex and age (though seemingly not to socioeconomic status), it also changes clinical expression and co-morbidity according to age and sex. Furthermore, there is no available laboratory marker for the disease, and we have to rely, for diagnostic purposes, on clinical criteria alone.

Despite the efforts of the International Headache Society (IHS),[4] these criteria are far from being perfect or even universally accepted: in particular their usefulness in specific age groups such as in children or adolescents is being questioned. Reliance on clinical criteria alone makes epidemiological enquiries

difficult and the use of questionnaires or any indirect recollection of data useless or outright wrong (see below). We do not know whether the different nosological categories of primary headaches listed by the IHS, from migraine to tension-type to cluster headache, represent just descriptions that are useful in the clinical evaluation of patients or separate diseases in their own right, e.g. the distinction between migraine with (MA) and without aura (MO) may be artificial and the two 'diseases' indeed often occur in the same family and in the same individual. There are, moreover, other clinical categories such as cyclical vomiting in infancy, periodic vertigo or acephalgic migraine, e.g. migraine without pain, which are considered as migraine 'equivalents' and may also run on their own in a familial form.[5] Should they be considered true migraine or not? The basic problem in the genetics of migraine lies in the fact that, as a result of our substantial ignorance of the pathogenic process, we must identify symptoms with disease. Indeed, migraine is a byword both for headache of a certain type occurring in attacks, and for the underlying process that produces these attacks (and other manifestations too). This problem is also shared by the epilepsies, which are manifested by recurrent crises, often varying in semeiology from one attack to another and according to age and sex; epilepsy, however, enjoys EEG markers and a basic understanding of pathogenesis.

All these difficulties compound to make migraine a difficult subject for the geneticist. As with many other diseases that have a high prevalence among the general population, such as diabetes mellitus, hypertension or affective disorders, migraine is widely conceived of as a multifactorial trait, i.e. it has both environmental and genetic causes, and is polygenic when it comes to heredity. The parallel with the epilepsies, however, helps to introduce a concept that, although accepted by migraine researchers, is difficult to incorporate into genetic analysis: the notion of threshold. Migraine can be considered a threshold characteristic[6] and, if we could know and determine this threshold in manifesting and non-manifesting individuals, we could probably overcome at least some of the difficulties in genetic analysis. It is hoped that clinical neurophysiologists and pharmacologists are moving close to the target and may ultimately help the geneticist by providing the long sought for laboratory marker for migraine.

In this chapter, I review the evidence behind the concept of migraine as a hereditary disorder, and consider familial hemiplegic migraine (FHM), the only type of migraine until now clearly delineated genetically. This isolated success in migraine genetics is the result of the usefulness of linkage analysis in FHM, a disease that behaves as a single mendelian trait and with an autosomal-dominant pattern of inheritance. Linkage analysis in typical migraine has not, however, proved so successful and association studies, more suited to a multifactorial disease, remain negative, provisional or controversial. They have nevertheless led to the identification of candidate genes that may be implicated in migraine, and are discussed here.

# Is migraine hereditary?

Traditional means employed in genetic studies of migraine have been, as for other diseases, the detailed analysis of migraine pedigrees: searching for evidence of particular patterns of hereditary transmission; the study of twins, by comparing prevalence rates of migraine among mono- and dizygotic twins, raised together or apart, in order to dissect the relative contribution of environmental and genetic influences; epidemiological studies of the disease risk among relatives of probands with migraine compared with that of the control population or spouses/partners of probands, again with the aim of apportioning environmental and genetic rates of causation and thus calculating a heritability index. The application of statistical models also gives useful insights about the genetic patterning of the disease.

Segregation analysis of family data performed in 128 patients with migraine showed that neither an autosomal dominant nor a recessive model of simple mendelian inheritance was supported by the data, thus suggesting that migraine is characterized by genetic heterogeneity.[7] Baier[8] examined 81 children with migraine and found that inheritance of the trait was mainly from the maternal side, irrespective of the sex of the index case; onset of migraine was earlier with higher familial impact of migraine. Again, however, the findings did not conform to simple mendelian inheritance, and a multifactorial pathogenesis was suggested. A series of papers from Russell and co-workers[1,9–14] have been dedicated to complex segregation analysis of MO and MA in a Danish population. Compared with the general population, first-degree relatives of probands with MO had a threefold increased risk of MO, whereas first-degree relatives of probands with MA had a twofold increased risk for both MA and MO; these findings strongly suggest a genetic determination of migraine. Complex segregation analysis was, however, in favour of a multifactorial inheritance. In further studies, spouses were compared to first-degree relatives, in addition to a control population: although no increased risk was found for spouses of MA probands (compared with a fourfold increase in first-degree relatives), spouses of MO probands showed a 1.5-fold increased risk for MO (compared with 1.9 for first-degree relatives); these findings suggest a strict genetic determination for MA but a mixed one, environmental and genetic, for MO. When further analysing 31 families with an apparently autosomal-dominant transmission of MA, a statistically significant lower risk than expected of MA in first- and second-degree relatives did not confirm a true autosomal-dominant pattern, and a recessive one was unlikely because of unequal sex distribution.

Maternal and X-linked transmissions could be likewise excluded, thus warranting the conclusion that, even in apparently autosomal-dominant families with MA, a multifactorial inheritance was likely.[1] Throughout their works these authors remarked on the several shortcomings hampering research into the genetic causes of migraine, such as selection of probands not from the general population but rather from selected clinics, a lack of distinction between MA and MO and, in particular, obtaining family history through questionnaires or from probands, instead of by direct interview.[15] Indeed, migraine assessment by proband report is not satisfactory, because the number of affected relatives is highly underestimated[15,16] and direct interviews with each relative are required.

These shortcomings notwithstanding, several previous studies had reached similar conclusions. A familial aggregation suggestive of a hereditary factor of migraine was found in 53% of urban and 39% of rural patients in a Mexican population,[17] and multifactorial inheritance was hypothesized as the most likely pattern in a Greek sample.[18] In a Finnish paediatric population, headache in the mother before pregnancy was predictive of headache in the child, and children with headaches more frequently had first- and second-degree relatives with headache.[19] In a US general population, the risk of migraine was 50% more likely in relatives of migraine probands, especially if migraine was disabling.[20] A high degree of heritability was found for both MO and MA in an Italian population; both maternal and X-linked transmission were excluded and, although an autosomal recessive pattern was considered the most likely, the presence of additional genetic and environmental factors was suggested.[6] According to D'Amico et al,[21] MO was significantly more frequent among relatives, especially females, of probands, and a sex-limited transmission mode the most likely pattern of transmission. Finally, a family history in the parents was reported as a favourable prognostic indicator in MA.[22] There is therefore universal agreement that the risk for migraine, whether MA or MO, is increased among relatives of probands with migraine, and the lower or absent risk in spouses is an indication of the scant effect of the environment.

Several studies in twins concur with this conclusion. Monozygotic twins, especially females, have higher concordance rates for lifetime migraine[23] and 40–50% of the liability to migraine was attributed to genetic factors in another population study of 2690 mono- and

5497 dizygotic pairs.[24] In 154 pairs of twins raised together and 43 raised apart since infancy, all analysed for zygosity, the heritability estimate came to 52%,[25] to 65% (similar in males and females) in a set of Danish twins with MA[26] and 61% in a similar set of twins with MO.[27] In Swedish twin children, inheritance for liability to headaches was estimated at 70%.[28] However, when 51 migraine concordant monozygotic twin pairs were analysed for clinical characteristics, 20 pairs were concordant for MA and 6 for MO, whereas 12 pairs were mixed, and thus discordant for the aura. Therefore not all of the phenotypic differences between MA and MO could be explained by genetic factors; these authors hypothesized that different liability loci account for aura and headache in migraine, and that the distribution of these different loci together with environmental factors accounts for the development of MA or MO.[29] Overall, these twin studies provide evidence that approximately half of the variability in migraine may be attributable to genetic factors, probably cumulative, with the remainder caused by environmental influences, probably not shared between the twins.[30]

Finally, it is intriguing to observe that genetic influences may be detected by electrophysiological techniques performed in migraine patients. Contingent negative variation slow potentials have a particularly high amplitude in migraine patients and may also be increased in asymptomatic siblings of migraine children, suggesting family-related cortical hypersensitivity.[31] Migraine patients display deficient habituation of visual evoked potentials and intensity dependence of auditory cortical evoked potentials: these traits were found to be common among related parents and children with migraine;[32] photo-

sensitivity is a trait found in migraine families even in asymptomatic members.[33] These initial studies augur well for the possibility of detecting a 'migraine threshold' by means of clinical neurophysiological techniques, thus providing the long sought for laboratory marker. On the other hand, induction of migraine attacks by means of nitroglycerine or *m*-chlorophenylpiperazine in normal individuals with a family history of migraine,[34] may indicate that there are pharmacological means of detecting such a 'migraine trait' and these should be explored.

## Familial hemiplegic migraine, episodic ataxia type 2, spinocerebellar ataxia type 6 and CACNA1A

Familial hemiplegic migraine is a subtype of MA characterized by some degree of hemiparesis during the aura.[4] FHM has been recognized as hereditary and indeed, for diagnosis, the presence of similar symptoms in at least another first-degree relative is required. The pattern of inheritance has also been identified since the first clinical descriptions as autosomal dominant; thus FHM constitutes a mendelian form of MA. Long before its genetic characterization, however, it was recognized that FHM was heterogeneous. In fact, some families with FHM displayed clinically relevant cerebellar symptoms such as ataxia or signs such as nystagmus, whereas in others these signs were absent. Other clinical expressions found in FHM were epileptic seizures, possibly during the attacks, and the triggering of the attacks by even trivial head trauma. In other cases, the phenotype was complicated by psychosis, coma or pleocytosis and neck stiffness during the attacks, simulating a meningoencephalitis.[35] Some of this phenotypic variability can now be explained on the basis of genetics. In 1993, linkage studies led to assignment of FHM to the short arm of chromosome 19p13,[36] and in 1996 further refinements identified the gene responsible for FHM in *CACNA1A* (also termed *CACNL1A4*).[37] *CACNA1A* defines a gene that specifies the $\alpha_1$-subunit of a neuronal P/Q type calcium channel and is composed of 47 exons in about 300 kilobases (kb). The $\alpha_1$-subunit forms the pore of the channel and seems to be implicated in the voltage regulation of the channel. The four missense mutations originally described, at codons 192, 666, 714 and 1181, were localized at the channel pore and were later shown to alter the electrophysiological characteristics and the density of the channels, although not all did so in the same manner.

Loss and gain of function were effects observed with different mutations, and there was no correlation between the resulting clinical phenotype and the electrophysiological characteristics of the mutations,[38] an indication of the complexities of the pathogenic mechanisms underlying FHM. An intriguing result of the linkage analysis was the demonstration that FHM is a disease allelic with episodic ataxia type 2 (EA2), which is characterized by attacks of variable duration of cerebellar ataxia with interictal nystagmus, and which was shown to be linked to mutations in the same *CACNA1A* gene, but now disrupting the reading frame and generating an abnormal protein.[37] Finally, spinocerebellar ataxia type 6 (SCA6) was also shown to map to the *CACNA1A* gene and to be caused by expansions in the CAG repeats at the 3′ terminus of the gene.[39] Thus, three different diseases,

FHM, EA2 and SCA6, were surprisingly found to result from mutations, albeit of different kinds, in the same gene, and all linked to episodic and progressive cerebellar ataxia with migraine. Later reports have vastly increased the number of mutations in the *CACNA1A* gene, and shown that the specificity of the types of mutation – missense for FHM, in the reading frame for EA2 and polyglutamine repeats in SCA6 – is not so strict; there is some, as yet not completely charted, degree of overlap in clinical expression among these three allelic diseases.[40] In fact, cerebellar ataxia may be a symptom in FHM families that seems to be related to some mutations only (666 and 583 in particular) and not to others, and the 715 mutation is associated with essential tremor occurring together with FHM. Why these particular mutations result in additional progressive cerebellar ataxia and atrophy is still unclear, and apparently unrelated to the electrophysiological characteristics in vitro of the mutated channel, as already described.

Familial hemiplegic migraine is genetically heterogeneous. In 1997 a new locus for FHM was mapped to 1q31 in a multigenerational American family,[41] and again to chromosome 1 but to 1q21–23 in three French families with FHM.[42] It is still unclear whether the two new loci of linkage are really separate or one and the same. A review of the clinical characteristics of these families mapping to chromosome 1 indicates that penetrance is lower than with the *CACNA1A* families, and that some patients may develop epileptic seizures during the attack, a feature not observed in FHM linked to chromosome 19. Ataxia, whether episodic or progressive, has not, however, been observed in families with FHM linking to chromosome 1, at least not until now. FHM families linking to chromosome 1 are rarer than FHM linked to *CACNA1A*, and there are still families that do not link to either locus. Even for so rare a disease as FHM, therefore, there is evidence for relevant genetic heterogeneity, and at least three genes and probably more must be implicated.

# Linkage and association studies in typical migraine

After the discovery that FHM maps to the *CACNA1A* gene on chromosome 19 and as obligate carriers in FHM families could display features of MO or MA only, several studies were devoted to the possibility that this gene could also involved in the pathogenesis of the more common forms of migraine, e.g. MO and MA. Even before the identification of the gene, a linkage study performed with markers near the FHM locus on 19p13 in four families from Finland, a population characterized by reduced genetic heterogeneity, gave negative results.[43] However, sib-pair analysis in one migraine family (out of 28) indicated that affected sibs shared the same marker allele D19S394 (highly informative for FHM), suggesting that the gene on 19p13 is involved in the aetiology of the common forms of migraine too.[44,45] Similar conclusions were reached in one family by Nyholt et al.[46] In a study of seven Italian families with MO and seven with MA, studied with linkage and sib-pair analysis, uniformly negative results were obtained, and the more common mutations in the *CACNA1A* gene were also excluded.[47] Kim et al[48] sequenced the whole *CACNA1A* gene, exons and introns, in nine American families with autosomal-dominant periodic vertigo and migraine (closely mimicking FHM features) and could not find any mutation.

Thus, until now, no family with only MO or MA has been conclusively shown to harbour mutations in the *CACNA1A* gene, and the role of this gene in the genetic determination of the most common forms of migraine is unclear, and unlikely to be highly relevant.

Recent linkage studies in two large Australian pedigrees led to significant linkage of migraine to Xq24–28.[49] Other linkage and association studies have instead been devoted to candidate genes chosen for their possible pathogenic involvement according to fashionable hypotheses. Pedigree analysis has never suggested any mitochondrial (mt) inheritance;[6] however, based on the striking clinical similarities between some mitochondrial encephalomyopathies such as MELAS (mitochondrial encephalomyopathy with lactic acidosis and stroke), and MA or migraine with prolonged aura or migraine stroke, several searches have been made for mtDNA mutations (e.g. the 3243, 3271, 11084, mitochondrial deletions) even in multigenerational female-transmitting families, with negative results.[2,50] The occasional cases of migraine harbouring mitochondrial mutations[51] should therefore be considered phenocopies. Interestingly, however, mitochondrial deletions have been reported in children with cyclical vomiting syndrome and migraine,[52] secondary LHON mutations 4216 and 13708 were more common in patients with stroke and MA,[53] and the U mitochondrial haplogroup has been associated with increased risk for occipital stroke in migraine.[54] It is therefore possible that mt DNA mutations act as phenotype modifiers or risk factors for vascular co-morbidity in migraine.

Allelic variation in serotonin (5HT) receptor genes has likewise been explored in migraine populations, based on the rationale of the efficacy of the triptans in the treatment of the attack and the prophylactic properties of serotoninergic drugs. The $5HT_{2A}$ and $5HT_{2C}$ genes were, however, found not to be involved[47,55–57] and variability at the $5HT_{1B}$ receptor, the one involved in the response to sumatriptan, did not account for the treatment effect.[58] An altered allelic distribution at the 5HT transporter gene in MO and MA was shown by Ogilvie et al[59] but not by Monari et al.[47] Negative or controversial results also apply to dopamine receptors chosen as candidate genes on the basis of the hypothetical involvement of dopamine in the pathogenesis of the migraine attack. Allele NcoI of the dopamine receptor gene 2 (DRD2) was found to be implicated in liability to MA and in the co-morbidity of MA with anxiety and depression,[60,61] and in liability to nausea and yawning during the attack of MO in a Sardinian sample of 50 nuclear families (the whole sample was negative, Del Zompo et al[62]). However, no allelic association with this allele could be found in MA or MO by other authors,[63,64] and dopamine receptors 3 and 4 and other dopamine metabolism enzymes such as MAO-A (monoamine oxidase A) and COMT were also excluded.[62,64]

Pro-thrombotic factors have also been investigated, in the hope of explaining the well-known co-morbidity of migraine with stroke. The factor V Leiden mutation, conferring resistance on activated protein C, has been widely investigated by means of association studies, with either negative[65–67] or positive results.[68,69] Negative associations have been reported with the 20210 prothrombin gene mutation,[66,70] the platelet HPA-1 and HPA-2 alloantigens and the decanucleotide insertion/deletion in factor VII promoter.[66] Positive associations have been described by Paterna et al[71] between angiotensin-converting enzyme gene deletion polymorphism and frequency of MO, and by Kowa et al[72] between migraine and methylenetetrahydrofolate reductase gene C677T mutation, responsible for hyperhomocysteinaemia. Linkage and association studies excluded a role for the endothelial nitric oxide synthase gene (NOS3) in migraine,[73] for complement C3F and C3S[74] and for cytochrome P450 2D6 and glutathione S-transferase M1 genotypes.[75] A protective association between HLA-DR2 antigens and MA was reported by Martelletti et al.[76]

All of these association studies suffer from recognized problems in epidemiological surveys: small samples, selection from populations that are not truly representative of the disease (clinic populations), problems in the choice of controls, insufficient clinical homogeneity, etc.; all therefore need replication in much larger and better controlled samples. Moreover, proof of genetics is not proof of pathogenic association. A more substantial problem is also implied: the extent to which association studies are capable of extricating the genetic influences of modifier genes from the truly 'causative' migraine 'genes' remains unclear. Indeed, migraine co-morbidity, possibly related to modifying genes (and most probably environmental influences too), is not migraine, and the clinical features of migraine are sufficiently homogeneous and stereotyped over different populations, occupational statuses and economic classes to warrant the existence of a 'core' of truly 'migrainous' genes. Assembling a bewildering variety of genetic associations, in the hope of finding the cause of a disease that remains similar and true to itself throughout the life of an individual, and throughout different members of the same family, different families of the same population and different populations of the world, is probably just a fancy, and anyway probably insufficient in the detection of the mechanisms specific for migraine.

## Migraine co-morbidity and syndromic migraine

Clinical and epidemiological observations confirm that migraines have significant co-morbidity; this has been subjected to genetic analysis. Psychiatric disorders, specifically anxiety and depression are particularly frequent in migraineurs and their relatives[77,78] and women with bipolar disorders are frequently affected by migraine.[79] Children with headache have a higher proportion of mothers with a history of depression; also, maternal depression and migraine correlate with abdominal migraine and pain in the child.[80] However, it is hard to discount environmental influences on this latter point, even though genetic associations have been reported with psychiatric co-morbidity of migraine and allelic distribution at the DRD2 gene.[61]

Co-morbidity of migraine with epilepsy is a well-known issue, and one that is implied by the genetics of FHM: in fact epileptic seizures occur in FHM families linked to chromosome 1, and CACNA1A is a gene that, when mutated, causes absence seizures in the mouse.[81] Epidemiological studies in humans, however, remain inconclusive, either excluding[82] or confirming[83] an association between migraine and epilepsy. There is little doubt that some epileptic syndromes – myoclonic epilepsy, and benign partial epilepsy of the rolandic or occipital type – are specifically associated with headache or migraine[84,85] and the same applies to some paroxysmal movement disorders, such as kine-

siogenic paroxysmal dyskinesia, which is also probably epileptic in origin.[86] The genetic mechanisms of these associations (if these can be said to be true genetic associations) remain unexplored. Recently, the CACNA1A gene was implicated in the pathogenesis of primary epilepsy based on association studies.

Parental history of migraine is a risk factor for allergic rhinitis, bronchial asthma and eczema in the child,[87,88] and migraine itself is particularly frequent in these children.[89] Rhinitis in children correlates with maternal migraine. These interesting correlations seem to implicate immunity or inflammation in the pathogenesis or at least co-morbidity of migraine but, except for HLA determinants,[76] there is still no genetic study of such associations. The same also holds for other reported co-morbid associations of migraine, e.g. with vertigo and essential tremor,[90,91] primary dyslipoproteinaemias,[92] and vomiting and motion sickness.[93] A final consideration must be given to the fact that migraine attacks, often indistinguishable from those encountered in typical migraines, may be part of the spectrum of other hereditary diseases, some of which are well characterized genetically (syndromic migraine). CADASIL (cerebral autosomal dominant arteriopathy with subcortical infarcts and leukoencephalopathy) is a well-known MA mimicker,[94] and related to mutations in the Notch3 gene, one of a family that is involved in the specification of the fate of neural cells and neural boundaries.[95] Other syndromes in which migraine attacks may recur are Chiari type I malformation,[96] paroxysmal exercise-induced dystonia,[97] familial alternating hemiplegia of childhood,[98] familial multiple cavernomatosis,[99] hereditary endotheliopathy with retinopathy, nephropathy and stroke (HERNS),[100] etc. The molecular basis of these syndromes, which might provide insights into the pathogenesis of the more common migraine headaches, are still unknown, except for familial cavernomatosis type 1, which is related to mutation in *KRIT1*, an ankyrin repeat-containing protein.[101]

## Conclusions

The genetics of migraine headaches is a fascinating but complex topic. In fact, the above review of the studies performed until now clearly shows that the only certain data pertain to FHM, a variety of MA that conforms to mendelian transmission. The success obtained with FHM probably resulted from the fact that FHM has a clearly delineated autosomal pattern of inheritance and a characteristic phenotypic expression. Yet, even FHM shows incomplete penetrance (from 80% to 60% in families mapping to chromosome 19 and 1, respectively) and there are monozygotic twins discordant for the trait.[102] The fact that mutations in a calcium channel subunit underlie FHM and other paroxysmal disorders, such as episodic ataxia type 2 and seizures (in the animal model), has led to the proposal that migraines be considered as channelopathies, and that migraine and seizures all belong to a spectrum of calcium-related channel disorders.[103] This concept certainly applies to FHM, but has still to be validated for the more common MA and MO types, because no family with pure MA and MO has yet been demonstrated to harbour mutations in the *CACNA1A* gene. Moreover, syndromic migraine (e.g. migraine in CADASIL or MELAS syndromes, etc.) is not related to genetic abnormalities in ion channel genes. The concept of migraine as a channelopathy is alluring, because it incorporates the notion of

a threshold that is consistently supported by electrophysiological findings. It is hoped that future studies will clarify this issue, and confirm in particular whether FHM mapping to chromosome 1 is also the result of genetically abnormal ion channel function.

Apart from FHM, however, the results of genetic investigations with the more common types of migraine are still under scrutiny, and many need confirmation in larger and different population sizes. Thus, migraine follows a pattern that is common to many so-called multifactorial diseases which have high prevalence rates in the general population. There are several considerations in favour of a multifactorial model for migraine: the recurrence risk for migraine increases according to the number of affected family members, and both age at onset occurs earlier and risk increases with increased severity of migraine attacks and number of affected relatives;[8] however, other conditions are not exactly respected, e.g. the ratio for recurrence risk in first-degree and second-degree relatives of migraine probands[8] and, from a more general point of view, there is no evidence that migraine is a quantitative trait with a normal distribution in the population. Considering migraine as a multifactorial disease does not unfortunately offer any clue to the possible genes involved or even evidence of the pattern of gene involvement. A multifactorial model implicates a threshold among the general population above which genetic liability gives rise to the disease and, more to the point, there is an implication that such genetic liability has a continuum distribution in the general population. This is unsubstantiated. It is highly unlikely that migraine, a self-consistent disease with a stereotyped expression for both features of the attacks and disease course for each affected individual and across populations with diverse genetic backgrounds, customs and mores, may be caused by the random assembly of a series of polymorphisms and mutations in unrelated genes. This 'harlequin' model does not provide for a coherent pathogenic explanation of the disease, and the risk of such an approach is that of searching for disparate genes for each phenotypic aspect of migraine and its co-morbidity (how many genes for aura – and for how many types of aura?, how many genes for nausea, for vomiting, how many for pain, how many for the response to triptans and other drugs, how many for rhythmicity of attacks, how many for oestrogen modulation?).

Such an approach does not make sense: migraine cannot be caused by a random collection of modifying characters, with nothing left to modify! In this respect, the heuristic value of association studies must be carefully evaluated for a more useful application. Most probably, the genetic liability to migraine relates to some selected genes acting in concert along one or a few biochemical pathways – a cohort of genes so to speak – and migraine is a composite term, indicating several mendelian characters that interact in families and of course modified in their expression by other related and unrelated genes (oligogenetic model). As migraine as a whole sets in during the interval years around puberty, genes coding for receptors and for modifiers of protein function are more probable candidates.[104] Moreover, as migraine represents a genetic trait that is seemingly not associated with increased overall mortality, and that apparently does not reduce life expectancy or reproduction (there are even data that migraine is associated with increased longevity[105]), we must conclude that migraine genes have some positive adaptive value. In this regard, it is remarkable that MA patients have been found to display higher visual perceptual abilities than controls.[106] If the oligogenic model is true, an effort should be made to dissect further the phenotypes of migraines, to verify their familial and twin concordance, and to apply genetic analysis to selected families and phenotypes.

# Acknowledgements

I thank Ms A. Laffi for help with the manuscript and the references, and Ms A. Collins for revising the English. The work was supported by CNR no. 99.02536.CT04, and MURST ex-60% 1999–2000 grants.

# References

1. Ulrich V, Russell MB, Ostergaard S, Olesen J, Analysis of 31 families with an apparently autosomal-dominant transmission of migraine with aura in the nuclear family. *Am J Med Genet* 1997; **74**: 395–7.
2. Buzzi MG, Di Gennaro G, D'Onofrio M et al, mtDNA A3243G MELAS mutation is not associated with multigenerational female migraine. *Neurology* 2000; **54**: 1005–7.
3. Launer LJ, Terwindt GM, Ferrari MD, The prevalence and characteristics of migraine in a population-based cohort: the GEM study. *Neurology* 1999; **53**: 537–42.
4. Headache Classification Committee of the International Headache Society, Classification and diagnostic criteria for headache disorders, cranial neuralgias and facial pain. *Cephalalgia* 1988; **8**(suppl): 19–28.
5. Shevell MI, Familial acephalgic migraines. *Neurology* 1997; **48**: 776–7.
6. Mochi M, Sangiorgi S, Cortelli P et al, Testing models for genetic determination in migraine. *Cephalalgia* 1993; **13**: 389–94.
7. Devoto M, Lozito A, Staffa G, D'Alessandro R, Sacquegna T, Romeo G, Segregation

analysis of migraine in 128 families. *Cephalalgia* 1986; **6**: 101–5.

8. Baier WK, Genetics of migraine and migraine accompagnee: a study of eighty-one children and their families. *Neuropediatrics* 1985; **16**: 84–91.

9. Russell MB, Olesen J, The genetics of migraine without aura and migraine with aura. *Cephalalgia* 1993; **13**: 245–8.

10. Russell MB, Hilden J, Sørensen SA, Olesen J, Familial occurrence of migraine without aura and migraine with aura. *Neurology* 1993; **43**: 1369–73.

11. Russell MB, Olesen J, Increased familial risk and evidence of genetic factor in migraine. *BMJ* 1995; **311**: 541–4.

12. Russell MB, Iselius L, Olesen J, Inheritance of migraine investigated by complex segregation analysis. *Hum Genet* 1995; **96**: 726–30.

13. Russell MB, Iselius L, Olesen J, Migraine without aura and migraine with aura are inherited disorders. *Cephalalgia* 1996; **16**: 305–9.

14. Gervil M, Ulrich V, Kaprio J, Olesen J, Russell MB, The relative role of genetic and environmental factors in migraine without aura. *Neurology* 1999; **53**: 995–9.

15. Russell MB, Fenger K, Olesen J, The family history of migraine. Direct versus indirect information. *Cephalalgia* 1996; **16**: 156–60.

16. Ottman R, Hong S, Lipton RB, Validity of family history data on severe headache and migraine. *Neurology* 1993; **43**: 1954–60.

17. Alonso Vilatela ME, Garcia Pedroza F, Ziegler DK, Gonzalez Mendez A, Familial migraine in a Mexican population. *Neuroepidemiology* 1992; **11**: 46–9.

18. Kalfakis N, Panas M, Vassilopoulos D, Malliara-Loulakaki S, Migraine with aura: segregation analysis and heritability estimation. *Headache* 1996; **36**: 320–2.

19. Aromaa M, Rautava P, Sillanpää M, Helenius H, Ojanlatva A, Familial occurrence of headache. *Cephalalgia* 1999; **19**(suppl 25): 49–52.

20. Stewart WF, Staffa J, Lipton RB, Ottman R, Familial risk of migraine: a population-based study. *Ann Neurol* 1997; **41**: 166–72.

21. D'Amico D, Leone M, Macciardi F, Valentini S, Bussone G, Genetic transmission of migraine without aura: a study of 68 families. *Ital J Neurol Sci* 1991; **12**: 581–4.

22. Cologno D, Torelli P, Manzoni GC, Possible predictive factors in the prognosis of migraine with aura. *Cephalalgia* 1999; **19**: 824–30.

23. Larsson B, Bille B, Pedersen NL, Genetic influence in headaches: a Swedish twin study. *Headache* 1995; **35**: 513–19.

24. Honkasalo ML, Kaprio J, Winter T, Heikkila K, Sillanpää M, Koskenvuo M, Migraine and concomitant symptoms among 8167 adult twin pairs. *Headache* 1995; **35**: 70–8.

25. Ziegler DK, Hur YM, Bouchard TJ Jr, Hassanein RS, Barter R, Migraine in twins raised together and apart. *Headache* 1998; **38**: 417–22.

26. Ulrich V, Gervil M, Kyvik KO, Olesen J, Russell MB, The inheritance of migraine with aura estimated by means of structural equation modelling. *J Med Genet* 1999; **36**: 225–7.

27. Gervil M, Ulrich V, Kyvik KO, Olesen J, Russell MB, Migraine without aura: a population-based twin study. *Ann Neurol* 1999; **46**: 606–11.

28. Svensson DA, Larsson B, Bille B, Lichtenstein P, Genetic and environmental influences on recurrent headaches in eight- to nine-year-old twins. *Cephalalgia* 1999; **19**: 866–72.

29. Kallela M, Wessman M, Farkkila M et al, Clinical characteristics of migraine concordant monozygotic twin pairs. *Acta Neurol Scand* 1999; **100**: 254–9.

30. Merikangas KR, Genetics of migraine and other headache. *Curr Opin Neurol* 1996; **9**: 202–5.

31. Kropp P, Kirbach U, Detlefsen JO, Siniatchkin M, Gerber WD, Stephani U, Slow cortical potentials in migraine: a comparison of adults and children. *Cephalalgia* 1999; **19**(suppl 25): 60–4.

32. Sandor PS, Afra J, Proietti-Cecchini A, Albert A, Schoenen J, Familial influences on cortical evoked potentials in migraine. *Neuroreport* 1999; **10**: 1235–8.

33. Lahat E, Nadir E, Barr J, Eshel G, Aladjem

M, Bistritze T, Visual evoked potentials: a diagnostic test for migraine headache in children. *Dev Med Child Neurol* 1997; **39**: 85–7.

34. Catarci T, Clifford Rose F, Migraine and heredity. *Pathol Biol* 1992; **40**: 284–6.

35. Fitzsimons RB, Wolfenden WH, Migraine coma. Meningitic migraine with cerebral oedema associated with a new form of autosomal dominant cerebellar ataxia. *Brain* 1985; **108**: 555–77.

36. Joutel A, Bousser MG, Biousse V et al, A gene for familial hemiplegic migraine maps to chromosome 19. *Nat Genet* 1993; **5**: 40–5.

37. Ophoff RA, Terwindt GM, Vergouwe MN et al, Familial hemiplegic migraine and episodic ataxia type-2 are caused by mutations in the $Ca^{2+}$ channel gene CACNL1A4. *Cell* 1996; **87**: 543–52.

38. Hans M, Luvisetto S, Williams ME et al, Functional consequences of mutations in the human alpha1A calcium channel subunit linked to familial hemiplegic migraine. *J Neurosci* 1999; **19**: 1610–19.

39. Zhuchenko O, Bailey J, Bonnen P et al, Autosomal dominant cerebellar ataxia (SCA6) associated with small polyglutamine expansions in the alpha 1A-voltage-dependent calcium channel. *Nat Genet* 1997; **15**: 62–9.

40. Montagna P, Molecular genetics of migraine headaches: a review. *Cephalalgia* 2000; **20**: 3–14.

41. Gardner K, Barmada MM, Ptacek LJ, Hoffman EP, A new locus for hemiplegic migraine maps to chromosome 1q31. *Neurology* 1997; **49**: 1231–8.

42. Ducros A, Joutel A, Vahedi K et al, Mapping of a second locus for familial hemiplegic migraine to 1q21-q23 and evidence of further heterogeneity. *Ann Neurol* 1997; **42**: 885–90.

43. Hovatta I, Kallela M, Farkkila M, Peltonen L, Familial migraine: exclusion of the susceptibility gene from the reported locus of familial hemiplegic migraine on 19p. *Genomics* 1994; **23**: 707–9.

44. May A, Ophoff RA, Terwindt GM et al, Familial hemiplegic migraine locus on 19p13 is involved in the common forms of migraine

with and without aura. *Hum Genet* 1995; **96**: 604–8.

45. Ophoff RA, Terwindt GM, Vergouwe MN, Frants RR, Ferrari MD, Wolff Award 1997. Involvement of a $Ca^{2+}$ channel gene in familial hemiplegic migraine and migraine with and without aura. Dutch Migraine Genetics Research Group. *Headache* 1997; **37**: 479–85.

46. Nyholt DR, Lea RA, Goadsby PJ, Brimage PJ, Griffiths LR, Familial typical migraine: linkage to chromosome 19p13 and evidence for genetic heterogeneity. *Neurology* 1998; **50**: 1428–32.

47. Monari L, Mochi M, Valentino ML et al, Searching for migraine genes: exclusion of 290 cM out of the whole human genome. *Ital J Neurol Sci* 1997; **18**: 277–82.

48. Kim JS, Yue Q, Jen JC, Nelson SF, Baloh RW, Familial migraine with vertigo: no mutations found in CACNA1A. *Am J Med Genet* 1998; **79**: 148–51.

49. Nyholt DR, Curtain RP, Griffiths LR, Familial typical migraine: significant linkage and localization of a gene to Xq24–28. *Hum Genet* 2000; **107**: 18–23.

50. Haan J, Terwindt GM, Maassen JA, Hart LM, Frants RR, Ferrari MD, Search for mitochondrial DNA mutations in migraine subgroups. *Cephalalgia* 1999; **19**: 20–2.

51. Bresolin N, Martinelli P, Barbiroli B et al, Muscle mitochondrial DNA deletion and $^{31}$P-NMR spectroscopy alterations in a migraine patient. *J Neurol Sci* 1991; **104**: 182–9.

52. Boles RG, Williams JC, Mitochondrial disease and cyclic vomiting syndrome. *Dig Dis Sci* 1999; **44**: 103S–7S.

53. Ojaimi J, Katsabanis S, Bower S, Quigley A, Byrne E, Mitochondrial DNA in stroke and migraine with aura. *Cerebrovasc Dis* 1998; **8**: 102–6.

54. Majamaa K, Finnila S, Turkka J, Hassinen IE, Mitochondrial DNA haplogroup U as a risk factor for occipital stroke in migraine. *Lancet* 1998; **352**: 455–6.

55. Nyholt DR, Curtain RP, Gaffney PT, Brimage P, Goadsby PJ, Griffiths LR, Migraine association and linkage analyses of

the human 5-hydroxytryptamine ($5HT_{2A}$) receptor gene. *Cephalalgia* 1996; **16**: 463–7.

56. Buchwalder A, Welch SK, Peroutka SJ, Exclusion of $5\text{-}HT_{2A}$ and $5\text{-}HT_{2C}$ receptor genes as candidate genes for migraine. *Headache* 1996; **36**: 254–8.

57. Burnet PW, Harrison PJ, Goodwin GM et al, Allelic variation in the serotonin 5-HT2C receptor gene and migraine. *Neuroreport* 1997; **8**: 2651–3.

58. Maassen VanDenBrink A, Vergouwe MN et al, Chromosomal localization of the 5-HT1F receptor gene: no evidence for involvement in response to sumatriptan in migraine patients. *Am J Med Genet* 1998; **77**: 415–20.

59. Ogilvie AD, Russell MB, Dhall P et al, Altered allelic distributions of the serotonin transporter gene in migraine without aura and migraine with aura. *Cephalalgia* 1998; **18**: 23–6.

60. Peroutka SJ, Wilhoit T, Jones K, Clinical susceptibility to migraine with aura is modified by dopamine D2 receptor (DRD2) NcoI alleles. *Neurology* 1997; **49**: 201–6.

61. Peroutka SJ, Price SC, Wilhoit TL, Jones KW, Comorbid migraine with aura, anxiety, and depression is associated with dopamine D2 receptor (DRD2) NcoI alleles. *Mol Med* 1998; **4**: 14–21.

62. Del Zompo M, Cherchi A, Palmas MA et al, Association between dopamine receptor genes and migraine without aura in a Sardinian sample. *Neurology* 1998; **51**: 781–6.

63. Dichgans M, Forderreuther S, Deiterich M, Pfaffenrath V, Gasser T, The $D_2$ receptor NcoI allele: absence of allelic association with migraine with aura. *Neurology* 1998; **51**: 928.

64. Mochi M, Monari L, Valentino ML et al, Migraine and dopamine metabolism related genes: a genetic association study. *Cephalalgia* 2000; **20**: 265–7.

65. Haan J, Kappelle LJ, de Ronde H, Ferrari MD, Bertina RM, The factor V Leiden mutation (R506Q) is not a major risk factor for migrainous cerebral infarction. *Cephalalgia* 1997; **17**: 605–7.

66. Corral J, Iniesta JA, Gonzalez-Conejero R, Lozano ML, Rivera J, Vicente V, Migraine and prothrombotic genetic risk factors. *Cephalalgia* 1998; **18**: 257–60.

67. Soriani S, Borgna-Pignatti C, Trabetti E, Casartelli A, Montagna P, Pignatti PF, Frequency of factor V Leiden in juvenile migraine with aura. *Headache* 1998; **38**: 779–81.

68. Kontula K, Ylikorkala A, Miettinen H et al, Arg506Gln factor V mutation (factor V Leiden) in patients with ischaemic cerebrovascular disease and survivors of myocardial infarction. *Thromb Haemost* 1995; **73**: 558–60.

69. D'Amico D, Moschiano F, Leone M et al, Genetic abnormalities of the protein C system: shared risk factors in young adults with migraine with aura and with ischemic stroke? *Cephalalgia* 1998; **18**: 618–21.

70. Haan J, Kappelle LJ, Ferrari MD, Bertina RM, The transition G to A at position 20210 in the 3′-untranslated region of the prothrombin gene is not associated with migrainous infarction. *Cephalalgia* 1998; **18**: 229–30.

71. Paterna S, Di Pasquale P, D'Angelo A et al, Angiotensin-converting enzyme gene deletion polymorphism determines an increase in frequency of migraine attacks in patients suffering from migraine without aura. *Eur Neurol* 2000; **43**: 133–6.

72. Kowa H, Yasui K, Takeshima T, Urakami K, Sakai F, Nakashima K, The homozygous C677T mutation in the methylenetetrahydrofolate reductase gene is a genetic risk factor for migraine. *Am J Med Genet* 2000; **96**: 762–4.

73. Griffiths LR, Nyholt DR, Curtain RP, Goadsby PJ, Brimage PJ, Migraine association and linkage studies of an endothelial nitric oxide synthase (NOS3) gene polymorphism. *Neurology* 1997; **49**: 614–17.

74. Peroutka SJ, Price SC, Jones KW, The comorbid association of migraine with osteoarthritis and hypertension: complement C3F and Berkson's bias. *Cephalalgia* 1997; **17**: 23–6.

75. Mattsson P, Bjelfman C, Lundberg PO, Rane A, Cytochrome P450 2D6 and glutathione S-

transferase M1 genotypes and migraine. *Eur J Clin Invest* 2000; **30**: 367–71.

76. Martelletti P, Lulli P, Morellini M et al, Chromosome 6p-encoded HLA-DR2 determination discriminates migraine without aura for migraine with aura. *Hum Immunol* 1999; **60**: 69–74.

77. Merikangas KR, Risch NJ, Merikangas JR, Weissman MM, Kidd KK, Migraine and depression: association and familial transmission. *J Psychiatr Res* 1988; **22**: 119–29.

78. Merikangas KR, Merikangas JR, Angst J, Headache syndromes and psychiatric disorders: association and familial transmission. *J Psychiatr Res* 1993; **27**: 197–210.

79. Blehar MC, DePaulo JR Jr, Gershon ES, Reich T, Simpson SG, Nurnberger JI Jr, Women with bipolar disorder: findings from the NIMH Genetics Initiative sample. *Psychopharmacol Bull* 1998; **34**: 239–43.

80. Mortimer MJ, Kay J, Jaron A, Good PA, Does a history of maternal migraine or depression predispose children to headache and stomach-ache? *Headache* 1992; **32**: 353–5.

81. Doyle J, Ren X, Lennon G, Stubbs L, Mutations in the Cacnl1a4 calcium channel gene are associated with seizures, cerebellar degeneration, and ataxia in tottering and leaner mutant mice. *Mamm Genome* 1997; **8**: 113–20.

82. Ottman R, Lipton RB, Is the comorbidity of epilepsy and migraine due to a shared genetic susceptibility? *Neurology* 1996; **47**: 918–24.

83. Guidetti V, Fornara R, Marchini R et al, Headache and epilepsy in childhood: analysis of a series of 620 children. *Funct Neurol* 1987; **2**: 323–41.

84. Saka E, Saygi S, Familial adult onset myoclonic epilepsy associated with migraine. *Seizure* 2000; **9**: 344–6.

85. Andermann F, Zifkin B, The benign occipital epilepsies of childhood: an overview of the idiopathic syndromes and of the relationship to migraine. *Epilepsia* 1998; **39**(suppl 4): S9–23.

86. Singh R, Macdonell RA, Scheffer IE, Crossland KM, Berkovic SF, Epilepsy and paroxysmal movement disorders in families: evidence for shared mechanisms. *Epileptic Disord* 1999; **1**: 93–9.

87. Gurkan F, Ece A, Haspolat K, Dikici B, Parental history of migraine and bronchial asthma in children. *Allergol Immunopathol (Madr)* 2000; **28**: 15–17.

88. Chen TC, Leviton A, Asthma and eczema in children born to women with migraine. *Arch Neurol* 1990; **47**: 1227–30.

89. Mortimer MJ, Kay J, Gawkrodger DJ, Jaron A, Barker DC, The prevalence of headache and migraine in atopic children: an epidemiological study in general practice. *Headache* 1993; **33**: 427–31.

90. Baloh RW, Foster CA, Yue Q, Nelson SF, Familial migraine with vertigo and essential tremor. *Neurology* 1996; **46**: 458–60.

91. Biary N, Koller W, Langenberg P, Correlation between essential tremor and migraine headache. *J Neurol Neurosurg Psychiatry* 1990; **53**: 1060–2.

92. Glueck CJ, Bates SR, Migraine in children: association with primary and familial dyslipoproteinemias. *Pediatrics* 1986; **77**: 316–21.

93. Jan MM, Camfield PR, Gordon K, Camfield CS, Vomiting after mild head injury is related to migraine. *J Pediatr* 1997; **130**: 134–7.

94. Verin M, Rolland Y, Landgraf F et al, New phenotype of the cerebral autosomal dominant arteriopathy mapped to chromosome 19: migraine as the prominent clinical feature. *J Neurol Neurosurg Psychiatry* 1995; **59**: 579–85.

95. Joutel A, Corpechot C, Ducros A et al, Notch3 mutations in cerebral autosomal dominant arteriopathy with subcortical infarcts and leukoencephalopathy (CADASIL), a mendelian condition causing stroke and vascular dementia. *Ann NY Acad Sci* 1997; **826**: 213–17.

96. Stovner LJ, Headache and Chiari type I malformation: occurrence in female monozygotic twins and first-degree relatives. *Cephalalgia* 1992; **12**: 304–7.

97. Munchau A, Valente EM, Shahidi GA et al, A new family with paroxysmal exercise induced

dystonia and migraine: a clinical and genetic study. *J Neurol Neurosurg Psychiatry* 2000; **68**: 609–14.

98. Andermann E, Andermann F, Silver K, Levin S, Arnold D, Benign familial nocturnal alternating hemiplegia of childhood. *Neurology* 1994; **44**: 1812–14.

99. Terriza F, Amrani Y, Asencio JJ, Goberna E, Casado A, Peralta JI, Familial multiple cavernomatosis. *Rev Neurol* 1997; **25**: 560–2.

100. Jen J, Cohen AH, Yue Q et al, Hereditary endotheliopathy with retinopathy, nephropathy, and stroke (HERNS). *Neurology* 1997; **49**: 1322–30.

101. Dubovsky J, Zabramski JM, Kurth J et al, A gene responsible for cavernous malformations of the brain maps to chromosome 7q. *Hum Mol Genet* 1995; **4**: 453–8.

102. Ducros A, Joutel A, Labauge P, Pages M, Bousser MG, Tournier-Lasserve E, Monozy-gotic twins discordant for familial hemiplegic migraine. *Neurology* 1995; **45**: 1222.

103. Terwindt GM, Ophoff RA, Haan J, Sandkuijl LA, Frants RR, Ferrari MD, Migraine, ataxia and epilepsy: a challenging spectrum of genetically determined calcium channelopathies. Dutch Migraine Genetics Research Group. *Eur J Hum Genet* 1998; **6**: 297–307.

104. Jimenez-Sanchez G, Childs B, Valle D, Human disease genes. *Nature* 2001; **409**: 853–5.

105. Waters WE, Campbell MJ, Elwood PC, Migraine, headache, and survival in women. *BMJ* 1983; **287**: 1442–3.

106. Mulleners WM, Chronicle EP, Palmer JE, Koehler PJ, Vredeveld JW, Suppression of perception in migraine: Evidence for reduced inhibition in the visual cortex. *Neurology* 2001; **56**: 178–83.

# 12

# Migraine: pathogenic concepts*

*Peter J Goadsby*

Our understanding of migraine has advanced considerably over the last century when compared to the previous 40 or so centuries.[2] This knowledge explosion has left a requirement to update physicians on the pathophysiology of migraine because understanding the disease can impact on diagnosis and management.[3] Time spent understanding the mechanisms of headache is well spent, given how common headache problems are and the expansion of migraine treatments that has taken place in the last few years.[4] If there is an age group in which the imperative for understanding the disease is most striking, it is in adolescents and children. This is because the clinical manifestations are more subtle and recognition of migraine requires a more searching clinical approach, although the patients can be no less disabled then their adult counterparts. Generally, the clinical features of migraine are less well developed in childhood: sometimes shorter attacks, perhaps fewer associated features, but still a life-disabling, biologically determined, manageable condition.

The following are essential elements to be considered (Table 12.1) in understanding migraine:

- Anatomy of head pain: the large intracranial vessels and dura mater, and their trigeminovascular innervation.

*This chapter has been modified from Goadsby.[1]

- Physiology and pharmacology of activation of the peripheral branches of the ophthalmic branch of the trigeminal nerve, as marked by plasma protein extravasation (PPE) and neuropeptide release.
- Physiology and pharmacology of the trigeminal nucleus, in particular its caudal-most part, the trigeminocervical complex.
- Central nervous system (CNS) activation in association with pain in the thalamus and cortical areas.
- Brain-stem and diencephalic modulatory systems that control trigeminal pain processing.

To understand migraine, we must integrate the anatomy and physiology that are presented here with the genetic predisposition (see Chapter 11) to have a full picture of the clinical problem. If nothing else, a family history helps patients and families alike to accept the basically biological nature of the disorder, and sometimes reduces often fruitless and pointless searches of psychopathology that is either not present or often simply co-morbid.

## Trigeminovascular anatomy: structures that produce pain

Surrounding the large cerebral vessels, pial vessels, large venous sinuses and dura mater is

| Target innervation | Structure | Comments |
|---|---|---|
| Cranial vessels | Ophthalmic branch of | |
| Dura mater | trigeminal nerve | |
|   First | Trigeminal ganglion | Middle cranial fossa |
|   Second | Trigeminal nucleus | Trigeminal nucleus caudalis |
| | *(quintothalamic tract)* | and C1/C2 dorsal horns |
|   Third | Thalamus | Ventrobasal complex |
| | | Medial nerve of posterior group |
| | | Intralaminar complex |
|   Final | Cortex | Insula |
| | | Frontal cortex |
| | | Anterior cingulate cortex |
| | | Basal ganglia |

**Table 12.1**
*Neuroanatomical processing of vascular head pain.*

a plexus of largely unmyelinated fibres that arise from the ophthalmic division of the trigeminal ganglion[5] and in the posterior fossa from the upper cervical dorsal roots.[6] Trigeminal fibres innervating cerebral vessels arise from neurons in the trigeminal ganglion, which contain substance P and calcitonin gene-related peptide (CGRP),[7] both of which can be released when the trigeminal ganglion is stimulated in either humans or cats.[8] Stimulation of the cranial vessels, such as the superior sagittal sinus, is certainly painful in humans.[9,10] Human dural nerves that innervate the cranial vessels consist largely of small-diameter myelinated and unmyelinated fibres, which almost certainly subserve a nociceptive function.[11]

A major question for migraine pathophysiology is what the source of the pain is. It must also be borne in mind that the pain process is likely to be a combination of direct factors, i.e. activation of the nociceptors of pain-produc-

ing intracranial structures, in concert with a reduction in the functioning of the endogenous pain control pathways that normally channel that pain.[12] Certainly, if the carotid artery is occluded ipsilateral to the side of headache in migraineurs, two-thirds of them will experience relief, although this does not account for the other one-third.[13] Moreover, distension of major cerebral vessels by balloon dilatation leads to pain referred to the ophthalmic division of the trigeminal nerve.[14–16] There is little doubt that sufficient changes in vascular diameter would produce pain. However, are the changes in migraine sufficient of themselves? When considering the contribution of the periphery and the brain, we must keep an open mind; we accept photophobia and phonophobia without any hint that there is peripheral change.

# *Trigeminovascular physiology*
## *Peripheral connections*

There is a considerable bulk of experimental animal and human work for understanding the physiology of activating trigeminal nociceptive afferents. These data allow us to build up a picture of what may happen during migraine and some plausible explanation of how the current acute anti-migraine compounds may work.[17]

### *Plasma protein extravasation*
Moskowitz[18] has provided an elegant series of experiments to suggest that some component of the pain of migraine may be a form of sterile neurogenic inflammation. Neurogenic plasma extravasation can be seen during electrical stimulation of the trigeminal ganglion in the rat.[19] Plasma extravasation can be blocked by ergot alkaloids,[20] indometacin,[21] acetylsalicylic acid,[21] and the serotonin $5HT_{1B/1D/1F}$ agonist, sumatriptan.[22] The pharmacology of the new abortive anti-migraine drugs, in the context of plasma protein extravasation, has recently been reviewed in detail.[23] In addition, there are structural changes seen in the dura mater which are seen with trigeminal ganglion stimulation, and these include mast cell degranulation[24] and changes in postcapillary venules, including platelet aggregation.[25] Although it is generally accepted that such changes, and particularly the initiation of a sterile inflammatory response, would cause pain,[26,27] it is not clear whether this is sufficient or requires other stimulators or promoters.

It has been shown that, although plasma extravasation in the retina, which can be blocked by sumatriptan, could be seen after trigeminal ganglion stimulation in the rat, no changes are seen with retinal angiography during acute attacks of migraine or cluster headache.[28] Clearly, blockade of neurogenic plasma protein extravasation is not completely predictive of anti-migraine efficacy in humans, as evidenced by the failure in clinical trials of substance P, neurokinin-1 antagonists,[29–32] specific PPE blockers, CP122,288[33] and 4991w93,[34] an endothelin antagonist[35] and the neurosteroid ganaxolone.[36] Indeed, substance P (neurokinin 1) receptor blockers also have no role in the preventive management of migraine.[37]

### *Neuropeptide studies*
Electrical stimulation of the trigeminal ganglion in both humans and cats leads to increases in extracerebral blood flow[38,39] and local cranial release of both CGRP and substance P.[8] In cats, stimulation of the more nociceptive specific structure, the superior saggital sinus, increases cerebral blood flow to a greater extent than trigeminal ganglion stimulation.[40] A substantial component of the trigeminovascular activation is mediated by a pathway traversing the superior salivatory nucleus[41] and projecting through the greater superficial petrosal branch of the facial nerve,[42] again releasing a powerful vasodilator peptide, vasoactive intestinal polypeptide (VIP).[43] It is of interest that the VIPergic innervation of the cerebral vessels is predominantly anterior rather than posterior.[44] This may contribute to this region's vulnerability to spreading depression and in part explain why the aura is so often seen to commence posteriorly. Stimulation of the superior sagittal sinus which more specifically produces vascular pain increases cerebral blood flow and jugular vein CGRP levels.[45] Human evidence is that CGRP

is elevated in the headache phase of migraine,[46,47] cluster headache,[48,49] chronic paroxysmal hemicrania[50] and throbbing exacerbations of chronic tension-type headache.[51] These data support the view that the trigeminovascular system may be activated in a protective role in these conditions. In this regard it is interesting that compounds that have *not* shown activity in human migraine, notably the conformationally restricted analogue of sumatriptan, CP122,288,[52] and the conformationally restricted analogue of zolmitriptan, 4991w93,[53] were both *ineffective* inhibitors of CGRP release after stimulation of the superior sagittal sinus in the cat. Current indications are that the CGRP antagonist BIBN4096,[54] a potent selective non-peptide antagonist, may answer the question of whether blockade of CGRP receptors can abort acute migraine. This is an exciting prospect, because it would usher in an age of acute medications that are not vasoconstrictors.

## Central connections

### The trigeminocervical complex

The sites within the brain stem that are responsible for craniovascular pain have been mapped in experimental animals up to monkeys. Using Fos immunohistochemistry, a method for looking at activated cells, after meningeal irritation with blood, Fos expression is reported in the trigeminal nucleus caudalis.[55] After stimulation of the superior sagittal sinus, Fos-like immunoreactivity is seen in the trigeminal nucleus caudalis and the dorsal horn at the C1 and C2 levels in cats[56] and monkeys.[57] Fos-like immunoreactivity can be observed bilaterally after unilateral stimulation of the peridural tissue around the meningeal artery.[58] Activation in the high cervical cord is consistent with similar data using 2-deoxyglucose measurements with superior sagittal sinus stimulation[59] and the early observations of Kerr.[60,61] Most recently, we have seen direct evidence for activation of neurons in the high cervical cord from both forebrain dura mater and regions innervated by the greater occipital nerve.[62] Taken together, these data contribute to our view of the trigeminal nucleus extending beyond the traditional nucleus caudalis to the dorsal horn of the high cervical region, in a functional continuum that includes a cervical extension which could be regarded as a trigeminal nucleus *cervicalis*. The entire group of cells could be regarded functionally as the *trigeminocervical* complex, and probably accounts for the largest part of the phenotype for the pain of primary headaches.

These data demonstrate that a substantial portion of the trigeminovascular nociceptive information comes by way of the most caudal cells. This concept provides an anatomical explanation for the referral of pain to the back of the head in migraine. Moreover, experimental pharmacological evidence suggests that some abortive anti-migraine drugs, such as dihydroergotamine,[63] acetylsalicylic acid,[64] sumatriptan after blood–brain barrier disruption,[65] eletriptan,[66] naratriptan,[67,68] rizatriptan[69] and zolmitriptan;[70] can have actions at these second-order neurons. Such an effect would reduce neuronal activity, providing a further site for therapeutic intervention in migraine.

# Higher-order processing

## Thalamus

After transmission in the caudal brain stem and high cervical spinal cord, information is relayed in a group of fibres (the quintothalamic tract) to the thalamus. Processing of vascular pain in the thalamus occurs in the ventroposteromedial thalamus, medial nucleus of the posterior complex and the intralaminar thalamus.[71] Zagami and Lambert[72] have shown, by application of capsaicin to the superior sagittal sinus, that trigeminal projections with a high degree of nociceptive input are processed in neurons, particularly in the ventroposteromedial thalamus and its ventral periphery. Human imaging studies have confirmed activation of the thalamus contralateral to pain in acute migraine,[73] cluster headache[74] and SUNCT (short-lasting unilateral neuralgiform headache with conjunctival injection and tearing).[75]

## Cortical processing

Pain in general is a complex phenomenon which is mediated by a network of neuronal structures, including cingulate cortex, insula and thalamus.[76–78] One framework proposes *medial* (thalamus, anterior cingulate cortex and prefrontal cortex) and *lateral* (primary and secondary somatosensory cortex) *pain systems* and these have been investigated using functional imaging techniques.[79] Most functional imaging studies demonstrate activation in these structures with clinical or experimental pain and recent reviews are available.[76,80] Recently, the amygdala,[76,81,82] basal ganglia[76,83] and posterior parietal cortex[84] have also been implicated in CNS responses to pain.

It has been shown in migraine that the anterior cingulate cortex, frontal cortex, and visual and auditory association cortex are activated during acute attacks.[73,85] Similarly, in cluster headache, cingulate cortex, insula, prefrontal cortex and basal ganglia are activated during

pain.[74] The activation of these non-specific areas during acute migraine and cluster headache is neither surprising nor unusual in pattern. How these areas relate to each other and the processing is unknown, and will require challenging and technically difficult experiments to untangle.

# Central modulation of trigeminal pain

A key observation, perhaps the crucial observation of functional imaging in migraine, has been that brain-stem areas are active during pain and after successful treatment this activation persists.[73,85] The activation corresponds with the brain region that Raskin et al[86] initially reported, and Veloso et al confirmed,[87] to cause migraine-like headache when stimulated in patients with electrodes implanted for pain control. Could these areas be pivotal in initiating or terminating the acute attack of migraine?

It has been shown in the experimental animal that stimulation of a discrete nucleus in the brain stem, nucleus locus ceruleus (the main central noradrenergic nucleus) reduces cerebral blood flow in a frequency-dependent manner[88] through an $\alpha_2$-adrenoceptor-linked mechanism.[89] This reduction is maximal in the occipital cortex.[90] Although a 25% overall reduction in cerebral blood flow is seen, extracerebral vasodilatation occurs in parallel.[88] In addition, the main serotonin-containing nucleus in the brain stem, the midbrain dorsal raphe nucleus, can increase cerebral blood flow when activated.[12] We have recently seen that, after stimulation of the superior sagittal sinus, Fos expression is increased in the ventrolateral periaqueductal grey matter (PAG) in cats and monkeys.[91] Similarly, we have also shown that stimulation of this region will inhibit sagittal sinus-evoked trigeminal neuronal activity in cats.[92] The ventrolateral PAG would certainly have been included within the area of activation on the human neuroimaging studies outlined above, so its physiology and interactions with the trigeminovascular system are of particular interest. These aminergic brain-stem neurons are an attractive site to host the basic defects in migraine, and they require detailed study and further human neuroimaging as we try to define the detail of the biology of migraine.

## Conclusions

An understanding of the basic anatomy and physiology of the cranial circulation facilitates the assessment and management of patients with migraine. Physiological processes clearly mature and change in childhood and adolescence, so it should not be a surprise that migraine evolves and changes, maturing to its adult form during adolescence. It seems likely that it is the brain control mechanisms that alter and mature; perhaps this explains why the disease has the same flavour all through life but runs at different temperatures. It has become clear that migraine is *not* a vascular headache *but* that the trigeminovascular and parasympathetic innervation of the cranial circulation drives the vascular changes of migraine, which is in essence neurovascular in expression. Migraine involves a disease process of the CNS at its core. Migraine may be considered an episodic aminergic system dysfunction with predominantly sensory consequences. As therapy evolves such a concept will drive new treatments and an understanding of the basic anatomy and physiology of headache will aid clinical management at

every level, from explaining the problem to the patient to initiating treatment.

## Acknowledgements

The work of the author has been supported by the Wellcome Trust and the Migraine Trust. He is a Wellcome Senior Research Fellow.

## References

1. Goadsby PJ, Migraine pathophysiology. In: Winner P, Rothner AD, eds, *Headache in Children and Adolescents*. Hamilton, Canada: BC Decker, Inc, 2001: 47–59.
2. Lance JW, Goadsby PJ, *Mechanism and Management of Headache*, 6th edn. London: Butterworth-Heinemann, 1998.
3. Goadsby PJ, Ferrari MD, Lipton RB, Migraine: current understanding and management. *N Eng J Med* 2001: in press.
4. Goadsby PJ, Silberstein SD, eds, Headache. In: Asbury A, Marsden CD, eds, *Blue Books in Practical Neurology*, vol 17. New York: Butterworth-Heinemann, 1997.
5. McNaughton FL, The innervation of the intracranial blood vessels and the dural sinuses. In: Cobb S, Frantz AM, Penfield W, Riley HA, eds, *The Circulation of the Brain and Spinal Cord*. New York: Hafner Publishing Co. Inc, 1966: 178–200.
6. Arbab MA-R, Wiklund L, Svendgaard NA, Origin and distribution of cerebral vascular innervation from superior cervical, trigeminal and spinal ganglia investigated with retrograde and anterograde WGA-HRP tracing in the rat. *Neuroscience* 1986; **19**: 695–708.
7. Uddman R, Edvinsson L, Ekman R, Kingman T, McCulloch J, Innervation of the feline cerebral vasculature by nerve fibers containing calcitonin gene-related peptide: trigeminal origin and co-existence with substance P. *Neurosci Lett* 1985; **62**: 131–6.
8. Goadsby PJ, Edvinsson L, Ekman R, Release of vasoactive peptides in the extracerebral circulation of man and the cat during activation of

the trigeminovascular system. *Ann Neurol* 1988; **23**: 193–6.

9. Feindel W, Penfield W, McNaughton F, The tentorial nerves and localisation of intracranial pain in man. *Neurology* 1960; **10**: 555–63.

10. McNaughton FL, Feindel WH, Innervation of intracranial structures: a reappraisal. In: Rose FC, ed., *Physiological Aspects of Clinical Neurology*. Oxford: Blackwell Scientific Publications, 1977: 279–93.

11. Cushing H, The sensory distribution of the fifth cranial nerve. *Bull Johns Hopkins Hosp* 1904; **15**: 213–32.

12. Goadsby PJ, Zagami AS, Lambert GA, Neural processing of craniovascular pain: a synthesis of the central structures involved in migraine. *Headache* 1991; **31**: 365–71.

13. Drummond PD, Lance JW, Extracranial vascular changes and the source of pain in migraine headache. *Ann Neurol* 1983; **13**: 32–7.

14. Nichols FT, Mawad M, Mohr JP, Hilal S, Adams RJ, Focal headache during balloon inflation in the vertebral and basilar arteries. *Headache* 1993; **33**: 87–9.

15. Nichols FT, Mawad M, Mohr JP, Hilal S, Stein B, Michelson J, Focal headache during balloon inflation in the internal carotid and middle cerebral arteries. *Stroke* 1990; **21**: 555–9.

16. Martins IP, Baeta E, Paiva T, Campo T, Gomes L, Headaches during intracranial endovascular procedures: a possible model of vascular headache. *Headache* 1993; **33**: 227–33.

17. Goadsby PJ, The pharmacology of headache. *Prog Neurobiol* 2000; **62**: 509–25.

18. Moskowitz MA, Basic mechanisms in vascular headache. *Neurol Clin* 1990; **8**: 801–15.

19. Markowitz S, Saito K, Moskowitz MA, Neurogenically mediated leakage of plasma proteins occurs from blood vessels in dura mater but not brain. *J Neurosci* 1987; **7**: 4129–36.

20. Buzzi MG, Moskowitz MA, Evidence for 5-HT$_{1B/1D}$ receptors mediating the antimigraine effect of sumatriptan and dihydroergotamine. *Cephalalgia* 1991; **11**: 165–8.

21. Buzzi MG, Sakas DE, Moskowitz MA, Indomethacin and acetylsalicylic acid block neurogenic plasma protein extravasation in rat

dura mater. *Eur J Pharmacol* 1989; **165**: 251–8.

22. Buzzi MG, Moskowitz MA, The antimigraine drug, sumatriptan (GR43175), selectively blocks neurogenic plasma extravasation from blood vessels in dura mater. *Br J Pharmacol* 1990; **99**: 202–6.

23. Cutrer FM, Limmroth V, Waeber C, Yu X, Moskowitz MA, New targets for antimigraine drug development. In: Goadsby PJ, Silberstein SD, eds, *Headache*. Philadelphia: Butterworth-Heinemann, 1997: 59–72.

24. Dimitriadou V, Buzzi MG, Moskowitz MA, Theoharides TC, Trigeminal sensory fiber stimulation induces morphological changes reflecting secretion in rat dura mater mast cells. *Neuroscience* 1991; **44**: 97–112.

25. Dimitriadou V, Buzzi MG, Theoharides TC, Moskowitz MA, Ultrastructural evidence for neurogenically mediated changes in blood vessels of the rat dura mater and tongue following antidromic trigeminal stimulation. *Neuroscience* 1992; **48**: 187–203.

26. Burstein R, Yamamura H, Malick A, Strassman AM, Chemical stimulation of the intracranial dura induces enhanced responses to facial stimulation in brain stem trigeminal neurons. *J Neurophysiol* 1998; **79**: 964–82.

27. Strassman AM, Raymond SA, Burstein R, Sensitization of meningeal sensory neurons and the origin of headaches. *Nature* 1996; **384**: 560–3.

28. May A, Shepheard S, Wessing A, Hargreaves RJ, Goadsby PJ, Diener HC, Retinal plasma extravasation can be evoked by trigeminal stimulation in rat but does not occur during migraine attacks. *Brain* 1998; **121**: 1231–7.

29. Diener HC, Substance-P antagonist RPR100893-201 is not effective in human migraine attacks. In: Olesen J, Tfelt-Hansen P, eds, *Proceedings of the VIth International Headache Seminar*. New York: Lippincott-Raven, 1996.

30. Goldstein DJ, Wang O, Saper JR, Stoltz R, Silberstein SD, Mathew NT, Ineffectiveness of neurokinin-1 antagonist in acute migraine: a crossover study. *Cephalalgia* 1997; **17**: 785–90.

31. Connor HE, Bertin L, Gillies S, Beattie DT, Ward P, The GR205171 Clinical Study Group, Clinical evaluation of a novel, potent, CNS penetrating NK$_1$ receptor antagonist in the acute treatment of migraine. *Cephalalgia* 1998; **18**: 392.

32. Norman B, Panebianco D, Block GA, A placebo-controlled, in-clinic study to explore the preliminary safety and efficacy of intravenous L-758,298 (a prodrug of the NK1 receptor antagonist L-754,030) in the acute treatment of migraine. *Cephalalgia* 1998; **18**: 407.

33. Roon K, Diener HC, Ellis P et al, CP-122,288 blocks neurogenic inflammation, but is not effective in aborting migraine attacks: results of two controlled clinical studies. *Cephalalgia* 1997; **17**: 245.

34. Earl NL, McDonald SA, Lowy MT, 4991W93 Investigator Group, Efficacy and tolerability of the neurogenic inflammation inhibitor, 4991W93, in the acute treatment of migraine. *Cephalalgia* 1999; **19**: 357.

35. May A, Gijsman HJ, Wallnoefer A, Jones R, Diener HC, Ferrari MD, Endothelin antagonist bosentan blocks neurogenic inflammation, but is not effective in aborting migraine attacks. *Pain* 1996; **67**: 375–8.

36. Data J, Britch K, Westergaard N et al, A double-blind study of ganaxolone in the acute treatment of migraine headaches with or without an aura in premenopausal females. *Headache* 1998; **38**: 380.

37. Goldstein DJ, Offen WW, Klein EG, Phebus LA, Lanepitant, an NK-1 antagonist, in migraine prophylaxis. *Cephalalgia* 1999; **19**: 377.

38. Tran-Dinh YR, Thurel C, Cunin G, Serrie A, Seylaz J, Cerebral vasodilation after the thermocoagulation of the trigeminal ganglion in humans. *Neurosurgery* 1992; **31**: 658–62.

39. Goadsby PJ, Duckworth JW, Effect of stimulation of trigeminal ganglion on regional cerebral blood flow in cats. *Am J Physiol* 1987; **253**: R270–4.

40. Goadsby PJ, Knight YE, Hoskin KL, Butler P, Stimulation of an intracranial trigeminally-innervated structure selectively increases cereb-ral blood flow. *Brain Res* 1997; **751**: 247–52.

41. Knight YE, Goadsby PJ, Distribution of c-Fos in cat medulla following superior sagittal sinus stimulation: Structures involved in craniovascular nociceptive transmission. *Eur J Neurosci* 2000; **12**: 71.

42. Lambert GA, Bogduk N, Goadsby PJ, Duckworth JW, Lance JW, Decreased carotid arterial resistance in cats in response to trigeminal stimulation. *J Neurosurg* 1984; **61**: 307–15.

43. Goadsby PJ, Macdonald GJ, Extracranial vasodilatation mediated by VIP (vasoactive intestinal polypeptide). *Brain Res* 1985; **329**: 285–8.

44. Matsuyama T, Shiosaka S, Matsumoto M et al, Overall distribution of vasoactive intestinal polypeptide-containing nerves on the wall of the cerebral arteries: an immunohistochemical study using whole-mounts. *Neuroscience* 1983; **10**: 89–96.

45. Zagami AS, Goadsby PJ, Edvinsson L, Stimulation of the superior sagittal sinus in the cat causes release of vasoactive peptides. *Neuropeptides* 1990; **16**: 69–75.

46. Goadsby PJ, Edvinsson L, Ekman R, Vasoactive peptide release in the extracerebral circulation of humans during migraine headache. *Ann Neurol* 1990; **28**: 183–7.

47. Gallai V, Sarchielli P, Floridi A et al, Vasoactive peptides levels in the plasma of young migraine patients with and without aura assessed both interictally and ictally. *Cephalalgia* 1995; **15**: 384–90.

48. Goadsby PJ, Edvinsson L, Human *in vivo* evidence for trigeminovascular activation in cluster headache. *Brain* 1994; **117**: 427–34.

49. Fanciullacci M, Alessandri M, Figini M, Geppetti P, Michelacci S, Increases in plasma calcitonin gene-related peptide from extracerebral circulation during nitroglycerin-induced cluster headache attack. *Pain* 1995; **60**: 119–23.

50. Goadsby PJ, Edvinsson L, Neuropeptide changes in a case of chronic paroxysmal hemicrania – evidence for trigemino-parasympathetic activation. *Cephalalgia* 1996; **16**: 448–50.

51. Ashina M, Bendsten L, Jensen R, Schifter S, Jansen-Olesen I, Olesen J, Plasma levels of cal-

citonin gene-related peptide in chronic tension-type headache. *Neurology* 2000; **55**: 1335–9.

52. Knight YE, Edvinsson L, Goadsby PJ, Blockade of CGRP release after superior sagittal sinus stimulation in cat: a comparison of avitriptan and CP122,288. *Neuropeptides* 1999; **33**: 41–6.

53. Knight YE, Connor HE, Edvinsson L, Goadsby PJ, Only $5HT_{1B/1D}$ agonist doses of 4991W93 inhibit CGRP release in the cat. *Cephalalgia* 1999; **19**: 401.

54. Doods H, Hallermayer G, Wu D et al, Pharmacological profile of BIBN-4096BS, the first selective small molecule CGRP antagonist. *Br J Pharmacol* 2000; **129**: 420–3.

55. Nozaki K, Boccalini P, Moskowitz MA, Expression of c-fos-like immunoreactivity in brainstem after meningeal irritation by blood in the subarachnoid space. *Neuroscience* 1992; **49**: 669–80.

56. Kaube H, Keay K, Hoskin KL, Bandler R, Goadsby PJ, Expression of c-*Fos*-like immunoreactivity in the caudal medulla and upper cervical cord following stimulation of the superior sagittal sinus in the cat. *Brain Res* 1993; **629**: 95–102.

57. Goadsby PJ, Hoskin KL, The distribution of trigeminovascular afferents in the non-human primate brain *Macaca nemestrina*: a c-fos immunocytochemical study. *J Anat* 1997; **190**: 367–75.

58. Hoskin KL, Zagami A, Goadsby PJ, Stimulation of the middle meningeal artery leads to bilateral Fos expression in the trigeminocervical nucleus: a comparative study of monkey and cat. *J Anat* 1999; **194**: 579–88.

59. Goadsby PJ, Zagami AS, Stimulation of the superior sagittal sinus increases metabolic activity and blood flow in certain regions of the brainstem and upper cervical spinal cord of the cat. *Brain* 1991; **114**: 1001–11.

60. Kerr FWL, Olafson RA, Trigeminal and cervical volleys. *Arch Neurol* 1961; **5**: 69–76.

61. Kerr FWL, A mechanism to account for frontal headache in cases of posterior fossa tumous. *J Neurosurg* 1961; **18**: 605–9.

62. Bartsch T, Goadsby PJ, Stimulation of the greater occipital nerve (GON) enhances responses of dural responsive convergent neurons in the trigemino-cervical complex in the rat. *Cephalalgia* 2001; **21**: in press.

63. Hoskin KL, Kaube H, Goadsby PJ, Central activation of the trigeminovascular pathway in the cat is inhibited by dihydroergotamine: a c-*Fos* and electrophysiology study. *Brain* 1996; **119**: 249–56.

64. Kaube H, Hoskin KL, Goadsby PJ, Intravenous acetylsalicylic acid inhibits central trigeminal neurons in the dorsal horn of the upper cervical spinal cord in the cat. *Headache* 1993; **33**: 541–50.

65. Kaube H, Hoskin KL, Goadsby PJ, Sumatriptan inhibits central trigeminal neurons only after blood–brain barrier disruption. *Br J Pharmacol* 1993; **109**: 788–92.

66. Goadsby PJ, Hoskin KL, Differential effects of low dose CP122,288 and eletriptan on Fos expression due to stimulation of the superior sagittal sinus in the cat. *Pain* 1999; **82**: 15–22.

67. Goadsby PJ, Knight YE, Naratriptan inhibits trigeminal neurons after intravenous administration through an action at the serotonin $(5HT_{1B/1D})$ receptors. *Br J Pharmacol* 1997; **122**: 918–22.

68. Cumberbatch MJ, Hill RG, Hargreaves RJ, Differential effects of the $5HT_{1B/1D}$ receptor agonist naratriptan on trigeminal versus spinal nociceptive responses. *Cephalalgia* 1998; **18**: 659–64.

69. Cumberbatch MJ, Hill RG, Hargreaves RJ, Rizatriptan has central antinociceptive effects against durally evoked responses. *Eur J Pharmacol* 1997; **328**: 37–40.

70. Goadsby PJ, Hoskin KL, Inhibition of trigeminal neurons by intravenous administration of the serotonin (5HT)-1-D receptor agonist zolmitriptan (311C90): are brain stem sites a therapeutic target in migraine? *Pain* 1996; **67**: 355–9.

71. Zagami AS, Goadsby PJ, Stimulation of the superior sagittal sinus increases metabolic activity in cat thalamus. In: Rose FC, ed., *New Advances in Headache Research: 2*. London: Smith-Gordon & Co. Ltd, 1991: 169–71.

72. Zagami AS, Lambert GA, Craniovascular application of capsaicin activates nociceptive

thalamic neurons in the cat. *Neurosci Lett* 1991; **121**: 187–90.

73. Bahra A, Matharu MS, Buchel C, Frackowiak RSJ, Goadsby PJ, Brainstem activation specific to migraine headache. *Lancet* 2001: 1016–17.

74. May A, Bahra A, Buchel C, Frackowiak RSJ, Goadsby PJ, Hypothalamic activation in cluster headache attacks. *Lancet* 1998; **351**: 275–8.

75. May A, Bahra A, Buchel C, Turner R, Goadsby PJ, Functional MRI in spontaneous attacks of SUNCT: short-lasting neuralgiform headache with conjunctival injection and tearing. *Ann Neurol* 1999; **46**: 791–3.

76. Derbyshire SWG, Jones AKP, Gyulai F, Clark S, Townsend D, Firestone LL, Pain processing during three levels of noxious stimulation produces differential patterns of central activity. *Pain* 1997; **73**: 431–45.

77. Jones AK, Brown WD, Friston KJ, Qi LY, Frackowiak RSJ, Cortical and subcortical localization of response to pain in man using positron emission tomography. *Proc R Soc Lon B* 1991; **244**: 39–44.

78. Melzack R, Casey KL, Sensory, motivational and central control determinants of pain. In: Kenshalo DR, ed., *The Skin Senses*. Springfield, IL: CC Thomas, 1968: 423–39.

79. Jones AK, Qi LY, Fujirawa T et al, *In vivo* distribution of opioid receptors in man in relation to the cortical projections of the medial and lateral pain systems measured with positron emission tomography. *Neurosci Lett* 1991; **126**: 25–8.

80. Chen AC, Human brain measures of clinical pain: a review. II. Tomographic imaging. *Pain* 1993; **54**: 133–44.

81. Bernard JF, Huang GF, Besson JM, Nucleus centralis of the amygdala and the globus pallidus ventralis: electrophysiological evidence for an involvement in pain processes. *J Neurophysiol* 1992; **68**: 551–69.

82. Hsieh JC, Stahle-Backdahl M, Hagermark O, Stone-Elander S, Rosenquist G, Ingvar M, Traumatic nociceptive pain activates the hypothalamus and the periaqueductal gray: a positron emission tomography study. *Pain* 1996; **64**: 303–14.

83. Chudler EH, Dong WK, The role of the basal ganglia in nociception and pain. *Pain* 1995; **60**: 33–8.

84. Dong WK, Hayashi T, Roberts VJ, Fusco BM, Chudler EH, Behavioral outcome of posterior parietal cortex injury in the monkey. *Pain* 1996; **64**: 579–87.

85. Weiller C, May A, Limmroth V et al, Brain stem activation in spontaneous human migraine attacks. *Nat Med* 1995; **1**: 658–60.

86. Raskin NH, Hosobuchi Y, Lamb S, Headache may arise from perturbation of brain. *Headache* 1987; **27**: 416–20.

87. Veloso F, Kumar K, Toth C, Headache secondary to deep brain implantation. *Headache* 1998; **38**: 507–15.

88. Goadsby PJ, Lambert GA, Lance JW, Differential effects on the internal and external carotid circulation of the monkey evoked by locus coeruleus stimulation. *Brain Res* 1982; **249**: 247–54.

89. Goadsby PJ, Lambert GA, Lance JW, The mechanism of cerebrovascular vasoconstriction in response to locus coeruleus stimulation. *Brain Res* 1985; **326**: 213–17.

90. Goadsby PJ, Duckworth JW, Low frequency stimulation of the locus coeruleus reduces regional cerebral blood flow in the spinalized cat. *Brain Res* 1989; **476**: 71–7.

91. Hoskin KL, Bulmer DCE, Lasalandra M, Jonkman A, Goadsby PJ, Fos expression in the midbrain periaqueductal grey after trigeminovascular stimulation. *J Anat* 2001; **197**: 29–35.

92. Knight YE, Goadsby PJ, Brainstem stimulation inhibits trigeminal neurons in the cat. *Cephalalgia* 1999; **19**: 315.

# 13

# Clinical features of migraine

*Paul Winner, Donald Lewis*

Migraine with or without aura is a common recurrent headache syndrome in children and adolescents. Determining an appropriate system for diagnosis and classification of migraine is an important priority for both clinical practice and clinical research. The criteria established by the International Headache Society (IHS)[1] in 1988 represent a marked advance, although the criteria were developed primarily for headache disorders in adults (Table 13.1). This classification has not been extremely useful in children. Revised criteria should provide an important tool for clinical practice, clinical trials and epidemiological research.

In the IHS system, migraine is defined on the basis of symptom profiles and the pattern of attack. The general medical examination and neurological evaluation, as well as diagnostic tests, serve primarily to exclude secondary headache.

Migraine is a heterogeneous disorder with attacks varying in pain intensity, duration and pattern of associated features. The headaches may have exacerbations or remissions in children and often vary by sex and age of the individual. In children aged 4–7, migraine is more frequent in boys than in girls. Between the ages of 7 and 11 the prevalence is equal. From about 11–12 on, the ratio changes to the classic three girls to one boy.[2]

## Migraine in children

Migraine is characterized by recurrent episodes of throbbing head pain of variable intensity, duration and frequency, with associated nausea and vomiting, as well as photophobia and/or phonophobia. In 1988, the IHS proposed a new set of criteria for childhood migraine based on international expert consensus (Table 13.2). Before this, Vahlquist[3]

---

A. ≥5 attacks fulfilling features B–D
B. Headache attack lasting *2–48 hours*[a]
C. Headache has at least two of the following four features:
   1. Unilateral location
   2. Pulsating quality
   3. Moderate-to-severe intensity
   4. Aggravated by routine physical activities
D. At least one of the following accompanies headache:
   1. Nausea and/or vomiting
   2. Photophobia and phonophobia

[a] differences from adult migraine are italicized: shorter duration

**Table 13.1**
*IHS classification: criteria for childhood migraine without aura[1]*

was one of the first to define childhood migraine as a paroxysmal headache separated by pain-free intervals and accompanied by at least two of the following four features: visual aura, nausea, unilateral pain and a family history of migraine. Prensky[4] redefined migraine as paroxysmal headache, with three of six associated symptoms: aura, abdominal pain, unilateral pain, throbbing quality, relief with sleep and family history of migraine. Even though there are minor variations, the common denominators are paroxysmal headache separated by symptom-free intervals and accompanied by other specific features. Although inclusion of family history is not a criterion in the IHS system, it is an important consideration when diagnosing childhood migraine. Since the IHS's proposal, there have been several studies looking at subtle changes in the criteria.[5,6] Authors have assessed the diagnostic utility of the IHS defining features of migraine and stressed that migraine tends to be of shorter duration in children and adolescents. The IHS criteria initially took this into account, permitting the length of headaches in children aged under 15 years to be changed to 2–48 hours. However, more recent findings have recommended a further decrease in the length of headaches from 2 h to 1 h.[5,6] Unilateral pain has also been challenged as a diagnostic criterion, because it is much more characteristic of adult migraine than childhood migraine. Although bilateral location (frontal/temporal) is common in children, unilateral headache has a high positive predictive value for migraine at 85%.[6] Thus, some physicians feel that unilateral pain should remain a migraine-defining feature in children.

Other migraine characteristics such as pain intensity and pulsating quality are difficult to ascertain in children. Once determined, they

E. ≥5 attacks fulfilling features B–D
F. Headache attack lasting *1–48 hours*[a]
G. Headache has at least two of the following four features:
   5. *Bilateral (frontal/temporal)* or unilateral location
   6. Pulsating quality
   7. Moderate-to-severe intensity
   8. Aggravated by routine physical activities
H. At least one of the following accompanies headache:
   3. Nausea and/or vomiting
   4. *Photophobia and/or phonophobia*

[a] differences from adult migraine are italicized: shorter duration

**Table 13.2**
*Proposed revised IHS classification: criteria for childhood migraine without aura[5]*

correlate well with the diagnosis of migraine. These pain features should remain part of the IHS definition in children.

The visual aura of migraine is reported in 14–30% of children and adolescents as disturbances, distortions, or obscuration before or as the headache begins. Children will present with complaints of seeing spots, colours or rainbows, but usually the symptoms need to be elicited by asking pointed questions. Hachinski et al[7] reported that children's visual symptomatology included three dominant visual phenomena: binocular visual impairment with scotoma (77%), distortion or hallucinations (16%), and monocular visual impairment or scotoma (7%). The diagnosis of migraine with aura requires two or more fully reversible symptoms, including visual, motor or sensory symptoms. The aura should develop gradually over at least 4 min, and usually lasts 20–30 min but may last as long as 60 min. In an aura that is short in duration or rapid in onset, an alternative paroxysmal event may be the aetiology. An atypical and/or prolonged event (> 60 min) may signal an organic disorder that requires further diagnostic assessment.

Multicentre perspective evaluation of a proposed childhood migraine revision has been performed.[5,6] The proposed revision includes: duration of 1–48 h; location (bifrontal, bitemporal) or unilateral; and symptoms including photophobia or phonophobia (see Table 13.2).

# Migraine variants

Migraine presents with dramatic neurological signs such as hemiparesis, ataxia, acute confusional states, ophthalmoparesis and vertigo. These clinical entities are often termed 'migraine variants'.

The abrupt appearance of such focal and ominous neurological signs, accompanying an excruciating headache with vomiting, will initially raise concerns of a life-threatening neurological aetiology such as a brain tumour, intracranial haemorrhage, hydrocephalus, CNS infection or intoxication. Only after careful history taking, physical and neurological examination and appropriate neurodiagnostic studies can the diagnosis of migraine variant (a diagnosis of exclusion) be entertained.

The transient deficits of the migraine variants are thought to result from a wave of depolarization migrating across the visual cortex and/or from regional oligaemia caused by a neuropeptide-mediated, sterile, neurogenic inflammation. There are frequently shared or overlapping clinical features with many of the migraine variants, and this observation suggests a common pathophysiology. Still incompletely explained are the cranial nerve signs associated with ophthalmoplegic and basilar migraine.

Some of the migraine variants are represented as part of the classification system of the IHS (Table 13.3).[1,8] Inclusion of hemiplegic and basilar migraine variants within the spectrum of migraine *with aura* reflects the contemporary view of their pathogenesis. The IHS system fails to include the clinical entities confusional migraine and cyclical vomiting, but both are reviewed. Also omitted is the Alice-in-Wonderland syndrome, which most probably represents an unusual form of visual aura with distortions, illusions, micropsia and macropsia.

## Familial hemiplegic migraine – IHS 1.2.3

Familial hemiplegic migraine (FHM) is an uncommon autosomal dominant form of

| |
|---|
| 1.1 Migraine without aura (common migraine) |
| 1.2 Migraine with aura (classic migraine) |
|     1.2.1 Migraine with typical aura |
|     1.2.2 Migraine with prolonged aura |
|     1.2.3 Familial hemiplegic migraine |
|     1.2.4 Basilar migraine |
|     1.2.5 Migraine aura without headache |
|     1.2.6 Migraine with acute-onset aura |
| 1.3 Ophthalmoplegic migraine |
| 1.4 Retinal migraine |
| 1.5 Childhood periodic syndromes |
|     1.5.1 Benign paroxysmal vertigo |
|     1.5.2 Alternating hemiplegia of childhood |

**Table 13.3**
*Migraine classification[1]*

migraine headache, in which the aura produces some degree of hemiparesis. There is a wide diversity of symptoms and signs that can accompany this migraine variant beyond motor deficits (hemiplegia, hemiparesis, monoplegia, monoparesis) including: sensory (hemidyaesthesia, hemianaesthesia, hemihypaesthesia), visual (hemianopia, quadrantanopia), confusion, aphasia, dysphasia and dysarthria. The IHS criteria clearly require that some degree of hemiparesis must be present, so the term will probably persist.[1]

A series of recent discoveries into the molecular genetics of FHM have broadened our understanding of the fundamental mechanisms of migraine. Genetic linkage to chromosome 19p13 has been identified in half of the known FHM pedigrees and, more recently, a separate pedigree with linkage to chromosome 1q31 has been reported.[9,10] The chromosomal 19 defect produces a missense mutation in a neuronal calcium channel gene, providing compelling evidence that FHM represents a channelopathy.[4] These discoveries have revolutionized our understanding of migraine and may open new territory for pharmacological interventions.

Hemiplegic migraine is characterized by transient (hours to days) episodes of focal neurological deficits, which precede the headache phase by 30–60 min, although occasionally, they extend well beyond the headache itself. The headache is often contralateral to the focal deficit.

The appearance of acute focal neurological deficits in the setting of headache in a child necessitates investigation for organic disorders. Neuroimaging (magnetic resonance imaging [MRI] and magnetic resonance angiography [MRA]) and EEG may be indicated. Investigations for embolic sources or hypercoagulable states are likewise appropriate.

Mitochondrial encephalomyopathy, lactic acidosis and stroke-like attacks (MELAS) warrant particular attention in the differential diagnosis of hemiplegic migraine because of the high frequency of migraine-like headache in MELAS patients. MELAS is caused by a point mutation in the mitochondrial DNA (A→G at 3243 in mitochondrial [mt] DNA) and clinically characterized by episodes of focal neurological deficits, with variable MRI changes that may not respect vascular territories. Although there is some overlap of symptoms with hemiplegic migraine, children with MELAS also have muscle weakness and atrophy, dementia and epilepsy. Serum lactic acid levels are usually quite elevated and the diagnosis is confirmed by specific mtDNA testing.

## Basilar migraine – IHS 1.2.4

Basilar migraine (BM) also known as basilar artery, vertebrobasilar or Bickerstaff migraine: it is the most frequent of the migraine variants and is estimated to represent 3–19% of all migraines.[11–14] This wide range of frequency relates to the rigorousness of the definition. Some definitions included any headache with dizziness to be within the spectrum of BM, whereas others require the presence of clear signs and symptoms of posterior fossa involvement before establishing this diagnosis. The IHS criteria require two or more symptoms (Table 13.4) and emphasizes bulbar and bilateral sensorimotor features.[1]

The age of onset of BM tends to be in younger children with a mean age of 7 years, although the clinical entity probably appears as early as 12–18 months as episodic pallor, clumsiness and vomiting (benign paroxysmal vertigo).

| Sign/symptom | Percentage |
|---|---|
| Vertigo | 73 |
| Nausea or vomiting | 30–50 |
| Ataxia | 43–50 |
| Visual field deficits | 43 |
| Diplopia | 30 |
| Tinnitus | 13 |
| Vertigo | 73 |
| Confusion | 20 |
| Weakness (hemiplegia, quadriplegia, diplegia) | 20 |

**Table 13.4**
*Basilar migraine: signs and symptoms*[9–12,38]

Affected children will have attacks of intense dizziness, vertigo, visual disturbances, ataxia and diplopia. These early transient features last minutes to an hour and are then followed by the headache phase. Unlike the more typical frontal or temporal location, however, the headache may be occipital in location. The quality of the pain may be difficult for the child to describe.

The pathogenesis of BM is unclear. Focal cortical processes, oligaemia or depolarization may explain the deficits in hemiplegic migraine, but what of the posterior fossa signs? There is a single case report of a 25-year-old woman with BM, wherein transcranial Doppler and single photon emission computed tomography (SPECT) were performed through the course of a BM attack. These data suggest decreased posterior cerebral artery perfusion through the aura phase, at a time when the described patient was experiencing transient bilateral blindness and ataxia.[15]

Sudden appearance of diplopia, vertigo and vomiting must prompt consideration of dis-orders within the posterior fossa, such as; arteriovenous malformations, cavernous angiomas, tumours (medulloblastoma, ependymoma, brain-stem glioma), congenital malformations (Chiari, Dandy–Walker) or vertebrobasilar insufficiency (vertebral dissection or thrombosis). Acute labyrinthitis or positional vertigo can mimic BM. Complex partial seizures and drug intoxications must be considered at any age. Rarely, metabolic diseases such as Hartnup's disease, hyperammonaemias (urea cycle or organic acidaemias), or disorders of pyruvate/lactate metabolism may present with episodic vertigo, but these inborn errors of metabolism usually have some degree of altered consciousness and/or coma.

## Ophthalmoplegic migraine – IHS 1.3

Ophthalmoplegic migraine (OM) is one of the least common migraine variants. Epidemiological data suggest an annual incidence of 0.7 per million.[16] The two key features are ophthalmoparesis and headache, although the headache may be mild or a nondescript retro-orbital discomfort. Although verbally sophisticated school-aged children may describe blurred vision or diplopia, young children may simply rub their eyes or have a slight head tilt. Attacks of OM have been reported during infancy, as early as 5–7 months of age.[17] Ptosis, adduction defects and skew deviations are the common objective findings. Symptoms and signs of oculomotor dysfunction may appear well into the headache phase, rather than at the onset of the headache. The signs may persist for days or even weeks after the headache has resolved.

The oculomotor nerve, or its divisions, are the most frequently involved, but pupillary involvement is inconsistent and controversial. In our experience of three cases, all had pupillary involvement. Some authors report pupillary involvement in only one-third of patients.[18] The third nerve involvement may be incomplete, with partial deficits in both the inferior and the superior divisions of the third nerve. Abduction defects, caused by abducens involvement, is the second most frequently reported variant of OM, and involvement of the trochlear nerve is the least common. The mechanism of OM is openly debated. The primary theories suggest ischaemic, compressive or inflammatory processes.[16] Lack of pupillary involvement supports an ischaemic mechanism, whereas a higher incidence of pupillary involvement suggests a compressive mechanism. Alternatively, recent reports have questioned whether OM may be an inflammatory process within the spectrum of the Tolosa–Hunt syndrome, particularly given the steroid responsiveness of many patients.[19] Furthermore, high-resolution neuroimaging has shown a reversible enhancement and even thickening of the oculomotor nerve during attacks, which lends further credence to an inflammatory mechanism.[20]

Aneurysm or mass lesion in or around the orbital apex and parasellar region should be aggressively sought. The differential diagnosis for OM is shown in Table 13.5. Neuroimaging with MRI or MRA is usually indicated. The performance of angiography is recommended by some authors and cautioned by others, because of the theoretical risk of vasospasm with contrast agents in migraine patients. In those children with external ophthalmoparesis, a test dose of edrophonium is recommended.

Repeated attacks of OM can lead to permanent deficits, so acute treatment with steroids

Ophthalmoplegic migraine
Head trauma
Thyroid disease (Grave's disease)
Myasthenia gravis, ocular myasthenia
Chronic progressive external
    ophthalmoplegia (Kearns–Sayre
    syndrome)
Miller–Fisher variant of Guillan–Barré
    syndrome
Orbital pseudotumour
Tolosa–Hunt syndrome
Sarcoidosis
Cerebral aneurysms (intracavernous carotid
    artery, posterior communicating)
Cavernous sinus thrombosis
Orbital tumours (lymphoma, sarcoma)
Orbital abscess
Post-infectious
Metabolic: diabetes, branched-chain
    aminoacidopathy, non-ketotic
    hyperglycinaemia
Idiopathic

**Table 13.5**
*Ophthalmoparesis in childhood[38]*

and prophylactic treatment should be considered.

## Retinal migraine – IHS 1.4

Retinal migraine (RM), also referred to as ocular, ophthalmic or anterior visual pathway migraine, is extremely uncommon in children and rarely seen in young adults. Unlike the descending curtain-like onset of amaurosis fugax, affected patients will report brief (from seconds to <60 min), sudden, monocular black or grey 'outs', or bright, blinding episodes (photopsia) of visual disturbance before, after or during the headache. A 60-min interval between visual symptom and headache may occur. As with ophthalmoplegic migraine, the pain is often described as retro-orbital and ipsilateral to the visual disturbance.

Examination of the fundus during an attack may disclose constriction of retinal veins and arteries with retinal pallor. An occasional patient may suffer significant visual sequelae (scotoma, altitudinal defects or monocular blindness) in retinal migraine, presumably as a result of vasoconstriction with retinal infarction. Using a rat model, May et al[21] demonstrated the evolution of a sterile neurogenic inflammation in both the retina and dura after stimulation of the trigeminal ganglion, but were unable to view the same phenomenon in the human retina in acute migraine.

Although the patient population with retinal migraine is generally much younger than those who experience amaurosis fugax from atheromatous carotid disease, evaluation for hypercoagualable states, embolic sources and vascular disruption (carotid dissection) must be considered.

# Childhood periodic syndromes (migraine equivalents)

Two clinical entities are included in this category by the IHS: benign paroxysmal vertigo and alternating hemiplegia of childhood.

## Benign paroxysmal vertigo – IHS 1.5.1

Benign paroxysmal vertigo (BPV) is reportedly common, although incidence figures are lacking. Typically, an unaffected young child (median 18 months) will be struck by a sudden unsteadiness on his or her feet. The child will anxiously grab on to a nearby table, chair or adult for stability or fall to the ground. Consciousness will not be lost but astute observers may notice nystagmus. Vomiting may be vigorous. The spells usually last minutes and afterwards the child will sleep. On awakening, the child returns to his or her normal baseline. The spells will occur in clusters over several days, then subside for weeks or months.[22,23]

These spells may represent the early evolution of basilar migraine and the differential diagnosis is similar. During a long-term follow-up of seven cases, Lanzi reported that five or seven BPV cases spontaneously resolved and six of seven patients later developed migraine and other migraine-related symptoms. The authors suggest that BPV can be interpreted as a migraine precursor.[24]

## Alternating hemiplegia of childhood – IHS 1.5.2

Alternating hemiplegia of childhood (AHC) is a rare syndrome which has traditionally been considered a variant of hemiplegic migraine.

The first symptoms start before 18 months of age. Affected children have attacks of paralysis: hemiparesis, monoparesis, diparesis, ophthalmoparesis, and bulbar paralysis which may be accompanied by variable tone changes (flaccid, spastic or rigid). A variety of paroxysmal involuntary movements, including chorea, athetosis, dystonia, nystagmus and respiratory irregularities (hyperpnoea), can be seen. The attacks of paralysis can be brief (minutes) or prolonged (days), and potentially life threatening during periods of bulbar paralysis. Curiously, the attacks generally subside after sleep. Affected children are frequently developmentally challenged.[25,26]

The link to migraine is based on the presence of a high incidence of migraine in the families of affected children and on cerebral blood flow data, which suggest a migrainous mechanism.

In 1997, an international workshop was conducted to address the various hypotheses surrounding AHC, and the proceedings have been reviewed by Rho.[27] Proposed mechanisms include channelopathy, mitochondrial cytopathy and cerebrovascular dysfunction, although the first seems to be the most likely hypothesis. The calcium channel blocker flunarezine can be remarkably effective in reducing attack frequency and severity.

This entity warrants aggressive evaluation for vascular disorders, inborn errors of metabolism, mitochondrial encephalomyopathies or epileptic variants.

Benign paroxysmal torticollis, cyclical vomiting syndrome and abdominal migraine are considered by most to be part of the childhood periodic syndromes.

## Benign paroxysmal torticollis

Benign paroxysmal torticollis (BPT) is a rare paroxysmal dyskinesia characterized by attacks of head tilt alone or tilt accompanied by vomiting and ataxia, which may last hours to days.[28] Other torsional or dystonic features, including truncal or pelvic posturing, were described by Chutorian.[29] Attacks first manifest themselves during infancy, between the ages of 2 and 8 months. The original descriptions of BPT by Snyder[30] suggested a form of labyrinthitis and demonstrated abnormal vestibular reflexes. Theoretically, paroxysmal torticollis may be an early onset variant of basilar migraine or a variant of benign paroxysmal vertigo. In addition, there is often a family history of migraine.

The differential diagnosis includes gastro-oesophageal reflux (Sandifer's syndrome), idiopathic torsional dystonia and complex partial seizure, although particular attention should be paid to the posterior fossa and craniocervical junction where congenital or acquired lesions may produce torticollis. Rarely, troclear nerve dysfunction produces compensatory head tilt.

## Cyclical vomiting syndrome

Cyclical vomiting syndrome (CVS) is a symptom complex in young infants and children, characterized by repeated, stereotyped bouts of pernicious vomiting, often to the point of dehydration. Over the past decade, over 60 articles have been added to the existing literature on CVS. Diagnostic criteria have been established. The qualitative clinical criteria for cyclical vomiting require episodic vomiting with interval wellness and quantitative requirement for high-peak intensity of emesis (four or more emeses/hour) and low episode frequency (two or fewer episodes/week).[31]

The mechanism of CVS is incompletely understood and migraine remains among the possible explanations. The link between CVS and migraine has traditionally been based on the strong family history of migraine, the episodic nature of CVS, and the shared list of provocative influences including stress and excitement. Further support has been presented recently with autonomic–neurocardic data, which show a commonality of sympathetic nervous system alterations between CVS and migraine.[32] The link has been further strengthened by the favourable clinical response of CVS patients to migraine prophylactic agents cyproheptadine and amitriptyline, with decreased frequency and severity of attacks.[33]

Li et al[34] examined the overlap between CVS and migraine in a population of 214 children with CVS, and found that 82% had migraine-associated CVS based on either a positive family history or the subsequent development of typical migraine attacks. The authors support a continuum, wherein migraine presents with different patterns at various ages: cyclic vomiting in toddlers, abdominal migraine in school-aged children and migraine headache in older children.

Before this clinical entity can be comfortably diagnosed, cautious and thorough investigations for gastrointestinal disturbances or obstruction (duplications, stenosis or intussception), intracranial hypertension (diencephalic tumours, subdural effusions, hydrocephalus), and inborn errors of metabolism, particularly urea cycle defects and organic acidaemias, should be considered.

Li et al[35] reported a series of 225 children aged less than 18 years who had experienced at least three episodes of vomiting before presenting to their gastroenterology clinic at Columbus Children's Hospital. Between attacks, these children were healthy; 88% were diagnosed as idiopathic CVS, but only after extensive negative evaluation. Critically, 41% had associated co-morbid disorders which were felt to be contributors to the vomiting. Their excellent study emphasized the point that CVS is not a single diagnostic entity, but rather a clinical presentation that can result from heterogeneous disorders.[35]

The treatment of CVS is empirical and parallels that of migraine, with the prudent use of prophylactic medications and intensive use of antiemetics, plus hydration, during attacks.

## Abdominal migraine

Abdominal migraine is characterized by repeated, stereotyped bouts of unexplained abdominal pain, with nausea and vomiting, in childhood. The diagnosis is entertained after exhaustive gastrointestinal and metabolic evaluations have not revealed anything. We could cautiously propose that abdominal migraine may be a variant of CVS. Headache is infrequently described, except in the course of long-term follow-up.

As abdominal pain is one of the key features of childhood migraine, few would argue that a small subset of children with recurrent unexplained abdominal pain may represent a spectrum of childhood migraine.

## Alice-in-Wonderland syndrome

Patients with Alice-in-Wonderland syndrome report that bizarre visual illusions and spatial distortions occasionally precede migraine headaches. As for Alice's visual distortions after eating mushrooms in *Alice Through the Looking Glass*, affected children will describe visual distortions before or as the headache is beginning. The children may describe bizarre or vivid visual illusions such as: micropsia – objects appear smaller; macropsia – objects appear larger; metamorphopsia – objects (such as faces) appear distorted; and teleopsia – objects appear far away.

Anecdotally, the children are not confused or frightened by these illusions and are able to relate the experience with detail. This unusual visual symptomatology is best considered as migraine with aura, although, historically,

Alice-in-Wonderland syndrome is included as a distinct variant. This type of visual–perceptual abnormality has been reported with infectious mononucleosis, complex partial seizures (particularly benign occipital epilepsy) and drug intoxications.

# Confusional migraine

Confusional migraine has been reported in children aged 8–16 years experiencing acute confusional states, lasting 4–24 hours, associated with agitation an aphasia as a presenting feature of juvenile migraine.[36] Ehyai and Fenichel[37] introduced the term 'acute confusional migraine'. Subsequent reports have broadened the clinical phenomenology to include blindness, paraesthesiae, hemiparesis and amnesia. Amnesia can be such a prominent feature that Jenson proposed the term 'transient global amnesia of childhood', although amnesia is just part of the spectrum.[37]

Affected patients, usually boys, become agitated, restless, disoriented and, occasionally, combative for minutes to hours. Once consciousness has returned to baseline, the patients will describe an inability to communicate, frustration, confusion and loss of orientation to time, and may not recall a headache phase at all. A strong family history of migraine is elicited in 75% of patients.

There is clear link to head trauma in many cases.[39] The term 'footballer's migraine' is applied in Europe when a soccer player, after 'heading' the ball, develops acute confusional state with headache. Similar phenomena may follow other causes of minor head injury. This should be viewed within the spectrum of trauma-triggered migraine.

There is a great deal of overlap between the migraine variants. Perhaps this entity of confusional migraine is a hybrid and should best be included within the spectrum of either basilar or hemiplegic migraine, dependent on which symptoms predominate in individual patients. Those with aphasia, hemiparesis and confusion are probably hemiplegic, and those with bilateral blindness, vertigo and confusion should be classified as basilar migraine.

Acute confusional states in children and adolescents warrant investigation for encephalitis, brain abscess, drug intoxication, cerebrovascular disease, vasculitis or metabolic encephalopathies.[40] Particular attention should be focused on the possibility of complex partial seizures or postictal states.

# Conclusion

Many adult patients with migraine report that their headaches began in childhood and adolescence. Most children and adolescents will have migraine without aura, manifesting as recurrent bilateral (frontal/temporal) or unilateral head pain, with nausea and pounding headaches. Migraine variants may present with dramatic neurological signs such as ataxia, vertigo, hemiparesis, ophthalmoparesis or acute confusional states, but should be considered diagnoses of exclusion. Careful anatomical, electrographic, metabolic, toxicological and haematological investigations are usually needed to exclude more ominous organic disorders.

The IHS is scheduled to introduce a revision of the 1988 classification, and changes are expected that will make the diagnosis of childhood migraine more specific. This will help with the clinical diagnosis as well as research studies in childhood migraine. A better understanding of diagnostic criteria, early diagnosis and more effective treatment may be the key to influencing the prevalence of headaches in adults. Continued research is the only answer to the questions raised by the most recent studies in this population.

# References

1. Headache Classification Committee of the International Headache Society, Classification and diagnostic criteria for headache disorders, cranial neuralgias and facial pain. *Cephalalgia* 1988; 8(suppl 7): 1096.

2. Mortimer J, Kay J, Jaron A, Epidemiology of headache and childhood migraine in an urban general practice using ad hoc, Vahlquist and ISH criteria. *Dev Med Child Neurol* 1992; **34:** 1095–101.

3. Vahlquist B, Migraine in children. *Int Arch Allergy* 1955; **7:** 348–55.

4. Prensky AL, Sommer D, Diagnosis and treatment of migraine in children. *Neurology* 1979; **23:** 506–10.

5. Winner P, Wasieswski W, Gladstein J, Linder S, Multicenter prospective evaluation of proposed pediatric migraine revisions to the ISH criteria. *Headache* 1997; **37:** 545–8.

6. Maytel J, Young M, Schechter A, Lipton RB, Pediatric migraine and the International Headache Society (HIS) criteria. *Neurology* 1997; **48:** 602–7.

7. Hachinski VC, Porchawka J, Steele JC, Visual symptoms in the migraine syndrome. *Neurology* 1973; **23:** 570–9.

8. Olesen J, Headache Classification Committee of the International Headache Society. Classification and diagnostic criteria for headache disorders, cranial neuralgia, and facial pain. *Cephalalgia* 1988; 8(suppl 7): 1–96.

9. Ophoff RA, Terwindt GM, Vergouwe MN et al, Involvement of a $Ca^{2+}$ channel gene in familial hemiplegic migraine and migraine with and without aura. *Headache* 1997; **37:** 479–85.

10. Gardner K, Barmada MM, Ptacek LJ et al, A new locus for hemiplegic migraine maps to chromosome 1q31. *Neurology* 1997; **49:** 1231–8.

11. Bickerstaff ER, Basilar artery migraine. *Lancet* 1961; **i:** 15–17.

12. Lapkin ML, Golden GS, Basilar artery migraine, a review of 30 cases. *Am J Dis Child* 1978; **132:** 278–81.

13. Barlow CF, Headaches and migraine in childhood. *Clin Dev Med* 1984; **91:** 103–9.

14. Golden GS, French JH, Basilar artery migraine in young children. *Pediatrics* 1975; **56:** 722–6.

15. La Spina I, Vignati A, Porazzi D, Basilar artery migraine: transcranial Doppler EEG and SPECT from the aura phase to the end. *Headache* 1997; **37:** 43–7.

16. Hansen SL, Borelli-Moller L, Strange P et al, Ophthalmoplegic migraine: diagnostic criteria, incidence of hospitalization, and possible etiology. *Acta Neurol Scand* 1990; **81:** 54–60.

17. Woody RC and Blaw ME, Ophthalmoplegic migraine in infancy. *Clin Pediatr* 1986; **25:** 82–4.

18. Vijayan N, Ophthalmoplegic migraine: Ischemic or compressive neuropathy? *Headache* 1980; **20:** 300–4.

19. Stommel EW, Ward TN, Harris RD, Ophthalmoplegic migraine or Tolosa–Hunt syndrome? *Headache* 1994; **34:** 177.

20. Mark AS, Casselman J, Brown D et al, Ophthalmoplegic migraine: reversible enhancement and thickening of the cisternal segment of the oculomotor nerve on contrast-enhanced MR images. *AJNR Am J Neuroradiol* 1998; **19:** 1887–91.

21. May A, Shepheard SL, Knorr M et al, Retinal plasma extravasation in animals but not in humans: implications for the pathophysiology of migraine. *Brain* 1998; **121:** 1231–7.

22. Fenichel GM, Migraine as a cause of benign paroxysmal vertigo of childhood. *J Pediatr* 1967; **71:** 114–15.

23. Basser LS, Benign paroxysmal vertigo of childhood. *Brain* 1987; **141:** 1964.

24. Lanzi G, Balottin U, Fazzi E et al, Benign paroxysmal vertigo of childhood: a long-term follow-up. *Cephalalgia* 1994; **14:** 458–60.

25. Verret S, Steele JC, Alternating hemiplegia in childhood: A report of eight patients with complicated migraine beginning in infancy. *Pediatrics* 1971; **47:** 675–80.

26. Aicardi J, Bourgeois M, Goutieres F, Alternating hemiplegia of childhood: clinical findings

and diagnostic criteria. In: Andermann F, Aicardi J, Vigevano F, eds, *Alternating Hemiplegia of Childhood*. New York: Raven Press, 1995: 3–18.

27. Rho JM, Chugani HT, Alternating hemiplegia of childhood: Insights into its pathogenesis. *J Child Neurol* 1998; **13**: 39–45.

28. Chaves-Carballo E, Paroxysmal torticollis. *Semin Pediatr Neurol* 1996; **3**: 255–6.

29. Chutorian AM, Benign paroxysmal torticollis, tortipelvis and retrocollis of infancy. *Neurology* 1974; **24**: 366–7.

30. Snyder CH, Paroxysmal torticollis in infancy. A possible form of labyrinthitis. *Am J Dis Child* 1969; **117**: 458–60.

31. Pfau BT, Li BUK, Murray RD et al, Differentiating cyclic vomiting from chronic vomiting patterns in children: quantitative criteria and diagnostic implications. *Pediatrics* 1996; **97**: 364–8.

32. To J, Issenman RM, Kamath MV, Evaluation of neurocardiac signals in pediatric patients with cyclic vomiting syndrome through power spectral analysis of heart rate variability. *J Pediatr* 1999; **135**: 363–6.

33. Andersen JM, Sugerman KS, Lockhart JR et al, Effective prophylactic therapy for cyclic vomiting syndrome in children using amitriptyline and cyproheptadine. *Pediatrics* 1997; **100**: 977–81.

34. Li BUK, Murray RD, Heitlinger LA et al, Is cyclic vomiting syndrome related to migraine? *J Pediatric* 1999; **134**: 567–72.

35. Li BUK, Murray RD, Heitlinger LA et al, Heterogeneity of diagnoses presenting as cyclic vomiting. *Pediatrics* 1998; **102**: 583–7.

36. Garcon G, Barlow CF, Juvenile migraine presenting as acute confusional states. *Pediatrics* 1970; **45**: 628–35.

37. Ehyai A, Fenichel G, The natural history of acute confusional migraine. *Arch Neurol* 1978; **35**: 368–9.

38. Jensen TS, Transient global amnesia in childhood. *Dev Med Child Neurol* 1980; **22**: 654–8.

39. Ferrera PC, Reicho PR, Acute confusional migraine and trauma-triggered migraine. *Am J Emerg Med* 1996; **14**: 276–8.

40. Amit R, Acute confusional state in childhood. *Child Nerv Syst* 1988; **4**: 255–8.

# 14

# Psychiatric co-morbidity
*Federica Galli, Vincenzo Guidetti*

## General issues in co-morbidity

The term 'co-morbidity' is a general medical word that dates back to Feinsten.[1] Initially, it related to the occurrence of two distinct diseases in the same patient – 'additional ailment in a patient with a particular index disease'.

The current conceptualization of the term implies an association, more than casual, but probably not causal, between an index disease or disorder and one, or more, coexisting physical or psychological pathologies.

The adoption of Feinstein's definition does not imply the assumption in itself of a hierarchy between the 'index disorder' and the 'additional' ones, if not in relation to our main focus, or consideration of a disease or disorder as the starting point of our analysis or in terms of a time sequence. In part, the applicability of the definition to the medical field has been facilitated by knowledge about biological mechanisms explaining the occurrence of some diseases (e.g. diabetes).

The transposition of the conceptualization to the psychiatric field is more recent in adulthood, although mainly in childhood and adolescence.[2] The contents and implications of the concept of 'co-morbidity' have suggested reconsiderations and re-framing over the time.

Co-morbidity refers to 'disorders' ('behavioural and psychological problems that are deviant from 'normality') and/or 'diseases' (well defined as clinical entities), not to the existence of related co-occurring symptoms (syndrome). However, recognition of co-morbidities may be an initial step for identifying 'new syndromes'.

In addition, clarification of the direction, meaning and the weight of co-morbidities has pathophysiological, nosological, course and treatment implications. The study of co-morbidity may, however, present a series of difficulties related to the current understanding of aetiology and pathophysiology of diseases at the centre of our attention. Sometimes, as happens in migraine topics, we proceed on a background that still needs clarification of many issues. The question is amplified in psychiatry, and even more troublesome when the co-occurrence of psychiatric and no psychiatric variables is analysed.

In the psychiatric field, we deal mainly with disorders and not diseases.[2] The psychiatric classification system presents weak points, even more so when age-related variables are taken into account. To date, knowledge about the aetiology and pathophysiology of most psychiatric disorders is inferential at best, and the problems increase with developmental age, in relation to specific, although not well-recognized, clinical characteristics, as well as to peculiarities in classification of psychiatric diseases. DSM-IV[3] provides a small number of diagnostic criteria for psychiatric disorders with the age of onset in childhood (see below).

The research and clinical approaches to co-morbidity need to consider several issues. First, it is very important to consider the 'time' factor. The inferences that can be drawn from the existence of specific, non-casual relationships between two or more disorders depend very much on the 'current' or 'lifetime' (even 'concurrent' or 'successive'[2]) coexistence of disorders. Current co-morbidity refers to the co-presence of two or more disorders in the same time span. Lifetime co-morbidity concerns the occurrence of disorders over a period of time that needs to be specified (it may be 6 months, 1 year or the individual's lifetime to date). The concept of 'successive' co-morbidity has been suggested with regards to two disorders that do not overlap in time.[2] When 'lifetime' co-morbidity is considered, the temporal margin should be carefully specified, in order to avoid biased conclusions.

Andrews[4] suggested preservation of the term 'co-morbidity' for the conditions in which the temporal sequence is not specified, and to apply the concept of 'co-occurrence' when two or more disorders occur at the same time.

In children, consideration and specification of the timing are very important to avoid confounding the time trend of age-related characteristics with the phenomenology of disorders. Dealing with co-morbidities allows us to describe clinical situations without inevitably assuming or embracing causal explanations, even if a better specification of the temporal interval may give us valid help in the comprehension and systematization of the subject.

The second issue is the concept of 'homo-typic' (continuity of disease phenomenology without strong changes over time) or 'heterotypic' (a continuous process assuming different forms over time) co-morbidity. Considering co-morbidity from different diagnostic groupings (such as migraine and anxiety and/or depression) or within a unique diagnostic grouping (such as dysthymia and major depression) additional and different questions arise about the co-occurrence pattern, aetiology, course and therapy. Could heterotypic co-morbidity represent a marker of severity and/or worst outcome? Could it represent a means of subtyping a disorder? What is the aetiology of heterotypic co-morbidity? Can we call it a syndrome? What are the causes? Are there correlated causes or shared common factors?

Third, we need to consider relating the use of general population or clinical studies in research on co-morbidity. Both present pros and cons. On the one hand, population-based studies avoid the so-called Berkson's bias, namely the tendency of self-selected patients to consult specialists. A major severity of illnesses, personality characteristics and the same co-morbidity may represent biased selection filters, altering the likely findings. Only population-based studies can provide prevalence and incidence rates, unbiased estimates of risk factors for co-morbidity. On the other hand, clinical studies may strengthen findings by population study, permit better monitoring of co-morbidity pattern and course over time, and give data about the better implementation of therapy interventions. Only clinical studies allow the study of rare disorders, even more when there is co-morbid presentation. The focus on potential risk factors, and the outcome and developmental trend of co-morbid patterns may be highlighted by the use of clinical studies.

The fourth important issue relates to the probable causes of co-morbidity. At present, the likelihood that co-morbidity is solely the result of methodological problems (a consequence of Berkson's bias, information-collection bias or lack of systematic diagnostic systems) seems to have been ruled out.[2] The concept of 'epiphenomenal' co-morbidity has been recently pointed out[2] as a reason for the co-morbid association of three conditions: one may be only the 'product' of the other two. However, it is difficult to tailor to our specific field issues; probably only more detailed quantitative and qualitative analysis can give us better framing of the topic.

## Psychiatric co-morbidity and migraine

A characteristic set of psychological features has been observed among migraine sufferers over the past (twentieth) century. Peters[5] stated that migraine occurs 'most frequently in delicate males and females of a highly nervous temperament ... apt to be reproduced by any unusual excitement, by joy, hope, fear, excessive pleasure, anxiety, fasting, fatigue, ...'. Anstie[6] suggested that migraine follows a period of bodily changes, and then 'the patient begins to suffer headache after any unusual fatigue or excitement'. Liveing[7] considered depression and drowsiness as characteristics of migraineurs. Emotional disturbance is one of three causes of migraine, together with gastric and menstrual disturbances. Moersch[8] reported mild mental and physical depression, anxiety, apathy, lack of energy and fatigue.

Wolff[9] proposed the definition of 'migraine personality'. Although his investigations concerned migrainous adults, he suggested that, as children, they were shy, withdrawn and obedi-

ent, but occasionally they could become inflexible, obstinate and rebellious. Several studies outlined the association of psychological factors and migraine among children (see Chapter 14).

Knopf[10] described patients who were well behaved and nervous as children. They portrayed themselves as unhappy in childhood, 'goody goody, ambitious, reserved and repressed'. Vahlquist[11] recorded neurovegetative instability, ambition and perfectionism among migrainous children. Bille[12] described migrainous children as more anxious, sensitive, cautious, fearful, vulnerable to frustration, tidy and less physically enduring than control group children. Among girls the differences were stronger.

Coch and Melchior[13] found signs of nervousness, mental instability and immaturity in both migraineur and non-migraineur patients. They suggested 'a decreased resistance to psychological stress and conflict situations, rather than overt psychological disorder, or endogenous disease'.

Guidetti et al[14] found feeling of being excluded from the family group, and repressed hostility towards important figures. Andrasik et al[15] found a greater number of somatic complaints in migraineurs and higher ratings of depression and anxiety among migrainous adolescents, compared with matched headache-free patients. The hypothesis that 'frequent, unexplainable and intense head pain would likely lead to heightened levels of depression and anxiety' is suggested.[15] Cunningham et al,[16] comparing migraine and chronic non-headache pain samples, found no difference in anxiety and depression levels between the two groups with chronic pain, compared with pain-free controls.

From the beginning of the 1990s, the

subject has turned to systematizing through conceptualization in terms of 'psychiatric co-morbidity' by prospective population-based studies on young adults.[17–22] Merikangas et al[19] suggested that many of the psychological features frequently related to migraine are more akin to psychopathological symptoms than personality characteristics, so much so that a syndromic relationship with a peculiar time sequence (anxiety, migraine and depression) has been suggested.[17,20] This remark had been supported by the population-based study by Breslau et al,[18] even though a bidirectional influence between migraine and depression has been suggested,[21,22] with one increasing the first onset of the other. Reviews on the topic have been carried out in both adults[23,24] and children and adolescents.[25,26]

There are two alternative putative proposal explanations: (1) migraine causes psychopathology or, vice versa, is caused by it; and (2) underlying pathological (genetic or environmental) mechanisms are shared by migraine and anxiety/depression. The greatest number of studies on psychiatric co-morbidity have been carried out on migraine, and less frequently on tension-type headache.[27] However, the International Headache Society (IHS) classification[28] lists, as potential 'causes' for tension-type headache, psychosocial stress, anxiety and depression. From the above brief references there emerges the ongoing systematization of the issue, even though the aetiological mechanisms remain at an inferential level.

The hypothesis of a shared biological predisposition between migraine and depression has been suggested on the basis of similarities in biological aspects (role of the serotoninergic system).[29,30]

The strict, but unclear, relationship of anxiety and depression (without the presence of migraine) is well recognized in the literature and should be taken into account before making any inference in the headache field. Co-morbidity of anxiety and depression seems to be more the rule than the exception:[31] children with anxiety disorders have co-morbid major depression with rates ranging from 47%[32] to 69%,[33] and 30–80% of patients with major depression, and 40% of patients with dysthymic disorder are also affected by at least one anxiety disorder.[34] Breslau and Davis[35] reported an increased risk of major depression only in people with a history of migraine plus anxiety.

The reference to developmental ages has been made by the same studies[17–22] through the suggestion that there is a time sequence in determining the occurrence of a probable syndromic relationship of anxiety in childhood and adolescence, followed by migraine and then depression. Clinical studies have strengthened these findings, stressing the negative prognostic meaning of the co-morbid association of psychiatric disorders and course of headache.[36]

Also population-based studies on the psychiatric side have suggested that 'the association of headaches with depression and anxiety may be distinct phenomena',[37] with 20.5% of children with a psychiatric diagnosis suffering headache, and 34.1% of girls with an anxiety disorder and 40.8% presenting with depression having headache (vs, respectively, 10% and 10.5% of girls without anxiety or depression); the more frequent and severe headache is experienced by depressed girls. However, the generic reference to 'headache' and the absence of a systematic evaluation of subtype specification[37,38] limit the generalization of the results to our field.

In developmental ages, however, analysis of the interplay of anxiety and/or mood disorders and migraine presents additional difficulties related to the absence of a strong classification system of childhood and adolescence psychopathology.

## Anxiety disorders

The implication of anxiety in migraine has been strongly outlined in both clinical and population-based studies (see above). However, the implication and meaning of co-morbid anxiety disorders in the headache field should have better empirical clarification and probably substantial consideration in diagnostic terms. The IHS classification[28]

considers anxiety as a possible 'cause' of tension headache, but no suggestions are given for migraine. Anxiety disorders have been found to predict the persistence of migraine over time[36] and to precede the onset of migraine.[17]

The American Academy of Child and Adolescent Psychiatry (AACAP)[34] classified migraine as a disease to consider in the differential diagnosis of anxiety, because it is 'a physical condition that may mimic anxiety disorders'. DSM-IV[3] diagnostic criteria for 'separation anxiety disorder' specifically refer to 'headaches' (Table 14.1). The topic requires

---

A.  Developmentally inappropriate and excessive anxiety concerning separation from home or from those to whom the individual is attached, as evidenced by three or more of the following:

    (1)  Recurrent excessive distress when separation from home or major attachment figures occurs or is anticipated
    (2)  Persistent or excessive worry about losing, or about possible harm befalling, major attachment figures
    (3)  Persistent or excessive worry that an untoward event will lead to separation from a major attachment figure (e.g. getting lost or being kidnapped)
    (4)  Persistent reluctance or refusal to go to school or elsewhere because of fear of separation
    (5)  Persistently and excessively fearful or reluctant to be alone or without major attachment figures at home or without significant adults in other settings
    (6)  Persistent reluctance or refusal to go to sleep without being near a major attachment figure or to sleep away from home
    (7)  Repeated nightmares involving the theme of separation
    (8)  Repeated complaints of physical symptoms (such as headaches, stomachaches, nausea or vomiting) when separation from major attachment figure occurs or is anticipated

B.  The duration of the disturbance is at least 4 weeks
C.  The onset is before 18 years
D.  The disturbance causes clinically significant distress or impairment in social, academic (occupational) or other important areas of functioning
E.  The disturbance does not occur exclusively during the course of pervasive developmental disorder, schizophrenia or other psychotic disorders, and in adolescents and adults, is not better accounted for by panic disorder with agoraphobia

**Table 14.1**
*DSM-IV diagnostic criteria for separation anxiety disorder*

more specific analyses, however, in order to clarify the role of any anxiety disorder in childhood headache sufferers. From the youngest age, anxiety presents high levels of co-morbidity,[39,40] so that whether anxiety should be conceptualized as an independent disorder, or as a residual or prodrome of other disorders, is questionable.[41] The general reference to anxiety helps a systematization of the subject very little. By developmental psychiatry, the issue presents weak points, lacking clear-cut boundaries between diagnostic categories that are often tailored for adults.

However, knowledge about the different manifestations that anxiety may assume in the developmental ages is, according to the current knowledge, of crucial importance for both clinical and research purposes.

The third, revised edition of the manual, DSM-III-R,[42] provided criteria for the child and adolescent categories of 'overanxious disorder' (OAD), 'avoidant disorder' (AD) and 'separation anxiety disorder' (SAD). OAD and AD have been eliminated in DSM-IV,[3] because there is no recognition of specific clinical relevance and they are considered to overlap with

---

A.  Excessive anxiety and worry (apprehensive expectation), occurring more days than not for at least 6 months, about a number of events or activities (such as work or school performance)
B.  The person finds it difficult to control the worry
C.  The anxiety and worry are associated with three (or more) of the following six symptoms (with at least some symptoms present for more days than not for the past 6 months). **Note:** only one item is required in children:

    (1)  Restlessness or feeling keyed up or on edge
    (2)  Being easily fatigued
    (3)  Difficulty concentrating or mind going blank
    (4)  Irritability
    (5)  Muscle tension
    (6)  Sleep disturbance (difficulty falling or staying asleep, or restless unsatisfying sleep)

D.  The focus of the anxiety and worry is not confined to features of an axis I disorder, e.g. the anxiety or worry is not about having a panic attack (as in panic disorder), being embarrassed in public (as in social phobia), being contaminated (as in obsessive–compulsive disorder), being away from home or close relatives (as in separation anxiety disorder), having multiple physical complaints (as in somatization disorder) or having a serious illness (as in hypochondriasis), and anxiety and worry do not occur exclusively during post-traumatic stress disorder
E.  The anxiety, worry and physical symptoms cause clinically significant distress or impairment in social, occupational or other important areas of functioning
F.  The disturbance is not due to the direct physiological effects of a substance (e.g. a drug of abuse, a medication) or a general medical condition (e.g. hyperthyroidism) and does not occur exclusively during a mood disorder, a psychotic disorder or a pervasive developmental disorder

**Table 14.2**
*DSM-IV diagnostic criteria for generalized anxiety disorder*

A.  A marked and persistent fear of one or more social or performance situations in which the person is exposed to unfamiliar people or to possible scrutiny by others. The individual fears that he or she will act in a way (or shows anxiety symptoms) that will be humiliating or embarrassing. **Note:** in children, there must be evidence of the capacity of age-appropriate social relationships with familiar people and the anxiety must occur in peer settings, not just in interactions with adults

B.  Exposure to the feared social situation almost invariably provokes anxiety, which may take the form of a situationally bound or situationally predisposed panic attack. **Note:** in children, the anxiety may be expressed by crying, tantrums, freezing or shrinking from social situations with unfamiliar people

C.  The person recognizes that the fear is excessive or unreasonable. **Note:** in children the feature may be absent

D.  The feared social or performance situations are avoided or else are endured with intense anxiety or distress

E.  The avoidance, anxious anticipation or distress in the feared social or performance situation(s) interferes significantly with the person's normal routine, occupational (academic) functioning, or social activities or relationships, or there is marked distress about having the phobia

F.  In individuals under 18 years of age, the duration is at least 6 months

G.  The fear or avoidance is not due to the direct physiological effects of a substance (e.g. a drug of abuse, a medication) or a general medical condition and is not better accounted for by another medical disorder (e.g. panic disorder with or without agoraphobia, separation anxiety disorder, body dysmorphic disorder, a pervasive developmental disorder or schizoid personality disorder)

H.  If a general medical condition or another mental disorder is present, the fear is not of stuttering, trembling in Parkinson's disease, or exhibiting abnormal eating behaviour in anorexia nervosa or bulimia nervosa

**Table 14.3**
*DSM-IV diagnostic criteria for social phobia*

other disorders;[43] therefore, they are respectively considered to be included in the categories of 'generalized anxiety disorder' (Table 14.2) and 'social phobia' (Table 14.3). Other anxiety disorders included in DSM-IV are 'panic disorder' and specific phobias.

Panic disorder (Table 14.4) most often begins in adolescence or early adult life, even though it may affect children.[44] It is interesting that children with early onset of separation anxiety are at increased risk of later development of panic disorder.[34,43]

The occurrence of specific phobias (Table 14.5) needs to consider the developmental perspective, to determine whether some fears are appropriate at some ages.[44] Other anxiety disorders affecting children and adolescents include obsessive–compulsive disorder and post-traumatic stress disorder.[34]

From the youngest age, the co-morbid presentation of anxiety disorders recurs frequently: one-third of children with anxiety meet the criteria for two or more additional anxiety disorders,[34] and the estimates of co-

A discrete period of intense fear or discomfort, in which four (or more) of the following symptoms developed abruptly and reached a peak within 10 minutes:

(1)  Palpitations, pounding heart, or accelerated heart rate
(2)  Sweating
(3)  Trembling or shaking
(4)  Sensations of shortness of breath or smothering
(5)  Feeling of choking
(6)  Chest pain or discomfort
(7)  Nausea or abdominal distress
(8)  Feeling dizzy, unsteady, lightheaded or faint
(9)  Derealization (feeling of unreality) or depersonalization (being detached from oneself)
(10)  Fear of losing control or going crazy
(11)  Fear of dying
(12)  Paraesthesias (numbness or tingling sensations)
(13)  Chills or hot flushes

**Note:** a panic attack is not a codable disorder. The presence or absence of agoraphobia needs to be coded

**Table 14.4**
*DSM-IV criteria for panic attack*

A.  Marked and persistent fear that is excessive or unreasonable, cued by the presence or anticipation of a specific, object or situation (e.g. flying, heights, animals, receiving an injection, seeing blood)
B.  Exposure to the phobic stimulus almost invariably provokes an immediate anxiety response, which may take the form of a situationally bound or situationally predisposed panic attack. **Note:** in children the anxiety may be expressed by crying, tantrums, freezing or clinging
C.  The person recognizes that the fear is excessive or unreasonable. **Note:** in children, this feature may be absent
D.  The phobic situation(s) is avoided or else is endured with intense anxiety or distress
E.  The avoidance, anxious anticipation or distress in the feared situation(s) interferes significantly with the person's normal routine, occupational or academic functioning, or social activities or relationships, or there is marked distress about having the phobia
F.  In individuals under 18 years, the duration is at least 6 months
G.  The anxiety, panic attacks, or phobic avoidance associated with the specific object or situation are not better accounted for by another mental disorder, such as obsessive–compulsive disorder (e.g. fear of dirt in someone with an obsession about contamination), post-traumatic stress disorder (e.g. avoidance of stimuli associated with a severe stressor), separation anxiety disorder (e.g. avoidance of school), social phobia (e.g. avoidance of school situations because of fear of embarrassment), panic disorder with agoraphobia or agoraphobia without history of panic disorder

**Table 14.5**
*DSM-IV diagnostic criteria for specific phobia*

morbid major depression range from 28% to 69%.[39] Merikangas[31] outlined that as many as 75% of depressed adolescents have one or more anxiety disorders.

Within anxiety disorders, particular attention should be paid to school refusal (or phobia). Clinical observations frequently suggest the weight of schooling in headache sufferers, ranging from excessive involvement in school achievement to relationship problems with teachers or schoolmates up to real school withdrawal.

School refusal is not a psychiatric diagnosis, and the DSM-IV[3] makes no specific reference to it, not as a diagnostic criterion for SAD (see Table 14.1). In addition, simple or social phobia and major depressive disorders are the most recurrent diagnoses for school refusers,[45] and often multiple diagnoses occur.[46] The boundaries between school phobia and SAD, social phobia or depression are not well recognized, and only an analysis case by case may give elements to decode the clinical situation and address the intervention.[47]

The frequent co-occurrence of somatic complaints (mainly gastrointestinal disorders and headache)[37,45,47] and school refusal needs clarifications.

## Mood disorders

Mood disorders have long been underdiagnosed in prepubertal children, because sufficient evidence has not been recognized. Only in the 1970s was the existence of depression in children first officially recognized.[48] Major depressive disorder (Table 14.6) and dysthymic disorder (Table 14.7) are the most relevant and recurrent of mood disorders affecting children and adolescents. Bipolar disorder (I and II) and cyclothymic disorder (DSM-IV) may start in adolescence or early adult life.

The clinical presentation of depression in prepubertal age presents differences compared with adolescents and adults. DSM-IV[3] represents a firm point of reference in the psychiatric field towards having a common shared language, even though the diagnostic parameters are not always adequate for the developmental age's characteristics. With reference to major depressive disorder (Table 14.6), children may present more symptoms such as phobias, anxiety separation and somatic complaints, whereas adolescents tend to display more sleep and eating disturbances, delusions and more impairment in functioning than younger children, although there are more behavioural problems or neurovegetative symptoms than in adults.[34]

Differential diagnoses should exclude the occurrence of disorders that cause alterations in mood tone: non-affective psychiatric disorders (such as separation anxiety, learning disabilities, disruptive disorders, substance use disorders, attention-deficit/hyperactive disorder, premenstrual dysphoric disorder, etc.), adjustment disorder with depressed mood, general medical conditions (such as cancer, hypothyroidism, lupus erythematosus, acquired immune deficiency syndrome, anaemia, diabetes and epilepsy) and bereavement.

## Overview

Over the last 10 years, the unquestionable relationship of migraine and psychiatric co-morbidity has been described. The challenge of the immediate future relates to the explanation of the mechanisms involved in the aetiology and pathophysiology, in order to draw the consequences in diagnostic (does co-morbid migraine represent a different subtype?) and

A.  Five (or more) of the following symptoms have been present during the same 2-week period and represent a change from previous functioning; at least one of the symptoms is either (1) depressed mood or (2) loss of interest or pleasure
**Note**: do not include symptoms that are clearly due to a general medical condition, or mood-incongruent delusions or hallucinations

(1)  Depressed mood most of the day, as indicated by either subjective report (e.g. feels sad or empty) or observation made by others (e.g. appeared tearful). **Note**: in children and adolescents, can be irritable mood
(2)  Markedly diminished interest or pleasure in all, or almost all, activities most of the day, nearly every day (as indicated by either subjective account or observation made by others)
(3)  Significant weight loss when not dieting or weight gain (e.g. a change of more than 5% of body weight in a month), or decrease or increase in appetite nearly every day. **Note**: in children, consider failure to make expected weight gains
(4)  Insomnia or hypersomnia nearly every day
(5)  Psychomotor agitation or retardation nearly every day (observable by others, not merely subjective feelings of restlessness or being slowed down)
(6)  Fatigue or loss of energy nearly every day
(7)  Feelings of worthlessness or excessive or inappropriate guilt (which may be delusional) nearly every day (not merely self-reproach or guilt about being sick)
(8)  Diminished ability to think or concentrate, or indecisiveness, nearly every day (either by subjective account or as observed by others)
(9)  Recurrent thoughts of death (not just fear of dying), recurrent suicidal ideation without specific plan, or a suicide attempt or a specific plan for committing suicide

B.  The symptoms do not meet criteria for a mixed episode
C.  The symptoms cause clinically significant distress or impairment in social, occupational or other important areas of functioning
D.  The symptoms are not due to the direct physiological effects of a substance (e.g. a drug of abuse, a medication) or a general medical condition (e.g. hypothyroidism)
E.  The symptoms are not better accounted for by bereavement, i.e. after the loss of a loved one, the symptoms persist for longer than 2 months, or are characterized by marked functional impairment, morbid preoccupation with worthlessness, suicidal ideation, psychotic symptoms or psychomotor retardation

**Table 14.6**
*DSM-IV criteria for major depressive episode*

therapeutic terms (how do we treat migraine in co-morbid association?). However, methodological problems limit research and interpretations of findings in this sphere. The use of clinical samples (Berkson's bias), non-standardized assessment techniques, the doubtful validity of retrospective data and the absence of control samples are weakening factors. The same research in the child and adolescent psychopathological field is difficult, lacking clear-cut criteria and instruments of diagnosis, with the influence of age-related

A. Depressed mood for most of the day, for more days than not, as indicated either by subjective account or observation by others, for at least 2 years. **Note**: in children and adolescents mood may be irritable and duration must be at least 1 year

B. Presence while depressed, of two (or more) of the following:

(1) Poor appetite or overeating
(2) Insomnia or hypersomnia
(3) Low energy or fatigue
(4) Low self-esteem
(5) Poor concentration or difficulty making decisions
(6) Feelings of hopelessness

C. During the 2-year (1 year for children or adolescents) disturbance, the person has never been without the symptoms in criteria A and B for more than 2 months at a time

D. No major depressive episode has been present during the first 2 years of the disturbance (1 year for children and adolescents), i.e. the disturbance is not better accounted for by chronic major depressive disorder, or major depressive disorder, in partial remission
**Note**: there may have been a previous major depressive episode provided there was a full remission (no significant signs or symptoms for 2 months) before development of the dysthymic disorder. In addition, after the initial 2 years (1 year for children and adolescents) of dysthymic disorder, there may be superimposed episodes of major depressive disorder, in which case both diagnoses may be given when the criteria are met for a major depressive episode

E. There has never been a manic episode, a mixed episode or a hypomanic episode, and criteria have never been met for cyclothymic disorder

F. The disturbance does not occur exclusively during the course of a chronic psychotic disorder, such as schizophrenia or delusional disorder

G. The symptoms are not due to the direct physiological effects of a substance (e.g. drug abuse, a medication) or a general medical condition (e.g. hypothyroidism)

H. The symptoms cause clinically significant distress or impairment in social, occupational or other important areas of functioning

**Table 14.7**
*DSM-IV criteria for dysthymic disorder*

differences or of social and environmental conditions still being unclear.

At present, the probability of an incidental association between migraine and co-morbid psychiatric disorders has been ruled out, and consequently the related issues need to be examined closely; several points need to be clarified:

• Direction of the relationship: Is migraine caused by or a cause of anxiety/mood disorders? Is migraine associated with anxiety/mood disorders the final, but unrelated result of factors other than themselves? Is the co-morbid association related to a specific moment ('current') of the life of the patient or 'lifetime'?

• Pathophysiological mechanisms: What are

the main factors involved? Are there shared common biological, genetic, environmental or psychological processes in migraine and such psychiatric disorders? What is the relative weight of each factor?

- Diagnostic consequence: Is migraine in psychiatric co-morbid association a different disease from migraine occurring alone? Should we start to make an additional differentiation in migraine subtypes according to the presence or absence of psychiatric co-morbidity?
- Therapeutic lines: How do we treat migraine with psychiatric co-morbid association?
- Influences on the outcome: What is the weight of psychiatric co-morbidity in relation to the evolution of migraine? What is the role of age at onset, sex, distressing life events, personality characteristics, etc.?

To date, the implications of psychiatric co-morbidity in relation to the course, outcome and classification system have not been drawn in either adults or mainly, childhood migraine.

Psychiatric co-morbidity may represent an obstacle for drug treatment effectiveness, but also another point on which to act when treating headaches. In fact, the occurrence of psychiatric disorders may address the treatment, e.g. by joining drug and non-drug therapy according to the specificities of the case.

Whether the occurrence of migraine in psychiatric co-morbid association is responsive to different treatments, compared with the 'pure' presentation, is not defined.

Another viewpoint concerns the possible role of external events as the stressful experiences. These could have a different impact, according to the presence or absence of a psychological basic profile, not excluding the fun-

damental role of predisposing biological factors. The consequences of headache crises on the patient's environment (secondary gains, the influence on parental or family relationships, etc.) or, vice versa, the potential effects of environmental factors on the patient's health have to be taken into account in a general model of headache.

More than ever in clinical practice, however, we must avoid framing the discussion only using a 'psychiatric' viewpoint. The dangerous effects of labelling a young headache sufferer as a 'psychiatric patient' exist. At the opposite end, the consequences of excluding from the analysis the involvement of pyschological factors are not always considered.

On the one hand, the meaning and the exact role of these co-occurring factors should be more closely analysed and a greater comparison made among different spheres of research (mainly neurology and psychiatry). On the other, determination of a clear distinction among personality traits, psychological factors (including attentional and cognitive elements, role of stress and emotional disposition as basic vulnerability or trigger factors) and psychiatric co-morbidity is crucial, to avoid a confounding overlap of these different factors.

As long as we have not established a clear difference among all these factors, the possibility of confounding overlapping and contradictory interpretations of our findings should be considered. A correct approach to diagnosis and treatment of headaches requires a comprehensive evaluation, considering the young patient as the whole of his or her neurobiological and psychological development.

# References

1. Feinsten AR, The pre-therapeutic classification of comorbidity in chronic disease. *J Chron Dis* 1970; **23**: 455–68.

2. Angold A, Costello JE, Erkanli A, Comorbidity. *J Child Psychol Psychiatry* 1999; **40**(1): 57–87.

3. American Psychiatric Association, *Diagnostic and Statistical Manual of Mental Disorders*, 4th edn. International Version with ICD-10 codes. Washington, DC: American Psychiatric Association, 1994.

4. Andrews G, Comorbidity and the general neurotic syndrome. *Br J Psychiatry* 1996; **168**(suppl 30): 76S–84S.

5. Peters JC, A treatise on headache. In: Merskey H, Psychological factors in migraine. In: Blau JN, ed., *Migraine*. London: Chapman & Hall: 1987; 367–86.

6. Anstie FE, *Neuralgia and Disease that Resemble It*. London: Macmillan, 1871. In: Blau JN, ed., *Migraine*. London: Chapman & Hall, 1987.

7. Liveing E, *On Migraine, Sick-Headache, and Some Allied Disorders: A contribution to the pathology of nerve storms*. London: J & A Churchill, 1978.

8. Moersch FP, Psychic manifestations in migraine. *Am J Psychiatry* 1924; **3**: 698–716.

9. Wolff HG, Personality features and reactions of subjects with migraine. *Arch Neurol Psychiatry* 1937; **37**: 895.

10. Knopf O, Preliminary report on personality studies in thirty migraine patients. *J Nerv Ment Dis* 1935; **82**: 270–85.

11. Vahlquist B, Migraine in children. *Int Arch Allergy* 1962; **7**: 348–52.

12. Bille B, Migraine in schoolchildren. *Acta Paediatr* 1962; **51**(suppl 136): 1–151.

13. Coch C, Melchior JC, Headache in childhood – a five year material from a pediatric university clinic. *Dan Med Bull* 1969; **16**: 109–14.

14. Guidetti V, Ottaviano S, Pagliarini N, Paolella A, Seri S, Psychological peculiarities in children with recurrent primary headache. *Cephalalgia* 1983; **41**(suppl 1): 215–17.

15. Andrasik F, Kabela E, Quinn S, Attanasio V, Blanchard AB, Rosenblum EL, Psychological functioning of children who have recurrent migraine. *Pain* 1988; **34**: 43–52.

16. Cunningham SJ, McGrath PJ, Ferguson HB et al, Personality and behavioural characteristics in pediatric migraine. *Headache* 1987; **27**: 16–20.

17. Merikangas KR, Angst J, Isler H, Migraine and psychopathology. Results of the Zurich cohort study of young adults. *Arch Gen Psychiatry* 1990; **47**: 849–53.

18. Breslau N, Davis GC, Andreski P, Migraine, psychiatric disorders and suicide attempts: an epidemiological study of young adults. *Psychiatry Res* 1991; **37**: 11–23.

19. Merikangas KR, Merikangas JR, Angst J, Headache syndromes and psychiatric disorders: association and familial transmission. *J Psychiat Res* 1993; **2**: 197–210.

20. Merikangas KR, Psychopathology and headache syndromes in the community. *Headache* 1994; **34**: S17–26.

21. Breslau N, Davis G, Migraine, physical health and psychiatric disorder: a prospective epidemiologic study in young adults. *J Psychiat Res* 1993; **2**: 211–21.

22. Breslau N, Davis GC, Schultz LR, Peterson EL, Migraine and major depression: a longitudinal study. *Headache* 1994; **34**: 387–93.

23. Haythornthwaite JA, Migraine headaches and psychopathology: future directions. *J Psychiat Res* 1993; **27**: 183–6.

24. Merikangas KR, Fenton B, Ramadan NM, Comorbidity and migraine. *Semin Headache Man* 1996; **1**(4): 1–10.

25. Galli F and Guidetti V, Psychiatric comorbidity. *Semin Headache Man* 1997; **2**(4): 5–7.

26. Karwautz A, Wöber C, Lang T et al, Psychosocial factors in children and adolescents with migraine and tension-type headache: a controlled study and review of the literature. *Cephalalgia* 1999; **19**: 32–43.

27. Andrasik A, Passchier J, Psychological aspects. In: Olesen J, Tfelt-Hansen P, Welch KMA, eds, *The Headaches*. New York: Raven Press, 1993: 489.

28. International Headache Society, Classification and diagnostic criteria for headache disorders,

cranial neuralgias, and facial pain. *Cephalalgia* 1988; (suppl 7): 1–96.

29. Glover V, Jarman J, Sandler M, Migraine and depression: biological aspects. *J Psychiat Res* 1993; **2**: 223–31.

30. Silberstein SD, Serotonin (5-HT) and migraine. *Headache* 1994; **34**: 408–17.

31. Merikangas KR, Genetic epidemiologic studies of affective disorders in childhood and adolescence. *Eur Arch Psychiatry Clin Neurosci* 1993; **243**: 121–30.

32. Bernstein GA, Comorbidity and severity of anxiety and depressive disorders in a clinical sample. *J Am Acad Child Adolesc Psychiatry* 1991; **30**: 43–50.

33. Kashani JH, Orvaschel H, Anxiety disorders in midadolescence: a community sample. *Am J Psychiatry* 1998; **145**: 960–4.

34. AACAP Official Action. Practice parameters for the assessment and treatment of children and adolescents with anxiety disorders. *J Am Acad Child Adolesc Psychiatry* 1998; **37**(10 suppl): 63S–83S.

35. Breslau N, Davis GC, Migraine, major depression and panic disorder. *Cephalalgia* 1992; **12**: 85–90.

36. Guidetti V, Galli F, Fabrizi P, Giannantoni AS, Napoli L, Bruni O, Trillo S, Headache and psychiatric comorbidity: clinical aspects and outcome in an 8-year follow-up study. *Cephalalgia* 1998; **7**: 455–62.

37. Egger HL, Angold A and Costello J, Headache and psychopathology in children and adolescents. *J Am Acad Child Adolesc Psychiatry* 1998; **37**: 951–8.

38. Pine DS, Cohen P, Brook J, The association between major depression and headache: results of a longitudinal epidemiologic study in youth. *J Child Adolesc Psychopharmacol* 1996; **6**: 153–4.

39. Kashani JH, Orvaschel H, A community study of anxiety in children and adolescents. *Am J Psychiatry* 1990; **147**: 313–18.

40. Strauss CC, Last CG, Social and simple phobias in children. *J Anxiety Dis* 1993; **7**: 141–52.

41. Wittchen HU, Zhao S, Kessler RC, Eaton WW, DSM-III-R generalized anxiety disorder in the National Comorbidity Survey, *Arch Gen Psychiatry* 1994; **51**: 355–64.

42. American Psychiatric Association, *Diagnostic and Statistical Manual of Mental Disorders*, 3rd edn, revised (DSM-III-R). International Version with ICD-10 codes. Washington, DC: American Psychiatric Association, 1987.

43. Bernstein GA, Rapoport JL, Leonard HL, Separation anxiety and generalized anxiety disorder. In: Wiener JM, ed. *Textbook of Child and Adolescent Psychiatry*. Washington, DC: American Psychiatric Press, 1997: 467–80.

44. Marks IM, *Fears, Phobias, and Rituals*. Oxford: Oxford University Press, 1987.

45. Elliot JG, Practitioner review: school refusal: issues of conceptualization, assessment, and treatment. *J Child Psychol Psychiatry* 1999; **40**: 1001–12.

46. King N, Ollendick TH, Tonge BJ, *School Refusal: Assessment and Treatment*. Needham Heights, MA: Allyn & Bacon, 1995.

47. Klein RG, School refusal. In: Noshpitz JD, ed., *Handbook of Child and Adolescent Psychiatry* New York: John Wiley & Sons, Inc., 1998: 120–1.

48. Schulterbrandt JG, Raskin A, *Depression In Childhood: Diagnosis, Treatment, and Conceptual Models*. New York: Raven, 1977.

# 15

# Menstrual migraine in adolescence
*Fabio Facchinetti, Laura Sgarbi*

## Sex hormones and migraine

### Theoretical links

Hormones and the brain are interrelated so that they can be considered a unique functional entity, the neuroendocrine system. In fact, hormones are influenced by the central nervous system (CNS) although they also exert several different actions on the brain. The key structure in which most of these influences occur is the hypothalamus. Here the vegetative, emotional and temporal functions essential for living and being, both in the environment and in time, are integrated and transduced into order signals that the endocrine system can execute.

With regard to primary headaches, the hypothalamic–pituitary–gonadal (HPG) axis seems to be the most interesting structure among the various endocrine systems. A reason for this could be that the reproductive system strongly conditions human life, because its integrity is absolutely necessary for the species to go on. The reproductive function, in fact, gives time to the crucial life events connected with the acquisition, presence and loss of fertility. The normal female life cycle is associated with a number of hormonal milestones: menarche, pregnancy, contraceptive use, menopause and the use of replacement sex hormones. The normal menstrual cycle induces changes not only in the genital tract but also in several other body systems, as a result of complex hormonal changes. Therefore, a two-way relationship is established between sex hormones of the HPG and central neurotransmitters believed to be involved in migraine pathophysiology.

Under the control of noradrenaline, serotonin, the opioids and other neurotransmitters, the hypothalamus secretes gonadotropin-releasing hormone (luteinizing hormone-releasing hormone or LHRH) in a pulsatile manner; this, in turn, stimulates pituitary luteinizing hormone (LH) and follicle-stimulating hormone (FSH) in the bloodstream and regulates the ovarian cycle. Some neurotransmitters, such as the catecholamines, acetylcholine and vasoactive intestinal peptide, stimulate LHRH synthesis. Conversely, the opioid peptides, corticotrophin-releasing factor, melatonin and γ-aminobutyric acid, have an inhibitory role. Dopamine and serotonin (5HT) exert both stimulatory and inhibitory effects, depending on the condition.[1]

Ovarian estradiol and progesterone feed back either to the pituitary to modulate the relative amounts of LH and FSH or to the hypothalamus to regulate LHRH itself. Both ovarian hormones display direct CNS effects through binding to receptors in opioidergic and other neuronal networks responsible for reproductive behaviour and gonadotrophin release.[2] In particular, the role of opioid peptides on the HPG axis has been established in humans as well as the modulation of ovarian hormones on opioid-related analgesic activity.[3]

Estradiol also increases the number of progesterone and muscarinic receptors and modulates 5HT and β-adrenergic receptors. Conversely, progesterone modulates the estrogen effects on the 5HT receptor.[4] Both estradiol and progesterone also affect indole metabolism through their effect on metabolizing enzymes. All the above changes justify the important changes of 5HT activity occurring throughout the menstrual cycle, either in pain-free or migraine patients.[5]

Estrogen-stimulated LH secretion may also be mediated by prostaglandins. Conversely, prostaglandin F2α inhibits gonadotrophin-stimulated progesterone production by luteinized cells. Prostaglandins, namely $E_2$, act as neurotransmitters. Some findings indicate that LHRH release may be regulated directly by intraneuronal $E_2$ production, which also mediates the effects of catecholamines on LHRH activity.[1] The role of prostanoids and leukotrienes in the pathogenesis of migraine is well known. Clinical studies have shown that injection of prostaglandin $E_1$ in humans can produce a migraine-type headache in non-migraineurs.[6] In low concentrations, the same compound is a potent vasoconstrictor, whereas in high concentrations it is a vasodilator. Moreover, drugs that inhibit prostaglandin synthesis had some efficacy in preventing menstrual migraine.[7] Overall, prostaglandins inhibit adrenergic transmission, sensitize nociceptors and promote the development of neurogenic inflammation through the release of substance P, vasodilatation, leakage of plasma proteins and inflammatory response. The neurogenic inflammation sustains part of the painful sensation of headache.[8]

## Clinical findings

The clinical findings supporting the concept of a sex hormone modulation of migraine attacks in women are in their hundreds. The basic considerations stem from the epidemiological data which allow the notion of migraine as a feminine disorder. Indeed, elegant, prospective, longitudinal studies performed in Finland demonstrated that, during adolescence, i.e. after pubertal maturation, the female to male ratio of migraine prevalence was 3:1 whereas in infancy, i.e. in prepubertal life, boys and girls showed similar figures of prevalence.[9]

Later in life, during the reproductive period, migraine attacks show a chronological pattern synchronous with that of the menstrual cycle: women have two to five attacks per month, almost constantly as a menstrually associated migraine; in some women migraine attacks occur exclusively in the perimenstrual period, leading to the diagnosis of menstrual migraine, a form of migraine without aura that is discussed below.[10] The physiological absence of menstrual cycle, which is associated with pregnancy, is followed by a definite relief from migraines, which completely disappear from the third month, reappearing almost certainly in the postpartum period.[11] Neither migraine with aura nor tension-type headache shows a hormonal modulation similar to that of migraine without aura. Indeed, migraine with aura does not change in pregnancy, patients reporting the constant number and quality of attacks.[12] Such forms of primary headache differ in their evolution also at the end of reproductive life although some contradiction exists as far as the effect of menopause on headache is concerned: for some authors there is a regression, for others a worsening.[13,14]

The menopause, involving a dramatic fall in the level of oestrogens, is expected to trigger a striking worsening or even an onset of migraine. However, this does not seem to be the case because the distribution of headache types at menopause is similar to that found in the fertile period.[15] Thus, it should be concluded that oestrogens are not the direct mediator between reproductive events and the headache course, and other factors of neural origin are possibly involved.

However, according to more controlled studies, migraines without aura undergo an improvement in most cases, whereas tension-type headaches show a trend towards a worsening, some cases reporting a switch from migraine to tension-type headache. All authors agree that the removal of the ovaries with the sudden reduction of their hormonal secretions is associated with a worsening of migraine, the surgical menopause thus representing a factor of the chronic nature of migraine.[12]

More doubtful are the data about the effect of hormone replacement on migraine course because no controlled studies could be found in the literature. Based on clinical experiences, the use of natural rather than synthetic oestrogens was advised, as well as the delivery of the lowest dose of hormones.[16] In a prospective, randomized study, we recently demonstrated that the transdermal route of estradiol delivery is preferred to the oral one: using the latter there was an increase both of attack frequency and of analgesic consumption (personal communication). Interestingly, only migraine patients are sensitive to hormone replacement, whereas those affected by tension-type headache did not show any change in the course of migraine.

The use of hormonal contraception was classically associated with a withdrawal from treatment just before the onset of headache.[17] By lowering oestrogen doses and changing the quality of progestogenic compounds, the prevalence of migraine suddenly decreased to less than 8% of contraceptive users. It should be pointed out that the onset of migraine on use of the contraceptive pill is more frequent in those women having a positive family history of migraine, thus supporting the idea that hormones do not induce migraine as such, but affect only those women with predisposing factors.[18]

## Menstrual migraine

Physical and psychological symptoms as well as behavioural disorders, have been linked to the menstrual cycle since ancient times, e.g. Hippocrates noted that 'shivering, lassitude and heaviness of the head denote the onset of menstruation'. It is well known that two-thirds of female migraineurs indicate the menstrual cycle as a factor conditioning their migraine attacks. According to various studies, 14–32% of attacks are exclusively perimenstrual (and they may be a part of the premenstrual syndrome, now a part of the *Diagnostic and Statistical Manual of Mental Disorders*, 4th edn [DSM-IV] criteria for premenstrual dysphoric disorder), whereas just 15% reported absolutely no correlation between headache and their menstrual cycle.[22] In an Italian study it was found that 92% of these women suffered from premenstrual syndrome;[20] 32 women had exclusively menstrual migraine and they described the premenstrual period as completely disabling. In contrast, in the group of women with migraine not associated with their menstrual cycle, their premenstrual syndrome consisted mostly of back pain, fluid retention and breast discomfort, but never in a disabling fashion. In terms of intensity, one-third of the population had the severest migraine attacks just in the premenstrual period: in a significant proportion they reported that analgesics completely relived the attacks only in the intermenstrual period, whereas drug use was less effective premenstrually. In a study by Metcalf et al,[21] observing seven moods and five physical symptoms daily throughout the course of 133 menstrual cycles in 44 premenstrual syndrome suffers, it was concluded that migraine was a menstrual rather than a premenstrual phenomenon. Therefore, migraine could be temporally distinguished from the other symptoms making up the premenstrual syndrome, although there is a strong co-morbidity between the two conditions.[22]

As far as the pathophysiology of menstrual migraine is concerned, Lundberg[23] reported that these women do not suffer from gross endocrine abnormalities or reduced fertility. On the other hand, he reported two Danish studies in which 67% of 50 women with polycystic ovary syndrome were migraineurs, whereas the frequency in the general population of the same city was 16.3%. Similarly, a study by Couch et al[24] reported that the incidence of migraine in the pathological ovulatory states, including polycystic ovary syndrome and galactorrhoea–amenorrhoea, was higher (50%) than in normally menstruating women. The authors suggested that these data may be explained through abnormalities of the hypothalamic–pituitary hormones (high levels of LH and low levels of FSH) or through the neural mechanism in the hypothalamus related to their secretion. The opioid theory of menstrual migraine agrees with the above studies. Data from our studies[25] provide convincing evidence that central opioid tonus (investigated through the neuroendocrine response of LH to naloxone) fluctuates abnormally in patients with menstrual migraine, consistent with its transient failure in the days before the menses. This pattern seems to be reversible because patients tested in the mid-luteal phase exhibited a naloxone-induced rise in LH similar to that of the control women. In these patients, there seems to be a common biochemical defect, which is a transient and reversible failure of central opioid tonus.[26] More recently, it has been reported that opioids exert a feedback on their own secretion, suggesting an opioid control of the hypothalamus–pituitary–adrenal axis. Patients with menstrual migraine also display a failure of this system. Indeed, the above-reported neuroendocrine response is lacking when women are tested premenstrually.[27] These findings indicate a failure of one of the endogenous systems subserving adaptive responses in patients with menstrual migraine.

## Menstrual migraine in adolescence

Adolescence is the period characterized by the onset of puberty, i.e. the period of becoming first capable of reproducing sexually, marked by maturation of genital organs, development of secondary sex characteristics and by the first occurrence of menstruation in the female. Puberty is recognized by the cascade of morphological, physiological and behavioural sequelae of increased ovarian activity at this time. The transition into puberty is tightly coupled with the initiation of a progressive increase in the overall secretory activity of the pituitary gonadotrophs. Then, the rise in FSH and LH secretions is the cause of activation of the gonads. The primary stimulus to pituitary gonadotrophs is generated within the central nervous system in the form of the episodic release of the LHRH.[1]

In a retrospective study, the relationships between reproductive life and headache among 1300 patients affected by common migraine (migraine without aura) were investigated. To evaluate the role exerted by the adolescence processes and considering that puberty is a milestone in the natural history of migraine, the population was subdivided into two groups according to the time of migraine appearance.[28] In 39.3% of girls, the onset of migraine was reported to occur during the adolescent period. In particular, 11.4% of the population refers to a time around menarche. However, throughout adolescence, there was no critical period and the distribution of migraine onset was similar in the 12–18 year range.

Interestingly, patients referred for onset of migraine at menarche had an actual coincidence of attacks with the menses which was double that of patients who had onset of migraine not linked to puberty. Moreover, the former group reported the disappearance of migraine during pregnancy (36.4%) in a significantly higher proportion than the latter (13.6%). As far as the family history of migraine was concerned, no differences between the two groups could be demonstrated. Similarly, the presence of an actual regular menstrual rhythm was similar between patients with and those without migraine

onset at menarche. On the contrary, a high prevalence of an invalidating primary dysmenorrhoea was reported in patients where migraine onset was unrelated to the adolescent period.

These findings indicate that the onset of migraine in the adolescent period, namely at menarche, is often associated with the particular kind of migraine that shows close clinical relationships with the hormonal environs. In particular, the onset of migraine at pubertal maturation easily predicts the development of a menstrual migraine later in life. On the contrary, perimenstrual migraine is quite uncommon during adolescence, possibly related to the fact that the first gynaecological years (3–5 years from menarche) are characterized by non-regular menstrual cycles. Indeed, because of maturational processes of the HPG axis, adolescent girls are characterized first by anovulatory menstrual cycles followed by ovarian cycle with a short and/or an inadequate luteal phase.

We have previously reported some observations about the role of ovulation in menstrual migraine.[29] In a case report, Holdaway et al[30] first described the successful use of chronic anovulation induced by an LHRH analogue in the treatment of a 38-year-old woman with severe menstrual migraine. Migraine totally disappeared during treatment and the patient decided to have definite surgical removal of the ovaries. More recently, a further five cases were reported on. The addition of hormone replacement during LHRH analogue treatment (which is mandatory for both skeletal and cardiovascular protection) did not interfere with the relief of menstrual migraine obtained through this form of chemical oophorectomy.[31]

The suppression of both ovulation and

menstrual flow aimed at the prophylaxis of perimenstrual migraine headaches, had been tried also through the use of tamoxifen, danazol or high-dose oestrogens. However, evidence suggested variable relief of migraine, although total disappearance was never achieved.[29] In the same way, the simple suppression of ovulation by using oral contraceptives also showed diverse effects over the course of migraine, without any consistency or proof of definite relief. It therefore seems evident that the total relief of menstrual migraine obtained through hypogonadism induced by LHRH agonist treatment is not the sole mechanism for explaining the efficacy of LHRH.

## Conclusions

Migraine in women is a phenomenon that is definitely sensitive to the hormone milieu and a significant proportion of migraineurs is affected only in relation to the menstrual cycle. Adolescence is the period of life where both the start of the menstrual cycle and the sensitivity to endocrine environment take place.

The origin of such a hallmark characterizing patients for their entire reproductive lives is unknown. However, several clinical and biological observations indicate that the hypothalamic secretion of LHRH is a crucial event. This decapeptide is the main driver of pubertal maturation and only transition into puberty makes the sex-related differences in migraine evident. On the other hand, LHRH is closely connected with networks involved in pain sensitivity, such as serotonin and opioids. Derangements of the above neuroendocrine pathways have been described in women with menstrual migraine and constitute a 'biochem-ical trait' predisposing them to hormone-related precipitation of migraine attacks.

In adolescent girls, the clinical expression of menstrual migraine is relatively low, whereas they are mainly disturbed by primary dysmenorrhoea. Menstrual migraine becomes evident in the 20s when menstrual cramps are no longer present. In those few teenagers with menstrual migraine, any hormonal approach should be avoided, in view of the developing maturation of the hypothalamus–pituitary–ovarian axis. Non-steroidal anti-inflammatory drugs should be the first choice of medication because of their efficacy in relieving uterine spasms.

## References

1. Yen SCC, Jaffe RJ, *Reproductive Endocrinology*, 3rd edn. Philadelphia: WB Saunders, 1991.
2. Pfaff DW, McEwen BS, Actions of estrogens and progestins on nerve cells. *Science* 1993; **219**: 808–14.
3. Petraglia F, Porro C, Facchinetti F et al, Differences in the opioid control of luteinizing hormone secretion between pathological and iatrogenic hyperprolactinemic states. *J Clin Endocrinol Metab* 1987; **64**: 508–12.
4. Biegon A, Reches A, Snyder L, McEwen BS, Serotononergic and noradrenergic receptors in the rat brain: modulation by chronic exposure to ovarian hormones. *Life Sci* 1983; **32**: 2015–28.
5. Fioroni L, Andrea GD, Alecci M, Cananzi A, Facchinetti F, Platelet serotonin pathway in menstrual migraine. *Cephalalgia* 1996; **16**: 427–30.
6. Carlson LA, Ekelund LG, Oro L, Clinical and metabolic effects of different doses of prostaglandin E1 in man. *Acta Med Scand* 1968; **183**: 423–30.
7. Peatfield RC, Gawel MJ, Rose FC, The effect of infused prostacyclin in migraine and cluster headache. *Headache* 1981; **21**: 190–5.

8. Moskowitz MA, The neurobiology of vascular head pain. *Ann Neurol.* 1984; **16**: 157–68.

9. Sillanpää M, Changes in the prevalence of migraine and other headaches during the first seven school years. *Headache* 1983; **23**: 15–19.

10. MacGregor EA, Menstruation, sex hormones and migraine. *Neurol Clin* 1997; **15**: 125–41.

11. Rubin PC, McCabe R, Postpartum migraine and severe preeclampsia. *Lancet* 1984; **ii**: 285–6.

12. Manzoni GC, Farina S, Granella F, Alfieri M, Busi M, Classic and common migraine. Suggestive clinical evidence of two separate entities. *Funct Neurol* 1986; **1**: 112–22.

13. Whitty CWM, Hockaday JM, Migraine: a follow-up study of 92 patients. *BMJ* 1968; **i**: 735–6.

14. Fettes I, Migraine in the menopause. *Neurology* 1999; **53**: S29–33.

15. Facchinetti F, Sternieri E, Nappi G et al, Clinical findings of headaches in postmenopausal age. In: Fioretti P et al, eds, *Postmenopausal Hormonal Therapy: Benefits and Risks.* New York: Raven Press, 1987: 67–70.

16. Neri I, Granella F, Nappi R, Manzoni GC, Facchinetti F, Genazzani AR, Features of headache at menopause: a clinico-epidemiological study. *Maturitas* 1993; **17**: 31–3.

17. Silberstein SD, Merriam GR, Estrogens, progestins and headache. *Neurology* 1991; **41**: 786–93.

18. Larson-Cohn U, Lundberg PO, Headache and treatment with oral contraceptives. *Acta Neurol Scand* 1978; **46**: 267–78.

19. Epstein MT, Hockaday TD, Migraine and reproductive hormones throughout the menstrual cycle. *Lancet* 1975; **1**: 543–8.

20. Martignoni F, Sances M, Facchinetti F et al, Emicrania e sindrome premestruale: osservazioni clinico epidemiologiche. In: Genazzani AR, eds, *Endocrinologia Ginecologica.* Bologna: Monduzzi editore, 1984: 441–64.

21. Metcalf MG, Livesey JH, Hudson SM, Wells EJ, The premenstrual syndrome: moods, headaches and physical symptoms in 1333 menstrual cycles. *J Psychosom Obstet Gynecol* 1988; **8**: 31–43.

22. Facchinetti F, Neri I, Martignoni L, Fioroni L, Nappi G, Genazzani AR, The association of menstrual migraine with the premenstrual syndrome. *Cephalalgia* 1993; **13**: 422–5.

23. Lundberg PO, Endocrinology of headache. A review. In: Pfaffenrath V, Lundberg PO, Sjaastad O, eds, *Updating in Headache.* Berlin: Springer Verlag, 1995: 334–40.

24. Couch JR, Wortsman J, Beares C, Anovulatory state as a factor in occurrence of migraine. In: Clifford Rose F, ed., *Migraine.* Basel: Karger, 1987: 50–5.

25. Facchinetti F, Nappi G, Petraglia F, Volpe A, Genazzani AR, Estradiol/progesterone imbalance and the premenstrual syndrome. *Lancet* 1983; **ii**: 1302.

26. Facchinetti F, Martignoni E, Sola D et al, Transient failure of central opioid tonus and premenstrual symptoms. *J Reprod Med* 1988; **33**: 633–8.

27. Facchinetti F, Martignoni M, Fioroni L, Sances G, Genazzani AR, Opioid control of the hypothalamus–pituitary–adrenal axis cyclically fails in menstrual migraine. *Cephalalgia* 1990; **10**: 51–6.

28. Facchinetti F, Neri I, Granella F, Manzoni GC, Martignoni E, Genazzani AR, Perimenstrual headache and adolescence. In: Gallai V, Guidetti V, eds, *Juvenile Headache.* Amsterdam: Elsevier Science, 1991: 93–4.

29. Facchinetti F, Sgarbi L, Piccinini F, Hypothalamic resetting at puberty and the sexual dimorphism of migraine. *Cephalalgia* 2000 (in press).

30. Holdaway IM, Parr CE, France J, Treatment of a patient with severe menstrual migraine using the Depot LHRH analogue Zoladex. *Aust NZ Obstet Gynecol* 1991; **31**: 164.

31. Murray SC, Muse KN, Effective treatment of severe menstrual migraine headaches with gonadotropin-realising hormone agonist and 'add-back' therapy. *Fertil Steril* 1997; **67**, **2**: 390–3.

# 16

# Prognosis of recurrent headaches in childhood and adolescence

*Bo Larsson*

Recurrent headache is one of the most common health problems in children as reported by parents and adolescents themselves.[1,2] Prevalence gradually increases from early school age throughout adolescence.[3] Over time, headaches can lead to considerable subjective discomfort, disrupt concentration, promote use of various medications and result in frequent school absences. As a consequence, it is important to identify those headaches most likely to be frequent, intense and sustained, because they are the ones most in need of treatment. The need for treatment is even stronger for those types of headaches associated with a poor prognosis. Effective treatments might also prevent young individuals from becoming chronic adult headache sufferers.

Historically, the prime interest of clinicians as well as researchers has been the study of various aspects of migraine headaches in children, whereas non-migrainous and tension-type headaches have been only sparsely addressed. Although migraine is more intense and socially handicapping in school-aged children than non-migrainous headaches (see, for example, Bille[3]) it should be emphasized that frequent tension-type headache is more common and that the most problematic

headaches – chronic daily or almost daily headaches – have important psychosocial consequences for adolescent girls in particular.

Existing information about the course of headaches in clinical or school populations of children and adolescents is based exclusively on global reports of headache activity. Research has shown that global reports provided by children and parents overestimate headache activity, compared with systematic headache recordings, e.g. daily diaries. In an epidemiological study, overall agreement between child and parent reports of headaches in the children was low to moderate.[4] Although higher rates of overall agreement have been found in clinic-based studies of school-aged children,[5,6] lower agreement was found for ratings of low intensity headaches.[5] Metsähonkala[7] found that prepubescent children with migraine or non-migrainous headaches reported similar frequencies of headaches when interviewed, compared with a longer time period of headache diary recordings (2–7 months) that were event based. However, duration of headache episodes was longer when estimated in the diary, compared with the interviews. Thus, the direction of the biases is mixed with regard to estimates of headache activity in these age groups.

This chapter provides an overview of the prognosis and course for unspecified headaches, migraine, non-migrainous and tension-type headaches (TTHs) in children and adolescents. The following review focuses on both clinic and school samples and examines short- and long-term outcome in studies where treatment has been provided.

## Clinic samples (Table 16.1)

In an early report on prognosis, conducted at the Mayo Clinic, 83% of the children with migraine attending still had migraine at a 1- to 2-year follow-up; however, half of them had improved.[8] A longer-term follow-up of the same sample 9–14 years later[9] found that about the same proportion of children had improved. One-third were headache free, but one-fifth were unchanged or had worsened. Similar outcomes were reported by Koch and Melchior[10] at a paediatric clinic in Copenhagen, Denmark, for 136 children with migraine or non-migrainous headaches after a mean follow-up period of 2.5 years (maximum 5 years). Overall improvement rates for children with non-migrainous headaches were 85%, compared with 70% for those with migraine. Information was gathered by means of questionnaires distributed to parents and private doctors. Using chart information available for 73 Canadian children with migraine, Tal and collaborators[11] found that overall outcome was encouraging and only about one-third still had migraine at a mean follow-up of 5.4 years. About half the children had become migraine free and 16% had mild attacks.

In a study by Congdon and Forsythe[12] conducted in Ireland and Leeds, UK, employing a similar period of follow-up, about one-third of the original sample of 300 children with

migraine had achieved remission after 8–11 years and many of the children had become free of headache between 9 and 16 years of age. Most of these children had attained a 2-year remission. The authors estimated the annual remission rate to be 3–14%. At a 9-year follow-up about one-third of the children had achieved an 8-year remission. Similar remission rates were found at an 11-year follow-up (about one-third reported experiencing a 10-year remission). None of these children had relapsed. Information on the outcomes was based on parental recording of the child's migraine attacks.

In a study of 77 Canadian children with migraine or TTH diagnosed with the International Headache Society (IHS) criteria,[13] Dooley and Bagnell[14] noted that 81% of the participants were 'much improved', whereas 27% were headache free. However, 73% still had persistent headaches. Of the children with TTH 50% were headache free, compared with 20% of those with migraine. TTH persisted in 40% of the children and 10% had changed into migraine. For children with migraine 56% had persistent attacks and 26% had turned into TTH. Headache severity decreased overall during the 10-year follow-up period. Although three-quarters of the sample reported their headaches to be moderate to severe at the start of the investigation, this was reduced to about half over time. Similarly, headache frequency decreased from 11 episodes per month to 2 at the follow-up and most participants with TTH or migraine stated that their headaches had improved.

In an 8-year follow-up study of 100 children aged 4–18 with migraine or TTH, conducted at a special headache clinic in Rome, Guidetti and Galli[15] noted that about one-third had achieved remission, 45% were

| Study | Year | Headache free (%) | Improved (%) | Unchanged or worsened (%) | Other headaches (%) |
|---|---|---|---|---|---|
| **Migraine** | | | | | |
| Burke and Peters[8] (1–2 years) | 1956 | – | 50 | – | |
| Hinrichs and Keith[9] (9–14 years) | 1965 | 33 | 47 | 20 | |
| Koch and Melchior[10] (<5 years; mean = 2.5 years) | 1969 | 39 | 40 | 21 | |
| Hockaday[16] (8–25 years)[a] | 1978 | 22 | 50 | 20 | |
| Congdon and Forsythe[12] (8–11 years) | 1979 | 34 | – | – | |
| Tal et al[11] (mean = 5.4 years) | 1984 | 48 | 22 | 23 | |
| Dooley and Bagnell[14] (10 years)[b] | 1995 | 19 | 81 | – | 26 TTH |
| Guidetti and Galli[15] (8 years) | 1998 | 28 | 50 | 22 | 27 ETTH |
| **TTH** | | | | | |
| Dooley and Bagnell[14] (10 years) | 1995 | 50 | 78 | – | 11 migraine |
| Guidetti and Galli[15] (8 years) | 1998 | | | | |
|   ETTH | | 54 | – | – | 11 migraine; |
| | | | 36 | 20 | 4 CTTH |
|   CTTH[c] | | 13 | – | – | 63 ETTH |

[a] Outcomes are summarized for common (no aura) and classic (with aura) migraine and 72 participants. For 8% outcome was unclear.
[b] Outcomes reported for migraine with and without aura.
[c] Figures based on eight participants only.
ETTH, episodic tension-type headache; CTTH, chronic tension-type headache.

**Table 16.1**
*Outcomes of follow-up evaluations in clinical samples of children and adolescents by headache type and follow-up time*

improved and about 20% were unchanged or had worsened. However, about 40% of the children with migraine still experienced attacks at the follow-up and a somewhat higher proportion of youngsters (47%) still had TTH episodes. A higher proportion of children with migraine had transformed to TTH (27%), compared with TTH turning into migraine (8%). A higher remission rate was found for boys (42%), compared with girls (18%). Further, the prognosis was better for boys than for girls in that 70% of the former were headache free at the follow-up compared with 27% of the girls. Overall, about half of the boys had achieved a remission, compared with 22% of the girls. The authors concluded that TTH has a better prognosis than migraine – 44% were headache free compared with 28% of those with migraine. However, when overall headache improvement was assessed, there was no difference in improvement rates between the two headache types.

In an extended 8- to 25-year follow-up of 102 children previously seen at a paediatric clinic, Hockaday[16] found that attacks had terminated in about one-third of the children with migraine without aura (common migraine), whereas about one-fifth of those who had migraine with aura had achieved remission. Substantial improvement in attack frequency and severity or both was found for about half of the total sample. In line with similar figures reported in other studies of headache prognosis for children and adolescents, about one-fifth of the children were unchanged or had become worse and boys had a better prognosis and outgrew their attacks more often than girls.

## School- or community-based samples (Table 16.2)

Although follow-up studies of children and adolescents attending paediatric or university clinics contribute valuable information about the prognosis for migraine or TTH, it should be emphasized that these subjects represent highly selected samples, e.g. Prensky and Sommer[17] noted that most children were referred to a clinic shortly after onset of severe headaches that were usually complicated by aura or after long-standing migraine headaches that had begun to deteriorate. Similarly, in a Finnish study children from clinic samples were found to have more frequent or severe headaches, in addition to having higher rates of school absence and complicated migraine symptoms such as aura and nausea.[18] The prognosis for children with less severe recurrent headaches in unbiased community or school-based samples might therefore be expected to be more favourable (see, for example, Bille[3]).

Aromaa and co-workers[19] obtained pre-pregnancy information from Finnish mothers and, on giving birth, 968 children were followed for 6 years until school entry. At that time 22% of parents reported that the child had headaches severe enough to disturb their daily activities. About 6% had had headaches previously, but not at the 6-year assessment. When predictors of outcome were examined, the authors found that pre-pregnancy headache history of mothers could predict headache in the 6-year-old child. At the age of 9 months, the mother's assessment of the child's health as poor and the presence of feeding problems predicted preschool headaches in the child. At the age of 3 years, sleep problems and nocturnal confusion

| Study | Year | Headache free (%) | Improved (%) | Unchanged or worsened (%) | Other headaches (%) |
|---|---|---|---|---|---|
| **Unspecified recurrent headaches** | | | | | |
| Sillanpää[21] (7 year follow-up) | 1983 | 22 | 37 | 41 | |
| Wännman and Agerberg[24] (2 year follow-up) | 1987 | | | | |
|    1-year follow-up | | 46 | | – | |
|    2-year follow-up | | 59 | | – | |
| Schmidt et al[22] (5–10 year follow-up) | 1992 | | | | |
|    8–13 year follow-up | | – | – | 73 | |
|    13–18 year follow-up | | – | – | 56 | |
|    8–18 year follow-up | | – | – | 47 | |
| Brattberg and Wickman[23] (2 year follow-up)[a] | 1993 | | | | |
|    Grade 4 | | | 12 | 25 | |
|    Grade 7 | | | 15 | 36 | |
|    Grade 10 (high school) | | | 16 | 30 | |
| Aromaa et al[25] (15 year follow-up) | 2001 | 27 | | | 12 migraine |
| **Migraine** | | | | | |
| Bille[3] (6 year follow-up) | 1962 | – | 50 | – | |
|    Pronounced (7–13 years) | | 34 | 51 | 15 | – |
|    Migraine (aged 7–15 years) | | 51 | 34 | 15 | – |
| Metsähonkala et al[20] (3 year follow-up) (aged 8–9 years) | 1997 | 5 | – | 63[c] | 8 ETTH |
| **Non-migrainous/TTH** | | | | | |
| **Frequent non-migrainous headaches** | | | | | |
| Bille[3] (6 year follow-up) | 1962 | 69 | 19 | 12 | 12 migraine |
| Metsähonkala et al[20] (3 year follow-up) (aged 8–9 years) | 1997 | 9 | – | 57[b] | 34 migraine |

[a] Improvement rates here refer to those subjects who reported recurrent headaches at first test vs at follow-up. Persistence rates reported for those who responded positively at both test occasions.
[b] Follow-up for children between 7 and 22 years of age.
[c] The authors report rates for stability but no information regarding improvement.
ETTH, episodic tension-type headache.

**Table 16.2**
*Outcomes of follow-up evaluations in cohort and school samples of children and adolescents by headache type and follow-up time*

seizures, in addition to headaches in family members and suspected headache episodes in the child, predicted headaches in the 6-year-old child. Finally, when the child was aged 5 headache episodes or TTH was highly predictive of headaches a year later.

In a follow-up study of prepubescent children with recurrent headaches from this sample, Metsähonkala[7] reported that about one-third of 8- to 9-year-old children with migraine also had had headaches at the age of 5, whereas the corresponding figure for TTH was slightly lower (29%). In a prospective study, the author found that about 80% of the 8–9 year olds still had migraine when they reached 11–12 years of age, and a small proportion (8%) had turned into ETTH (episodic TTH), but only 5% were free of migraine.[20] More than half of those with TTH still had the same headaches at the 2- to 3-year follow-up evaluation, one-third had transformed to migraine and 9% had become headache free. Thus, the prognosis was found to be better for TTH, and it was more common for TTH to change into migraine than for changes to occur in the opposite direction. Somewhat surprisingly, the prognosis for boys was found to be worse than for girls in that their frequency of attacks was higher. The number of attacks also correlated positively with school absence, use of drugs and parental divorce rates.

In a longitudinal study of a large cohort of Finnish children starting school, Sillanpää[21] noted that boys who experienced any type of headache at school entry were twice as likely to develop migraine at the age of 14 as boys who were headache free at the start of school. The risk for girls was six times higher. The prognosis was better for boys than for girls: 26% of boys were free of headaches at the 7-year-follow-up, whereas the corresponding

figure for girls was 17%. However, about one-third of both sexes showed improvement and the overall improvement rate (including remission) was 60%.

In a similar study with a smaller cohort of German children living in the city of Mannheim, Schmidt and collaborators[22] assessed headache status by interviewing parents and older children. The authors reported a strikingly high 5-year stability (73%) of headache complaints in 8- to 13-year-old children, but this was less so for adolescents aged 13–18 years (56%). The 10-year stability was also high (47%).

The prognosis for recurrent headaches in schoolchildren and adolescents has been examined in two longitudinal Swedish studies. In the first, Brattberg and Wickman[23] examined 471 schoolchildren living in a moderately large city attending grades 4 (age about 11 years) and 7 (age about 14 years), and first grade in junior high school (age 16–17 years); they reassessed the participants 2 years later. In a questionnaire the children were asked whether they usually had headaches and about one-third reported recurrent headaches at both test points. In all three grades, about twice as many girls as boys reported such headaches (32–46% vs 18–25%). Overall, 14% of those reporting headaches at test 1 were free from headaches at the follow-up 2 years later. Small differences between the sexes were found among the older children, in contrast to those in the youngest age group in which twice as many girls as boys had improved. In the second study, focusing on older adolescents (17–19 years of age), 11% reported recurrent unspecified headaches.[24] One year later about 50% still had such headaches, whereas the figure was slightly lower for stability between the first and second year of follow-up (41%).

The authors concluded that there seems to be a 'major transient' and a 'chronic recurrent headache' group who may have different needs and demands for treatment.

In an extended follow-up study, Aromaa and collaborators[25] found that 27% of 1205 school children who had headaches at the age of 7 were free of headache at the age of 22. Of the children who were headache free at school entry, 33% were still headache free at the age of 22. At this age, 5% of those who were headache free at the age of 7 had migraine, whereas the corresponding figure was 12% for those who had recurrent headaches at the age of 7. As expected, headache at preschool age predicted frequent headaches in young adulthood.

The longest follow-up of the course of 'pronounced' migraine (occurring at least once a month for an hour or more and disturbing daily activities, or requiring the child to lie down; most of the children had two to three attacks per month) has been conducted by Bille[26] who reported outcomes for older school-aged children over a 40-year time period. In his first follow-up, which occurred at year 6, about one-third of these children were free of migraine (they had no attacks for at least 1 year), half of them had improved and 15% were unchanged or had become worse. Comparisons were also made with a group of schoolchildren with less severe migraine and a group of children with frequent non-migrainous headaches. In the first comparison group, half of the children had become migraine free (same criteria as above) and a third had improved, whereas in the latter group a higher proportion of children (70%) had not experienced headaches for at least 1 year and 20% were noted as improved. About the same proportions of children were unchanged or had deteriorated (12–15%). In the non-migrainous headache group, 12% of the children had instead become migraine sufferers. It should be noted that about one-third of the children in the pronounced migraine group also had frequent non-migrainous headaches. With regard to the 6-year follow-up status, it was clear that children with less severe migraine or non-migrainous headaches also had a better prognosis. The annual persistence rate was 90%, corresponding to a 10% recovery rate for the ages 7–20 years; no sex differences were found.

In his extended follow-up evaluations conducted by telephone, Bille[26] noted that many of the children became migraine free or had improved during adolescence, but then relapsed in adulthood. At his 22-year follow-up evaluation, 40% of the participants overall had become migraine free. A smaller group had been free of migraine for certain time periods but had then relapsed (22%), and 38% had migraine attacks annually since the original study. These figures were only slightly changed at subsequent 30-year and 40-year follow-up evaluations, when the subjects were aged 37–43 years and 47–53 years, respectively. Males had become free of migraine significantly more often than females (34% and 15%, respectively). About one-third had had attacks at least once a year over a 40-year time period. Overall, the subjects experienced the attacks as less frequent than in childhood, although the intensity was reported to be similar. More than half of the subjects also reported suffering from TTH related to or in between the migraine attacks.

## Conclusion

Overall, studies of outcomes for clinical samples of children clearly show that about one-third of these individuals become headache free after short (1–5 years) as well as extended time periods (5–25 years), 40–54% reveal improvement, but about one-fifth still suffer from migraine or show deterioration. However, it should be emphasized that these outcomes often include subjects who have received various types of treatments delivered at clinics or by paediatricians, e.g. Dooley and Bagnell[14] reported that about two-thirds of the 77 patients followed for a 10-year period had received some form of treatment, with the most common being various types of non-prescribed drugs and relaxation. Although outcome rates have been strikingly consistent in most studies of prognosis, estimates of headache improvement have generally been based on global reports, such as questionnaires or interviews conducted by clinicians.

Only one study used a prospective, systematic approach to gather information about children's headaches.[12] In this study outcomes were comparable to results of studies in which other types of assessment methods have been used, so varying the methods of data collection may not be problematic. Again, it should be underlined that children attending a clinic typically display more severe forms of migraine and also have more neurological symptoms and, thus, represent highly selected cases.[18] In follow-up evaluations of large-size cohorts, fairly strong stability has been found between late preschool and early school years.[19] Frequent headaches in pre-school-aged children predicted more frequent headaches at school entry compared with those with no headaches. Although most school-aged children who have frequent migraines improve over extended time periods, about one-third continue to have annual attacks in adulthood. For unspecified recurrent headaches in school-aged children, there seems to be a fairly high

stability, in particular among adolescents, with about 50% of them continuing to have such complaints over a period of 1 year. Overall, the prognosis seems to be better for frequent non-migrainous headaches, which are most probably episodic TTH. The course for the most severe form of TTH (chronic) in children and adolescents remains unclear. Retrospective information suggests that such headaches have a shorter history than migraine among adolescents who want help because of their recurrent headaches.[27] In particular, adolescent girls with this headache type are most likely to face a high risk of continuing to experience chronic TTH and also to develop psychosocial consequences, such as higher levels of anxiety, depression or other somatic complaints.

Other factors that are important in predicting outcomes for child and adolescent headache sufferers in longitudinal studies are sex, prepregnancy family loadings of headaches and various types of behavioural problems in preschool children.[19] Prepubescent boys with migraine have been reported to have a worse prognosis than girls;[20] however, in adulthood women continue to suffer from attacks more often than men. Recurrent headaches in mothers predict the development of headaches in preschool children as do various types of behavioural problems in the child during these ages. However, suspected headache episodes reported by parents among 5-year-olds were found to be the most important predictor of headache occurrence at school entry.

## Short- and long-term prognosis after treatment

Prensky and Sommer[17] stated that about half of children with migraine have more than a

50% reduction of headaches within 6 months of visiting a neurology clinic. There were no differences in outcome related to palliative or prophylactic drug treatment – about 40% of the children had achieved at least a 50% headache reduction. Frequency of headaches had decreased regardless of treatment.

Since the Prensky and Sommer study[17] (1979), more than 30 published controlled outcome studies have examined the short- and long-term outcomes for various forms of psychological treatments for children and adolescents with migraine, TTH or both headache types.[28] Outcomes in these experimental studies have been based on more conservative measures, such as systematic headache recordings in diaries collected both before and after treatment (in contrast to retrospective and global information often used in early clinical studies). Thus, the estimates of headache reduction in such follow-up studies provide better and more reliable measures of outcome.

In one of the first follow-up studies, Werder and Sargent[29] found that children with migraine, non-migrainous headaches or the two combined had achieved a sizeable reduction for headache and medication consumption (87%) after a 5-day intensive treatment programme which included biofeedback, relaxation and autogenic training, and continued with 8–10 weekly subsequent sessions. Children with migraine improved more (71%) than those with non-migrainous headache (39%). In general, those children who had attained a substantial headache reduction at a 1-year follow-up also continued to improve. Age at onset was not found to be an important predictor of outcome.

In the first controlled treatment study, Labbé and Williamson[30] found that improvement after autogenic and biofeedback training was greater at a 1-month follow-up than at a subsequent 6-month follow-up evaluation, at which time it was found that headache activity had increased. At the first follow-up, 87% of the children achieved a 50% of greater reduction of headache, but this figure dropped at the later follow-up (62%). It should be noted, however, that these figures are only suggestive in that the follow-up sample was small and only eight children participated (57% of the original sample).

Results of several other clinical studies show that outcomes after relaxation and biofeedback training or cognitive coping approaches are well maintained for 6–12 months after treatment (see, for example, the literature[31–37]). In several of those studies medication usage has also been found to decrease after treatment.[30,34] Osterhaus and her collaborators[36] noted that a higher use of avoidant coping before treatment predicted a worse outcome for headache frequency at a 7-month follow-up. In a subsequent clinic study, Osterhaus et al[37] reported that treatment gains were well maintained for both migraine and TTH at a 1-year follow-up. Higher levels of mother reward for illness behaviour was negatively related to headache reduction. Most of the children and adolescents treated with relaxation or biofeedback training procedures have identified relaxation practices as the most important treatment component,[31,32,38] although this finding has not always held true. Waranch and Keenan[39] found that relaxation practices decreased during the 0.5- to 2-year follow-up period, but most participants remained headache free or reported only mild headaches. Maintenance of achieved headache improvement has also been found to be substantial for adolescents with frequent TTH or non-migrainous headache.

In school-based studies, more than 50% of adolescents (aged 10–18 years) who have chronic TTH (for at least a year) have well-maintained improvement at short-term follow-up evaluations[40,41] and 3–4 years after treatment.[42] Overall, the 5- to 6-month outcome has been found to be worse for migraine headaches (often combined with TTH) in adolescents than for TTH. However, at the extended follow-up evaluations, no differences in outcomes were found with regard to headache or treatment type, or to headache history. Headache severity, anxiety levels and home satisfaction predicted outcome at the first follow-up; however, at the latter evaluation, only higher levels of headache severity predicted a worse outcome.

## Untreated participants and attention control

In a few studies, outcomes for untreated participants in experimental school-based treatment studies have been examined for a time period of about 8–9 months.[40,42] The adolescents maintained diaries in which headache recordings were made for about a month at the beginning and the end of this time period. Improvements in headache activity were found to be negligible for the adolescents (aged 10–18 years) who had frequent migraine or TTH. Although adolescents treated with various attention-control approaches did show some improvements after a 5- to 6-month period,[42,43] a substantial improvement was found at the 3- to 4-year follow-up after treatment.[42] Interestingly, Bussone and collaborators[43] noted that a group of adolescents with TTH treated with a pseudo-relaxation training approach ('sitting quietly for an extended period in the laboratory') achieved a smaller improvement at later follow-ups than those treated with relaxation and biofeedback procedures. These improvements were obtained in the absence of asking subjects to practise relaxation at home. However, it should be noted that, in the largest outcome study, McGrath and co-workers[33] found that children and adolescents treated with relaxation training or a credible attention-control procedure had achieved very similar headache reductions, at both 3-month and 1-year follow-up evaluations. The authors suggest that natural variation of migraine activity in the child, in addition to brief reassurance and assistance provided at a clinic, may be sufficient to give relief.

## Conclusion

In most studies of children and adolescents with migraine or TTH, once headache improvement has been achieved after relaxation, biofeedback training or cognitive therapy, the reduction is typically well maintained for most subjects over a time period of between 6 months and 4 years. However, untreated subjects with migraine or TTH who perform headache recordings show only minor improvements over a time period of 8–9 months. These outcomes, which generally have been based on global parent or adolescent reports, are in contrast to clinical studies for similar follow-up periods in which much higher improvements have been presented. Given that children and adolescents often seek help at the peak of their headache complaints, the outcomes of various psychological treatments, short term as well as long term, are highly encouraging. Except for headache severity before treatment, few headache characteristics have been found to be useful in the prediction of outcomes for children and adolescents. This is an important area to address in future research so that treatments can be further developed and better tailored to children experiencing recurring migraines and/or TTH.

## Acknowledgement

This chapter was written in honour of professor Bo Bille, Uppsala, a pioneer of research on childhood headaches and their prognosis, a mentor and a good friend.

## References

1. Goodman JE, McGrath PJ, The epidemiology of pain in children and adolescents: a review. *Pain* 1991; **46**: 247–64.
2. Berg Kelly K, Erhvér M, Erneholm T, Gundevall C, Wennerberg I, Wettergren L, Self-reported health status and use of medical care by 3500 adolescents in Western Sweden. *Acta Paediat Scand* 1991; **80**: 837–43.
3. Bille B, Migraine in schoolchildren. *Acta Paediat Scand Suppl* 1962; **51**(136): 1–151.
4. Deubner DC, An epidemiologic study of migraine and headache in 10–20 year olds. *Headache* 1977; **17**: 173–80.
5. Richardson GM, McGrath PJ, Cunningham SJ, Humphreys P, Validity of the headache diary for children. *Headache* 1988; **23**: 184–7.
6. Andrasik F, Burke EJ, Attanasio V, Rosenblum EL, Child, parent, and physician reports of a child's headache pain: Relationships prior to and following treatment. *Headache* 1985; **25**: 421–5.
7. Metsähonkala L, *Migraine in Childhood*. Medica-odontologica Turku University, 266, Thesis, 1997.
8. Burke EC, Peters GA, Migraine in childhood. A preliminary report. *Am J Dis Child* 1956; **92**: 230–6.
9. Hinrichs WL, Keith HM, Migraine in childhood: a follow-up report. *Mayo Clin Proc* 1965; **40**: 593–6.
10. Koch C, Melchior JC, Headache in childhood. A five year material from a pediatric university clinic. *Dan Med Bull* 1969; **16**: 109–14.
11. Tal Y, Dunn G, Chrichton JU, Childhood migraine – a dangerous diagnosis? *Acta Paediat Scand* 1984; **73**: 55–9.
12. Congdon PJ, Forsythe WI, Migraine in childhood: a study of 300 children. *Dev Med Child Neurol* 1979; **21**: 209–16.
13. The Headache Classification Committee of the International Headache Society, Classification and diagnostic criteria for headache disorders, cranial neuralgias and facial pain. *Cephalalgia* 1988; **8**(suppl 7): 1–96.
14. Dooley J, Bagnell A, The prognosis and treatment of headaches in children – a ten year follow-up. *Can J Neurol Sci* 1995; **22**: 47–9.
15. Guidetti V, Galli F, Evolution of headache in childhood and adolescence: an 8-year follow-up. *Cephalalgia* 1998; **18**: 449–54.
16. Hockaday JM, Late outcome of childhood onset migraine and factors affecting outcome, with particular reference to early and late EEG findings. In: Greene R, ed., *Current Concepts in Migraine Research*. New York: Raven Press, 1978.
17. Prensky AL, Sommer D, Diagnosis and treatment of migraine in children. *Neurology* 1979; **19**: 506–10.
18. Metsähonkala L, Sillanpää M, Tuominen J, Use of health care services in childhood migraine. *Headache* 1996; **36**: 423–8.
19. Aromaa M, Rautava P, Helenius H, Sillanpää M, Factors of early life as predictors of headache in children as school entry. *Headache* 1998; **38**: 23–30.
20. Metsähonkala L, Sillanpää M, Tuominen J, Outcome of early school-age migraine. *Cephalalgia* 1997; **17**: 662–5.
21. Sillanpää M, Changes in the prevalence of migraine and other headaches during the first seven school years. *Headache* 1983; **23**: 15–19.
22. Schmidt MH, Blanz B, Esser G, Häufigkeit und Bedeutung des Kopfschmerzes im Kindes- und Jugendalter. *Kindheit und Entwicklung* 1992; **1**: 31–5.
23. Brattberg G, Wickman V, Longitudinell studie av skolelever. Rehabilitera tidigt vid ryggont

och huvudvärk (A longitudinal study of school children). *Läkartidningen* 1993; **90**: 1452–60.

24. Wänman A, Agerberg G, Recurrent headaches and craniomandibular disorders in adolescents: a longitudinal study. *J Craniomand Dis Facial Oral Pain* 1987; **1**: 227–36.

25. Aromaa M, Sillanpää M, Aro H, A population-based follow-up study of headache from age 7 to 22. *J Head Child Pain* 2000; **1**: 11–15.

26. Bille B, A 40-year follow-up of school children with migraine. *Cephalalgia* 1997; **17**: 488–91.

27. Larsson BS, The role of psychological, health behaviour and medical factors in adolescent headache. *Dev Med Child Neurol* 1988; **30**: 616–25.

28. Holden EW, Deichmann MM, Levy JD, Empirically supported treatments in pediatric psychology: recurrent pediatric headaches. *J Ped Psychol* 1999; **24**: 91–109.

29. Werder DS, Sargent JD, A study of childhood headache using biofeedback as a treatment alternative. *Headache* 1984; **24**: 122–6.

30. Labbé EE, Williamson DA, Treatment of childhood migraine using autogenic feedback training. *J Consult Clin Psychol* 1984; **52**: 968–76.

31. Fentress DW, Masek BJ, Mehegan JE, Bensen H, Biofeedback and relaxation-response training in the treatment of pediatric migraine. *Dev Med Child Neurol* 1986; **28**: 139–46.

32. Mehegan JE, Masek BJ, Harrison RH, Russ DC, Leviton A, A multicomponent behavioral treatment for pediatric migraine. *Clin J Pain* 1987; **2**: 191–6.

33. McGrath PJ, Humphreys P, Goodman JT, Keene D, Relaxation prophylaxis for childhood migraine: A randomized placebo-controlled trial. *Dev Med Child Neurol* 1988; **30**: 626–31.

34. Allen KD, McKeen LR, Home-based multicomponent treatment of pediatric migraine. *Headache* 1991; **31**: 467–72.

35. McGrath PJ, Humphreys P, Keene D et al, The efficacy and efficiency of a self-administered treatment for adolescent migraine. *Pain* 1992; **49**: 321–4.

36. Osterhaus SOL, Passchier J, van der Helm Hylkema H, de Jong KT, Effects of behavioral psychophysiological treatment on schoolchildren with migraine in a nonclinical setting: predictors and process variables. *J Ped Psychol* 1993; **18**: 697–711.

37. Osterhaus SOL, Lange A, Linssen WHJP, Passchier J, A behavioral treatment of young migrainous and nonmigrainous headache patients: prediction of treatment success. *Int J Behav Med* 1997; **4**: 378–96.

38. Engel JM, Rapoff MA, Pressman AR, Long-term follow-up of relaxation training for pediatric headache disorders. *Headache* 1992; **32**: 152–6.

39. Waranch HR, Keenan DM, Behavioral treatment of children with recurrent headaches. *J Behav Ther Exp Psychiat* 1985; **16**: 31–8.

40. Larsson B, Carlsson J, A school-based, nurse-administered relaxation training for children with chronic tension-type headache. *J Ped Psychol* 1996; **21**: 603–14.

41. Larsson B, Recurrent headaches in children and adolescents. In: McGrath PJ, Finley GA, eds, *Chronic and Recurrent Pain in Children and Adolescents. Progress in Pain Research and Management*, vol. 13. Seattle: IASP Press, 1999: 115–40.

42. Larsson B, Melin L, Follow-up on behavioral treatment of recurrent headache in adolescents. *Headache* 1989; **29**: 249–53.

43. Bussone G, Grazzi L, D'Amico D, Leone M, Andrasik F, Biofeedback-assisted relaxation training for young adolescents with tension-type headaches. *Cephalalgia* 1998; **18**: 463–7.

# 17

# Equivalents, variants and precursors of migraine
*David NK Symon*

It has long been recognized that migraine is not merely a syndrome of headache, but that the headache is associated with a range of other symptoms. Migraine is the most common cause of headache in the prepubertal child,[1] but headache is not its only manifestation. It figures prominently in the causation of periodic abdominal pain, cyclical vomiting and other aspects of the 'periodic syndrome', as well as in the differential diagnosis of vertigo and the less frequent clinical syndromes of complex migraine. In many cases, the associated symptoms are more prominent than the headache and often these occur in the absence of headache. These associated symptoms form several recognized clinical syndromes such as abdominal migraine and cyclical vomiting, although it is not unusual to see a degree of overlap clinically between these syndromes. The outstanding feature of migraine in any of its manifestations is its paroxysmal or periodic occurrence. There is always a return to baseline with resulting symptom-free intervals. Without this feature it is not migraine.

## Abdominal migraine

Recurrent episodes of abdominal pain are a common problem in childhood. Apley and Naish[2] studied 1000 schoolchildren and reported recurrent abdominal pain in 108. A similar frequency of recurrent abdominal pain was found by Oster[3] in a series of 2200 children and adolescents. Two large population studies showed an even higher prevalence: in the UK, the National Child Development study[4] found a history of periodic abdominal pain in 14% of 7-year-old boys and 15.7% of girls, and the Newcastle 1000 family study[5] found a continuing complaint of abdominal pain in 18% of children. Abu-Arafeh and Russell,[6] in a schools survey, studied more severe episodes of abdominal pain – severe enough to interfere with normal activities – and found that 32% of children had had at least one such episode in the past year and 8% had had two or more episodes.

An organic cause for recurrent abdominal pain, such as a surgically correctable lesion or a urinary tract problem, is found in only a small minority (approximately 7%) of children.[7] The others are usually described as functional abdominal pain, a term that reflects our ignorance of the aetiology. Many paediatricians regard children with recurrent abdominal pain in the absence of demonstrable organic disease as suffering from emotional stress, such as home or school problems, but there is no evidence from controlled studies to support the hypothesis of a psychological cause of recurrent abdominal pain. McGrath et al[8] found no statistically significant differences between children with recurrent abdominal pain and pain-free children with regard to various psychological variables thought to be associated with psychogenicity. Heinild et al[9] described evidence of maladjustment in 87.7% of children with recurrent abdominal pain but also found similar maladjustment in 64.1% of their controls.

Abdominal symptoms are common in children and adults with migraine headaches.[10,11] Recurrent abdominal pain is common in adults with migraine, although rare in adults with tension-type headaches.[12,13] Abdominal pain probably related to migraine but occurring in the absence of headache was first described in adults by Buchanan in 1921,[14] but the term 'abdominal migraine' was not introduced until the following year by Brams.[15] In children, the association between migraine and episodic pain has long been recognized and this is frequently referred to as the 'periodic syndrome'. Wyllie and Schlesinger, in 1933,[16] coined the phrase 'periodic disorders of childhood' to describe episodic pyrexia, headache, vomiting and abdominal pain in childhood, and suggested that the symptoms might persist into adult life as vomiting, migraine or both. The syndrome was further described by Cullen and Macdonald[17] who noted the frequency of migraine in adult relatives of children with periodic syndrome. Barlow,[18] in his monograph describing 20 years' experience as a paediatric neurologist, noted that the periodic syndrome frequently developed into migraine headaches, and stated that the periodic syndrome should be viewed as an incident in the longitudinal history of juvenile migraine.

From clinical experience it has been possible to derive diagnostic criteria for abdominal migraine. This syndrome has been described by various clinicians in remarkably similar terms over several decades.[18–21] Apart from the location of the pain, abdominal migraine bears a close resemblance to migraine headache. The syndrome consists of recurrent episodes of midline abdominal pain lasting for many hours and occurring in discrete attacks, with complete recovery between episodes. The pain is sufficiently severe to make the children unable to continue with their normal activities, and they are forced to stop playing and may be sent home from school. Most children wish to lie down in a darkened room and attempt to sleep, which may relieve the symptoms. They most definitely wish to remain undisturbed, and this easily distinguishes them from the attention-seeker who appreciates parental attention and concern. The pain is nearly always associated with vasomotor symptoms, usually pallor but occasionally facial flushing. Over half the parents comment on the presence of dark rings under or around the eyes during an attack. Attacks are almost invariably accompanied by anorexia and nausea and in half the children by vomiting. Phonophobia and photophobia are common features and dizziness may be reported by some children. The attack of abdominal migraine may be preceded by a prodromal period of listlessness or drowsiness. The onset of abdominal pain may be at any time of day but occurs most frequently first thing in the morning on wakening. The symptoms continue for a minimum of 2 hours and frequently all day, and may persist for up to 72 hours in a few individuals.

In a hospital-based study of migraine and associated syndromes, we identified 120 children with abdominal migraine.[11,22] They presented at a mean age of 7.2 years. In hospital practice the average duration of attack was 26 hours, although shorter attacks may not be referred to hospital. Abdominal migraine is not a rare condition. A survey in general practice found abdominal migraine in 2.4% of children,[23] whereas in a community-based study abdominal migraine had a prevalence of 4.1%.[6] The symptoms of abdominal migraine commonly appear in childhood before puberty, reaching a peak at the age of 10 years and thereafter falling rapidly.[6] In most children with abdominal migraine the symptoms will settle with time, although they may be followed by the development of migraine headaches in adolescence. In many others the symptoms of headache and abdominal pain will overlap for a period. Although abdominal migraine is largely a disease of childhood, it was first described in adults[14,15] and there are several reports of abdominal migraine in adults.[13,24] The symptoms in adults appear to be similar to those found in children, but it is not known if there is any difference in the underlying pathology.

There is a considerable clinical overlap between children presenting with abdominal migraine and those presenting with migraine headache. In Bille's study of 9000 schoolchildren in Uppsala,[41] he found attacks of abdominal pain in 20.5% of children with pronounced migraine. In our hospital-based study,[11,22] 58% of the 120 children who presented with abdominal migraine also suffered from migraine headaches simultaneously, whereas 25% of 150 children presenting with migraine headaches also suffered from abdominal migraine. In nearly all cases of abdominal migraine, there is a family history of migraine headaches in either first- or second-degree relatives.[11] A family history of migraine is found as commonly in abdominal migraine as in migraine headache, and 65% of the children

with abdominal migraine had a family history of migraine headaches in a first-degree relative. As is the case in migraine headache, a family history of migraine is much more common in the mother than in the father.[6,11,23] Mortimer et al[25] found similar changes in the visual evoked responses of children with periodic syndrome and migraine headaches.

The diagnosis of abdominal migraine is not yet universally accepted by neurologists,[26,27] although it appears to be gaining greater acceptance. Objections include the supposed derivation of the word migraine from hemicrania, suggesting that only headaches qualify for the term, and the lack of any test or marker to prove the migrainous nature of the attacks – a criticism that could equally be applied to all migraine headaches. It is important to recognize that abdominal migraine is a relatively uncommon cause of recurrent abdominal pain in children and that most children with recurrent abdominal pain will have other conditions that may or may not be found on investigation. It is important to make a definite specific diagnosis of abdominal migraine and only those children who fit the diagnostic criteria for abdominal migraine should be diagnosed as such.

There is little evidence-based treatment for abdominal migraine. In most children, the attack will subside if they are allowed to lie down undisturbed in a quiet and darkened room and go to sleep. Vomiting also frequently gives relief. In many children, the symptoms may improve after medical consultation and reassurance, without any specific treatment being given. Trigger factors for abdominal migraine are similar to those for migraine headache in children and should be avoided where possible. Common triggers include stress, both pleasant (i.e. excitement) and unpleasant, travel, exposure to bright or flickering lights, and a variety of foodstuffs. Fizzy drinks, especially cola drinks, are frequent triggers and their avoidance may be sufficient to abolish symptoms. Other foodstuffs that are occasionally seen as triggers include chocolate, cheese, wheat products and baked beans. The foods may not always trigger an attack, but tip the balance when the child is vulnerable. Excluded foods should be reintroduced if there is no significant improvement. Some clinicians recommend a much wider exclusion diet, gradually reintroducing foods after symptoms resolve. This may be difficult to achieve in practice. Missing meals may also trigger attacks later in the day.

Analgesic drugs are frequently given but are not always effective in relieving pain. This may be because gastric stasis prevents their absorption. If symptoms are frequent and severe despite the measures described above, drug prophylaxis may be indicated. Pizotifen has been shown in a double-blind trial to be highly effective.[28] If treatment is continued for 6 months, many of the responders will remain well after treatment is stopped.[29] Both propranolol and cyproheptadine have also been used for prophylaxis,[30] but there is no evidence yet from controlled clinical trials to support their use.

## Cyclical vomiting

Cyclical vomiting is another recurrent condition seen mainly in children that is believed to be related to migraine. The syndrome was first described by Lombard in 1861[31] and again by Gee[32] in 1882, although there is an earlier case report from 1843 which probably describes cyclical vomiting.[33] Many paediatricians would include cyclical vomiting within the umbrella diagnosis of the periodic syndrome.

Cyclical vomiting typically has an on–off pattern which is stereotypical within individuals.[34,35] The episodes are similar in time of onset, duration and symptomatology specific for each patient. There is a rapid onset, more often during the night or early morning. The principal feature is recurrent, discrete episodes of vomiting lasting hours or days with intense nausea being a prominent feature. There is a high peak frequency of vomiting every 10–15 min. In community studies the average attack duration is 24 h but longer attacks are reported from hospital studies.[11] The attacks are self-limited and at the end of the attack there is rapid resolution to normality. Patients are completely well and free of nausea and vomiting between attacks. Individual attacks are usually diagnosed as gastroenteritis when they first occur, but over time a pattern emerges which can be identified as cyclical vomiting syndrome.

Before the attack some patients may experience a prodrome minutes to hours in length and consisting usually of malaise, anxiety or mild nausea. The onset of the attack is most frequently seen during the night or on awakening in the morning. The child will then have continuing frequent bouts of vomiting and retching. Initially, the vomiting is seen four to six times per hour, although the frequency may gradually decrease as the attack progresses. If prolonged and untreated, the attack may cause life-threatening dehydration. Nausea is constant throughout the episode and is frequently intense, although the intensity varies from patient to patient. Attacks are accompanied by vasomotor symptoms, usually intense pallor but occasionally facial flushing,[11] and dizziness is seen as commonly as in abdominal migraine. Other associated symptoms include headache, abdominal pain and photophobia.[36] The cessation of the attack is as abrupt as its onset and shortly afterwards the child is likely to be demanding food.

The frequency of attacks ranges from 1 to 70 per year, with a mean of 12 attacks per year.[34] They occur fairly regularly in about half the patients and sporadically in others. Most patients can identify experiences or conditions that may precipitate attacks, the most common being heightened emotional states and infections.[34,37] Both unpleasant emotional stress and pleasant excitement such as birthdays, parties and holidays may trigger episodes. Other reported triggers include tiredness, hot weather, motion sickness, fasting and specific foods. It may be possible to reduce the number of attacks by identifying and avoiding these trigger factors.

The initial presentation of cyclical vomiting usually occurs at a younger age than abdominal migraine (mean 5.1 years),[11] although the onset of symptoms may be at any age. Although cyclical vomiting syndrome is commonly a disease of children, the syndrome is also seen in adults.[38] In some adults the symptoms have persisted since childhood, and in others the onset may have been in adult life. It is not known whether these adult patients have the same underlying condition, or whether they may have similar symptoms of different aetiology. In most children with cyclical vomiting the attacks will subside after several years.[34] Many will become symptom free whereas others will develop migraine headaches.[39-43]

There is considerable overlap between the symptoms of cyclical vomiting and other migraine syndromes. Abdominal pain typical of abdominal migraine is reported by 76% of children with cyclical vomiting and 38% also had migraine headaches.[11,22,39] Similarities in the visual evoked response patterns and electroencephalograms of children with migraine and cyclical vomiting have been reported, with these groups being different from normal controls.[44,45] A family history of migraine headaches is common in children with cyclical vomiting,[46] and is found as frequently as in children with migraine headaches.[39] The similarities between the presentation, pattern of attacks, associated symptoms and family histories of children with migraine headaches and of those with cyclical vomiting has led many clinicians to conclude that cyclical vomiting is a condition related to migraine.[39,46,47]

Cyclical vomiting is considered by most clinicians to be a rare disease, and few cases are seen in hospital practice. However, in a community-based study in Scotland using clear diagnostic guidelines, the prevalence rate of cyclical vomiting in schoolchildren was estimated at 1.9%.[48] In many cases the children and their parents had not sought medical attention, or the condition had not been recognized.

Although most cases of cyclical vomiting are believed to be related to migraine, there are patients with similar symptoms with different aetiologies. These may be difficult or impossible to distinguish clinically. The diagnosis should be reviewed with each attack, and particularly if the patient does not return to a completely symptom-free state between acute episodes. The differential diagnosis[37] includes a number of gastrointestinal disorders causing bowel obstruction, including intermittent volvulus associated with malrotation, duodenal webs and duplication cysts. Disorders of gastrointestinal motility may cause similar symptoms, and chronic intestinal pseudo-obstruction typically causes recurrent episodes of vomiting. Obstructive uropathies may also be a cause of recurrent vomiting. Cerebral tumour with vomiting, as a result of intermittent raised intracranial pressure, may be mistaken for cyclical vomiting.

Vomiting is the primary manifestation of a number of inborn errors of metabolism and may be precipitated in these disorders, as in episodes of cyclical vomiting syndrome, or by intercurrent infection, fasting or specific food substances. Vomiting episodes may also be recurrent. The disorders most likely to be incriminated are the disorders of amino acid metabolism such as the urea cycle defects, particularly heterozygous ornithine transcarbamylase deficiency, the organic acidurias such as propionic acidaemia and methylmalonic acidaemia, the fatty acid oxidation defects such as medium-chain acyl-CoA dehydrogenase, the disorders of carbohydrate metabolism such as hereditary fructose intolerance, and acute intermittent porphyria. A mitochondrial DNA deletion has also been reported in a child with symptoms similar to cyclical vomiting syndrome, but who had some additional symptoms.[49]

Treatment of cyclical vomiting remains controversial and unsatisfactory. There are no double-blind controlled studies of the various treatments that have been used, although there are anecdotal reports of marked success with a variety of agents. As the acute episodes are so devastating for many of the patients, it is desirable to prevent these if possible. The first action should be to identify and where possible to avoid trigger factors. Unfortunately this is impossible in many cases and many patients are treated with drugs normally used for migraine prophylaxis. There are reports that pizotifen[11,50] and β blockers such as propranolol[46,51] have been successful in reducing the frequency of cyclical vomiting episodes in many patients, and cyproheptadine[46] has also been used. One report has suggested that barbiturates[52] may provide effective prophylaxis and it has also been suggested that erythromycin,[53] which acts as a motilin agonist, may have a role in some patients.

Despite the above measures many patients continue to have acute attacks of cyclical vomiting. Many of these patients will require hospital admission for intravenous rehydration and supportive nursing care. The drug used most commonly to relieve nausea and vomiting is intravenous ondansetron.[46,54] If this is unsuccessful some physicians will give lorazepam,[54] a benzodiazepine with antiemetic and sedative properties. There is a report of the use of the anti-migraine drug sumatriptan.[54] Where attacks are prolonged, ranitidine is frequently given to prevent oesophagitis.[54]

Children and their parents may also benefit from the support of others with the condition. There is a well-established support group for patients and parents, the Cyclical Vomiting Syndrome Association. This is based in North America, but has numerous groups in all parts of the world. They have an internet web site and produce regular newsletters, as well as holding meetings with medical experts.

## Paroxysmal vertigo

Vertigo is a common symptom in childhood. About 20% of all schoolchildren will have an episode of vertigo over a 1-year period.[56] Most of these episodes occur during self-limiting intercurrent infections or are associated with trauma. A smaller number of children will have recurrent episodes of vertigo. Vertigo caused by underlying neurological or auditory disorders is rare in children.

Paroxysmal vertigo is a disorder characterized by recurrent transient episodes of an unreal sensation of rotation of the patient or his or her surroundings with no loss of consciousness, no associated neurological or auditory abnormalities, and with complete recovery between attacks.[56]

Idiopathic vertigo in children is usually classified into two forms depending on the age of presentation. Benign paroxysmal vertigo of children commonly affects young children aged between 1 and 4,[57,58] although onset may be found also in older children.[59] It is a specific disorder characterized by severe sudden and brief recurrent episodes of unsteadiness, nystagmus and pallor, with no headache or loss of consciousness. The child may be nauseated and vomit. The attack often lasts only a few seconds and less commonly a few minutes. The child appears completely well between attacks. Benign paroxysmal vertigo is often regarded as a variant of migraine or a migraine equivalent.[60]

In schoolchildren idiopathic vertigo may occur in association with migraine. Most children with migraine headaches may report vertigo either just before or during the migraine headache.[56] In a population-based study, attacks of vertigo occurred on average 11 times per year and each attack lasted for a mean of 6 min.[56] The prevalence of paroxysmal vertigo in a school-aged population was estimated at 2.6%.[56]

The most common trigger factor reported for paroxysmal vertigo is tiredness. During the episode, pallor and nausea are commonly reported with attacks of vertigo. Relief is reported from lying or sitting down or from sleep. A family history of migraine is found in

paroxysmal vertigo as commonly as in migraine headaches.[56] Children with paroxysmal vertigo may have other features of the periodic syndrome including cyclical vomiting and abdominal pain.[59] Motion sickness and atopic disease are more common in children with paroxysmal vertigo than in the general population.[56]

The attacks of paroxysmal vertigo are brief and self-limiting and no treatment is usually given. Some authors have used anti-migraine drugs,[59] but there are no controlled trials of therapy. The condition usually settles spontaneously with age.

Paroxysmal vertigo has many features in common with childhood migraine headaches, including mode of presentation, triggering and relieving factors, vasomotor symptoms during attacks and associated gastrointestinal symptoms. There is a marked overlap between the conditions and their family histories. These features confirm the strong relationship between paroxysmal vertigo and migraine.[56,59]

# Recurrent limb pain

Limb pain is common in children and most cases are related to trauma or to viral or flu-like illnesses.[61] A number of specific orthopaedic problems may also cause limb pain, including arthritis, osteochondritis, irritable hip and Perthes' disease.

There is also a group of children who have recurrent short episodes of limb pains lasting for less than 72 hours and with complete normality between attacks. The pain is severe enough to disrupt normal daily activities and is often localized deeply in the arms and legs.[62] There is no abnormality on clinical examination and no identifiable underlying organic cause. The condition runs a benign and self-limiting course. It is often referred to as 'growing pains'. Many of these children have limb pain as their only symptom, but about one-third also complain of abdominal pain and headache.[3]

In a population-based study, recurrent limb pains were found in 2.6% of schoolchildren.[61] Episodes of limb pain occurred on average 12 times per year and each episode lasted on average 10 hours. The most common trigger factor was tiredness. Associated features included anorexia and nausea. The pain was relieved by rest, simple analgesics or sleep, and in some children by counterirritation such as applying hot water bottles or rubbing the affected limb.

A history of migraine in a first-degree relative is as common in children with recurrent limb pain as in children with migraine headache, and much more common than in a matched control group of children.[61]

Non-specific limb pain is common in children with migraine[41] and there are marked similarities between recurrent limb pain and migraine in the trigger factors for attacks, the associated symptoms during attacks and the relieving factors. These indicate a strong relationship between recurrent limb pains and migraine.

## Basilar migraine

Basilar migraine was previously known as basilar artery migraine but the preferred term is now 'basilar migraine' because spasm of the basilar artery may not be the mechanism of the attacks.[63] It is a variety of migraine with aura, with the aura symptoms clearly originating either from the brain stem or from both occipital lobes. The entity of basilar artery migraine was first described by Bickerstaff[64] who suggested that occurrence was most typically in adolescent and preadolescent girls. Barlow[18] has, however, suggested that the age of onset can range from infancy to middle adult years, with a strong female predominance from puberty onwards, but lesser female bias in the younger prepubertal patients. The symptoms and signs that make up basilar migraine are those that are related to the tissue supplied by the basilar–vertebral system. With many migraine attacks, there will be some symptoms that could be attributable to the basilar artery territory and there is enormous variability in the clinical presentation of basilar migraine. Thus, estimates of incidence vary widely and depend largely on the definition used in individual studies.

Although the clinical presentation is very variable, within individuals the presentation of attacks is similar. In most children specific neurological signs precede headache, which may occur only as specific features of the attack resolve. Many of the symptoms of basilar migraine are open to misinterpretation because they may occur together with anxiety and hyperventilation. Visual symptoms, including tunnel vision, total amblyopia and positive or negative hallucinations, are common in children. Commonly flashes or blobs of light are seen rather than more formed fortification spectra.[65] Ataxia may then appear, often accompanied by vertigo and perhaps tinnitus. Dysarthria may be mistaken for intoxication with drugs or alcohol. Numbness and tingling around the face, mouth and tongue, and bilaterally in the hands and feet, is common, typically occurring early in an attack. There may be weakness related to the bulbocorticospinal system, and this may be hemiplegic, diplegic or quadriplegic. Other symptoms and signs may include nystagmus, diplopia, third and seventh nerve lesions, and pyramidal dysfunction. Consciousness is impaired in some patients.

Nausea and vomiting are severe and frequently prostrating, and pallor, lethargy and drowsiness are very common during attacks. This may lead to a diagnostic overlap between symptoms of basilar migraine and of parts of the periodic syndrome including cyclical vomiting and paroxysmal vertigo.

The specific symptoms of basilar migraine usually last only minutes and seldom more than an hour. In most cases they are followed by headache, which may be occipital in a minority of patients. The headache may be absent, particularly in younger prepubertal patients.[66]

The differential diagnosis of basilar migraine includes posterior fossa tumours which may sometimes produce intermittent symptoms, although most will produce symptoms and signs of raised intracranial pressure, and congenital abnormalities at the base of the brain. Several metabolic disorders may also simulate attacks similar to basilar migraine, including homocystinuria, pyruvate carboxylase deficiency, ornithine transcarbamylase deficiency, some organic acidaemias and disorders of the urea cycle. In most of these metabolic diseases there is evidence of persisting neurological dysfunction between attacks.

Where there is a clear history of basilar migraine, specific investigations are seldom indicated. If the history is less specific, intracranial structural abnormality may be excluded by magnetic resonance imaging (MRI). Metabolic screening may also be indicated where a metabolic abnormality is suspected.

It is usual for the complex episodes of basilar migraine to be interspersed with other episodes of migraine, although the basilar episode may be the first migraine attack or the first few attacks. They usually become a lesser problem when the adult pattern of headache for the individual evolves.

## Hemiplegic migraine

The development of unilateral neurological signs and symptoms, including hemiparesis and unilateral numbness associated with migraine headaches, has been known for many years.[67] Aphasia, usually together with hemiparesis, may be found when there is involvement of the hemisphere dominant for speech. These symptoms usually occur as part of the prodrome or as a manifestation of the migrainous aura, and are confined to this phase of the migraine sequence. The symptoms are then replaced by contralateral hemicranial headache, although the headache may be bilateral, diffuse or ipsilateral.[18] Where this occurs the symptoms are frequently categorized as 'type 1'.[68] Other symptoms such as nausea, vomiting and light-headedness are common. Random alternation between sides is most common, although in some patients there is a tendency for recurrence on the same side. Some alteration of consciousness may occur during attacks.

It is usual for the patient with hemiplegic migraine to have other types of migraine as well, either with or without aura. The prognosis is generally benign. In many patients, the frequency and severity of hemiplegic attacks decrease with age and they may be replaced by other forms of migraine attack. Hemiplegic migraine is a disorder of young people and the condition is relatively common in adolescent patients.[18] The prevalence of the condition is not known and no community studies have been reported.

A second variety of presentation is the less common and more troublesome 'type 2'.[68] In this variety hemiparesis continues into the headache phase or develops during the period of headache. In some patients, the symptoms have a biphasic expression during a single episode. The hemisyndrome may persist for one to several days, and may continue after the headache has subsided.[69] The onset is commonly in adolescents and young adults, although occasionally it is seen in children. The attacks are infrequent and confined to a relatively brief period in the lifespan of migraine in a given period. Migraine episodes without aura may occur with greater frequency between attacks.

The differential diagnosis of hemiplegic migraine includes the serious problems of vascular malformation or a tumour. Careful clinical evaluation is indicated and most patients will have cranial imaging by MRI. If, however, there is a clear-cut history of recurrent migrainous attacks, with or without aura, together with a positive family history, then no investigation may be required.

A common feature of this form of complex migraine is the occurrence of families with hemiplegic migraine.[67–69] Most of these families have a stereotyped syndrome of hemiplegia that occurs quite suddenly during the headache phase, and may be accompanied by impaired consciousness. In some, the hemiplegia regularly occurs on the same side in various members of the family.[68,69]

Familial hemiplegic migraine is an autosomal dominant condition, with half of the families being assigned to chromosome 19p13. Missense mutations have been identified in a brain-specific calcium channel $\alpha_{1A}$-subunit (CACNA1A) gene on 19q13 segregating with familial hemiplegic migraine.[70] One family has also been described where the locus for familial hemiplegic migraine maps to chromosome 1q31.[71]

A further syndrome of alternating hemiplegia of childhood has also been described.[72] The onset is usually before 18 months of age and children have repeated episodes of hemiplegia lasting from a few minutes to several days. Other features of the condition include tonic or dystonic attacks, nystagmus, dyspnoea and other autonomic phenomena, and the development of cognitive impairment and a choreoathetoid movement disorder.[73] The condition was originally described as a variety of hemiplegic migraine[72] but is probably not related to migraine.[73] Flunarizine has been shown to reduce the frequency and duration of attacks in many children,[73] and this may be combined with acetazolamide and acetylsalicylic acid.[74]

# References

1. Abu-Arafeh I, Russell G, Prevalence of headache and migraine in schoolchildren. *BMJ* 1994; **309**: 765–9.
2. Apley J, Naish N, Recurrent abdominal pains: a field survey of 1000 schoolchildren. *Arch Dis Childh* 1958; **33**: 165–70.
3. Oster J, Recurrent abdominal pain, headache and limb pains in children and adolescents. *Pediatrics* 1972; **50**: 429–36.
4. Pringle MLK, Butler NR, Davie R, *11,000 Seven-year-olds*. London: Longman, 1966: 184.
5. Miller FJW, Court SDM, Knox EG, Brandon S, *The School Years in Newcastle upon Tyne*. London: Oxford University Press, 1974: 280.
6. Abu-Arafeh I, Russell G, Prevalence and clinical features of abdominal migraine compared with those of migraine headache. *Arch Dis Childh* 1995; **72**: 413–17.
7. Dodge JA, Recurrent abdominal pain in children. *BMJ* 1976; **i**: 385–7.

8. McGrath PJ, Goodman JT, Firestone P, Shipman R, Peters S, Recurrent abdominal pain: a psychogenic disorder? *Arch Dis Childh* 1983; **58**: 888–90.

9. Heinild S, Malver E, Roelsgaard G, Worning B, A psychosomatic approach to recurrent abdominal pain in childhood. *Acta Paediatr* 1959; **48**: 361–70.

10. Krupp GR, Friedman AP, Migraine in children. A report of 50 children. *Am J Dis Childh* 1953; **85**: 146–50.

11. Symon DNK, Russell G, The general paediatrician's view of migraine – a review of 250 cases. In: Lanzi D, Balottin U, Cernibori A, eds, *Headache in Children and Adolescents*. Amsterdam: Elsevier Science Publishers, 1989: 61–6.

12. Blumenthal LS, Fuchs M, Abdominal migraine. *Am J Proctol* 1957; **8**: 370–9.

13. Lundberg PO, Abdominal migraine – diagnosis and therapy. *Headache* 1975; **15**: 122–5.

14. Buchanan JA, The abdominal crises of migraine. *J Nervous Ment Dis* 1921; **54**: 406–12.

15. Brams WA, Abdominal migraine. *JAMA* 1922; **78**: 26–7.

16. Wyllie WG, Schlesinger B, The periodic group of disorders in childhood. *Br J Child Dis* 1933; **30**: 1–21.

17. Cullen KJ, Macdonald WB, The periodic syndrome: its nature and prevalence. *Med J Aust* 1963; **2**: 167–73.

18. Barlow CF, *Headaches and Migraine in Childhood*. Oxford: Spastics International Medical Publications, 1984.

19. Lundberg PO, Abdominal migraine. *Triangle* 1978; **17**: 81–4.

20. McCormick J, Recurrent abdominal pain in childhood. *BMJ* 1980; **280**: 1377.

21. Symon DNK, Russell G, Abdominal migraine: a childhood syndrome defined. *Cephalalgia* 1986; **6**: 223–8.

22. Symon DNK, Russell G, Clinical features of abdominal and headache migraine in children. In: Galli V, Guidetti V, eds, *Juvenile Headache*. Amsterdam: Elsevier Science Publishers, 1991: 213–14.

23. Mortimer MJ, Kay J, Jaron A, Clinical epidemiology of childhood abdominal migraine in an urban general practice. *Dev Med Child Neurol* 1993; **35**: 243–8.

24. Santoro G, Curzio M, Venco A, Abdominal migraine in adults. Case reports. *Funct Neurol* 1990; **5**: 61–4.

25. Mortimer MJ, Good PA, Marsters JB, Addy DP, Visual evoked responses in children with migraine: a diagnostic test. *Lancet* 1990; **335**: 75–7.

26. Symon DNK, Is there a place for 'abdominal migraine' as a separate entity in the IHS classification? Yes! *Cephalalgia* 1992; **12**: 345–6.

27. Hockaday JM, Is there a place for 'abdominal migraine' as a separate entity in the IHS classification? No! *Cephalalgia* 1992; **12**: 346–8.

28. Symon DNK, Russell G, A double blind placebo controlled trial of pizotifen syrup in the treatment of abdominal migraine. *Arch Dis Childh* 1995; **72**: 48–50.

29. Symon DNK, Russell G, Continued benefit after stopping pizotifen therapy in childhood migraine. *Cephalalgia* 1989; **9**(suppl 10): 422–3.

30. Worawattanakul M, Rhoads JM, Lichtman SN, Ulshen MH, Abdominal migraine: prophylactic treatment and follow-up. *J Pediatr Gastroenterol Nutrition* 1999; **28**: 37–40.

31. Lombard HC, Description d'une névrose de la digestion, caractérisée par des crises périodiques de vomissements et une profonde modification de l'assimilation. *Gaz Méd Paris* 1861: 312–15.

32. Gee S, On fitful or recurrent vomiting. *St Bartholomew's Hospital Reports* 1882; **18**: 1–6.

33. Gruère N, Observation de vomissements périodiques, sans signes d'inflammation ni de lésion organique. *Précis analytique des traveaux de la Société Médicale de Dijon* 1843: 71–4.

34. Fleisher DR, The cyclic vomiting syndrome described. *J Pediatr Gastroenterol Nutrition* 1995; **21**(suppl 1): 1–5.

35. Fleisher DR, Matar M, The cyclic vomiting syndrome: a report of 71 cases and literature review. *J Pediatr Gastroenterol Nutrition* 1993; **17**: 361–9.

36. Li BUK, Cyclic vomiting: new understanding of an old disorder. *Contemp Pediatr* 1996; **13**: 48–62.
37. Forbes D, Withers G, Silburn S, McKelvey R, Psychological and social characteristics and precipitants of vomiting in children with cyclic vomiting syndrome. *Dig Dis Sci* 1999; **44**(suppl): 19–22.
38. Prakash C, Clouse R, Cyclic vomiting syndrome in adults: clinical features and response to tricyclic antidepressants. *Am J Gastroenterol* 1999; **94**: 2856–60.
39. Symon DNK, Is cyclical vomiting an abdominal form of migraine in children? *Dig Dis Sci* 1999; **44**(suppl): 23–5.
40. Marfan AB, Les vomissements périodiques avec acétonémie. *Arch Méd Enfants* 1921; **24**: 5–28.
41. Bille B, Migraine in school children. A study of the incidence and short-term prognosis, and a clinical, psychological and encephalographic comparison between children with migraine and matched controls. *Acta Paediatr* 1962; **51**(suppl 136): 1–151.
42. Hammond J, The late sequelae of recurrent vomiting of childhood. *Dev Med Child Neurol* 1974; **16**: 15–22.
43. Salmon MA, The evolution of adult migraine through childhood migraine equivalents. In: Lanzi D, Balottin U, Cernibori A, eds, *Headache in Children and Adolescents*. Amsterdam: Elsevier Science Publishers, 1989: 27–32.
44. Good PA, Neurologic investigations of childhood abdominal migraine: a combined electrophysiologic approach to diagnosis. *J Pediatr Gastroenterol Nutrition* 1995; **21**(suppl 1): 44–8.
45. Jernigan SA, Ware LM, Reversible quantitative EEG changes in a case of cyclic vomiting; evidence for migraine equivalent. *Dev Med Child Neurol* 1991; **33**: 80–5.
46. Li BUK, Murray RD, Heitlinger LA, Robbins JL, Hayes JR, Is cyclic vomiting syndrome related to migraine? *J Pediatr* 1999; **134**: 567–72.
47. Lanzi G, Balottin U, Ottolini A, Rosano Burgio F, Fazzi E, Arisi D, Cyclic vomiting and recurrent abdominal pains as migraine or epileptic equivalents. *Cephalalgia* 1983; **3**: 115–18.
48. Abu-Arafeh I, Russell G, Cyclical vomiting syndrome in children. A population based study. *J Pediatr Gastroenterol Nutrition* 1995; **21**: 454–8.
49. Boles RG, Chun N, Senadheera D, Wong LJC, Cyclic vomiting syndrome and mitochondrial DNA mutations. *Lancet* 1997; **350**: 1299–300.
50. Salmon MA, Walters DD, Pizotifen in the prophylaxis of cyclical vomiting. *Lancet* 1985; **i**: 1036–7.
51. Forbes D, Withers G, Prophylactic therapy in cyclic vomiting syndrome. *J Pediatr Gastroenterol Nutrition* 1995; **21**(suppl 1): 57–9.
52. Gokhale R, Huttenlocher PR, Brady L, Kirschner BS, Use of barbiturates in the treatment of cyclic vomiting during childhood. *J Pediatr Gastroenterol Nutrition* 1997; **25**: 64–7.
53. Vanderhoof JA, Young R, Kaufman SS, Ernst L, Treatment of cyclic vomiting in childhood with erythromycin. *J Pediatr Gastroenterol Nutrition* 1995; **21**(suppl 1): 60–2.
54. Fleisher DR, Management of cyclic vomiting syndrome. *J Pediatr Gastroenterol Nutrition* 1995; **21**(suppl 1): 52–6.
55. Benson JM, Zorn SL, Book LS, Sumatriptan in the treatment of cyclic vomiting. *Ann Pharmacotherapy* 1995; **29**: 997–9.
56. Abu-Arafeh I, Russell G, Paroxysmal vertigo as a migraine equivalent in children: a population based study. *Cephalalgia* 1995; **15**: 22–5.
57. Dunn DW, Snyder CH, Benign paroxysmal vertigo of childhood. *Am J Dis Child* 1976; **130**: 1099–100.
58. Koenigsberger MR, Chutorian AM, Gold AP, Schvey MS, Benign paroxysmal vertigo of childhood. *Neurology* 1970; **20**: 1108–13.
59. Lanzi G, Balottin U, Fazzi E, Mira E, Piacentino G, Benign paroxysmal vertigo in childhood: a longitudinal study. *Headache* 1986; **26**: 494–7.
60. Fenichel GM, Migraine as a cause of benign paroxysmal vertigo of childhood. *J Pediatr* 1967; **71**: 114–15.
61. Abu-Arafeh I, Russell G, Recurrent limb pain in schoolchildren. *Arch Dis Childh* 1996; **74**: 336–9.

62. Naish JM, Apley J, 'Growing pains': a clinical study of non-arthritis limb pains in children. *Arch Dis Childh* 1951; **26**: 134–40.

63. Headache Classification Committee of the International Headache Society, Classification and diagnostic criteria for headache disorders, cranial neuralgias and facial pain. *Cephalalgia* 1988; 8(suppl 7): 23–4.

64. Bickerstaff ER, Basilar artery migraine. *Lancet* 1961; **i**: 15–17.

65. Bickerstaff ER, The basilar artery and the migraine–epilepsy syndrome. *Proc R Soc Med* 1962; **55**: 167–9.

66. Lapkin ML, Golden GS, Basilar artery migraine: a review of 30 cases. *Am J Dis Child* **132**: 278–81.

67. Clarke JM, On recurrent motor paralysis in migraine, with a report in which recurrent hemiplegia accompanied the attacks. *BMJ* 1910; **i**: 1534–8.

68. Whitty CWM, Familial hemiplegic migraine. *J Neurol Neurosurg Psychiatry* 1953; **16**: 172–7.

69. Bradshaw P, Parsons M, Hemiplegic migraine, a clinical study. *Q J Med* 1965; **34**: 65–85.

70. Terwindt GM, Ophoff RA, Haan J et al, Variable clinical expression of mutations in the P/Q-type calcium channel gene in familial hemiplegic migraine. *Neurology* 1998; **50**: 1105–10.

71. Gardner K, Barmada MM, Ptacek LJ, Hoffman EP, A new locus for hemiplegic migraine maps to chromosome 1q31. *Neurology* 1997; **49**: 1231–8.

72. Verret S, Steele JC, Alternating hemiplegia in childhood: a report of eight patients with complicated migraine beginning in infancy. *Pediatrics* 1971; **47**: 675–80.

73. Bourgeois M, Aicardi J, Goutières F, Alternating hemiplegia of childhood. *J Pediatr* 1993; **122**: 673–9.

74. Siemes H, Casaer P, Alternierende Hemiplegie des Kindesalters. Klinischer Bericht und SPECT-Studie. *Monatsschrift Kinderheilk* 1988; **136**: 467–70.

# 18

# Relationship between migraine and stroke

*Livia Nicoletta Rossi*

In this chapter, we examine the following: Do strokes occur in the course of a migraine attack in children and cause true migraine-induced cerebral infarction? Can this event occur only in the presence of other risk factors?

## Definition and classification

It is well known that cerebral infarcts can develop in the course of migraine-like attacks in young adults. These infarctions have been termed 'migrainous strokes'.[1–6] The criteria usually used for the diagnosis of migrainous strokes by the authors who reported these cases were:

(1) Presence of acute neurological deficit
(2) Association of this acute event with headache or other symptoms that are characteristic of a migraine attack
(3) History of migraine
(4) Evidence of infarction on neuroradiological examinations
(5) No other known cause of stroke.

According to the International Headache Society (IHS) classification of 1988, 'migrainous cerebral infarction' is described as one or more migrainous aura symptoms not fully reversible within 7 days and/or associated with neuroimaging confirmation of ischaemic infarction. The following conditions should be present:

(1) Patients should have had previously fulfilled criteria for migraine with neurological aura.
(2) The present attack should be typical of previous attacks.
(3) Other causes of infarction should be ruled out by appropriate investigation.

In this way, the IHS definition of migraine-induced stroke is more restrictive because it does not allow the diagnosis in patients who previously had migraine without aura.

In relation to stroke migraine is an intriguing and perplexing problem,[7,8] which results in confusing terminology in the literature. In 1994, in his paper 'Relationship of stroke and migraine', Welch[7] proposed a classification and a redefinition of migraine-related stroke, distinguishing four different migraine-related stroke syndromes. The classification is reported in Table 18.1. 'Coexisting stroke and migraine' indicates a clinical stroke syndrome that occurs remotely in time from a typical migraine attack. 'Stroke with clinical features of migraine' indicates a structural lesion that is unrelated to migraine pathogenesis and presenting with clinical features of a migraine attack. It can be 'symptomatic', e.g. secondary to a vascular malformation or 'migraine mimic'

| Category | Feature |
|----------|---------|
| I | Coexisting stroke and migraine |
| II | Stroke with clinical features of migraine |
|   | (A) Symptomatic migraine |
|   | (B) Migraine mimic |
| III | Migraine-induced stroke |
|   | (A) Without risk factors |
|   | (B) With risk factors |
| IV | Uncertain |

**Table 18.1**
*Classification of migraine-related stroke (from Welch[7])*

(stroke caused by acute progressive structural disease with symptoms typical for migraine). The third category is 'migraine-induced' stroke in which the following criteria must be fulfilled:

(1) The neurological deficit must be identical to the migraine symptoms of previous attacks
(2) The stroke must occur during the course of a typical migraine attack
(3) All other causes of strokes have been excluded, although stroke risk factors may be present.

In the remainder of this chapter, the term 'migrainous stroke' is used, using the definition given at the beginning of this chapter.

## Epidemiology and characteristics of migrainous stroke in adults

Prospective studies have shown migraine to be an independent risk factor for ischaemic stroke, at least among women aged less than 45 years.[9–12] In some studies by Bogousslavsky et al,[4,13] migrainous stroke accounted for 10.4–15% of strokes in young adults. In a series of 4874 patients with migraine, studied by Broderick and Swanson,[14] 20 (0.4%) had an infarct during an attack of migraine. Connor[15] collected a total of 17 patients with migrainous stroke in a series of migraine cases; according to Barlow[16] the series consisted of 500 patients, so that the percentage of migrainous stroke would be 3.4%.

In general, strokes are more common in patients with migraine with aura.[6,13] However, Rothrock et al[6] found this association to be of little value in attempting to distinguish patients destined for migrainous stroke in a general migraine population. In his study, patients with migraine who had a stroke during a migraine attack were more likely to have recurrent strokes; among his 28 patients with migrainous stroke, 6 had a recurrence in the following 2 years, once again associated with migraine.

Could the concomitant presence of other risk factors determine the occurrence of strokes in patients with migraine? Silvestrini et al[17] investigated the prevalence of migraine and antiphospholipid antibodies in 162 patients with stroke. He found that migraine was present in 6 of 10 patients with antibodies and only in 5 of 152 patients without antibodies. Bogousslavsky et al[4] and Rothrock et al[6] did not find any association with stroke in migraine when considering the following factors: smoking, oral contraception, hypertension and mitral valve prolapse. In his study, Bogousslavsky et al[4] found that 91% of patients who had a stroke during a migraine attack had no cardiac or arterial lesions, as opposed to 9% of patients with migraine with aura who had a stroke remote from a migraine attack and 18% of patients with stroke without migraine. The patients with stroke during migraine attacks had had longer previous attacks of migraine and their infarct was more frequent in the territory involved during the attacks, thereby supporting the hypothesis, in his opinion, that a prolongation of the migraine process beyond its usual limits may explain most migraine strokes.

Even if epidemiological data are in favour of migraine as a causal factor for ischaemic stroke, in the individual patient the diagnosis is very difficult and it is necessary to rule out other known causes of stroke. However, once again, in this case, diagnosis of migrainous stroke can only be presumptive and there have been cases with stroke from other aetiologies masquerading as migrainous strokes.[18]

In migrainous stroke, frequently the area of infarct was in the posterior cerebral artery territory.[4,14-15] It is quite reasonable to think that the vascular territories of the posterior cerebral artery are frequently involved because they correspond to the territories involved in migraine with aura. In many cases, however, although the deficit fits the posterior cerebral artery distribution, the clinical features suggest a more widespread involvement. Hemiplegia and aphasia in fact usually indicate ischaemia in the middle cerebral artery territory.[14]

In most cases, angiography (performed 2–8 days after the event, when specified) was normal, suggesting that an occlusive or stenosing phenomenon was unlikely to play a major role.[3-5,14] In some cases, however, a transient segmental narrowing was found.[3,16,19] In the opinion of some authors,[19,20] the cause of this anatomical characteristic could be a vessel wall oedema caused by release of vasoactive peptides or a vasospasm.

Adult patients have been reported to have residual deficit of varying degrees of severity in many cases.[3,5,14]

# Epidemiology and characteristics of migrainous stroke in children

In the study on migrainous stroke in adults by Broderick and Swanson,[14] three children were included. In other studies on adults,[1,5,15,21,22] a total of five patients aged 16 years or less were included. There are few studies on migrainous stroke in children. In Barlow's book,[16] 300 children affected by migraine are reported: five (1.7%) had proven or presumed infarct (one with retinal infarct) during an attack of migraine; two had an anatomical lesion of a valve or the great vessels.

Another study was carried out by Rossi et al[23] on a group of seven children affected by migrainous stroke and collected from four different children's hospitals in Europe. A total of 600 migraine patients was examined in one of these hospitals during the same period, with three cases with migrainous stroke (0.5%) being found. Epidemiological data from the other hospitals are not available.

More recently, two children with cerebral infarction and headache have been reported by Wöber-Bingöl et al.[24] The first case had a cerebral infarction during a migraine-like episode and, in his medical history, there were migraine attacks with neurological deficit always on the same side; however, he also had a cardiac abnormality predisposing to cardioembolism. In the second case, the attack was accompanied by seizures, which is quite atypical for migraine; furthermore, the child had a learning disorder and had neither a previous nor a subsequent history of migraine.

Recently two other children with migrainous stroke were described by Ebinger et al.[25]

Among all these children with proven infarction on computed tomography (CT) or with presumed infarction (one case described by Barlow[16] with long-lasting neurological deficit – no CT scan performed), 11 who had the infarction during migraine-like attacks and were without other known risk factors for stroke were described in detail by their authors.[16,23,25] The children's history of migraine was characterized by paroxysmal episodes of headache, in some cases associated with vomiting or photophobia, and recurrent after symptom-free intervals. The principal feature of the migrainous stroke was a focal deficit that lasted beyond the headache, from a few hours to several days (usually 1–3 days). Three children had had multiple episodes of motor deficit at the time of their examination and these had always occurred on the same side. For all children, among their siblings and parents, none had had episodes of complicated migraine and in no case was there a family history of stroke at a young age.

Computed tomography showed an infarction in the posterior cerebral artery territories in four cases and in the middle artery territories in others. In the three children who had had multiple episodes of motor deficit at the time of examination, a CT scan had not been performed after each episode.[22] Angiography was performed in five cases; in three a segmental narrowing was found and in the other cases it was normal. It was also normal in the children reported by Broderick and Swanson.[14]

After the acute event, some of the 11 children reported in detail were treated with aspirin or anti-migrainous drugs for variable intervals of time. With the exceptions of one patient reported by Barlow,[16] who showed a residual mild-to-moderate hemiplegia, and of one child described by Rossi et al,[23] with hemianopia, the others had minimal or no residual deficit. Nine cases had a follow-up lasting from 1 year to $6\frac{1}{2}$ years. During the follow-up, other episodes of migraine were observed in six cases; two of these had neurological deficit on alternating sides during some attacks, but without infarction on CT scan and one case showed some recurrences of headache with hemiplegia, but he had no further CT scans. The patient described by Barlow[16] with retinal infarction had permanent field deficit.

## Case report

One of the cases reported by Rossi et al[23] is described here as a clinical example.

The patient was a 10-year-old boy with a family history of non-complicated migraine but with a personal history of migraine. The episode with stroke occurred with a severe headache on the left side, followed by dysarthria and, 2 hours later, by vomiting, aphasia, hemianopia, paraesthesia and paresis of the extremities on the right side. Improvement began to appear 24 hours later. A CT scan performed 4 days after the event showed an infarct in the area of the left posterior cerebral artery. Other laboratory examinations were negative. He was not given any drug treatment. After the episode, the boy showed a residual minimal motor deficit. During follow-up over $4\frac{1}{2}$ years, he had rare attacks of severe headache with photophobia.

## Comment on cases involving children

All the children reported had at least one episode of infarction with symptoms that were characteristic for migraine. In agreement with what is usually observed in adults, some children had more than one episode with either stroke or neurological deficit and presumed stroke, and these episodes were all on the same side. Therefore, it is quite reasonable to presume that an infarct tends to occur more easily when the same cerebral area is recurrently involved.

Frequently the area of infarct was in the posterior cerebral artery, which is in contrast to what is usually found in stroke of idiopathic origin in children; angiography showed a transient segmental narrowing in some of the cases. These characteristics are in agreement with what is frequently observed in adults.[4,14,15]

In contrast to what is observed in adults, in almost all cases involving children[16,23,25] recovery was complete or almost complete. Children affected by migrainous stroke do not perhaps have as severe migrainous strokes as adults. In fact, adults with severe migrainous stroke have not usually had a history of stroke during childhood.[1-5] In two cases reported by Barlow[16] and one observed by Wöber-Bingöl et al,[24] an anatomical lesion of a valve or the great vessels was found. In the other cases reported in children, illnesses that are well-known causes of stroke (such as arteritis or MELAS disease) can be excluded on the basis of clinical history and known risk factors for stroke were not found. One cannot, however, exclude the possibility that some of the patients had risk factors for thrombotic diseases. In fact some of the reported cases have been described in 1990 or previous years, and the children were not investigated for those risk factors that have been described more recently for stroke. Furthermore, not all children reported with migrainous stroke underwent complete laboratory investigations including angiography.

The IHS criteria for migrainous stroke were not fulfilled for those cases in which an exclusion of other causes of stroke was inadequate. Furthermore, children reported in the literature as having migrainous stroke do not fulfil all the IHS criteria for migrainous cerebral infarction, because most of them did not have migraine with aura and some of them had not had preceding migraine attacks at all. On the other hand, it is well known that an attack of complicated migraine in children can be the first indication of a migraine history. Therefore, various authors think that the IHS criteria seem to be too restrictive for children[23-25] and probably need to be revised. Also the criteria suggested by Welch[7] seem too restrictive for children, and, from a practical point of view, the distinction between 'causes' and 'risk factors' of stroke can be very difficult in the individual patient.

## Pathogenesis

According to Welch,[7] the pathogenesis of migraine-related stroke would be a combination of reduced blood flow in brain tissue and slow flow in large intracerebral vessels, together with factors predisposing to coagulopathy. The result would be an intravascular thrombosis.

According to the theory of the cortical spreading depression (see Pathophysiology section), the spread of the neuronal depression produces the neurological symptoms; the accompanying oligaemia could contribute to the neurological disabilities. Therefore, two mechanisms could be at the source of migrainous strokes: the calibre changes in arterioles and capillaries associated with a reduction in perfusion and changes in cellular metabolism. Some authors[21,22,26] think that an arterial spasm could also be the source of the neurological event.

An alternative hypothesis is that a migraine attack is triggered by an ischaemic event in susceptible individuals. According to this hypothesis, however, some peculiarities would be difficult to understand: the higher prevalence of strokes in patients with migraine; the tendency of recurrences in these patients; and the frequent involvement of the posterior cerebral arteries.

## Management in children

Management should be the same as that for idiopathic stroke. The association of long-term acetylsalicylic acid with an anti-migrainous drug (such as propranolol) for some months after the event is probably appropriate, although the efficacy of this prevention has not been proved in strokes in children.

## Conclusion

In adults, migraine is an intriguing problem in relation to stroke; however, there seems to be a casual relationship between migraine and stroke. As patients who are children have been observed with strokes in the course of migraine-like attacks, it is reasonable to think that there is also a causal relationship between the two conditions in children, although this relationship cannot be demonstrated. Migraine probably represents a contributory risk factor for strokes in childhood and should be considered in the differential diagnosis of stroke. Migraine is probably a risk factor when associated with other risk factors for stroke. In any case, stroke during a migraine attack is very uncommon in children. Of course, the diagnosis of migraine-related stroke can only be presumptive and it must be based on the exclusion of other known causes of stroke. Furthermore, new causes of stroke can be detected in the future. Various authors think that the definition of migrainous cerebral infarction in the IHS classification of 1988 is too restrictive for children and needs revision.

## References

1. Dorfman LJ, Marshall WH, Enzmann DR, Cerebral infarction in migraine: clinical and radiological correlations. *Neurology* 1979; **29**: 317–22.
2. Spaccavento LJ, Solomon GD, Migraine as an etiology of stroke in young adults. *Headache* 1984; **24**: 19–22.
3. Featherstone HJ, Clinical features of stroke in migraine: a review. *Headache* 1986; **26**: 128–33.
4. Bogousslavsky J, Regli F, Van Melle G, Payot M, Uske A, Migraine stroke. *Neurology* 1988; **38**: 223–7.
5. Rothrock JF, Walicke P, Swenson MR, Lyden PD, Logan WR, Migrainous stroke. *Arch Neurol* 1988; **45**: 63–7.
6. Rothrock JF, North J, Madden K, Lyden P, Fleck P, Dittrich H, Migraine and migrainous stroke: Risk factors and prognosis. *Neurology* 1993; **43**: 2473–6.
7. Welch KMA, Relationship of stroke and migraine. *Neurology* 1994; **44**(suppl 7): S33–6.
8. Dayno JM, Silberstein SD, Migraine-related stroke versus migraine-induced stroke. *Headache* 1997; **37**: 463 (letter).
9. Bartleson JD, Transient and persistent neurological manifestations of migraine. *Stroke* 1984; **15**: 383–6.
10. Merikangas KR, Fenton BT, Cheng SH, Stolar MJ, Risch N, Association between migraine and stroke in a large-scale epidemiological study of the United States. *Arch Neurol* 1997; **54**: 362–8.
11. Tzourio C, Iglesia S, Hubert J-B et al, Migraine and risk of ischemic stroke: a case–control study. *BMJ* 1993; **307**: 289–92.

12. Buring JE, Hebert P, Romero J et al, Migraine and subsequent risk of stroke in the physicians' health study. *Arch Neurol* 1995; **52**: 129–34.

13. Bogousslavsky J, Regli F, Ischemic stroke in adults younger than 30 years of age. *Arch Neurol* 1987; **44**: 479–82.

14. Broderick J, Swanson JW, Migraine-related strokes. Clinical profile and prognosis in 20 patients. *Arch Neurol* 1987; **44**: 868–71.

15. Connor RCR, Complicated migraine: a study of permanent neurological and visual defects caused by migraine. *Lancet* 1962; **ii**: 1072–5.

16. Barlow CF, *Headaches and Migraine in Childhood*. Clinics in Developmental Medicine, No. 91. (London: SIMP with Heinemann Medical; Lippincott: Philadelphia), 1984: 138–54.

17. Silvestrini M, Cupini ML, Matteis M, De Simone R, Bernardi G, Migraine in patients with stroke and antiphospholipid antibodies. *Headache* 1993; **33**: 421–6.

18. Shuaib A, Stroke from other etiologies masquerading as migraine-stroke. *Stroke* 1991; **22**: 1068–74.

19. Schon F, Harrison MJH, Can migraine cause multiple segmental cerebral artery constrictions? *J Neurol Neurosurg Psychiatry* 1987; **50**: 492–4.

20. Rothrock JF, Migrainous stroke. *Cephalalgia* 1993; **13**: 231.

21. Caplan LR, Migraine and vertebrobasilar ischemia. *Neurology* 1991; **41**: 55–61.

22. Buckle RM, Du Boulay G, Smith B, Death due to cerebral nasospasm. *J Neurol Neurosurg Psychiatry* 1964; **27**: 440–4.

23. Rossi LN, Penzien JM, Deonna Th, Goutières F, Vassella F, Does migraine-related stroke occur in childhood? *Dev Med Child Neurol* 1990; **32**: 1005–21.

24. Wöber-Bingöl Ç, Wöber C, Karwautz A, Feucht M, Brandtner S, Scheidinger H, Migraine and stroke in childhood and adolescence. *Cephalalgia* 1995; **15**: 26–30.

25. Ebinger F, Boor R, Gawehn J, Reitter B, Ischemic stroke and migraine in childhood: coincidence or casual relationship? *J Child Neurol* 1999; **14**: 451–5.

26. Olsen TS, Migraine-related stroke in childhood. *Lancet* 1991; **337**: 1546–54.

# 19

# Migraine and diet
*Livia Nicoletta Rossi, Maria Bardare, Gianfranco Brunelli*

## *Food allergy and intolerance*

### *Some historical data*

Hippocrates first described adverse reactions to foods over 2000 years ago, followed by other Greek scholars and then by many other physicians up to 1800.

It was not until 1950, however, that dietetic proof was employed (food allergen versus placebo) and only in the 1960s did Goldman et al[1,2] state that to diagnose food allergy three successive challenges should be positive after the elimination of the suspected food. This was the start of an era of scientific approach to food allergy, based on undeniable proof. In 1976, May[3] proposed double-masked placebo-controlled, oral food challenges for the diagnosis of food allergy and these tests are now accepted worldwide.

### *The problems of nomenclature*

The general term 'food allergy' grouped together the true allergic reactions and the non-immunologically mediated ones. As this created confusion, it was decided at first to use the term 'intolerance' for both the allergic (and pseudoallergic) and the non-allergic reactions.

Later, in 1995, the European Academy of Allergy and Clinical Immunology[4] proposed defining 'adverse food reactions' as any aberrant reaction after the ingestion of a food or food additive.

Adverse food reactions may be the result of toxic or non-toxic reactions. The non-toxic reactions may be immunologically mediated (allergic or hypersensitive reactions) or non-immunologically mediated (intolerance). The allergic reactions can be mediated by immunoglobulin E (IgE) (type I mechanism) or by immune complexes (type III mechanism), whereas intolerance reactions can be the result of susceptibility of the host (enzyme deficiency, idiosyncratic response) or of pharmacological properties of food.

### *Pathogenesis*

The enteric barrier is physiologically immature in the first months of life and this is one of the reasons for the frequency of adverse food reactions in childhood.[5] The gut barrier is (1) intraluminal and within the walls (secretory IgA and lamina propria plasma cells) and (2) within the walls (macrophages, glycoprotein secretions, enterocyte lysosomes).

In newborn babies for the first 6 weeks of life, this barrier does not work properly (allowing the macromolecules to penetrate across the enteric walls) as a result of the immaturity of the immunological mechanisms. After week 6, the gut barrier can be altered by the selective deficiency of secretory IgA or by an inflammation that can destroy the mucosa and damage the enteric flora. This flora is an important cofactor in the release of histamine and the damage of the mucosa, and it has a metabolic activity on the ingested food. So, a secretory IgA deficiency, as well as an early introduction of foreign food substances (in a period of enteric permeability), can predispose to *sensitivity* and, subsequently, to adverse food reactions. The quantity, quality and number of meals may play a major role.

In conclusion, the gut barrier alteration, secretory IgA deficiency and early weaning can favour sensitivity, especially in genetically predisposed infants.

Three mechanisms may play a pathogenic role: IgE-mediated (the most frequent), immune complex mediated and delayed hypersensitivity.

## Food allergens

A relatively small number of foods account for the adverse food reactions, given the enormous quantity of food substances present in our everyday diet.

Among adults, nuts, peanuts, fish and shellfish are responsible for the majority (85%) of the reactions, whereas among children it is milk, egg, wheat, soya and peanuts that account for 90% of adverse food reactions. The data are reported by Sampson,[6] but in some countries such as Italy allergy to soya and peanuts is less common, because of less consumption of these products.

## Diagnosis

The medical history is one of the most important diagnostic tools. The child's parents are asked about the dietary habits of the child, the period of weaning, the relationship of clinical symptoms to a particular food intake, and the length of time between ingestion and the appearance of symptoms. A diary for noting food ingestion, symptoms and signs can be advisable.

If an IgE-mediated reaction were present, prick tests with commercially available extracts or fresh food items (prick by prick) would be mandatory. The search for IgE antibodies in serum using a radioimmunological or immunoenzymatic assay is an alternative to the prick tests, but this is expensive and probably less sensitive.

Release of histamine from basophils has not been approved for routine use and immunoassays for determination of eosinophil-derived proteins should be regarded as research tools. However, none of these tests satisfied the criteria of reproducibility and specificity, and the diagnosis of adverse food reactions (whether or not immunologically mediated) can be established only with elimination–reintroduction diets.

The elimination diet is given for 2 weeks and, if symptoms improve, is followed by a challenge in a double-masked, placebo-controlled fashion. Three challenges are necessary in Goldman's opinion[1,2] for a conclusive evidence of food allergy.

## Symptoms and signs

There is a wide range of signs and symptoms caused by food allergy, affecting many parts of the body (Table 19.1). Even if rare, however,

| Skin | Urticaria/angio-oedema |
| | Flushing |
| | Erythematous pruritic rash |
| | Atopic dermatitis |
| Gastrointestinal tract | Pruritus and/or swelling of the lips, tongue or oral mucosa |
| | Nausea |
| | Abdominal cramping or colic |
| | Vomiting or reflux |
| | Diarrhoea |
| Respiratory tract | Nasal congestion |
| | Rhinorrhoea |
| | Pruritus/sneezing |
| | Laryngeal oedema, cough and/or dysphonia |
| | Wheezing/repetitive cough |
| Cardiovascular | Hypotension/shock |
| | Dizziness |
| Urogenital | Vulvovaginitis, eosinophil cystitis, haematuria, urinary tract infections |
| CNS | Headache, irritability, stress–fatigue syndrome |

**Table 19.1**
*Symptoms and signs of food-induced allergic reactions in various target organs*

there can be systemic symptoms such as severe anaemia, acute asthma and a true anaphylactic shock.

There are symptoms of immediate type, which appear soon after the ingestion of food and do not disappear through the years such as allergic rhinitis, asthma, vomiting, diarrhoea and angio-oedema. Other symptoms are delayed (or partially delayed), appear at a variable distance from the ingestion of large quantities of food and improve as time goes by: abdominal colic, arthritis, bronchiolitis, nervous system involvement, gastrointestinal disorders, atopic dermatitis.

## Management

In the therapy for food-induced allergic disorders, $H_1$ and $H_2$-receptor antihistamines have minimal efficacy, whereas oral corticosteroids are generally effective, especially in atopic dermatitis, asthma and non-IgE-mediated gastrointestinal disorders, although having unacceptable side effects. Some anecdotal results have been reported with sodium cromoglicate, but were not confirmed in controlled trials.[7]

The only proven therapy in an established allergy/intolerance is the elimination of the offending food(s). However, the elimination diet may have severe side effects, especially in very young individuals: 6–8% of the food allergies are seen in infants aged up to 1 year. So, the elimination of a large number of foods may lead to malnutrition, and the elimination of a single food can be very difficult, because that particular substance can be found in different commercially available foods (e.g. milk and egg).

| | Food | Cross-reaction | Percentage |
|---|---|---|---|
| Animal | Egg | Chicken meat | <5 |
| | Cow milk | Beef/veal | 10 |
| | Cow milk | Goat milk | 90 |
| | Beef/veal | Lamb | 50 |
| | Fish | Other fish species | >50 |
| Plant | Peanut | Legumes (except lentil) | <10 |
| | Soybean | Legumes | <5 |
| | Wheat | Other cereal grains | 25 |
| | Peanuts | Tree nuts | 35 |
| | Tree nuts | Other nuts | >50 |

It should be noted that patients frequently have positive PST or RAST results to other members of a plant family or animal species (>80%), but this does not correlate with clinical reactivity. Clinical reactivity is typically very food-allergen specific. PST, prick skin test; RAST, radioallergosorbent test.

**Table 19.2**
Clinical crossreactivity among members of plant and animal species (from Sampson[8])

Clinical reactivity to food allergens is very specific and crossreactivity rare (Table 19.2), so it is not necessary to exclude food families, only the offending food. Moreover, some subjects outgrow their sensitivity within a few years (except the sensitivity to nuts, peanuts, fish and shellfish), which makes it advisable to repeat allergic tests and dietetic challenges every 2–3 years.

As compliance to a diet (especially if very strict) is poor, many trials have been done to 'desensitize' the patients (reviewed by Sampson[8]): mutations of IgE-binding epitopes, protocols of DNA-based immunization, use of oligonucleotide immunostimulatory sequences (activating the secretion of cytokines and promoting a T-helper cell [Th1] response) and use of humanized anti-IgE antibodies. All these procedures are, however, still confined to research.

# Relationship between migraine and allergy: epidemiological data

There have been several studies on the prevalence of atopic disorders such as asthma, eczema and hay fever among patients with migraine, when compared with patients with non-specific headaches or historical controls.

Waters,[9] in a questionnaire survey of a community population of about 400 adults, found a significantly higher past history of eczema among subjects with migraine, when compared with subjects with non-specific headaches or no headache. In other studies, however, an epidemiological relationship between headache and allergy was not proved.[10,11] Studies on children showed conflicting results. Bille[12] found a positive family history of allergy in 31.5% of the migraine group and 21.9% of controls, and an individual history of allergic disorders in 24.7% of children with migraine and 12.1% of controls. The sample is, however, small and these figures are not statistically significant.

Congdom and Forsythe[13] studied 300 children with migraine (118 with classic migraine and 182 with common migraine) referred by general practitioners or paediatricians. Only in 7% of these children was there a personal history of asthma, hay fever or eczema.

The prevalence of headache and migraine was examined in a study of Mortimer et al,[14] in an unselected sample of atopic children from a general practice population of 1077 3- to 11-year-old children. He found that the prevalence of both headache and migraine was significantly higher in children with atopic disorders compared with those without. Not only was migraine more common in atopic, but atopy was more frequent in migraineurs.

# Foods as precipitating factors of headaches

It is necessary to make a distinction between headaches caused by gastrointestinal problems and those precipitated by foods. Neither form is recognized in the classification of the International Headache Society.[15]

The field of headache precipitated by food is difficult to understand, because one should know: (1) which foods are responsible, (2) the pathogenic mechanisms and (3) how to make a diagnosis. None of these aspects is well known. In various studies with adult patients, specific foods were reported to precipitate headache attacks.

Burr and Merrett[16] identified 15 people who reported headaches caused by foods among 475 subjects who answered a questionnaire; the foods implicated were cheese and chocolate. Paulin et al[17] identified 20 subjects who reported headaches caused by foods; among 568 who were affected by headaches, the most commonly implicated foods were chocolate, cream and cheese. These results were also based on responses to a questionnaire.

Other studies were performed on subjects affected by headaches. In a group of 490 patients affected by migraine and personally interviewed by the authors, Peatfield et al,[18] 19% reported that their headaches could be precipitated by foods – 18% indicated cheese as responsible and 11% citrus fruit. A highly significant majority of the patients were sensitive to more than one food.

In adults, alcohol was reported as a trigger of headache attacks. A sensitivity to alcohol was reported in Paulin's and Peatfield's studies. In Peatfield's study, 29% of the patients reported sensitivity to alcohol, and this was significantly associated with food sensitivity, although several patients were sensitive to alcohol but not to foods. Patients with affected relatives were significantly more likely to report sensitivity to alcohol and chocolate and less likely to report it to cheese and citrus fruit.

More recently, Peatfield[19] carried out another study on 577 patients with headaches, by questioning them about dietary precipitants of their headaches. For migraine patients, he found a statistical association between sensitivity to cheese or chocolate (prevalence of 16.5% in this population) and sensitivity to red wine and beer, but none between diet sensitivity and sensitivity to alcoholic drinks in general (prevalence 18.4%). None of the patients with tension-type headache reported sensitivity to food, and only one of these was sensitive to alcoholic drinks. The author concluded that cheese, chocolate and red wine sensitivity have closely related mechanisms, whereas separate mechanisms play a role in the sensitivity to alcoholic drinks in general (see also Pathogenesis section).

In adult patients with various disturbances, whose belief that they have a food allergy could not be confirmed, a psychiatric disorder may be the basis of their belief.[20]

Epidemiological studies on foods as precipitating factors in childhood migraine are scarce. Bernstein and Del Tredici[21] studied 52 children. A neurologist evaluated each child and a nutritionist did a thorough interview with each child and at least one parent. Patients were instructed on how to complete specially designed food questionnaires whenever they had a headache, recalling all foods consumed 12–24 hours before the onset of the migraine. The patients served as their own controls by filling out the same food questionnaire on non-migraine days. An increased risk of migraine was found on days when processed meat products (containing nitrates), chocolate, cheese and nuts were consumed. The risk varied form 30% (for nuts) to 70% (processed meat). The role of sodium content, food additives and other diet factors (not well specified) was also evaluated and no association with headaches was found.

In a study on children by Dalton and Dalton[22] (mentioned by Peatfield[23]), cheese, chocolate and citrus fruit were found to be more likely to have been consumed on the day of a headache attack.

# Other dietary components as triggers of migraine attacks

## Additives

Additives have been considered specifically associated with headache; they include sodium nitrite (in meat products, 'hot-dog headache'[24]), tartrazine and benzoic acid,[25] very high doses of aspartame[26] and monosodium glutamate ('Chinese restaurant syndrome'[27]). The 'Chinese restaurant syndrome' arose from reports of discomfort experienced after eating in Chinese restaurants; monosodium glutamate was implicated. However, various studies have failed to reveal signs accompanying the abnormal sensations that some individuals experience after the experimental ingestion of monosodium glutamate and, when some common food materials have been used in the same experimental setting, similar symptoms were observed in some people. Furthermore, the role of monosodium glutamate as a trigger of headaches has not been confirmed in double-masked tests. Therefore it seems that the 'Chinese restaurant syndrome' has no validity.[27]

As for monosodium glutamate, the role of the other substances also considered to be provocative agents of migraine attacks may not be specific. These substances seem to provoke attacks inconstantly.

## Hypoglycaemia as trigger of migraine attacks

The International Headache Society[15] recognized the existence of headaches secondary to hypoglycaemia. However, although it is well known that missing a meal can provoke headache, it is almost impossible to distinguish the effects of hypoglycaemia from those of stress linked to fasting. Hockaday[28] found no occurrence of migraine attacks provoked by hypoglycaemia in 14 patients with diabetes who also had migraine.

# Clinical studies on food as a trigger of migraine attacks: elimination diet and challenges

In most studies in which elimination diets were employed, there were various limitations which made any judgement of the effects of the diets difficult. Most studies were performed in adult patients. Medina and Diamond[11] studied the effects on 24 migraineurs of three different diets during an 18-week period. Diet A contained tyramine, exclusive of tyramine-free foodstuff, whereas diet B included tyramine-free foods and excluded those containing tyramine; diet C subjects ate freely. The results of this study showed that daily intake of foods containing high amounts of tyramine, phenylethylamine, dopamine or nitrates did not cause an increase in the severity of migraine. However, some headaches were time related to the intake of alcoholic drinks and chocolate, and less so to citrus, and the latter two foods had been mentioned most often by these patients as precipitants of migraine before the start of the study.

Grant[29] did an open study on 60 migraine patients who completed an elimination diet. When an average of 10 common foods was avoided, there was a dramatic fall in the number of headaches during the following period of observation, which lasted 3 months. Before testing, the patients had been under observation for the previous 3 months. Before the diet, all patients had been advised to avoid the following triggering factors: cheese, chocolate, citrus fruit, alcohol, other people's smoke, hunger and excessive stress. However, there was no favourable response to this avoidance. Thirty-four other patients who had shown a favourable response after following the same advice were excluded from the diet study.

Monro et al[30] investigated food allergy in a group of 47 severely affected migraine patients. Rotation and elimination diets were performed during a 2-year phase; 33 patients completed this phase and 23 of them incriminated a variety of specific foods. At the end of this phase, levels from radioallergosorbent tests (RASTs) confirmed the relevance of the foods that had been found to cause headaches. The author used the RAST values prospectively in 26 patients to predict which food should be eliminated and a response was observed in 23. Ten patients were pre-treated with oral sodium cromoglicate before challenge with the suspected food, and a protection from the symptoms was found. Monro's study received a lot of criticism from other colleagues, who in this report found technical errors inherent in the RAST determination, and felt that several questions were left unanswered.[31,32] In Monro's study, the results are unconvincing because the elimination diet apparently was not done with masking; the temporal relationship of the provocation to the headaches, and also the duration of the favourable response, were not clear and it was not specified whether the diets were done under medical supervision.

In another study by Monro et al,[33] the results of a double-masked study investigating the protection by sodium cromoglicate were reported. Nine patients were given either this drug or a placebo, together with foods previously identified as provocative. Five subjects reported a complete, and three a partial, protection with sodium cromoglicate. Objections to these results are that the size of the study is small and, furthermore, that the symptoms reported were mainly intestinal.

Mansfield et al[34] carried out a study on patients with migraine referred to an allergy–immunology service; 43 patients underwent skin tests to a battery of food allergens. Response to a food was considered positive when the response was greater than that to the negative control (saline). In the 16 patients with a positive response, the corresponding food was eliminated from the diet for 1 month on an open basis – during this period the subjects recorded in a diary their meals and their headache attacks. The 11 subjects who improved by more than a 66% reduction in headache frequency participated in a double-masked study with food and placebo challenge on different days. Five developed a headache attack after food challenges, whereas all the placebo challenges were negative. Among the 27 patients who had all negative skin tests, only two improved when four kinds of food were eliminated from the diet. Much criticism can be raised against these results: the patients were highly selected, the study was open, and the patients were challenged only with foods for which skin tests had been found to be positive.

Moffett et al[35] performed a study on chocolate as a trigger of headache attacks and obtained no definite demonstration of the effect of this food when compared with placebo. Furthermore, when the study was repeated in some of the subjects, results were reproducible only in a few.

Gibb et al[36] carried out a trial with patients who claimed that chocolate was a trigger for their headaches. They were divided into two groups and were respectively fed real and mock chocolate of similar taste, which they were unable to distinguish. A significant proportion of those who ate the authentic chocolate (5 of 12) developed headaches, when compared with those who received placebo (0 of 8); the lag period between ingestion and headache onset was 22 hours. A similar trial,[36] performed with red wine compared with a mixture of vodka of the same alcohol content, showed a significant effect of red wine as a trigger of migraine attacks; the lag period between ingestion and headache onset was approximately 3 hours.

In a recent, provocative, double-masked study by Marcus et al,[38] chocolate was used as the active agent and carob as the placebo: 63 women with headaches (50% migraine, 37.5% tension headache, 12.5% combined migraine and tension-type headache) participated in the study. After 2 weeks following a diet that restricted vasoactive amine-rich foods, each subject underwent double-masked provocative trials with two samples of chocolate and two of carob presented in random order. During the study, the subjects monitored diet and headache with a diary. The results demonstrated that chocolate did not appear to play a significant role when compared with carob in triggering headaches in any headache group; interestingly, these results were independent of subjects' believes about the role of chocolate as a trigger of their headaches.

Challenge studies with phenolic amines have not been reported in migraine patients. Very few studies have been performed with elimination diets in childhood migraine.

Egger et al[39] carried out a large-scale, double-masked trial of an elimination diet on children. Of the 99 children referred to his centre with severe frequent migraine, 88 kept an oligoantigenic diet for 3 or 4 weeks. Some children had begun drug treatment at least 4 weeks before the start of the study. Of the 88 children, 48 were atopic, 41 had behavioural disturbances (mostly hyperkinetic) and 14 had seizures. In 82 cases, there was a favourable response to an open diet, i.e. no headache or only one during the previous 2 weeks; 74 had a relapse when re-exposed to one or more specific foods in an open judgement – 17 had symptoms with only one, but most reacted to several foods (up to 24), from which one was selected for the double-masked phase of the trial. Children responding to placebo in this open phase of the study were eliminated from the following study. Of the 74 children, 40 completed the double-masked phase of the trial. The food was given repeatedly for at least a week and it was considered a positive response if the child developed abdominal pain, distension or behavioural disorders over the next 2–7 days. Of the 40 children, 26 responded with headaches only when challenged, on the double-masked basis, by the previously identified foods; two responded only to placebo, eight to neither and four to both. Patients with epilepsy remained seizure free under this diet after the withdrawal of the antiepileptic drugs. Prick tests were also performed on the patients and no relationship was found between positive tests and responses to diet. This study has various limitations: the challenge was not made under medical supervision and not with all the suspect foods. To be considered a positive response to the challenge, a long interval of time from ingestion of the food and the symptom was accepted; not all subjects developed a headache after the challenge and, furthermore, the patients of this study were not typical children affected by migraine.

Salfield et al[40] carried out an open-controlled study on 39 children with migraine. For the first 8 weeks, families had to record all disturbances in a diary; then, the children were randomly allocated to either a merely high-fibre diet or a high-fibre diet eliminating 'dietary vasoactive amines' such as chocolate, cheese, citrus fruit, cola, strong tea and coffee. The diet was maintained for a further 8-week period, during which the record of meals and headaches was continued. Both groups of children showed a remarkable decrease in headache frequency with no significant difference between the two groups. In both groups, at least half of the children showed at least a 50% improvement. The improvement could be the result of a spontaneous remission of migraine, a placebo effect or a diet with regular meals (some of the children before the study received a poor diet with irregular meals).

MacDonald[41] (cited by Peatfield[23]) reported that, in his study on 52 children with migraine, only 7 were shown to have food intolerance and 13 obtained no benefit from an elimination diet during a 3-week period. The results in the remainders were inconclusive because of the poor compliance, spontaneous remission or unpredictable response on re-challenge.

## Laboratory investigations

Some data about specific IgE were mentioned earlier when discussing studies on challenges. From these data, no clear relationship between IgE increase and dietary migraine emerges.

Other studies showed no elevation of serum IgE in patients with migraine, even when the patients were specifically selected for history of food-precipitated headaches. In 208 adults (74 with dietary migraine, 45 with non-dietary migraine, 29 with cluster headache and 60 controls), Merret et al[42] found no significant differences in serum level of food-related antibodies – IgE and IgG4 – with the exception that cluster headache patients had significantly increased levels of total serum IgE. However, in the author's opinion, this difference was perhaps explained by the high proportion of smokers.

In the study by Mansfield et al,[34] there was a relationship between specific IgE for foods and favourable response from elimination diet. However, as already stated, this study produced a lot of criticism.

High levels of IgE were found in the minority of subjects who were atopic. In the study by Pradalier et al,[43] total IgE, specific IgE against common foods, and prick tests with 11 common food allergens performed on 50 adult consecutive migraine sufferers, rendered abnormal results only in a few of them, almost all of these being atopic.

In a study of 12 children, aged between 5 and 15 years, with a clinical diagnosis of abdominal migraine, Bentley et al[44] found that 10 children became free of, or had diminished symptoms as a result of, a dietary regimen, but in none of the cases were the current serological tests (total or specific IgE) helpful.

In addition, investigations of complement activation in migraine during attacks provided conflicting results.[45–48] The studies examined various aspects such as differences between migraineurs both during or between attacks and controls. Most studies showed values in the normal range.

However, Jerzmanowski and Klimek[49] in a study with migraine patients and controls found that the C3 fraction level was significantly decreased in migraine patients, whereas the C4 fraction level and the total complement activity remained in a normal range. The immunoglobulin levels were also normal, except for the IgA level which was lower in the migraine patients. In the author's opinion, these data suggested an alternative pathway of the complement system.

Thonnard-Neumann and Neckers[50] found significantly fewer circulating T lymphocytes and basophils in migraine patients during attacks. The meaning of these results was not clear. Martelletti[51] studied the course of a cytokine panel (interleukins IL-4 and IL-6, interferon γ [IFN-γ], granulocyte–monocyte colony-stimulating factor [GM-CSF]) in plasma or samples from dietary migraine patients. The data obtained during the challenged migraine attacks were compared with the baseline values. A quantitative analysis of cytokine concentration showed a fall after challenge tests for IL-4 and IL-6 plasma levels and an opposite trend for IFN-γ and GM-CSF levels. In the author's opinion, considering the close link between ILs and other cytokines and the neuromediators of pain such as histamine and 5-hydroxytryptamine (serotonin or 5-HT), this study might show that dietary migraine may be the result of a disturbance of the homoeostasis operating between the immune and the central nervous systems.

## Pathogenesis

The finding that patients with dietary migraine are sensitive to different foods rather than to only one of them has suggested that some common chemical constituent could be responsible.

Tyramine liberates endogenous aromatic amines, e.g. serotonin from blood platelets. For many years, it was thought that tyramine was responsible for the headaches that follow ingestion in some migraineurs. This hypothesis was formulated by Hanington in 1967.[52] The same author later published a series of reports in which he showed that oral tyramine produces headache attacks. Peatfield et al[53] found that intravenous tyramine administration was followed by a slight headache in a number of subjects without a sufficient rise in blood pressure to account for.

Several other authors raised doubts, however, on the specificity of tyramine as a precipitating factor of headaches. Moffett[35] and Ryan[54] found that oral tyramine did not produce headaches more frequently than placebo.

In a double-masked study carried out by Ziegler and Stewart[55] on 80 migraine patients, headaches were precipitated by ingestion of 200 mg tyramine and not placebo in eight individuals. But, while re-testing seven of these patients, the same results were not produced. Placebo produced a severe headache as tyramine and in an even larger number of patients.

Forsythe and Redmond[56] performed two trials of tyramine on children with migraine. In the first trial of 59 children, 12 children developed headaches after taking tyramine: in 10, after taking a placebo and in 4 after ingestion of both tyramine and placebo. In the second trial of 38 children, 5 developed headaches after taking tyramine, 11 after taking a placebo, 4 after taking both tyramine and placebo. The author concluded that tyramine is not an important aetiological factor in childhood migraine.

Kohlenberg[57] tried to evaluate these conflicting results and made a comparison of the methodological differences used in the various studies. He found that the methodological differences among studies preclude direct comparison of the results. However, he found that the tyramine hypothesis appears to have some validity. He also remarked that, in several of the reported studies, the administration of placebo may precipitate a headache in up to 39% of the times in the general migraine population and 7% of the times in a non-

migraine population. Therefore, he recognized the importance of psychological factors as a trigger.

A variety of chemical agents other than tyramine has been considered as triggering factors of headaches, including reserpine[58] and *m*-chlorophenylpiperazine.[59]

It was shown by Sandler et al[60] that red wine is a powerful releaser of serotonin from preloaded platelets. However, this beverage has other chemical properties, which could be important in its role as a trigger of headaches. Phenolic flavonoids have been considered by Sandler et al as plausible candidates; they were found to be inhibitors of phenolsulphotransferase. Without the detoxicating effect of this enzyme, noxious phenols present in the alimentary tract could be in sufficient concentration to provoke a migraine attack.

Very recently, it has been found that red wine strongly inhibits the binding of 5HT to $5HT_1$ receptors, whereas white wine possesses this ability to a much lesser extent – the triggering action of red wine on migraine could be the result of this mechanism.

Contrary to what is commonly believed, chocolate contains little tyramine and phenolic molecules may be much more important. Phenolic amines have been found in other foods such as citrus fruits[61] – considered to be a trigger of migraine attacks.

## Conclusions

The effect of foods as a trigger of headache attacks is very difficult to evaluate. Most of the challenge studies performed have several limitations such as diet done without medical supervision, absence of controlled periods of time without elimination of the implicated foods, small size of patients, selected patients and study performed on an open basis. The results of the challenge studies that claim to demonstrate a relationship between migraine and allergy are unconvincing. From these studies, it appears that, in some individuals, a few foods trigger migraine attacks. However, there is a high variety of confounding variables that should be taken into account: quantity of ingested food, various associations of different foods, timing of ingestion (at lunch or at dinner), presence of other headache triggers, psychological aspects such as appearance of foods and common beliefs of the subjects.

Epidemiological studies do not show a link between migraine and allergy, and dietary factors do not seem to have a major role as provocative agents of migraine attacks. Perhaps their importance is greater when associated with other factors. Contrary to common belief, chocolate does not appear to have a major role in triggering headaches.

However, from many studies it emerges that, in some patients, adults or children, headache attacks can be precipitated by specific foods on some occasions. Laboratory investigations have no role in predicting headaches related to food.

Pathogenic mechanisms are not well understood; they are probably different for various substances or groups of substances. As biologically different foods seem to precipitate attacks in the same individuals, this suggests that the response is chemically mediated rather than immunologically mediated.

On a practical point of view, the following suggestions can be followed. If the history of a patient raises suspicion of dietary factors as a trigger of headache attacks, the patient should avoid ingesting this food for a period of 4 weeks, and should then take it again. If a clear association between ingestion of the specific food and headaches appears, the patient should avoid the suspected food for a long period (ranging from 1 to 2 years). Afterwards, a new challenge should be performed, because some allergies/intolerances disappear as the time goes by. If the personal history does not raise suspicion of dietary headaches, the patient should be warned to pay attention to foods that are possible causative agents of the attacks, whereas other evident triggers should be eliminated.

# References

1. Goldman AS, Anderson DW, Sellers WA, Saperstein A, Kniker WT, Halpern SR, Milk allergy I: oral challenge with milk and isolated milk proteins in allergic children. *Pediatrics* 1963; 32: 425–43.
2. Goldman AS, Sellers WA, Halpern SR, Anderson DW, Furlow TE, Johnson CH, Milk allergy II: skin testing of allergic and normal children with purified milk proteins. *Pediatrics* 1963; 32: 572–9.
3. May CD, Objective clinical and laboratory studies of immediate hypersensitivity reactions to food in asthmatic children. *J Allergy Clin Immunol* 1976; 58: 500–15.
4. Bruijnzeel-Koomen C, Ortolani C, Aas K et al, Adverse reactions to food. *Allergy* 1995; 50: 623–35.
5. Sampson HA, Food allergy. In: Kay AB, ed., *Allergy and Allergic Diseases*. London: Blackwell Science, 1997: 1517–49.
6. Sampson HA, Food allergy. Part 1: Immunopathogenesis and clinical disorders. *J Allergy Clin Immunol* 1999; 103: 717–28.
7. Burks AW, Sampson HA, Double-blind placebo-controlled trial of oral cromolyn in children with atopic dermatitis and documented food hypersensitivity. *J Allergy Clin Immunol* 1988; 81: 417–23.
8. Sampson HA, Food allergy. Part 2: Diagnosis and management. *J Allergy Clin Immunol* 1999; 103: 981–9.
9. Waters WE, Migraine and symptoms in child-

hood: bilious attacks, travel sickness and eczema. *Headache* 1972; **12**: 55–61.

10. Selby G, Lance JW, Observations on 500 cases of migraine and allied vascular headache. *J Neurol Neurosurg Psychiatry* 1960; **23**: 23–32.

11. Medina JL, Diamond S, The role of diet in migraine. *Headache* 1978; **18**: 31–4.

12. Bille B, Migraine in schoolchildren. *Acta Paediatr* 1962; **51**(suppl 136): 1–151.

13. Congdon PJ, Forsythe WI, Migraine in childhood: a study of 300 children. *Dev Med Child Neurol* 1979; **21**: 209–16.

14. Mortimer MJ, Kay J, Gawkrodger DJ, Iaron A, Barker DC, The prevalence of headache and migraine in atopic children: an epidemiological study in general practice. *Headache* 1993; **33**: 427–31.

15. The Headache Classification Committee of the International Headache Society, Classification and diagnostic criteria for headache disorders, cranial neuralgias and final pain. *Cephalalgia* 1988; **8**(suppl 7): 1–96.

16. Burr ML, Merrett TG, Food intolerance: a community survey. *Br J Nutr* 1983; **49**: 217–19.

17. Paulin JM, Waal-Manning HJ, Simpson FO, Knight RG, The prevalence of headache in a small New Zealand town. *Headache* 1985; **25**: 147–51.

18. Peatfield RC, Glover V, Littlewood JM, The prevalence of diet-induced migraine. *Cephalalgia* 1984; **4**: 179–83.

19. Peatfield RC, Relationships between food, wine, and beer-precipitated migrainous headaches. *Headaches* 1995; **35**: 355–7.

20. Pearson DJ, Rix KJB, Bentley SJ, Food allergy: how much in the mind? A clinical and psychiatric study of suspected food hypersensitivity. *Lancet* 1983; **i**: 1259–61.

21. Bernstein AL, Del Tredici AM, Migraine in children – a report of a dietary study. *Headache* 1983; **23**: 142 (abstract).

22. Dalton K, Dalton M, Food intake before migraine attacks in children. *J R Coll GP* 1979; **29**: 662–5.

23. Peatfield RC, Pathophysiology and precipitants of migraine. In: Hockaday JM, ed., *Migraine in Childhood*. London: Butterworths, 1988: 105–21.

24. Henderson WR, Raskin NH, 'Hot-dog' headache: individual susceptibility to nitrite. *Lancet* 1972; **ii**: 1162–3.

25. Hanington E, Migraine. In: Lessof MH, ed., *Clinical Reactions to Food*. Chichester: John Wiley, 1983: 155–80.

26. Johns DR, Migraine provoked by aspartame. *N Engl J Med* 1986; **315**: 456.

27. Kenney RA, The Chinese restaurant syndrome: an anecdote revisited. *Food Chemistry Toxicol* 1986; **24**: 351–4.

28. Hockaday JM, Anomalies of carbohydrate metabolism. In: Pearce J, ed., *Modern Topics in Migraine*. London: William Heinemann Medical, 1975: 124–37.

29. Grant ECG, Food allergies and migraine. *Lancet* 1979; **i**: 966–9.

30. Monro J, Brostoff J, Carini C, Zilkha K, Food allergy in migraine. *Lancet* 1980; **ii**: 1–4.

31. Speight JW, Atkinson P, Food allergy in migraine. *Lancet* 1980; **ii**: 532 (letter).

32. Merrett TG, Gawel MJ, Peatfield RC, Food allergy in migraine. *Lancet* 1980; **ii**: 532 (letter).

33. Monro J, Carini C, Brostoff J, Migraine is a food-allergic disease. *Lancet* 1984; **ii**: 719–21.

34. Mansfield LE, Vaughan TR, Waller SF, Haverly RW, Ting S, Food allergy and adult migraine: double-blind and mediator confirmation of an allergic etiology. *Ann Allergy* 1985; **55**: 126–9.

35. Moffet AM, Swash M, Scott DF, Effect of chocolate in migraine: a double-blind study. *J Neurol Neurosurg Psychiatry* 1974; **37**: 445–8.

36. Gibb CM, Davies PTG, Glover V, Steiner TJ, Clifford Rose F, Sandler M, Chocolate is a migraine-provoking agent. *Cephalalgia* 1991; **11**: 93–5.

37. Littlewood JT, Gibb C, Glover V, Sandler M, Davies PTG, Clifford Rose F, Red wine as a cause of migraine. *Lancet* 1988; **i**: 558–9.

38. Marcus DA, Scharff L, Turk D, Gourley LM, A double-blind provocative study of chocolate as a trigger of headache. *Cephalalgia* 1997; **17**: 855–62.

39. Egger J, Carter CM, Wilson J, Is migraine food allergy? A double-blind controlled trial of oligoantigenic diet treatment. *Lancet* 1983; **ii**: 865–9.

40. Salfield SAW, Wardley BL, Houlsby WT et al, Controlled study of exclusion of dietary vasoactive amines in migraine. *Arch Dis Childh* 1987; **62**: 458–60.

41. MacDonald A, Forsythe WI, Minford AMB, Practical problems associated with the dietary management of migraine. In: Rose FC, ed., *Current Problems in Neurology: 4. Advances in Headache Research*. Proceedings of the Sixth International Migraine Symposium. London: John Libbey, 1987: 113–16.

42. Merret J, Peatfield RC, Rose FC, Merret TG, Food related antibodies in headache patients. *J Neurol Neurosurg Psychiatry* 1983; **46**: 738–42.

43. Pradalier A, Weinman S, Launay JM, Total IgE, specific IgE and prick tests against foods in common migraine – a prospective study. *Cephalalgia* 1983; **3**: 231–4.

44. Bentley D, Katchburian A, Brostoff J, Abdominal migraine and food sensitivity in children. *Clin Allergy* 1984; **14**: 499–500.

45. Lord GDA, Duckworth JW, Complement and immune complex studies in migraine. *Headache* 1978; **18**: 255–60.

46. Sovak M, Kunzel, M, Dalessio DJ, Lang JH, C-1 inhibitor levels in migraineurs and normals. *Headache* 1980; **20**: 132–3.

47. Moore TL, Ryan RE, Pohl DA, Roodman ST, Ryan RE, Immunoglobulin, complement, and immune complex levels during a migraine attack. *Headache* 1980; **20**: 9–12.

48. Visintini D, Trabattoni G, Manzoni GC, Lechi A, Bortone L, Behan PO, Immunological studies in cluster headache and migraine. *Headache* 1986; **26**: 398–402.

49. Jerzmanowski A, Klimek A, Immunoglobulin and complement in migraine. *Cephalalgia* 1983; **3**: 119–23.

50. Thonnard-Neumann E, Necker LM, T-lymphocytes in migraine. *Ann Allergy* 1981; **47**: 325–7.

51. Martelletti P, Stirparo G, Rinaldi C, Frati L, Giacovazzo M, Disruption of the immunopeptidergic network in dietary migraine. *Headache* 1993; **33**: 524–7.

52. Hanington E, Preliminary report on tyramine headache, *BMJ* 1967; **ii**: 550–1.

53. Peatfield R, Littlewood JT, Glover V, Sandler R, Clifford Rose F, Pressor sensitivity to tyramine in patients with headache: relationship to platelet monoamine oxidase and to dietary provocation. *J Neurol Neurosurg Psychiatry* 1983; **46**: 827–31.

54. Ryan RE, A clinical study on tyramine as an aetiological factor in migraine. *Headache* 1974; **14**: 43–8.

55. Ziegler DK, Stewart R, Failure of tyramine to induce migraine. *Neurology* 1977; **27**: 725–6.

56. Forsythe WI, Redmond A, Two controlled trials of tyramine in children with migraine. *Dev Med Child Neurol* 1974; **16**: 794–9.

57. Kohlenberg RJ, Tyramine sensitivity in dietary migraine: a critical review. *Headache* 1982; **22**: 30–4.

58. Curzon G, Barrie M, Wilkinson MIP, Relationship between headache and amine changes after administration of reserpine to migrainous patients. *J Neurol Neurosurg Psychiatry* 1969; **32**: 555–61.

59. Brewerton TD, Murphy DL, Mueller EA, Jimerson DC, Induction of migraine-like headaches by the serotonin agonist *m*-chlorophenyl-piperazine. *Clin Pharmacol Ther* 1988; **43**: 605–9.

60. Sandler M, Li N-Y, Jarret N, Glover V, Dietary migraine: recent progress in the red (and white) wine story. *Cephalalgia* 1995; **15**: 101–3.

61. Perry TL, Hansen S, Hestrin M, Macintyre L, Exogenous urinary amines of plant origin. *Clin Chim Acta* 1965; **11**: 24–34.

# 20

# Medical prophylaxis in childhood migraine
*Raymund Pothmann*

Only very few controlled studies on pharmacological prophylaxis in childhood migraine are available. Many paediatricians have used dihydroergotamine for more than 30 years with no scientific background and uncertain results, especially in German-speaking countries. Given that migraine is one of the most common children's diseases that affects up to 10% of adolescents, evidence-based results of different prophylactic pharmacological regimens are necessary.[1–4]

## Indications

It is commonly accepted that at least two to three migraine attacks per month are necessary for the indication of long-term medical prophylaxis. Other prerequisites are single attacks of high severity or duration with neurological symptoms for more than 48 hours. Otherwise, the relationship between benefit and risk would not be justified. A condition should, in any case, be to document frequency, duration and intensity of migraine attacks for at least 1 month in a diary before the start and over the first 3 months of prophylaxis for treatment control purposes.

## Medical prophylactic regimen

The principles of medical prophylaxis are quite different. For every step in the pathophysiology of migraine, there is another possibility of stabilizing the migraine cascade. No one can say to date why and which pharmacological prophylaxis has a better rationale or predictable result in the single case. Most of the indications are therefore developed on the basis of clinical experience.

The most common substances are explained based on the literature and our own clinical data.

## Calcium antagonists: low-dose acetylsalicylic acid

As a result of the good results with the calcium antagonist flunarizine in adults[5,6] and encouraging experience in children,[7] an additional double-masked controlled study was designed comparing this substance with acetylsalicylic acid (ASA) in low concentrations.[8] ASA is widely used in children, and even studies in adults have shown a certain prophylactic effect in migraine.[9]

Thirty children aged between 7 and 17 years who had at least two migraine attacks/month for more than 1 year were studied. Most of them had migraine without aura. The attack frequency seems to be higher and the duration shorter than those in adults. Age, body measurements and sex did not differ in the two treatment groups (t-test: $p < 0.05$).

After clinical exclusion of symptomatic headaches, data were gathered for 4 weeks by means of a migraine diary. Flunarizine or ASA was administered in a double-masked design over 3 months. Dosage was given once in the evening: 100–200 mg ASA (thromboxane A – inhibiting doses of approximately 2–5 mg/kg) or 5–10 mg flunarizine depending on body weight; the deciding weight was 40 kg.

Documented attack frequency, intensity and duration of migraine, drug intake and side effects were determined at monthly intervals. The final results showed no differences between the different therapeutic approaches: a significant comparable reduction of migraine attack frequency occurred in both treatment groups (Fig. 20.1).

The initial frequency of seven to eight attacks was reduced after 3 months of prophylaxis to one to two attacks/month. In the overall clinical rating, including frequency,

intensity and accompanying symptoms, 73.3% of the ASA patients and 71.4% of the flunarizine patients improved by more than 50% or even completely (Fig. 20.2).

Minor side effects were registered in both groups without any significant difference: ASA was associated with abdominal discomfort of short duration, and flunarizine sometimes with periods of daytime tiredness. Only one patient was excluded as a result of general noncompliance.

For the first time, the effectiveness of migraine prophylaxis with flunarizine and low-dose ASA in middle European children has been shown under controlled conditions. The value of both substances seems to be greater than in adults,[5,6] especially with ASA.[9] The two drugs possibly have the prophylactic potency to prevent in particular the accumulating ischaemic brain damage of repeated migraine attacks with aura, which could occur during the later decades of life.[10] The study has confirmed the results of Sorge and Marano

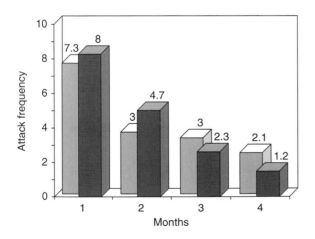

**Figure 20.1**
*Improvement of Migraine attacks under low-dose ASA (▨) or calcium antagonist flunarizine (▩).[8]*

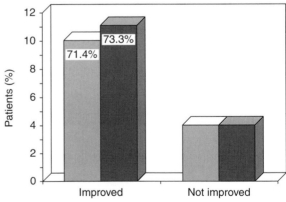

**Figure 20.2**
*Clinical improvement under migraine prophylaxis with low-dose ASA (▨) or the calcium antagonist flunarizine (▩).*

using flunarizine in childhood migraine.[7]

In cases of insufficient response to the first drug, the second should be tried. The long-term prognosis after 6–12 months was mostly excellent in the improving patients.

## Dihydroergotamine

Dihydroergotamine (DHE) is one of the drugs prescribed most often in middle European countries for childhood migraine prophylaxis. Until now controlled studies showing clinical improvement in children are lacking. Our purpose was to find out whether the widespread use of dihydroergotamine is justified under placebo-controlled conditions (see Figs 20.3–20.6).

Therefore 36 children aged between 6 and 14 years were investigated. After a run-in period of 4 weeks documented by diary, DHE was administered as drops over 3 months. The dosage was 1.5 mg twice daily for children with a body weight of 20–39 kg, and 2 mg

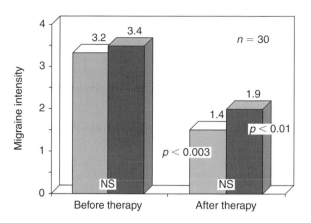

**Figure 20.4**
*Influence of the prophylaxis of dihydroergotamine (▨) drops on the intensity of migraine attacks. (■) Placbo. NS, not significant*

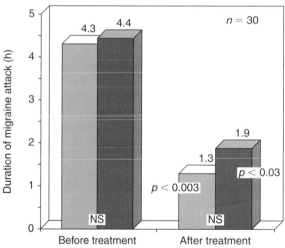

**Figure 20.5**
*Influence of dihydroergotamine and placebo drops on the duration of the migraine attack. (DHE ▨, Placebo ■)*

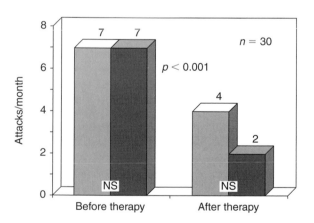

**Figure 20.3**
*Effect of prophylaxis with dihydroergotamine (▨) drops on migraine frequency. (■) Placebo. NS, not significant.*

twice daily for those over 40 kg. The clinical course was documented in a diary following duration and frequency. If the improvement was insufficient during the first month, the dosage was increased to 1.5 vs 2 mg three times daily. After treatment, the children were followed for 1 month.

No statistical difference was found between placebo and DHE with regard to improvement of duration or frequency of migraine attacks. Both DHE and placebo showed the same effect. No side effects were observed.

## Conclusion

Dihydroergotamine drops in the dosage used are of no value for migraine prophylaxis in children. A matter for further research would be whether a higher dosage or another form, such as tablets, is more effective.

## Serotonin antagonists

Serotonin antagonism has been a well-established principle of migraine prophylaxis in Anglo-American countries over the last decades. Pizotifen (Sanomigran) was the most common drug in adult migraineurs. In 1986, a placebo-controlled study in children did not reveal significant improvement for the active substance.[11] A more recent report showed more convincing results.[12] In addition, side effects such as tiredness and raised appetite/weight gain are limitations for primary and broad-based use. The same drug is used in Germany under another name as an appetizer.

## β Blocker

The blockade of sympathetic β receptors is the pharmacological approach of choice in adult migraine. The underlying action of a few types of β blockers such as propranolol and metoprolol, which probably penetrate the brain, is

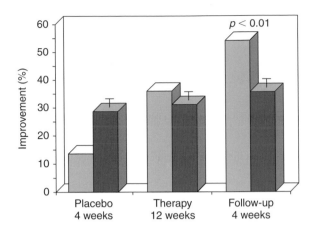

**Figure 20.6**
*Development of headache-free days during prophylaxis with metoprolol ( ) and dihydroergotamine ( ).[1]*

the inhibition of the noradrenaline (norepinephrine) effect of stress and fear. Propranolol was introduced as the first substance in the treatment of childhood migraine. In a double-masked study, Ludvigsson[13] showed significant improvement using propranolol compared with placebo. In comparison to self-hypnosis, however, propranolol was inferior in childhood migraine.[14] The specific β$_1$ blocker metoprolol has proved superior to propranolol in adult migraine.[15]

In our own double-masked study, its value for children was investigated vs placebo and DHE capsules. The dosage for both drugs was 1–1.5 mg/kg body weight once in the evening, with the duration of treatment 3–6 months. During the pre-study period, about 10% of the as yet untreated children were excluded from the study because of the spontaneous remission of their migraine. The results in 24 children revealed a significant advantage for metoprolol in migraineurs. Children with

| Substance | Dosage | Side effects |
|---|---|---|
| Metoprolol | 1–2 mg/kg | Nausea, vomiting |
| Propranolol | Single evening dose | Hypotonia, |
|  | 1 week: ½ dose | bradycardia, bronchial asthma, |
|  |  | diabetes mellitus, heart diseases |
| Flunarizine | 5 mg > 20 kg | Tiredness, increased |
|  | 10 mg > 40 kg | appetite |
|  | Single evening dose |  |
|  | After 2 weeks: every 2 days |  |
| Acetylsalicylic acid | 2(–5) mg/kg | Abdominal pain |
|  | single evening dose | *Contraindications:* |
|  |  | bronchial asthma, influenza, |
|  |  | chickenpox |
| Drugs with possible therapeutic action (second choice) | | |
| Dihydroergotamine | 2 × 1.5 mg: 20–40 kg | Dry mouth, |
|  | 2 × 2 mg: >40 kg | tachycardia, paraesthesia |
| Pizotifen | 20–40 kg: 0.5–1 mg | Weight gain, |
|  | >40 kg: 1 mg | tiredness |
|  | In the evening | *Contraindication:* |
|  |  | glaucoma |

**Table 20.1**
*Pharmacological prophylaxis of childhood migraine*

mixed headache, including autonomic (possibly circulatory) symptoms such as vertigo, obtained a comparable benefit when treated with DHE tablets. Clinically relevant side effects could not yet be registered.[16,17]

## Conclusion

The few drugs that could be recommended for medical prophylaxis of childhood migraine are: a retarded form of the β-blocking substance metoprolol given as a single dose in the evening. In cases of therapeutic resistance, the relatively best studied substance, flunarizine, should be given every second day in order to reduce side effects such as tiredness and weight gain.

Limited long-term results of drug regimens should encourage paediatricians to focus on a combination of pharmacological and behavioural treatment strategies. Only a few studies are available comparing directly relaxation strategies with medical treatment in childhood migraine.[14,18] Further research should focus especially on a therapeutic strategy combining the propagated short improvement of drugs and the late-onset effect of a behavioural treatment.

# References

1. Bille B, Migraine in schoolchildren. *Acta Paediatr Scand Suppl* 1962; **51**(136): 1–151.
2. Bille B, Migraine in childhood and its prognosis. *Cephalalgia* 1981; **1**: 71–5.
3. Oster J, Recurrent abdominal pain, headache and limb pains in children and adolescents. *Pediatrics* 1972; **50**: 429–36.
4. Sillanpää M, Changes in the prevalence of migraine and other headaches during the first seven school years. *Headache* 1983; **23**: 15.
5. Diamond S, Schenbaum H, Flunarizine, a calcium channel blocker, in the prophylactic treatment of migraine. *Headache* 1983; **23**: 38–42.
6. Peroutka St J, Bongart SB, Allen BS, Relative potency and selectivity of calcium antagonists used in the treatment of migraine. *Headache* 1984; **24**: 55–8.
7. Sorge F, Marano E, Flunarizine vs. placebo in childhood migraine. A double blind study. *Cephalalgia* 1985; **5**(suppl 2): 145–8.
8. Pothmann R, Migräneprophylaxe mit Flunarizin und Azetylsalizylsäure. Eine Doppelblindstudie. *Monatsschr Kinderheilkd* 1987; **135**: 646–9.
9. Grotemeyer KH, Viand R, Beykirch K, Klinische und laborchemische Ergebnisse zur Prophylaxe der Migräne mit Azetylsalizylsäure. *Med Welt* 1984; **23**: 762–7.
10. Olesen J, Larsen B, Lauritzen M, Focal hyperemia followed by spreading oligemia and impaired activation of rCBF in classic migraine. *Ann Neurol* 1981; **9**: 344–52.
11. Gillies D, Sills M, Forsythe I, Pizotifen (Sanomigran) in childhood migraine. A double-blind controlled trial. *Eur Neurol* 1986; **25**: 132–5.
12. Symon DNK, Russel G, Continued benefit after stopping pizotifen therapy in childhood migraine. *Cephalalgia* 1989; **9**(suppl 10): 422–3.
13. Ludvigsson J, Propranolol in treatment of migraine in children. *Lancet* 1973; **ii**: 799.
14. Olness K, MacDonald JT, Uden L, Comparison of self-hypnosis and propranolol in the treatment of juvenile classic migraine. *Pediatrics* 1987; **79**: 593–7.
15. Scholz E, Gerber WD, Diener HC, Langohr HD, Reinecke M, Dihydroergotamine vs flunarizine vs nifedipine vs metropolol vs propranolol: A comparative study based on time series analysis. In: Rose FC, ed., *Current Problems in Neurology 4 – Advances in Headache Research*. London: John Libbey, 1987: 139–46.
16. Pothmann R, Auch Kinder haben Migräne. Was ist zu tun? In: Dominiak P, Hjalmarson A, Kendall MJ et al. *Betablocker im Mittelpunkt der Forschung*. Heidelberg: Springer, 1998: 281–8.
17. Pothmann R, *Kopfschmerz im Kindesalter. Betablocker*. Stuttgart: Hippokrates, 1999: 99–102.
18. Headache Classification Committee of the International Headache Society. Classification and diagnostic criteria for headache disorders, cranial neuralgias and facial pain. *Cephalgia* 1988; **8**(7): 1–93.

# V

## Cluster headache

# 21

# Cluster headache

*Licia Grazzi, Massimo Leone, Domenico D'Amico, Susanna Usai,
Gennaro Bussone*

Cluster headache is the most severe form of essential head pain. In the episodic form of the condition, the pain crises occur within cluster periods lasting weeks or months, separated by periods of spontaneous remission lasting months or years. In about 10% of patients the headaches recur chronically and there is no remission. The crises are unilateral, located orbitally or periorbitally,[1] last 15–180 min, and recur with a frequency that varies from every other day to eight times a day. The severity of the pain is such that the patient becomes very anxious and cannot remain still. Homolateral autonomic symptoms necessarily accompany the crises and include one or more of the following: lacrimation, conjunctival injection, nasal congestion, rhinorrhoea, miosis, ptosis, facial sweating and palpebral oedema. The prevalence is around 0.1–0.4%, but men are more frequently affected than women in the ratio of about 5–6 : 1.[2] Onset is generally from 18 to 40 years. The headaches typically recur at fixed times of the day or night, whereas the cluster periods often begin in the spring or autumn when the rates of change of the amount of daylight are high.[3] There is evidence of a genetic component in some cases[4] and these are not as rare as was once thought.[5,6]

## Classification

The term 'cluster headache' was introduced by Kunkle in 1952.[7] Before that, numerous terms were used to refer to the condition: ciliary neuralgia, Horton's headache, Vidian's neuralgia and others.

Cluster headache is placed in group 3 of the International Headache Society (IHS) classification[1] together with chronic paroxysmal migraine (Table 21.1). Episodic and chronic cluster headache are the two main forms recognized. The episodic form is by far the most common (80–90% of cluster headache

| Cluster headache and chronic paroxysmal migraine | |
|---|---|
| 3.1 | Cluster headache |
| 3.1.1 | Cluster headache of undetermined periodicity |
| 3.1.2 | Episodic cluster headache |
| 3.1.3 | Chronic cluster headache |
| 3.1.3.1 | Chronic at onset |
| 3.1.3.2 | Evolves form episodic form |
| 3.2 | Chronic paroxysmal migraine |
| 3.3 | Cluster-like headache not fulfilling the above |

**Table 21.1**
*Category 3 of the IHS headache classification.*

diagnoses) and is characterized by cluster periods during which the headaches occur, separated by headache-free remission periods. A cluster period may last from 7 days to a year. Outside cluster periods, patients are generally free of cluster headaches, although sometimes there may be isolated attacks or brief periods of attacks (mini-bouts).

In the chronic form of cluster headache there is no remission and the condition is diagnosed after a year without remission or if the remission lasts less than 14 days. Chronic cluster headache may onset as such or develop from the episodic form.

There are also atypical forms of cluster headache placed in category 3.3 of the IHS classification; these are distinguished from cluster headache in the strictest sense by their differing clinical course or symptomatology (Table 21.1).

## Epidemiology

In marked contrast to migraine and tension-type headache, clinical experience is that cluster headache is uncommon. The incidence of all forms of cluster headache is around 0.4–0.8%.[8,9] However, the incidence of cluster headache remains controversial and even recent studies vary considerably in their incidence estimates, although this may result partly from differences in estimation methods rather than real differences between populations. Two studies have been published that study the general population. Ekbom et al[10] found a prevalence of 92 per 100 000 in the Swedish population and D'Alessandro et al[2] reported a prevalence of 69 per 100 000 in their San Marino survey. It must be noted that many cluster headache cases do not come to the attention of doctors so that, in any case,

incidence figures are likely to be underestimated. Furthermore, although in its usual presentation cluster headache is unmistakable, atypical forms may be confused with migraine and vice versa. Cluster headache is the only form of primary headache that shows a male preponderance. The male : female ratio is about 5 : 1, although the difference between the sexes seems to decrease progressively in the last decades of life.[11]

## Current status of genetic discoveries

Although cluster headache is not usually considered to be inherited, recent studies have shown that a positive family history for the condition is fairly common. In 1182 probands analysed, 47 first-degree relatives had cluster headache. As a result of the rarity of the condition[12] and its male predominance (4–5 : 1), it is likely that this relatively frequent familial occurrence is indicative of an inherited predisposition to the disease.

A genetic epidemiological study carried out in Denmark on 350 cluster headache patients found that their first-degree relatives had a significantly increased risk for the disease, amounting to 14 times that of the general population, after standardization for age and sex.[12]

A study on 330 mainly white probands in the USA found that the risk of cluster headache in first-degree relatives was 46 times that of the general population after standardization for sex, although the diagnosis in these relatives was not confirmed by interview.[12] The significantly increased risk of cluster headache among family members of cluster headache patients suggests an important genetic component to the disease.

Five pairs of monozygotic twins have been reported with cluster headache, again pointing to genetic factors in the disease.

## Possible mode of inheritance

A sporadic model for cluster headache emerged from a complex segregation analysis, even though an autosomal dominant gene may play a role in some families with cluster headache.[13] A Japanese man with cluster headache was found to have a point mutation in the mitochondrial leucine-tRNA at nucleotide pair 3243.[14] There was no family history of Mitochrodrial myopathy, Encephalopathy, Lactic Acidosis Strokelike episodes (MELAS) or cluster headache. This mutation had not been detected in Italian cluster headache sufferers, and so it cannot have a role in the aetiology of the disease in Italy.[15]

Multiple mitochondrial DNA deletions have been found in another Japanese man with cluster headache; however, at least two associations between deletion and cluster headache are necessary to hypothesize a causal relationship.[16]

## Clinical presentation

The clinical presentation of cluster headache is so distinctive that it may be diagnosed with confidence from the clinical examination and history (Table 21.2). The clinical characteristics of the chronic form are closely similar to those of the episodic form, although the latter tends to have a later age at onset. Males also seem to predominate among chronic cluster headache sufferers, although not in all studies.[8,11]

There are usually between one and five headaches per day during the cluster period, according to Ekbom et al,[17] but the IHS[1] give the range as from one every other day to up to eight per day. Each attack lasts 15–180 min. Attacks lasting longer than 180 min are not considered to be cluster headaches by the IHS.[1] Typically the attacks occur at fixed times of the day or night, more often at night.

The pain is severe and localized unilaterally in the orbital and periorbital regions, sometimes spreading to the brow, temporal region, jaw and ear and, more rarely, to the neck and shoulder. Attacks often begin with a vague sense of unease; the pain then develops and increases rapidly in intensity to become extremely severe. A defining characteristic of cluster headache attacks is that they are accompanied by homolateral symptoms of autonomic activation. Lacrimation and conjunctival injection are the most common symptoms; ptosis and miosis (Horner's syndrome) are also frequent and may persist between headaches in long-term sufferers. Homolateral rhinorrhoea during an attack is reported by many patients. Increased brow sweating, particularly during severe attacks, is seen in a minority of patients; there may also be changes in heart rate, with an increased rate at the beginning of the headache and a reduced one at the end. Occasionally, there are labile increases in diastolic and systolic pressure. Nausea is not uncommon but vomiting is rare. Some patients also experience photophobia and phonophobia.

Behaviour during a cluster headache is characteristic, although it varies with headache severity. Patients generally seek solitude and always become agitated, constantly changing position in an attempt to diminish the pain.

Cluster periods generally last 1–2 months,

---

**3.1 Cluster headache**

*Previously used terms:* erythroprosopalgia of Bing, ciliary or migrainous neuralgia (Harris), erythromelalgia of the head, Horton's headache, histaminic cephalalgia, petrosal neuralgia (Gardner), sphenopalatine, Vidian and Sluder's neuralgia, hemicrania periodica neuralgiformis.

*Description:* attacks of severe strictly unilateral pain orbitally, supraorbitally and/or temporally, lasting 15–180 min and occurring from once every other day to eight times a day. Are associated with one or more of the following: conjunctival injection, lacrimation, nasal congestion, rhinorrhoea, forehead and facial sweating, miosis, ptosis, eyelid oedema. Attacks occur in series lasting for weeks or months (so-called cluster periods) separated by remission periods usually lasting months or years. About 10% of patients have chronic symptoms.

*Diagnostic criteria:*

A. At least five attacks fulfilling B-D.
B. Severe unilateral orbital, supraorbital and/or temporal pain lasting 15–180 min untreated.
C. Headache is associated with at least one of the following signs which have to be present on the pain side:
   1. Conjunctival injection
   2. Lacrimation
   3. Nasal congestion
   4. Rhinorrhoea
   5. Forehead and facial sweating
   6. Miosis
   7. Ptosis
   8. Eyelid oedema
D. Frequency of attacks: from one every other day to eight per day.
E. At least one of the following:
   1. History, physical and neurological examinations do not suggest one of the disorders listed in groups 5–11.
   2. History and/or physical and/or neurological examinations do suggest such disorder, but it is ruled out by appropriate investigations.
   3. Such disorder is present, but cluster headache does not occur for the first time in close temporal relation to the disorder.

**Table 21.2**
*Cluster headache in the classification of the International Headache Society.*

but as noted this may vary from a few days to a year.[17-19] Most patients have one or two cluster periods a year, which occur typically when the seasons change. Remission periods generally last from 6 months to several years, with considerable variation between patients.

# Neurophysiological approach to diagnosis

Neurophysiological methods, especially in combination with drugs that modify electro-physiological responses, are useful for investigating the function of the trigeminovascular system. Such non-invasive methods may be expected to provide new information on both the central and peripheral abnormalities that characterize diseases such as cluster headache.

Various neurophysiological methods have been used to assess the processing of pain information at the spinal and trigeminal levels in cluster headache.

## The electrically elicited corneal reflex

A study on 15 cluster phase and 6 remission phase cluster headache patients found a significant reduction in the pain threshold, more evident on the pain side, during the cluster period. This finding was interpreted as indicating sensitization of the pars caudalis of the trigeminal nucleus, perhaps associated with reduced anti-nociceptive control as a result of disturbed limbic control.[20]

## Blink reflex

Taken together, the results of blink reflex studies in cluster headache patients indicate that the neurons of the spinal trigeminal complex are hyperexcitable on the pain side.[21] This may be the result of irritation or inflammation of the ophthalmic division of the trigeminal nerve in the region of the cavernous sinus, which has been proposed as the underlying cause of cluster headache.[22] Perhaps central opioid activity is reduced in the cluster period, contributing to lack of activation of the reticular nuclei.

The finding of increased latency of the P300 wave in cluster periods is a further indication of a possible perturbation in the processing of cognitive information.[23]

## R III reflex

It has been reported that pain threshold and reflexes (R III reflex) are lowered on the pain side in patients with episodic cluster headache in the active phase of their illness.[24] This is consonant with the view that a dysfunction of the descending inhibitory system can affect responses to noxious stimuli at the trigeminal and spinal levels.

## Pupillary response

Studies of the pupillary response (the ciliospinal reflex) to painful stimuli applied to the cornea and sural nerve found an impaired mydriatic response on both sides, even in remission patients. This suggests a dysfunction in the integrative neural system controlling autonomic activity and pain perception. The dysfunction could be the result of permanent sympathetic hypofunction.[25]

## Cardiovascular reflex

Investigations of the autonomic nervous system function in cluster headache, e.g. by cardiovascular reflex and Holter electrocardiography, suggest that the system is disturbed and in particular that the relationship between the sympathetic and parasympathetic arms is upset.[26,27]

# Pathophysiology
## The trigeminofacial reflex

A satisfactory hypothesis of the pathophysiology of cluster headache must explain the unilaterality of the pain, the accompanying autonomic disturbances, the predominance in men, and above all the periodic recurrence of the headaches and the cluster periods (in the episodic form). It has been proposed that the trigeminovascular system, which consists of the branches of the fifth cranial nerve innervating the cranial blood vessels and meninges, becomes activated during cluster headache.[28] Stimulation of these nerves can cause the release of neuropeptides, including calcitonin gene-related peptide (CGRP), both peripherally – in the blood vessel and meninges (antidromic conduction) – and centrally – in the pars caudalis of the trigeminal ganglion (orthodromic conduction). These neuropeptides may give rise to pain signals originating in the blood vessels, whereas centrally they are likely to facilitate the passage of pain signals. Increased CGRP and vasoactive intestinal polypeptide (VIP) levels have been reported in the homolateral external jugular vein during a cluster headache attack.[29,30] The increased VIP levels also suggest that the seventh cranial nerve parasympathetic fibres, originating from the superior salivatory nucleus of the pons, could be activated. Plausibly, this would be secondary to activation of the trigeminofacial reflex,[31] itself a consequence of trigeminovascular activation. It is interesting that increased CGRP levels have also been observed during migraine, but VIP was unchanged.[32]

## Involvement of the hypothalamus

This account ignores the problem of how the trigeminovascular system might become activated in cluster headache. It seems that it is not the result of a peripheral derangement, except perhaps in rare cases of cluster headache-like symptomatic headaches. Neuroendocrine findings provide fairly persuasive evidence that the hypothalamus may be involved in trigeminal system activation in cluster headache.[33]

Before reviewing this evidence, we emphasize that the periodic character of the condition suggests a connection with the biological pacemaker, known to be located in the hypothalamus, although the selective accumulation in the hypothalamus of lithium[34] – an effective prophylactic for cluster headache[35] – also implicates this structure. Lithium is also effective in manic depressive illness – a periodic and often seasonally recurring condition – whereas verapamil is effective in both cluster headache[36] and manic depression.[37]

One of the best-known functions of the hypothalamus is to modulate the neuroendocrine system by producing and secreting releasing and inhibiting factors that control the rhythmic and phasic release of the adenohypophyseal hormones. Neurohormone levels have been investigated in patients with cluster headache, as a means of obtaining information on the functional state of the hypothalamus.[33]

### Melatonin
Melatonin is the principal product of the pineal gland.[38] Plasma levels of this hormone are low during the day when retinal photoreceptors are hyperpolarized, and high at night when retinal signals reach the suprachiasmatic nuclei of the hypothalamus. These signals pass on to sympathetic centres in the thoracic spine, the cervical plexus and the pericarotid plexus; they terminate in the pineal gland where they stimulate the release of noradrenaline (norepinephrine). Noradrenaline activates arylalkylamine *N*-acetyltransferase and hydroxyindol-*O*-methyltransferase, to catalyse the transformation of serotonin to melatonin[38]. In this way light levels influence the circadian rhythm of melatonin, which is also influenced by other environmental factors; however, the rhythm itself is generated

endogenously within the suprachiasmatic nucleus.

In cluster headache patients in cluster period, 24-hour plasma levels of melatonin are reduced, and plasma peaks are shifted (anticipated or delayed).[39–43] Excretion of the principal metabolite of melatonin (6-sulphatoxymelatonin) is also reduced over 24 hours, and the reduction does not correlate with illness duration, or duration of cluster period in course, time since last headache or frequency of headaches within the cluster period.[44] Cluster headache patients in remission excrete less 6-sulphatoxymelatonin than normal, and in some of these patients the rhythm of excretion is completely deranged.[44] A similar derangement could be present in the cluster period, but is masked by the considerable overall reduction in melatonin levels.[43] These alterations point to a hypothalamic derangement in cluster headache that is independent of the pain.

### The hypothalamo-hypophyseal–adrenal axis

Circulating hormones under direct control of the hypothalamic releasing and inhibiting factors are also altered in cluster headache patients.[33] Specific anomalies of the hypothalamus–hypophysis–adrenal (HPA) axis are increased basal plasma cortisol,[40,42,45,46] as well as reduced cortisol and ACTH responses to insulin-induced hypoglycaemia and challenge with ovine corticotrophin-releasing hormone.[46,47] These anomalies are present during the cluster period and remission, but are not found in other painful conditions. A similar pattern of responses has been reported in patients in multisystem atrophy.[48]

Serotonin (5HT) is an important modulator of HPA activity, although other peptide and classic neurotransmitters are involved. Hypo-thalamic serotonin is concerned with the regulation of biological rhythms, and it has been suggested that lithium may act in cluster headache by increasing serotonin levels in the hypothalamus. Therefore, the possibility that the serotoninergic system is involved in the genesis of the altered HPA axis responses in cluster headache was investigated. m-Chlorophenylpiperazine (mCPP) was administered to cluster headache patients; mCPP causes an increase in serum cortisol and prolactin (PRL) by stimulating serotonin $5HT_{2C/1A}$ receptors and is also able to trigger migraine-like headaches.[49] We found a reduced cortisol response to mCPP both in the cluster period[50] and in remission,[51] as well as no PRL increase during remission.[51] The reduced cortisol response to mCPP seems to be specific to cluster headache because it is not observed in other painful conditions, such as migraine and low back pain.[52] Plausibly, downregulation of the $5HT_{2C}$ receptors in the paraventricular nucleus of the hypothalamus can explain the reduced hormonal responses to mCPP in cluster headache patients, because stimulation of these receptors normally results release of corticotrophin-releasing factor (CRF). A positron emission tomography (PET) study on cluster headache patients during a headache showed that the hypothalamus is activated on the side homolateral to the pain,[53] and the same area has been shown to have an increased neuronal density that is pain and age independent.[54]

In conclusion, the findings reviewed above clearly implicate the hypothalamus in the pathogenesis of cluster headache. However, the exact mechanisms by which this structure triggers both the cluster period and the individual headaches are not understood. Elucidation of the connections between the hypothalamus and the principal nucleus of the trigeminal nerve (in particular the circuit concerned with trigeminofacial reflex), and also the hypothalamic connections to the serotoninergic and noradrenergic brain-stem neuron systems that regulate cranial vascularization and pain modulation, would be expected to shed light on this problem.

## Prognosis and follow-up

Knowledge is sparse about the spontaneous course of cluster headaches.[55] The best prognostic factor derives from a recent investigation of 189 consecutive patients with a disease duration of over 10 years.[56] Based on the temporal course of onset during the year, patients were classified as having either episodic or chronic cluster headache. Episodic patients maintained the episodic form in about 80% of cases, shifted towards the chronic form (secondary chronic) in 12.9% of cases or shifted towards an intermediate pattern ('combined' form) in 6% of cases. Chronic cluster headache was still chronic (primary chronic form) after 10 years or more in 53.1% of cases, whereas it had turned into episodic headache in 32.6% of cases and into a 'combined' form in 14.3% of cases.

Nineteen patients (10%) had not had any attack for the last 3 years. It seems that, in all its forms, cluster headache is a chronic disease lasting in most cases for many years or even for the rest of the patient's life.

However, it is also striking that 'active' cluster headache is seldom seen after the age of 75 years. Episodic cluster headache tends to worsen from year to year, but the opposite pattern may also be experienced. The prognosis of the chronic form appears to be better than was previously thought, changing in many patients into an episodic form.[56,57] Pharmacotherapy (especially lithium) may be a reason for a change from chronic to episodic cluster headache, but it does not otherwise influence the outcome. Late onset, male sex and a history of episodic cluster headache for more than 20 years seem to be related to a negative course.

## Triggering and pain-relieving factors

It is established that alcohol consumption during cluster periods, but not during remission, can trigger a cluster headache. Histamine and glyceryl trinitrate (GTN) are known to be able to induce attacks, and are used to do so for diagnostic purposes.[58–61]

Several procedures have been proposed as useful for alleviating the pain of a cluster headache, but these are mostly anecdotal and have not been studied systematically. Ekbom et al[62] confirmed that compression of the homolateral superficial temporal artery can reduce the pain in spontaneous and GTN-induced crises.

## Diagnosis

Cluster headache is diagnosed by careful and thorough determination of the characteristics and history of the headache. Neurological examination is essential to exclude any underlying cause, but otherwise does not contribute to the diagnosis. The clinical characteristics of cluster headache are:

- unilaterality
- very severe pain
- orbital–periorbital location
- brief duration (maximum 3 hours)

- accompanying autonomic manifestations on the same side as the pain (lacrimation, conjunctival injection, rhinorrhoea, miosis, ptosis and brow sweating)
- strong tendency to occur at the same time of day or night.

Furthermore, during an attack the patient becomes very agitated and restless, continually changing position in an attempt to find relief. Although the autonomic manifestations are important diagnostic clues, they may be absent in certain cases.[63,64]

Computed tomography or magnetic resonance imaging (MRI) is useful only for excluding a symptomatic cluster headache-type

headache. Onset in advanced age, atypical attacks, and association with loss of consciousness, mental confusion or convulsions all mandate for more extensive diagnostic investigations.

## Differential diagnosis

The differential diagnosis is from other craniofacial pain conditions (Table 21.3). Migraine is distinguished from cluster headache by the characteristics of the pain, absence of the homolateral autonomic symptoms that usually accompany cluster headache, and the fact that nausea and vomiting are common in migraine.

| | Chronic paroxysmal hemicrania | Episodic paroxysmal hemicrania | SUNCT* | Hemicrania continua | Hypnic headache | Cluster headache |
|---|---|---|---|---|---|---|
| Female : male ratio | 3 : 1 | 1 : 1 | 1 : 8 | 1.8 : 1 | 1.7 : 1 | 1 : 9 |
| Pain quality | Piercing, throbbing, boring | Piercing, throbbing, boring | Piercing, searing | Basic pain with superimposed throbbing/piercing pain | Throbbing | Piercing, boring |
| Pain severity | Very severe | Very severe | Moderate | Moderate to severe | Moderate | Very severe |
| Site of major pain intensity | Orbit, temple | Orbit, temple | Periorbital | Orbit, temple | Generalized | Orbit, temple |
| Frequency of attacks | 1–40/day | 3–30/day | 1/day-30/h | Variable | 1–3/night | 0–8/day |
| Duration of headache | 2–45 min | 1–30 min | 15–20 seconds | Minutes to days | 15–30 min | 15–180 min |
| Autonomic disturbances | Yes | Yes | Yes | Yes (but less marked than in cluster headache) | No | Yes |
| Attacks triggered by alcohol | Yes | Yes | Yes | No | No | Yes |
| Attacks at night | Yes | Yes | Yes | Yes | Yes | Yes |
| Response to indometacin | Yes | Yes | No | Yes | No | Variable |

**Table 21.3**
*Clinical characteristics of cluster headache variants. *Short lasting unilateral neuralgiform headache with conjunctival injection and tearing.*

Chronic paroxysmal hemicrania (CPH) is considered the female equivalent of cluster headache (F : M, 6 : 1); in this condition the pain attacks are unilateral, last 2–45 min and may recur up to or even exceeding five times a day. Like cluster headache, CPH is characterized by autonomic manifestations; furthermore the attacks are always resolved by indometacin 100–150 mg.

In trigeminal neuralgia, the pain attacks are sudden, last just a few seconds and are localized in the distribution of the fifth cranial nerve. They may be triggered by brushing the teeth, speaking or mastication.

Sinusitis is usually characterized by bilateral continuous pain, associated with purulent nasal secretions.

Glaucoma must be considered in the differential diagnosis of cluster headache. The pain is severe and continuous, sometime bilateral, and is associated with visual loss and increased intraocular pressure.

## Unilateral headache in children

The IHS[1] criteria must be applied with caution in childhood headache, because headache characteristics often differ from those in adults. In general attacks are shorter lasting, less frequently unilateral, and photophobia and phonophobia are present less often, suggesting the need for revision of the IHS diagnostic criteria as they apply to children.

In any case, the unilateral location of pain is not a specific feature of juvenile migraine. The younger the patient, the more alternative diagnoses should be taken into account. Unilateral head pain seems to be more frequent in adolescents than in children, in whom the pain is frequently bilateral, becoming unilateral with increasing age.[65,66] Age-related difficulties in the description of pain location have been implicated in this difference.[67–69] Furthermore, unilateral headache does not exclude episodic tension-type headache. Briefly, in children the item 'location of pain' cannot be considered a specific differential parameter distinguishing migraine from tension-type headache. Conversely, it opens up other diagnostic possibilities.

The unilaterality of pain in children, especially when small, is not a common typical event of migraine forms. If headache is always present unilaterally before a diagnosis of migraine is given, secondary forms must be excluded. Anamnestic data, a careful neurological examination and instrumental examinations are needed.

Particularly in children, cluster headache represents an occasional case of severe unilateral head pain. Although it is rare in childhood, occasional cases have been reported in the literature,[8,70] with a prevalence of 0.09–0.4% for boys – much less common than migraine. Childhood-onset cluster headaches resemble the adult form with regard to the site and type of pain, the predominance in males and the associated symptoms. The most common symptom in childhood is lacrimation on the ipsilateral side and then conjunctival injection.[71] Cluster headache in children is rarely recognized and children have such headaches for years before receiving a correct diagnosis and treatment.[71] Some authors have detected high levels of histamine in the blood during the attacks;[72,73] although treatment with antihistamine drugs has been described as useless in such cases,[74] this treatment can be considered efficacious in cases with clinical evidence of histamine involvement.[75]

Moreover, in the differential diagnosis of

unilateral head pain in childhood, the following forms have to be excluded:

- Chronic paroxysmal hemicrania: CPH was first described in 1973,[76] but few cases have been reported in children.[77] However, many adult patients report onset in childhood.[78] Although the clinical features are similar to those of cluster headache, CPH is totally relieved by indometacin, and is much more (80–90% of the cases) frequent among girls.

- Malignant and benign tumours: headache is a common presenting symptom in children with brain tumours and can mimic migraine as reported in the literature.[79,80] Posterior fossa tumours, more frequent in children than in adults, can cause obstruction of the cerebrospinal fluid with consequent headache; only a minority of these patients had no headache with increased intracranial pressure.[81] Headache is also the most common symptom of colloid cysts of the third ventricle; this is a benign tumour that causes severe headache but rarely death.[82] The location of head pain is variable – any time, unilateral, typically severe and intense and throbbing in quality – and the attacks generally occur only during the day.

In conclusion the younger patient, the more the presence of unilateral head pain should alert the clinician to consider diagnoses other than migraine.

# References

1. Headache Classification Committee of the International Headache Society, Classification and diagnostic criteria for headache disorders, cranial neuralgias and facial pain. *Cephalalgia* 1988; **8**(suppl 7): 1–96.

2. D'Alessandro R, Gamberini G, Benasi G et al, Cluster headache in the Republic of San Marino. *Cephalalgia* 1986; **6**: 159–62.

3. Kudrow L, The cyclic relationship of natural illumination to cluster period frequency. *Cephalalgia* 1987; **7**(suppl 6): 76–7.

4. Russell MB, Andersson PG, Familial occurrence of cluster headache. *J Neurol Neurosurg Psychiatry* 1995; **58**: 341–3.

5. D'Amico D, Leone M, Moschiano F, Bussone G, Familial cluster headache: report of three families. *Headache* 1996; **36**: 41–3.

6. Montagna P, Mochi M, Prologo G et al, Heritability of cluster headache. *Eur J Neurol* 1998; **5**: 343–5.

7. Kunkle EC, Pfeiffer Jr, JB, Willhoit WM, Hamrick Jr, LW, Recurrent brief headache in cluster pattern. *Trans Am Neurol Assoc* 1952; **85**: 75–9.

8. Kudrow L, *Cluster Headache. Mechanism and management.* New York: Oxford University Press, 1980.

9. Nappi G, Manzoni GC, *Guidelines of Headache.* London: John Liberty Eurotext, 1993.

10. Ekbom K, Ahlborg B, Schèle R, Prevalence of migraine and cluster headache in Swedish men of 18. *Headache* 1978; **18**: 9–19.

11. Manzoni GC, Terzano MG, Bono G, Micieli G, Martucci N, Nappi G, Cluster headache: clinical findings in 180 patients. *Cephalalgia* 1981; **3**: 21–30.

12. Russell MB, Current status of genetic discoveries in cluster headache. *Ital J Neurol Sci* 1999; **20**: S7–9.

13. Russell MB, Andersson PG, Thomsen LL, Iselius L, Cluster headache is an autosomal dominantly inherited disorder in some families: a complex segregation analysis. *J Med Genet* 1995; **32**: 954–6.

14. Shimomura T, Kitano A, Marukawa H et al, Point mutation in platelet mitochondrial tRNA (Leu(UUR)) in patient with cluster headache. *Lancet* 1994; **344**: 625.

15. Cortelli P, Zacchini A, Barboni P, Malpassi P, Carelli V, Montagna P, Lack of association between mitochondrial tRNA (Leu(UUR)) point mutation and cluster headache. *Lancet* 1995; 345; 1120–1.

16. Odawara M, Tamaoka A, Mizusawa H, Yamashita K, A case of cluster headache associated with mitochondrial DNA deletions. *Muscle Nerve* 1997; **20**: 394–5.

17. Ekbom K, De Fine Olivarius B, Chronic migrainous neuralgia: diagnostic and therapeutic aspects. *Headache* 1971; **11**: 97–101.

18. Lovshin LL, Clinical caprices of histaminic cephalalgia. *Headache* 1961; **1**: 3–6.

19. Manzoni GC, Micieli G, Granella F, Martignoni E, Farina S, Nappi G, Cluster headache in women: clinical findings and relationship with reproductive life. *Cephalalgia* 1988; **8**: 37–44.

20. Sandrini G, Alfonsi E, Ruiz L et al, Impairment of corneal pain perception in cluster headache. *Pain* 1991; **47**: 299–304.

21. Lozza A, Schoenen J, Delwaide PJ, Inhibition of the blink reflex R2 component after supraorbital and index finger stimulations is reduced in cluster headache: an indication for both segmental and suprasegmental dysfunction? *Pain* 1997; **71**: 81–8.

22. Hardebo JH, Moskowitz MA, Synthesis of cluster headache pathophysiology. In: Olesen J, Tfelt-Hansen P, Welch KMA, eds, *The Headaches*. New York: Raven Press, 1993: 569–76.

23. Evers S, Bauer B, Suhr B, Husstedt I-W, Grotemyer KH, Cognitive processing in primary headache: a study on event-related potentials. *Neurology* 1997; **48**: 108–13.

24. Sandrini G, Proietti Cecchini A, Pucci E, Milanov I, Nappi G, Neurophysiological approach to the study of cluster headache. *Ital J Neurol Sci* 1999; **20**: S31–3.

25. Micieli G, Tassorelli C, Ruiz L, Sandrini G, Nappi G, The trigemino-pupillary response in cluster headache. *Cephalalgia* 1993; **13**: 338–42.

26. Boiardi A, Munari L, Milanesi I, Paggetti C, Lamperti E, Bussone G, Impaired cardiovascular reflexes in cluster headache and migraine patients: evidence for an autonomic dysfunction. *Headache* 1988; **28**: 417–22.

27. Micieli G, Cavallini A, Bosone D et al, Imbalance of heart rate regulation in cluster headache as based on continuous 24 h recordings. *Clin Auton Res* 1993; **3**: 291–8.

28. Moskovitz MA, The trigeminovascular system. In: Olesen J, Tfelt-Hansen P, Welch KMA, eds, *The Headaches*. New York: Raven Press, 1993: 97–104.

29. Goadsby PJ, Edvinsson L, Human in vivo evidence of trigeminovascular activation in cluster headache. Neuropeptide changes and effects of acute attack therapies. *Brain* 1994; **117**: 427–34.

30. Fanciullacci M, Alessandri M, Figini M, Geppetti P, Michelacci S, Increase in plasma calcitonin gene-related peptide from the extracerebral circulation during nitroglycerin-induced cluster headache attack. *Pain* 1995; **60**: 119–23.

31. Goadsby PJ, Lipton R, A review of paroxysmal hemicranias, SUNCT syndrome and other short-lasting headaches with autonomic feature, including new cases. *Brain* 1997; **120**: 193–209.

32. Goadsby PJ, Edvinsson L, Ekman R, Vasoactive peptide release in the extracerebral circulation of humans during migraine headache. *Ann Neurol* 1990; **28**: 183–7.

33. Leone M, Bussone G, A review of hormonal findings in cluster headache. Evidence for hypothalamic involvement. *Cephalalgia* 1993; **13**: 309–17.

34. Ghoshdastidar D, Dutta RN, Poddar MK, In vivo distribution of lithium in plasma and brain. *Indian J Exp Biol* 1989; **11**: 950–4.

35. Bussone G, Leone M, Peccarisi C et al, Double blind comparison of lithium and verapamil in cluster headache prophylaxis. *Headache* 1990; **30**: 411–17.

36. Leone M, D'Amico D, Frediani F et al, Verapamil in the prophylaxis of episodic cluster headache: a double-blind study *vs.* placebo. *Neurology* 2000; **54**: 1382–5.

37. Giannini AJ, Taraszewski R, Loiselle RH, Verapamil and lithium in maintenance therapy of manic patients. *J Clin Pharmacol* 1987; **27**: 980–2.

38. Brezinski A, Melatonin in humans. *N Engl J Med* 1997; **16**: 186–95.

39. Chazot G, Claustrat B, Brun J, Sassolas G, Schott B, A chronobiological study of mela-

tonin, cortisol growth hormone and prolactin secretion in cluster headache. *Cephalalgia* 1984; **4**: 213–20.

40. Waldenlind E, Gustafsson SA, Ekbom K, Wetterberg L, Circadian secretion of cortisol and melatonin in cluster headache during active cluster periods and remission. *J Neurol Neurosurg Psychiatry* 1987; **50**: 207–13.

41. Leone M, Frediani F, D'Amico D et al, Dexamethasone suppression test, melatonin and TRH-test in cluster headache. *Ital J Neurol Sci* 1992; **13**: 227–32.

42. Leone M, Lucini V, D'Amico D et al, Twenty-four hour melatonin and cortisol plasma levels in relation to timing of cluster headache. *Cephalalgia* 1995; **15**: 224–9.

43. Leone M, Bussone G, Melatonin in cluster headache: rationale for use and possible therapeutic potential. *CNS Drugs* 1998; **9**: 7–16.

44. Leone M, Lucini V, D'Amico D et al, Abnormal 24-hour urinary excretory pattern of 6-sulphatoxymelatonin in both phases of cluster headache. *Cephalalgia* 1998; **18**: 664–7.

45. Facchinetti F, Nappi G, Cicoli C et al, Reduced testosterone levels in cluster headache: a stress-related phenomenon? *Cephalalgia* 1986; **6**: 29–34.

46. Leone M, Zappacosta MB, Valentini S, Colangelo AM, Bussone G, The insulin tolerance test and the ovine corticotrophin releasing hormone test in episodic cluster headache. *Cephalalgia* 1991; **11**: 269–74.

47. Leone M, Maltempo C, Gritti A, Bussone G, The insulin tolerance test and the Ovine corticotrophin releasing hormone test in episodic cluster headache II: comparison with low back pain patients. *Cephalalgia* 1994; **14**: 57–64.

48. Polinsky RJ, Braun RT, Lee GK et al, Beta-endorphin, ACTH and catecholamine responses in chronic autonomic failure. *Ann Neurol* 1987; **21**: 573–7.

49. Brewerton TD, Murphy DL, Mueller EA, Jimerson DC, Induction of migrainelike headaches by the serotonin agonist meta-chlorophenylpiperazine. *Clin Pharmacol Ther* 1988; **43**: 605–9.

50. Leone M, Attanasio A, Croci D et al, The *m*-chlorophenylpiperazine test in cluster headache: a study on central serotoninergic activity. *Cephalalgia* 1997; **17**: 666–72.

51. Leone M, Attanasio A, Croci D et al, Neuroendocrinology of cluster headache. *Ital J Neurol Sci* 1999; **2**: S18–20.

52. Leone M, Attanasio A, Croci D et al, Serotonin$_{1A}$ receptor hypersensitivity in migraine is suggested by the *m*-chlorophenylpiperazine test. *NeuroReport* 1998; **9**: 2605–8.

53. May A, Bahra A, Buchel C, Frackowiak RSJ, Goadsby PJ, Hypothalamic activation in cluster headache attacks. *Lancet* 1998; **352**: 275–8.

54. May A, Ashburner J, Buchel C et al, Correlation between structural and functional changes in brain in an idiopathic headache syndrome. *Nature Medicine* 1999; **5**: 836–8.

55. Kudrow L, Natural history of cluster headache – part 1. Outcome of drop-out patients. *Headache* 1982; **22**: 203–6.

56. Manzoni GC, Micieli G, Granella F, Tassorelli C, Zanferrari C, Cavallini A, Cluster headache-course over ten years in 189 patients. *Cephalalgia* 1991; **11**: 169–74.

57. Krabbe A, The prognosis of cluster headache. In: Clifford Rose F, ed., *New Advances in Headache Research 2*. London: Smith Gordon, 1991: 289–91.

58. Drummond PD, Anthony M, Extracranial responses to sublingual nitroglycerin and oxygen inhalation in cluster headache patients. *Headache* 1985; **25**: 70–4.

59. Ekbom K, *Studies on Cluster Headache*. Stockholm: Solna tryckeri, 1970.

60. Horton BT, Histaminic cephalalgia. *JAMA* 1956; **160**: 468–9.

61. Peters GA, Migraine: diagnosis and treatment with emphasis on the migraine tension headache, provocative tests and use of rectal suppositories. *Mayo Clinic Proc* 1953; **28**: 673–86.

62. Ekbom K, Some observation on pain in cluster headache. *Headache* 1975; **14**: 219–25.

63. Ekbom K, Evaluation of clinical criteria for cluster headache with special reference to the classification of the International Headache Society. *Cephalalgia* 1990; **10**: 195–7.

64. Nappi G, Micieli G, Cavallini A, Zanferrari C, Sandrini G, Manzoni GC, Accompanying symptoms of cluster attacks: their relevance to the diagnostic criteria. *Cephalalgia* 1992; **12**: 165–8.

65. Silberstein SD, Twenty questions about headaches in children and adolescents. *Headache* 1990; **30**: 716–24.

66. Prensky AL, Sommer D, Diagnosis and treatment of migraine in children. *Neurology* 1979; **29**: 506–10.

67. Rothner AD, Headache in children: a review. *Headache* 1979; **19**: 156–62.

68. Guidetti V, Bruni O, Cerutti R et al, How and why childhood headache and migraine differ from that of the adults. In: Gallai V, Guidetti V, eds, *Juvenile Headache*. Amsterdam: Excerpta Medica, 1991: 27.

69. Bille B, Migraine in schoolchildren. *Acta Paediatr Scand Suppl* 1962; **51**(136): 1–151.

70. Linett MS, Stewart WF, Migraine headache: epidemiologic perspectives. *Epidemiol Reviews* 1984; **6**: 107–39.

71. Maytal J, Lipton RB, Solomon S, Shinnar S, Childhood onset cluster headache. *Headache* 1992; **32**: 275–9.

72. Anthony M, Lance JW, Histamine and serotonin in cluster headache. *Arch Neurol* 1971; **25**: 225–31.

73. Medina JL, Diamond S, Fareed J, The nature of cluster headache. *Headache* 1979; **19**: 309–22.

74. Russel D, Cluster headache: trial of combined histamine H1 and H2 antagonist treatment. *J Neurol Neurosurg Psychiatry* 1979; **42**: 668–9.

75. Neubauer D, Kuhar M, Ravnik I, Antihistamine responsive cluster headache in a teenage girl. *Headache* 1997; **37**: 296–8.

76. Sjaastad O, Dale I, evidence for a new (?) treatable headache entity. *Headache* 1976; **14**(2): 105–8.

77. Gladstein J, Holden EW, Peralta L, Chronic paroxysmal hemicrania in a child. *Headache* 1994; **34**: 519–20.

78. Sjaastad O, Apfelbaum R, Caskew W et al, Chronic paroxysmal hemicrania (CPH). The clinical manifestations. *Ups J Med Sci* 1980; **31**: 27–35.

79. Edgeworth J, Bullock P, Bailey A, Gallagher A, Crouchman M, Why are brain tumors still being missed? *Arch Dis Child* 1996; **74**: 148–51.

80. Battistella PA, Naccarella C, Soriani S, Perilongo G, Headache and brain tumors: different features versus primary forms in juvenile patients. *Headache Q* 1998; **9**: 245–8.

81. Forsyth PA, Posner JB, Intracranial neoplasm. In: Olesen J, Tfelt-Hansen P, Welch KMA, eds, *The Headaches*. New York: Raven Press, 1993: 705–14.

82. Young WB, Silberstein SD, Paroxysmal headache caused by colloid cyst of the third ventricle: case report and review of the literature. *Headache* 1997; **37**: 15–150.

# VI

## Tension-type headache

# 22

# Tension-type headache
## Liisa Metsähonkala

In adults, tension-type headache represents the most common type of primary headache. Children also have tension-type headaches but astonishingly there are few data on the prevalence, features and prognosis of this headache type in children. Before the classification by the International Headache Society (IHS),[1] several different terms were used for tension-type headache, such as muscle contraction headache, idiopathic headache, tension headache and psychogenic headache. The heterogeneity of the terminology indicates the unknown, and possibly also the heterogeneous aetiology of tension-type headache and the vague limits to other types of primary and secondary headaches. The reasons for the lack of research work on tension-type headache in children could be the difficulty in defining it, and also that it is commonly considered to be less severe and disabling than migraine. However, because a tension-type headache presents a frequent problem in adults and some patients with an episodic tension-type headache become patients with a chronic headache, it would be important to know which factors contribute to the pathogenesis of tension-type headache in children, which factors provoke and sustain the episodes, and which factors contribute to continuation of this disorder into adulthood and to the increasingly chronic nature of this disorder.

## Classification

Before the IHS classification of headaches was published in 1988,[1] there were no universally accepted and strict criteria for tension-type headache. In the definition by the Ad Hoc Committee on Classification of Headache,[2] tension-type headache or muscle contraction headache was described as an 'ache or sensations of tightness, pressure or constriction, widely varied in intensity, frequency and duration, sometimes longlasting, commonly suboccipital and associated with sustained contraction of skeletal muscles in the absence of permanent structural change, usually as a part of the individual's reaction during life stress'.

In the headache classification by the IHS,[1] tension-type headache is defined by its typical characteristics and subdivided into episodic (<180 days per year and <15 days per month) and chronic tension-type headache, and further into tension-type headache associated or unassociated with a disorder of the pericranial muscles. In addition, several possible causative factors are listed, including oromandibular dysfunction, psychosocial stress, anxiety and depression, muscular stress and drug overuse. The pericranial disorder should be detected by manual palpation, a pressure algometer or an increased electromyographic (EMG) level of pericranial muscles at rest or during physiological tests.[1] However, manual palpation seems to be the most specific and sensitive test for pericranial muscular disorders.[3]

In the Tenth Revision of the *International Classification of Diseases and Related Health Problems* (ICD-10), the classification of headaches follows the principles of the IHS's criteria. An additional diagnostic category should be used for persistent somatoform pain disorder (F45.4) or for psychological and behavioural factors (F54), when appropriate, in association to tension-type headache. So, in contrast to migraine, even according to the diagnostic criteria, tension-type headache is considered to be more of a symptom initiated by many different causes, rather than a separate disease or disorder.

The criteria for tension-type headache have not been evaluated in population-based studies in children. It seems that the present criteria apply to children, but it is not known how reproducibly and reliably these criteria define a separate and identifiable entity of headaches in children. In the studies using the IHS criteria for tension-type headache, several children were included in the group of tension-type headache that did not quite fulfil the criteria. The proportion of these children is 26–33% of all patients with tension-type headache in clinic-based studies[4,5] and 4% in a population-based study of 12-year-old children.[6] Nor do all adults totally fulfil the criteria of tension-type headache in population-based studies.[7] In a clinic-based analysis of children, the criteria for tension-type headache seemed to be highly sensitive but non-specific.[5] The most specific criteria for tension-type headache in this study were mild intensity of pain and absence of nausea, and the most sensitive diagnostic criterion for tension-type headache was absence of vomiting.[5] The IHS criteria for tension-type headache will probably be revised and the division into subclasses will be more accurate as research work in this field expands. Certain revisions for childhood tension-type headache, as well as for childhood migraine, may be adequate.

## *Epidemiology*

In adults the life-time prevalence of episodic tension-type headache, according to the IHS criteria, is 40–70%[7–9] and the prevalence of chronic tension-type headache is 2–3%.[7,9,10] Tension-type headache, both episodic and chronic, seems to be more prevalent in females[8,9] and the prevalence decreases in elderly adults,[9] even though these trends are clearer with migraine.[7]

In children, tension-type headache occurs in clinic patients, representing about 35% of patients in specialized headache clinics.[4,5] In clinic-based studies, the proportion of chronic tension-type headache out of all tension-type headache in children is 15–20%.[4,5] Population-based prevalence data on tension-type headache in children is sparse. Some guidelines have provided thorough studies on non-migrainous primary headache. Even when the IHS criteria have been applied, the results of different studies are not comparable. The prevalence of tension-type headache was 0.9% in 5- to 15-year-old-children in the study by Abu-Arefeh and Russell,[11] most probably representing the chronic tension-type headache with a psychogenic background. In the study by Barea et al,[12] the 1-year prevalence of tension-type headache was 73% in 10- to 18-year-old children, with female predominance in the adolescents. Their tension-type headache group also included children with tension-type headache that did not quite fulfil the criteria.

In a recent study from Sweden, the prevalence of tension-type headache fulfilling the IHS criteria was 10% in children aged 7–16 years.[13] This prevalence rate is very similar to the study in Finland, where the prevalence of tension-type headache in 12-year-old children was 12%.[6] In a population-based study on first-born children, the proportion of tension-type headache among all headaches was 36% at the age of 6.[14] In the study by Frankenberg et al,[15] 49.7% of headache was tension-type headache in children in grades 3, 6 and 9.

In 12-year-old children in the Finnish study, there was no sex difference.[6] In the Swedish study by Laurell et al,[13] there was a small predominance of girls in the tension-type headache group in 7- to 16-year-old children. In addition, in the study by Barea et al,[12] adolescent girls had tension-type headache more often than boys. Based on these results and on the data for non-migrainous primary headache, it seems that until adolescence the prevalence of tension-type headache in children does not differ much between girls and boys. The female predominance emerges in adolescence.

One of the problems in defining and evaluating the prevalence of tension-type headache is that one person can have several different types of headache episodes, and he or she may have difficulties in differentiating between the types. The proportion of children with mixed headaches is about 10% according to interviews, but based on headache diary data the number is much higher.[16]

There is no clear association between tension-type headache and social class in either adults or children.[17,18] However, in some studies, overall headache has been associated with lower social stratum of the family in preschool-aged children[19] and in girls.[20] In the clinic-based material of Holden et al,[21] social status was lower in children with chronic daily headache, in comparison to patients with chronic daily headache and migraine. There was a trend for lower education in the parents of children with migraine and children with non-migrainous headache, in comparison to control children with no headache in the study by Metsähonkala et al.[22] Overall headache and tension-type headache have been associated with a higher rate of divorced parents and fewer peer relationships.[18,23,24] In a population-based study on 8- to 9-year-old children, both boys and girls with non-migrainous headache reported stress in school, bullying in school and problems in relation to other children significantly more often than children with no headache. However, these factors were also associated with migraine.[22]

## Clinical features

The typical features of tension-type headache according to the IHS criteria are mild or moderate intensity, a pressing or tightening quality and bilateral pain, the absence of vomiting and nausea, and the absence of photophobia and phonophobia. The pain was described to be occipital in the Ad Hoc Definition of tension-type headache,[2] but is more often frontal or temporal in children. In clinic-based material with an age range of 3–19 years,[5] episodic tension-type headache was unilateral in 22%, non-pulsating in 74%, mild in 83%, and associated with photophobia in 8% and with phonophobia in 12%. The mean duration of episodic tension-type headache was

7.9 ± 15.0 hours. Of those who did not fulfil the criteria for tension-type headache, 30% had a duration of the headache episode of less than 30 min, which indicates the limiting role of the minimum duration limit for tension-type headache. The mean frequency of episodes was 1.5/week. Chronic tension-type headache episodes were longer than the episodic tension-type headache episodes (mean 11.8 ± 17.5 h) and were sometimes associated with nausea. Those who did not quite fulfil the criteria of tension-type headache more frequently had migrainous features in their headache than those who fulfilled the criteria.[5]

In another clinic-based study,[4] participants in the tension-type headache group who did not quite fulfil the criteria had headache episodes that were shorter than 30 min. The most typical duration of tension headache episodes was, however, 30 min to 2 h. The pain was described as pressing or tightening by 74%, pulsating by 16%, piercing by 5% and burning by 1% of their patients. The intensity of the pain was moderate in 49%, mild in 26%, severe in 24% and bilateral in 87% of their participants. Nausea was reported by 24%, photophobia by 30% and phonophobia by 29% of the patients.[4]

Little is known about the changes by age and by sex in the features of tension-type headache. In a clinic-based study, the frequency of the headache episodes, their duration, variability of headache location and frequency of nausea increased with age.[25] In clinic-based material, girls with tension-type headache more often reported mild headaches in comparison to boys.[25]

# Aetiopathogenetic theories

Genetic factors do not seem to be as important for tension-type headache as for migraine. However, there is an increased risk of chronic tension-type headache among first-degree relatives of chronic tension-type headache patients.[26] The aetiology of tension-type headache is most probably multifactorial with a genetic predisposition.

The exact aetiopathogenesis of tension-type headache is not known. Most probably both peripheral and central mechanisms are involved, including pericranial muscular tension, peripheral nociception, and trigeminal tract and supraspinal pain-modulation systems. It has been proposed, especially with the increasingly chronic nature of tension-type headache, that central mechanisms apply.[27]

The previously used expression for tension-type headache – muscle contraction headache – as well as several clinical findings indicate that muscle tension in the pericranial musculature might be of importance in the pathogenesis. The pain in tension-type headache resembles pain from myofascial tissues, being dull, pressing and difficult to localize. Muscle spasm of the pericranial muscles is a clinical finding in many adults and children with tension-type headache. However, there is not a muscular disorder in all patients with tension-type headache and such a disorder does not seem to be an important factor in defining the response to therapy.[28]

The pericranial muscular disorder can be studied by palpation or EMG. Standardized palpation points are used to evaluate the tenderness in pericranial muscles in research work. Furthermore, to increase the reliability of the tenderness evaluation, pressure-controlled palpation equipment has been developed[29] as well as a method of measuring muscle hardness.[30] Increased tenderness in the pericranial muscles, on manual palpation, is found in adults with episodic and even more often in those with chronic tension-type headache.[31–35] Tenderness is also found in several patients with migraine and especially during a migraine attack.[32,34,35] Tenderness of the pericranial muscles seems to be influenced by the recent occurrence of the headache episode.[34] As the tenderness of muscles outlasts the headache, it cannot be the only source of pain in tension-type headache.[32]

Normal as well as increased activity in pericranial muscle EMG has been found in the resting state in patients with tension-type headache.[36] Increased amplitudes of EMG have been found, particularly in patients with chronic tension-type headache.[28,37] Decreased activation was noticed during maximal voluntary activation in patients with chronic headache and those with current headache.[37,38] These findings could support the pain adaptation hypotheses; changes in the motor function of the muscles aim to protect the tissue from further damage.[27]

There is some evidence for an association of tension-type headache with altered perception of pain. The children with headache are more prone to other types of pain and to other somatic symptoms.[23,24] Thermal pain detection and thermal pain tolerance thresholds are decreased during a tension-type headache episode and unaltered interictally.[39] The peripheral myofascial pain sensitivity is measured as the pressure pain threshold and pressure pain tolerance with standardized algometers. In these studies, no consistent results have been obtained in adults with tension-type headache. In some studies, the participants with tension headache had

decreased thresholds in comparison to healthy controls and others with headache,[40,41] but in other studies no differences between headache groups or between headache groups and controls were observed.[34,42,43] In the study by Bendtsen et al,[43] there was no difference between the headache groups and healthy controls, but instead there was a significant difference between those with chronic tension-type headache and pericranial muscular tension and those without pericranial muscular tension. Any headache present seems to have no importance in pressure pain thresholds.[34]

The involvement of central mechanisms in the pathogenesis of tension-type headache is suggested by studies of the influence of mental states on the occurrence of tension-type headache, studies indicating changes in the pain detection in patients with tension-type headache and animal studies on central sensitization through myofascial stimulation.[44,45] In humans, the exteroceptive silent period of temporalis muscle activity was shortened in patients with chronic tension-type headache.[46,47]

Tension-type headache has been initiated experimentally by sustained tooth clenching. After the clenching those who developed headache had increased tenderness pericranially. The pressure pain thresholds increased in those who did not develop headache and remained stable in those who did.[48]

There are only few studies on the muscular findings in children with tension-type headache. Increased EMG levels have been observed in children with headache.[49] It seems that the subjective findings of pain and tension in the neck–shoulder area are more typical for children with migraine than for children with non-migranous headache.[6]

# Prognosis and follow-up studies

Little is known about the prognosis of tension-type headache in children. In a recent study from Italy,[50] tension-type headache on 12–26 year olds showed a high improvement rate through 8 years of follow-up. Out of children who had tension-type headache in 1988, 36.1% were headache free and headache occurred less than once a month in 44.4% in 1996. Worsening of headaches had occurred in only 2.7% of the patients with tension-type headache. The prognosis of tension-type headache was better than that for migraine and was not dependent on the age at onset of headache. Overall, the prognosis was poorer for females in all headache groups.

# Differential diagnosis

Tension-type headache does not have highly specific characteristics. Diagnosis of tension-type headache requires careful exclusion of possible causative or related factors. A thorough evaluation of the psychosocial environment and functioning of the child is also recommended because disorders in these can be provoking factors for tension-type headache. As the importance of muscular tension of the pericranial muscles in tension-type headache is not clear, this finding cannot be considered definite proof of tension-type headache or be a reason for less effort being made to exclude other possible causes.

# Psychological factors

In adults, episodic tension-type headache is not connected with either anxiety or depression, in contrast to patients with migraine who have both of these disorders more often than people with no headache.[51] Few studies analyse particularly the association of tension-type headache with psychological disorders in children. Most of the existing studies deal with overall headache or separate migraine and non-migrainous headache; this group, however, includes a highly heterogeneous population of children with tension-type headache, migrainous headache and miscellaneous headaches, with different associations with psychological factors.

In the clinic-based study by Puca et al,[52] there was anxiety in 51% of the children with episodic tension-type headache and in 56% of the patients with chronic tension-type headache. The corresponding figures were 29% and 38% for depression, and 17% and 27% for somatoform disorders. Stress, anxiety and depression have been reported to occur more often in children with any headache, in comparison to children with no headache.[23,24,53,54] Psychiatric co-morbidity was higher in children with chronic daily headache, in comparison with children with migraine in the study by Holden et al.[21]

# References

1. Headache Classification Committee of the International Headache Society, Classification and diagnostic criteria for headache disorders, cranial neuralgias and facial pain. *Cephalalgia* 1988; 8(suppl 7): S1–96.
2. Ad Hoc Committee on Classification of Headache, Classification of headache. *Arch Neurol* 1962; **6:** 173–6.
3. Jensen R, Rasmussen BK, Muscular disorders in tension-type headache. *Cephalalgia* 1996; **16:** 97–103.
4. Gallai V, Sarchielli P, Carboni F et al, Applicability of the 1988 IHS criteria to headache patients under the age of 18 years attending 21

Italian headache clinics. *Headache* 1995; **35**: 146–53.

5. Wöber-Bingöl C, Wöber C, Karwautz C et al, Diagnosis of headache in childhood and adolescence: a study in 437 patients. *Cephalalgia* 1995; **15**: 13–21.

6. Anttila P, Metsähonkala L, Aromaa M et al, Epidemiology of pediatric tension-type headache. In: *IVth International Congress on Headache in Childhood and Adolescence*, 1999.

7. Göbel H, Petersen-Braun M, Soyka D, The epidemiology of headache in Germany: a nationwide survey of a representative sample on the basis of the headache classification of the International Headache Society. *Cephalalgia* 1994; **14**: 97–106.

8. Nikoforow R, Epidemiological studies on headache in Northern Finland. A survey of an urban and a rural area. Department of Neurology, University of Oulu, 1981.

9. Rasmussen BK, Jensen R, Schroll M, Olesen J, Epidemiology of headache in a general population – a prevalence study. *J Clin Epidemiol* 1991; **44**: 1147–57.

10. Schwartz BS, Stewart WF, Simon D, Lipton RB, Epidemiology of tension-type headache. *JAMA* 1998; **279**: 381–3.

11. Abu-Arafeh I, Russell G, Prevalence of headache and migraine in schoolchildren. *BMJ* 1994; **309**: 765–9.

12. Barea LM, Tannhauser M, Rotta NT, An epidemiologic study of headache among children and adolescents of southern Brazil. *Cephalalgia* 1996; **16**: 545–9.

13. Laurell K, Eeg-Olofson O, Larsson B, Tension-type headache in children. In: *IVth International Congress on Headache in Childhood and Adolescence*, 1999.

14. Aromaa M, Sillanpää ML, Rautava P, Helenius H, Childhood headache at school entry. A controlled clinical study. *Neurology* 1998; **50**: 1729–36.

15. Frankenberg S, Pothmann R, Muller B, Sartory G, Wolff M, Hellmeier W, Prevalence of headache in schoolchildren. In: Gallai F, Guidetti V, eds, *Juvenile Headache*. Oxford: Elsevier Science, 1991: 113–17.

16. Metsähonkala L, Sillanpää M, Tuominen J, Headache diary in the diagnosis of childhood migraine. *Headache* 1997; **37**: 240–4.

17. Rasmussen BK, Migraine and tension-type headache in a general population: psychosocial factors. *Int J Epidemiol* 1992; **21**: 1138–43.

18. Karwautz A, Wöber C, Lang T et al, Psychosocial factors in children and adolescents with migraine and tension-type headache: a controlled study and review of the literature. *Cephalalgia* 1999; **19**: 32–43.

19. Sillanpää M, Piekkala P, Kero P, Prevalence of headache at preschool age in an unselected child population. *Cephalalgia* 1991; **11**: 239–42.

20. Kristjansdottir G, Wahlberg V, Sociodemographic differences in the prevalence of self-reported headache in Icelandic school children. *Headache* 1993; **33**: 376–80.

21. Holden W, Gladstein J, Trulsen M, Wall B, Chronic daily headache in children and adolescents. *Headache* 1994; **34**: 508–14.

22. Metsähonkala M, Sillanpää M, Tuominen J, Social environment and headache in 8 to 9 year-old children – a follow-up study. *Headache* 1998; **38**: 222–8.

23. Larsson B, The role of psychological health-behaviour and medical factors in adolescent headache. *Dev Med Child Neurol* 1988; **30**: 616–25.

24. Carlsson J, Larsson B, Mark A, Psychosocial functioning in schoolchildren with recurrent headaches. *Headache* 1996; **36**: 77–82.

25. Wöber-Bingöl C, Wöber C, Wagner-Ennsgraber C, Zebenholzer K, Vesely C, Geldner J, Karwautz A, IHS criteria and gender: a study on migraine and tension-type headache in children and adolescence. *Cephalalgia* 1996; **16**: 107–12.

26. Russell MB, Ostergaard S, Bendtsen L, Olesen J, Familial occurrence of chronic tension-type headache. *Cephalalgia* 1999; **19**: 207–10.

27. Jensen R, Pathophysiological mechanisms of tension-type headache: a review of epidemiological and experimental studies. *Cephalalgia* 1999; **19**: 602–21.

28. Schoenen J, Gerard P, dePasqua V, Sianard-Gainko J, Multiple clinical and paraclinical

analyses of chronic tension-type headache associated or unassociated with disorder of pericranial muscles. *Cephalalgia* 1991; **11**: 135–9.

29. Bendtsen L, Jensen R, Jensen NK, Olesen J, Muscle palpation with controlled finger pressure: new equipment for the study of tender myofascial tissues. *Pain* 1994; **59**: 235–9.

30. Ashina M, Bendtsen L, Jensen R, Sakai F, Olesen J, Measurement of muscle hardness: a methodological study. *Cephalalgia* 1998; **18**: 106–11.

31. Langemark M, Olesen J, Pericranial tenderness in tension headache. *Cephalalgia* 1987; **7**: 249–55.

32. Drummond PD, Scalp tenderness and sensitivity to pain in migraine and tension headache. *Headache* 1987; **27**: 45–50.

33. Hatch JP, Moore PJ, Cyr-Provost M, Boutros NN, Seleshi E, Borcherding S, The use of electromyography and muscle palpation in the diagnosis of tension-type headache with and without pericranial muscle involvement. *Pain* 1992; **49**: 175–8.

34. Jensen R, Rasmussen BK, Pedersen B, Olesen J, Muscle tenderness and pressure pain thresholds in headache. a population study. *Pain* 1993; **52**: 193–9.

35. Lipchik GL, Holroyd KA, Talbot F, Greer M, Pericranial muscle tenderness and exteroceptive suppression of temporalis muscle activity: a blind study of chronic tension-type headache. *Headache* 1997; **37**: 368–76.

36. Pikoff H, Is the muscular model of headache still viable? A review of conflicting data. *Headache* 1984; **24**: 186–98.

37. Jensen R, Fuglsang-Frederiksen A, Olesen J, Quantitative surface EMG of pericranial muscles in headache. A population study. *Electroencephalogr Clin Neurophysiol* 1994; **93**: 335–44.

38. Van Boxtel A, Goudsward P, Absolute and proportional resting EMG in chronic headache patients in relation to the state of headache. *Headache* 1984; **24**: 259–65.

39. Jensen R, Mechanisms of spontaneous tension-type headaches: an analysis of tenderness, pain thresholds and EMG. *Pain* 1995; **64**: 251–6.

40. Schoenen J, Bottin D, Hardy F, Gerard P, Cephalic and extracephalic pressure pain thresholds in chronic tension-type headache. *Pain* 1991; **47**: 145–9.

41. Kim HS, Chung SC, Kim YK, Lee SW, Pain–pressure threshold in the head and neck region of episodic tension-type headache patients. *J Orofacial Pain* 1995; **9**: 357–64.

42. Bovim G, Cervicogenic headache, migraine and tension-type headache. Pressure pain threshold measurements. *Pain* 1992; **51**: 169–73.

43. Bendtsen L, Jensen R, Olesen J, Decreased pain detection and tolerance thresholds in chronic tension-type headache. *Arch Neurol* 1996; **53**: 373–6.

44. Hu JW, Sessle BJ, Raboisson P, Dallel R, Woda A, Stimulation of craniofacial muscle afferents induces prolonged facilitatory effects in trigeminal nociceptive brainstem neurones. *Pain* 1992; **48**: 53–60.

45. Mense S, Nociception from skeletal muscle in relation to clinical muscle pain. *Pain* 1993; **54**: 241–89.

46. Schoenen J, Jamart B, Gerard P, Leanrduzzi P, Delwaide PJ, Exteroceptive suppression of temporalis muscle activity in chronic headache. *Neurology* 1987; **37**: 1834–6.

47. Wallasch TM, Reinecke M, Langohr HD, EMG analysis of the late exteroceptive suppression period of temporal muscle activity in episodic and chronic tension-type headaches. *Cephalalgia* 1991; **11**: 109–12.

48. Jensen R, Olesen J, Initiating mechanisms of experimentally induced tension-type headache. *Cephalalgia* 1996; **16**: 175–82.

49. Pritchard D, EMG levels in children who suffer from severe headache. *Headache* 1995; **35**: 554–6.

50. Guidetti V, Galli F, Evolution of headache in childhood and adolescence: an 8-year follow-up. *Cephalalgia* 1998; **18**: 449–54.

51. Merikangas KR, Angst J, Isler H, Migraine and psychopathology. *Arch Gen Psychiatry* 1990; **47**: 849–53.

52. Puca F, Genco S, Prudenzano MP et al, Psychiatric comorbidity and psychosocial stress in patients with tension-type headache from headache centers in Italy. *Cephalalgia* 1999; **19**: 159–64.

53. Egger HL, Angold A, Costello EJ, Headaches and psychopathology in children and adolescents. *J Am Acad Child Adolesc Psychiatry* 1998; **37**: 951–8.

54. Langevel JH, Koot HM, Loonen MCB, Haze-broek-Kampschreur AAJM, Passchier J, A quality of life instrument for adolescents with chronic headache. *Cephalalgia* 1996; **16**: 183–96.

# VII

## Chronic daily headache

# 23

# Chronic daily headache

*Paul Winner, Jack Gladstein*

Chronic daily headache (CDH) is a diagnostic term describing a patient who has recurrent headache, with an average frequency of 15 days/month without an underlying serious medical condition. It was described in adults by Mathew et al in 1987.[1] Estimating the incidence and prevalence of this disorder has been difficult, because strict uniform definitions have not been formed. Nevertheless, the prevalence rate for severe or recurrent headache in children and adolescents has been reported as 0.2%, 0.8% and 2.5% by Newachek and Taylor,[2] Sillanpää et al,[3] and Abu-Arafeh and Russell,[4] respectively. For the sufferers and their families, this condition is a source of concern and disability. It may mask depression, and may cause a tremendous amount of dysfunction for the youngster and his or her family.

## Classification

In adults, Mathew et al[1] described CDH as chronic recurrent headache that transformed from either episodic migraine or tension-type headache. Solomon et al[5] in 1992, and Messinger et al[6] in 1991, attempted to use International Headache Society (IHS) criteria to classify consecutive adults in their series, and were not able to in over a third of cases. This led to the work of Silberstein et al[7] in 1994, who defined four types of CDH, each with or without medication overuse. In his proposed criteria, a person would have transformed migraine (chronic migraine) if he or she had a history of episodic migraine, which has now become a daily or almost daily experience. Headache duration would be more than 4 hours/day, and this progression with increasing frequency and decreasing severity occurred over at least 3 months. In chronic tension-type headache, the patient would have an average headache frequency of 15 days/month (180 days/year) for 6 months. The headache would have two of the following pain characteristics: pressing/tightening quality, bilateral location, mild or moderate severity, aggravated by walking up or down stairs or similar routine physical activity, and no autonomic characteristics. There would also be a history of episodic tension-type headache. Again there would be a transformation period of at least 3 months. In new persistent daily headache, headache lasts more than 4 hours/day for more than 1 month. There is no history of episodic migraine or tension-type headache. In hemicrania continua, headaches present for at least 1 month. It is strictly unilateral, and responds to indomethacin. Pain is continuous but fluctuating, of moderate severity and lacks precipitating mechanisms.

We attempted to apply these criteria to a consecutive cohort of children and adolescents who presented to a tertiary referral clinic in 1996.[8] We found that 45% of children and adolescents in our population did not fit neatly into these categories. By adding a category called co-morbid (migraine and tension-type headache, mixed headache), all but one of our 37 patients could be classified according to Silberstein's 1994 criteria. In this type, it is as if two headache patterns exist independently of each other, without any transformation. There is an underlying tension-type headache, with intermittent full-blown migraine. In 1996,[9] Silberstein modified his criteria, loosening the diagnostic criteria for transformed migraine (chronic migraine), thereby capturing a lot of his patients with co-morbid headache (mixed headache). We have continued with the 1994 criteria, because we feel that the lack of transformation in so many of our youngsters merits a separate category for those with co-morbid headache (mixed headache).

## History

For patients with chronic headache, a skilled and careful history is the most important step in making the diagnosis and preparing an appropriate treatment plan. To arrive at the diagnosis of CDH, one must rule out serious medical diseases. We use the 1994 Silberstein criteria,[7] with the addition of co-morbid pattern (mixed headache), for those youngsters who have underlying tension-type headache with independent superimposed migraine. While obtaining a careful headache history to rule out chronic illness or tumor, we should explore coping mechanisms and disability.[10] For adolescent headache sufferers, it is critical to interview the youngster and

parent(s) together and separately. By starting the interview together, we gain critical information about how they interact with each other. Does the mother answer all the questions for the teenager? Is there a lot of conflict? By separating them later, we learn about what each person perceives to be the problem and the disability, and show all involved the practitioner's endorsement of their views. If the youngster will not separate, or if the parent will not let go, we learn a lot about the problem. By bringing the parties together at the end of the session, we can then summarize the situation, while not betraying anyone's confidence. This approach takes time, so patients with chronic headache often require increased scheduling time by office staff.

While obtaining the history, it is necessary to discuss symptoms and disability, and rule out the possibility of infections, sinus disease, trauma, hypertension, cerebrospinal pressure abnormalities and ocular disorders, as well as the possibility of factitious disorders or somatization.[11] A careful look at psychosocial factors is also crucial. Dietary, sleep and medication histories may help to pinpoint aggravating factors. A family history of headache and/or psychiatric disease may shed additional light on to the problem. Psychiatric co-morbidity of depression or anxiety disorders has been reported to occur more frequently in patients with CDH than in patients with migraine or tension-type headaches alone.[12] The presence or absence of daily medication overuse plays a big part in treatment options. Assessing disability for a youngster can be measured by days of school missed, days of school requiring early dismissal, visits to the nurses for medication, a drop in grades, and/or the inability to participate in after-school activities. A disparity between parent-

and patient-endorsed severity is suspicious for either child–parental conflict or parental overestimation of symptoms. In the younger child, we can glean helpful information from a careful description of how the parents react to the child when a headache is acknowledged. 'Is all OK at home?' and 'What is your home like?' are open-ended questions that can be answered by the youngster and the parents separately.

## Physical examination

The approach to the youngster with chronic headache demands a thorough physical examination to convince both the practitioner and the patient of benign aetiology, before proceeding with a treatment plan. Having the patient undressed facilitates a good dermatological examination, and the ability to assess Tanner staging in the adolescent. Vital signs help to rule out increased intracranial pressure as well as hypertension. Skin examination helps rule out neurofibromatosis as well as tuberous sclerosis. Palpation of the sinuses and the jaw help to rule out sinusitis and temporomandibular jaw (TMJ) dysfunction, respectively. A careful neurological examination goes without saying, stressing visual fields and fundoscopic examination. By emphasizing normalcy along the way, the examination can be made into a teaching experience for the youngster. A thorough mental status examination may help to diagnose depression or somatization. When there is mood incongruence, a patient may describe horrific symptoms, but show 'la belle indifférence'.

## Physiology

There is a great deal of literature about the physiology of migraine; however, studies related to the aetiology and physiology of tension-type headache have been more sparse. There are no studies that look at the physiology of CDH as an entity in itself; studies focus on recurrent migraine or tension-type headache. Nevertheless, in tension-type headache, patients have been shown to respond to stress with stronger muscle contraction than patients with no headaches.[13] Jensen suggested that prolonged muscle contraction may sensitize the central nervous system (CNS) to a lower general sensitivity to pain.[14]

## Aetiological factors

The role of stress has been considered an important factor in chronic headache since the work of Bille in 1962.[15] Stress has been shown to be more common in headache sufferers than in matched controls.[16] Bille[15] pointed out, and many headache centres report, that school stress-induced headaches are gone in the summertime. Anxiety, depression and chronic somatic complaints are more common in headache sufferers; however, we do not know whether the headaches cause the other complaints or are the consequences of having long-standing headaches.[17] It is interesting to note, however, that various psychological symptoms are elevated only when a patient had a headache at the time of measurement, so data interpretation of such studies may be biased by the intensity of pain.[18,19]

Familial patterns of headache do exist, especially for recurrent migraine.[19] Familial aggregation is lower in tension-type headache.[20] More important than family history, the response of the family to headache behaviour may influence the transformation from acute to chronic conditions.[21]

# Diagnostic work-up

Patients with suspicious histories or abnormal physical findings need an appropriate work-up. For patients with growth delay, or pubertal delay or arrest, medical work-up is indicated. For patients with dermatological examinations that are suspicious of a neuro-cutaneous disorder, neuroimaging is indicated (magnetic resonance imaging [MRI] with and without contrast, preferred). Sinus tenderness (computed tomography [CT] of the sinuses) or painful, limited jaw opening may warrant further dental investigation. Most patients with CDH have been imaged at some point, as their headache progression went from acute to chronic. The exception would be those patients with new persistent daily headache, where chronic headache started at the onset. Studies of children with recurrent headache with no significant change in severity or frequency over the previous 4 months, and an absence of physical examination abnormalities, do not require further imaging.[22] The role of EEGs is similarly not helpful in the vast majority of cases, unless there is a history of an atypical aura or concern over a paroxysmal event.[23]

# Treatment

A rational approach based on a careful consideration of headache type, the presence or absence of medication overuse, and a consideration of functional disability will assure that patients get judicious use of medications. Assessment of the youngster's ability to comply with relaxation training will help optimize outcome, because only those who will practise will succeed.

For patients with daily headache, it is important to find out whether there are intermittent migraine-like headaches superimposed on chronic tension-type headache (mixed headache). These migraine-like headaches can be treated with appropriate acute management. Careful instruction in the use of acute medications will aim to prevent inappropriate use of these agents. The presence of daily medication overuse makes treatment more complicated. Abrupt withdrawal of these medications may briefly precipitate more severe headache symptoms. Therefore we must be cautious about recommending cessation of medication until some preventive measure is in place.

Although there are many studies demonstrating efficacy of preventive agents in adults, few well-designed controlled studies have been performed specifically in children. Even fewer have been done with CDH. Nevertheless, there are studies of children or combinations of adults and adolescent that use β blockers,[24–26] tricyclic antidepressants,[27] calcium channel blockers,[28] and valproate.[29] Studies on this subject do not rigorously define chronic headache. Nevertheless, practitioners have been using these medications for years.

Behavioural treatment shows promise for patients with chronic headache.[30] Obvious advantages include the absence of medication with side effects, and helping youngsters gain control of their chronic pain. Disadvantages are in patient selection, because it does not work if it is not practised regularly. For both behavioural and pharmacological prevention of recurrent headache, no study has used rigorous definitions of headache type. Do patients with chronic tension-type headache respond differently from patients with transformed migraine (chronic migraine) or co-morbid headache (mixed headache)?

## Conclusion

Chronic daily headache in children and adolescents is currently receiving attention. Using a rigorous classification scheme, we now have the possibility of multicentre studies to elucidate whether the clinical patterns seen by experienced observers translate into rational differentiation of treatment approaches. If the entities are indeed different, then preventive and behavioural trials could guide us in offering a more evidence-based approach to the treatment.

## References

1. Mathew NT, Reuveni U, Perez F, Transformed or evolutive migraine. *Headache* 1987; **27**: 102–6.
2. Newachek PW, Taylor WR, Childhood chronic illness: Prevalence, severity, and impact. *Am J Public Health* 1992; **82**: 364–71.
3. Sillanpää M, Piekkala P, Kero P, Prevalence of headache in preschool age in an unselected child population. *Cephalalgia* 1991; **11**: 239–42.
4. Abu-Arafeh I, Russell G, Prevalence of headache and migraine in schoolchildren. *BMJ* 1994; **34**: 508–14.
5. Solomon S, Lipton RB, Newman LC, Evaluation of chronic daily headache – comparison to criteria for chronic tension-type headache. *Cephalalgia* 1992; **12**: 365–8.
6. Messinger HB, Spierings ELH, Vincent AJP, Overlap of migraine and tension-type headache in the International Headache Society classification. *Cephalalgia* 1991; **11**: 233–7.
7. Silberstein SD, Lipton RB, Solomon S, Mathew NT, Classification of daily and near-daily headaches: proposed revisions to the IHS criteria. *Headache* 1994; **34**: 1–7.
8. Gladstein J, Holden EW, Chronic daily headache in children and adolescents: a 2 year prospective study. *Headache* 1996; **36**: 349–51.
9. Silberstein SD
10. Holden EW, Levy JD, Deichmann MM, Gladstein J, Recurrent pediatric headaches: Assessment and intervention. *Devel Behav Pediatr* 1998; **19**: 109–16.
11. Gladstein J, Holden EW, Winner P et al, Chronic daily headache in children and adolescents: Current status and recommendations for the future. *Headache* 1997; **37**: 626–9.
12. Guidetti V, Galli F, Fabrizi P et al, Headache and psychiatric comorbidity: clinical aspects and outcome in an 8 year follow-up study. *Cephalalgia* 1998; **18**: 455–62.
13. Martin PR, *Psychological Management of Chronic Headaches*. New York: Guilford Press, 1993.
14. Jensen R, Berndtsen L, Olesen J, Muscular factors are of importance in tension-type headache. *Headache* 1998; **38**: 10–17.
15. Bille B, Migraine in schoolchildren. *Acta Paediatr Scand suppl* 1962; **51**(136): 1–151.
16. Larsson BS, The role of psychological, health behaviour and medical factors in adolescent headache. *Dev Med Child Neurol* 1988; **30**: 616–25.
17. Larsson B, Recurrent headaches in children and adolescents. In: McGrath PJ, Finley GA eds, *Chronic and Recurrent Pain in Children and Adolescents. Progress in Pain Research and Management*, Vol 13. Seattle: IASP Press, 1999: 115–40.
18. Holroyd KA, France JL, Nash JM, Hursey KG, Pain state as artifact in the psychological assessment of recurrent headache sufferers. *Pain* 1993; **53**: 229–35.
19. Ziegler DK, Hur Y-Mi, Bouchard TJ, Hassanein RS, Barter R, Migraine in twins raised together and apart. *Headache* 1998; **38**: 417–22.
20. Metsähonkala L, Sillanpää M, Touminen J, Outcome of early school age migraine. *Cephalalgia* 1997; **17**: 662–5.
21. Wall BA, Holden EW, Gladstein J, Parent responses to pediatric headache. *Headache* 1997; **37**: 65–70.
22. Chu ML, Shinnar S, Headaches in children younger than seven years of age. *Arch Neurol* 1992; **49**: 79–82.

23. Daly DD, Markland OM, Focal brain lesion. In: Daly DD, Pedley TA, eds, *Current Practice of Clinical Electroencephelography*. New York: Raven Press, 1990.

24. Ludvigsson J, Propranolol used in prophylaxis of migraine in children. *Acta Neurol Scand* 1974; **50**: 109–15.

25. Forsythe WI, Gillies D, Sills M, Propranolol in the treatment of childhood migraine. *Dev Med Child Neurol* 1984; **26**: 737–41.

26. Olness K, MacDonald JT, Uden DL, Comparison of self-hypnosis and propranolol in the treatment of juvenile classic migraine. *Pediatrics* 1984; **79**: 593–7.

27. Diamond S, Baltes BJ, Chronic tension headache treated with amitriptyline – a double blind study. *Headache* 1971; **11**: 110–16.

28. Solomon GD, The action and uses of calcium channel blockers in migraine and cluster headache. *Headache Quarterly* 1990; **10**: 111–16.

29. Sorensen KV, Valproate: a new drug in migraine prophylaxis. *Acta Neurol Scand* 1988; **78**: 346–8.

30. Engel JM, Rapoff MA, Pressman AR, Long-term follow-up of relaxation training for pediatric headache disorders. *Headache* 1992; **32**: 152–6.

# VIII

## 'Psychogenic' headache

# 24

# 'Psychogenic' headache
*Federica Galli, Vincenzo Guidetti*

When Charmides asked me if I knew the cure for his headache ... I replied it was partly a certain herb and partly a chant in addition to the herb: if one were to recite the chant at the same time as using the herb there would be a complete cure, but if the herb were used on its own there would be no benefit at all ... 'It is not able to heal the head in isolation,' I said, 'To think you could heal the head all by itself without taking care of the body also would be the height of folly' ... (Plato, *Charmides* 155e–156c)

## *'Psychosomatic' framing*

Since Socrates' and Hippocrates' times, physicians have dealt with the complex interaction between mind and body. Complex epistemological questions arise, starting from Descartes' perspective of mind–body dualism, which deeply influenced Western culture. The dichotomous logic 'or organic or psychological' is the direct consequence of this perspective, and it represents the background to the development of psychosomatic theories.

Over time, the term 'psychosomatic' has been used as an all-inclusive category embracing disorders for which organically determined factors had not been found. However, the indefinite border between the insufficiency of our understanding of pathophysiological mechanisms of physical diseases and the real weight of psychological determinants could be better considered when a disorder is labelled 'psychosomatic'. Having no clear and definitive understanding of the physical diseases does not necessarily open the psychological way, as an alternative. The matter is probably more difficult and embedded than it is thought to be. Currently, to categorize a disease as 'psychosomatic' tells us about the probable involvement of mind and body in determining a certain disease, but nothing about the direction of the influence (all physical diseases have influences on the psychological condition) on the pathophysiological mechanisms and on the specific determinants.

The conceptualization of psychosomatic disorders displays a growth in complexity and number of involved factors and levels, opening up an integrated and multifactorial approach.[1] Historically, psychosomatic theories show a trend going from the focus on a particular cause to a multifactorial approach.

Freud was the first to use the term 'conversion' in allusion to the substitution of a somatic symptom for a repressed idea.[2] An important change in the conceptualization of psychosomatic theory came about through the supposition of a specific involvement of the somatic symptom and psychological determinants. Alexander's theory[3] connected unconscious conflicts with specific somatic disorders, which symbolically represent the underlying conflict. The ways and modalities of the connection, and the role of developmental psychosocial factors and biological or genetic variables are not taken into account.

Selye[4] proposed the specific vulnerability theory: stress leads to autonomic arousal of a vulnerable target organ through physiological mechanisms. This perspective led to a significant number of studies on stress responses and illness in both adulthood and childhood and adolescence. Attention to the connection of physiological mechanisms and psychological variables begins to emerge, even though the roles of personality, and social, cognitive or affective variables were not taken into account.

Other theories suggested mechanisms for explaining psychosomatic disorders. Hollander[5] considered illness as the expression of forbidden ideas or feelings, when the normal means of communication is prohibited.

Specific conflict theory represents the focal point of the above conceptualizations. This view has been progressively replaced by wider approaches, which considered the implication of different levels in influencing psychosomatic disorders, beyond unidirectional and one-dimensional explanations. Engel[6] focused attention on the interaction of biological, psychological and social factors in determining psychosomatic symptoms (biopsychosocial model). The most important element to draw from this perspective is the importance given to a sum of factors in determining illnesses.

Currently, psychosomatic theories outline the complexity and non-linearity of the mind–body relationship. Genetic, physiological, social and psychological variables seem to be differently involved in determining the individual response to diseases. Psychosomatic disorders are defined as those in which psychological factors are thought to contribute significantly to the development, exacerbation or maintenance of the illness.[7] The role of psychological processes is substantial in at least some of the patients with a specific illness.[8]

On the one hand, it is very difficult not to consider any illness as influencing the psychological state, and consequently being 'psychosomatic'. On the other, psychological factors may play an important role in determining, modulating or maintaining physical diseases. In this way, all disorders risk being psychosomatic in origin or at some stage. The consequence has been an inflation of the term 'psychosomatic'. At this point, it is deprived of a clear meaning, if not a generic reference to the involvement of mind and body in such disease.

The term 'psychosomatic' is increasingly being replaced by terms such as 'biopsychosocial', 'biobehavioural', 'psychophysiological', 'psychoneuroimmunological', etc. These changes denote the multiple causality lying beneath illnesses, and the importance of genetic, biological, physiological, environmental, social and cultural factors.

Recently, Kandel[9] stressed the importance of learning and experience even in the regulation of gene expression. Each gene has a double function: the *template* function that guarantees the fidelity of replication and the *transcriptional* function that 'is responsive to environmental factors'.

The mere transposition of the above-cited models to the developmental age presents additional obstacles. The frequent lack of attention to developmental factors led to a transposition of adult-based models to childhood diseases, which represents a restrictive view for the comprehension of child or adolescent health problems.

The mind–body relationship raises additional questions when we refer to the developmental age. The difficulty of explaining psychological disease by words can facilitate the 'body way' of communicating it to the environment, to obtain attention or to avoid fearful situations. We do not know *if* and *how* the 'primary way' of communication can influence the probable subsequent patterns, or the 'choice' of the body as the first way of expressing its own diseases.

Clarification of the relationship between psychological factors and headaches could represent a significant aid for psychosomatic research, which often considers as an established assumption the 'psychosomatic' nature of headaches,[10] even though, often, the established criteria for defining headache sufferers are not systematized.

Consideration of the difficulty and questions arising from the use of the concept of 'psychosomatic', and reference to the concept of 'somatization', may in some measure give us a better framework for understanding somatic complaints with childhood onset. The concept of somatization overlaps to some extent with terms such as 'functional', 'psychogenic' or 'unexplained'. When explanatory organic factors are lacking, the term indicates the probable role of psychological factors in influencing the illness's onset, course and maintenance. In part, this definition may be pertinent and applicable to the headache field.

'Somatization' is the term used to denote psychological difficulty or distress that is shown through somatic symptoms, a tendency to experience and communicate somatic distress, and symptoms unaccounted for by pathological findings, to attribute them to physical illness and to seek medical help.[11] The symptoms are real and not consciously used to manipulate or control others or the situation. Physical symptoms have no pathophysiological basis or greatly exceed what one would expect on the grounds of objective medical findings.

To date, the agreement among authors prevails around Lipowsky's definition of somatization,[11] even though it is not in absolute accord on this matter.[7,12–15]

The concept of somatization has been employed to refer to a wide spectrum of symptoms in both adults and children or adolescents. It is a central feature of 'somatoform disorders' according to the *Diagnostic and Statistical Manual of Mental Disorders*, 4th edn (DSM-IV)[16] and the *International Classification of Disease*, 10th edn (ICD-10)[17] classifications. DSM-IV[16] provides for diagnostic criteria of somatoform disorder (somatization disorder, conversion disorder, pain disorder, hypochondriasis and body dismorphic disorder). The diagnostic criteria were established for adults and child-specific research is lacking.[18]

Most commonly seen in children and adolescents are persistent somatoform pain disorder, dissociative/conversion disorder and chronic fatigue syndrome (neurasthenia in ICD-10).[19] In children, and according to the DSM criteria, the diagnosis of somatization appears to be rare,[20] despite 'functional' aches and pain being very diffuse, ranging from 2% to 10% of children.[21] Developmentally appropriate criteria are lacking, because the existing diagnostic parameters have been calibrated on adults, e.g. the diagnosis of somatization disorder requires 13 physical symptoms from a list of 35, 8 of which are appropriate only for postpubertal or sexually active patients.[22]

In addition, polysymptomaticity is the main feature of somatization disorder. In developmental ages, the expression of pain and somatic symptoms appears to follow a developmental sequence, with initial monosymptomaticity, mainly in the youngest. Polysymptomatic somatization is more common in adolescence.[23]

## 'Psychogenic' headache

The International Headache Society (IHS) classification[24] does not provide criteria to classify the so-called 'psychogenic' headache, which is considered to be a 'previous term' used to name the current 'episodic' or 'chronic' 'tension-type headache without tenderness of pericranial muscles'. Chronic daily headache, chronic non-progressive headache, muscle contraction headache and psychogenic headache have often been used interchangeably. Headaches may occur alone or in association with migraine.

The concept of 'psychogenic' is related to the major role of psychological factors in determining headaches. Studies on psychological factors influencing headaches have been carried out from both the psychiatric and the neurological perspective. Anxiety, depression and stress are thought to play a major role in determining the so-called 'psychogenic headache', but the pathogenesis, the clinical characteristics and the exact role of psychological determinants are not clear.

Rothner[25] stated that 'psychogenic' headache is the most common type of headache occurring in the developmental age. The tendency of 'psychogenic' headache to increase in prevalence with age (after puberty) has been outlined.[26]

The IHS classification[24] lists, as potential 'causes' for tension-type headaches, psychosocial stress, anxiety and depression. No suggestions are given for other headache subtypes. The concept of 'masked depression', namely the tendency of depression to exhibit symptoms other than mood disorders, has been frequently related to the occurrence of psychogenic or chronic headaches.[15,25]

On the other hand, research from a psychopathological perspective outlines the association of psychological factors (from generic 'stressors' to psychiatric disorders) and headache,[27] although a clear-cut distinction of headaches' subtypes and systematic diagnostic evaluation according to international criteria are lacking.

In a similar way, studies from the psychiatric perspective ask for valid measures of psychiatric symptoms in clinical and population childhood and adolescence headache sample.[27] Often, research in child and adolescent psychopathology refers to 'somatic complaints' (e.g. 'abdominal pain or headaches') such as co-occurring symptoms in young psychiatric patients. Livingston et al[28] found that between 25% and 30% of children admitted to a psychiatric hospital had physical symptoms, including headache, food intolerance, abdominal pain, nausea and dizziness. Community studies on somatization[20] reported headaches in 10–30% of children and adolescents.

It is clear that, in spite of substantial agreement in findings, a better systematization of the studies and the acquisition of the reciprocal contents and tools of research and clinical practice may give important information about the subtle link that seems to connect psychological and somatic factors in children.

However, the high prevalence of headache, the tendency to change over the time, together with age-related clinical characteristics not well acknowledged and to date not recognized by the IHS classification[24] render the attempts to systematize this subject troublesome. Many studies continue to distinguish generically between migraine and non-migraine headaches; others deal with generic headache patients.

Aspects related to the implication of psychological factors in influencing the course of headache have been found in both migraine (see Chapter 6) and non-migraine headache, even if at the moment clear-cut differences by headache subtypes are not available.

Coch and Melchior[29] found signs of nervousness, mental instability and immaturity in migraineur and non-migraineur patients. They suggested 'a decreased resistance to psychological stress and conflict situations, rather than overt psychological disorder, or endogenous disease'. A positive history of depression has been found in migrainous and non-migrainous headache patients in child neurology patients.[30] Maratos and Wilkinson[31] found higher rates of anxiety and depression associated with conflicting parental relationships. They suggested a disturbed physiological constitution and emotional upset as triggering factors of headaches. Millichap[32] found symptoms of depression, anxiety, and emotional and personality disorders in half the children with chronic recurrent headaches. Kowal and Pritchard[33] carried out an investigation of a population sample of 23 children with headaches and 23 controls. It provided no support either of a higher prevalence of anxiety and depression or that headache children have experienced greater life stresses in the previous year or that their parents have a greater degree of achievement orientation. Partial support was found for the hypothesis that 'headache children were more shy and sensitive and had more psychosomatic problems'.

Guidetti et al[34,35] found feelings of being excluded from the family group and repressed hostility towards important figures. No differences in number of psychopathological disorders have been found between migraine and tension-type headache patients, even though the occurrence of multiple psychiatric symptoms has been found to predict the persistence of headache 8 years later.[36]

School problems, family problems, conflicts and expectations have been seen as significant 'psychological stressors' or 'triggering factors' for headache.[37-42] Different interpretations have been suggested. Andrasik et al[43] found a greater number of somatic complaints in migraineurs and higher ratings of depression and anxiety among migrainous adolescents, compared with matched headache-free individuals. The hypothesis suggested is that 'frequent, unexplainable and intense head pain would likely lead to heightened levels of depression and anxiety'. Cunningham et al,[44] comparing migraine, chronic non-headache pain and pain-free samples, found no difference in anxiety and depression levels between the two groups with chronic pain, compared with pain-free controls. Recently, it has been outlined that chronic illness in general, and not as a specific disorder, may explain variations in psychological functioning between chronically ill and healthy children.[45]

The literature on somatization in childhood and adolescence considers commonly recurrent abdominal pain and headaches (without subtype specification) as the most common forms of somatization.[19,20] An age-related trend in the development of somatization, with recurrent abdominal pain more common in early childhood, has been postulated, followed by headache and limb pain becoming more prevalent with increasing age.[46] Recurrent abdominal pain (RAP) reaches a peak in prevalence at the age of 9, and headaches at age 12, opening up the possibility of a developmental onset sequence.[20]

Broadening the analysis to children's somatic complaints other than headache, we note partly overlapping findings. The term 'psychogenic' has usually been used to refer to somatic complaints for which no organic causes have been found. Studies by others found an implication of psychological factors in maintaining somatic complaints over the time. Analysis of the probable risk factors for persistence of stomachache and headache, in a longitudinal study (4–10-year-old children), found that co-occurrence of the two diseases seemed to constitute a separate entity strongly associated with emotional problems and 'closer to developmental psychopathology'; emotional problems at 4 years, together with low maternal support and behavioural problems, predicted the co-occurrence syndrome. In a similar way, 'persistent problems of worrisomeness, fearfulness, poor appetite and unhappiness' at 10 years were again associated with the co-occurrence syndrome.[47]

A 1-year follow-up study on the persistence of non-specific musculoskeletal pain in pre-adolescents suggested that 'psychological distress' is 'one cause or aggravating factor' of persisting pain.[48] It is also important to note that 56% of subjects with musculoskeletal pain had co-occurring 'headache' and 38% had abdominal pain. The association of multiple psychiatric disorders and migraine or tension-type headache predicted the persistence of both headache subtypes 8 years later.[36]

The so-called 'recurrent pain syndromes' are common in children.[49] In these syndromes (headaches, abdominal pain, limb pain), pain occurs periodically, with symptom-free intervals and lack of organic causes. Children with headaches report more somatic complaints than headache-free controls.[50] Recurrent (cyclic) vomiting, RAP, recurrent headaches and recurrent limb pain are also considered to be 'periodic syndromes' of childhood.[49] Periodic syndromes represent a group of disorders characterized by limited periods of illness that recur regularly for years, in otherwise healthy individuals. The implication of stress, 'depression, poor psychosocial adjustment, or a reaction to negative life events' had been outlined for each of them,[49] and 'psychogenic framing' is often brought about.

Cycles of similar duration, a generally benign course and onset in infancy with persistence for years are the most common characteristics. Most of the peculiarities of periodic syndromes are applicable to headache, even though this risks confusions emerging. Sometimes periodic syndromes have been considered to be 'precursors of migraine' and all are included in the term 'abdominal migraine'.[37] Occasionally 'abdominal migraine' and 'recurrent headaches' have been considered as 'periodic syndromes'.[49] In the history of migraine sufferers, periodic syndromes (cyclic vomiting, recurrent abdominal pain, kinetosis, dizziness, sleep disorders, hyperactivity, growth pain) have been found.[51] The IHS classification[24] classifies only benign paroxysmal vertigo and alternating hemiplegia of infancy as diseases that 'may be precursors of migraine'. Currently, the existence of a real association, the likely direction that is taken and the related factors represent a diagnostic problem and therapeutic challenge.

With an awareness of the obstacles and

weaknesses of modern-day knowledge about this matter we outline the importance of broadening the background on which to frame headaches. There is a need for a better comparison among fields dealing with this matter, to avoid confusion and misunderstanding.

Systematization of the concept of 'stress', clarification of the role of biological predisposition (basic vulnerability?, pain-prone child?) and triggering factors (precipitants), and determination of the role and the different meanings of personality traits, specific psychological factors (including attentional and cognitive elements, the role of stress and emotional disposition) and psychiatric co-morbidity should avoid any confounding overlap among these different elements in the framing of headache.

Another viewpoint to take into account concerns the possible role of external events as the stressful experiences. These could have a different impact according to the presence or absence of a psychological basic profile, not excluding the fundamental role of predisposing biological factors.

We stress that the implication of psychological factors does not mean the exclusion of a biological predisposition (genetic or acquired), but psychological factors could graft on to a predisposed field. How this happens is a point of focus, and only a sort of 'rage of explanation' could induce consideration of the psychological factors as a 'cause' of headaches.

In clinical practice, individual or familial problems in children or their families need to consider the existence of somatic expression of such psychological factors. A temporal relationship between a probable life event and the onset or recrudescence of headache opens up a closer analysis of psychological determinants, such as the occurrence of concurrent psychiatric disorder or severe disability unaccounted for by the recognizable pathophysiology. The presence of a high number of somatic complaints (other than headache) in parents and relatives of children with functional complaints is another predisposing factor to the development of somatic expression of psychological disease.[15]

## Conclusion

In conclusion, we can say that, at our current state of knowledge, the role of psychological factors in influencing at least some headache subtypes is unquestionable, but the term 'psychogenic' says little about the real weight and direction of involvement of psychological factors in influencing headache. Probably there are different paths and modulating factors in influencing headache, which are in accord with predisposing biological field, genetic, environmental, familial and social factors.

Avoiding issues that are too speculative, it is crucial to stress the role of psychological assessment in the onset of headache at the developmental age. Headache is always 'a symptom', with the need to be framed and decoded. If this matter is not taken into account, we risk limiting our approach to organic factors, in a sort of 'scotomic view', limiting the possibilities of relieving headaches through the identification of psychological triggering factors.

In spite of the absence of a clear-cut diagnostic system to classify somatization (more than ever in children), such concepts may represent a valid framework to deal with some headache subtypes. Dealing with this matter is difficult, because we have few definitive points of reference. We move in a weak field, where the assumptions are often at best inferential.

We think that awareness of such difficulties may represent the best starting point to avoid the risks of giving diagnoses that we are uncertain about, in our natural desire to help our patients and their parents and to resolve their 'painful' worries and doubts.

# References

1. Kager VA, Arndt EK, Kenny TJ, Psychosomatic problems of children. In: Walker CE, Roberts MC, eds, *Handbook of Clinical Child Psychology*, 2nd edn. New York: John Wiley & Sons, 1992: 303–17.
2. Jones E, *The Life and Work of Sigmund Freud.* New York: Basic Books, 1953.
3. Alexander F, *Psychosomatic Medicine.* New York: Norton, 1950.
4. Selye H, *The Stress of Life.* New York: McGraw Hill, 1956.
5. Hollander MH, Conversion hysteria. *Arch Gen Psychol* 1972; **26**: 311–14.
6. Engel G, The clinical application of the biopsychosocial model. *Am J Psychiatry* 1980; **137**: 535–44.
7. Bridges KW, Goldberg DP, Somatic presentation of DSM-III psychiatric disorders in primary care. *J Psychosom Res* 1985; **29**: 563–9.
8. Kellner R, Psychosomatic syndromes, somatization and somatoform disorders. *Psychotherapy Psychosom* 1994; **61**: 4–24.
9. Kandel ER, A new intellectual framework for psychiatry. *Am J Psychiatry* 1998; **155**: 457–69.
10. Greene JD, Walker LS. Psychosomatic problems and stress in adolescence. *Pediatr Clin North Am* 1997; **44**: 1557–72.
11. Lipowsky ZJ, Somatization: The concept and its clinical application. *Am J Psychiatry* 1988; **145**: 1358–68.
12. Katon W, Kleinman A, Rosen G, Depression and somatization: A review. Part I. *Am J Med* 1982; **72**: 127–35.
13. Kleinman A, Kleinman J, The interconnections among culture, depression experience, and the meaning of pain. In: Kleinman A, Good B, eds, *Culture and Depression.* Berkeley, CA: University of California Press, 1986.
14. Ford CV, The somatizing disorders. *Psychosomatics* 1986; **27**: 327–37.
15. Garralda ME, Somatisation in children. *J Child Psychol Psychiatry* 1996; **1**: 13–33.
16. American Psychiatric Association, *Diagnostic and Statistical Manual of Mental Disorders, Fourth Edition* (DSM-IV). International Version with ICD-10 codes. Washington, DC: American Psychiatric Association, 1994.
17. World Health Organization, *International Classification of Diseases, 10th Revision.* Geneva: World Health Organization, 1990.
18. Fritz GK, Fritsch S, Hagino O, Somatoform disorders in children and adolescents: a review of the past 10 years. *J Am Acad Child Adolesc Psychiatry* 1997; **36**: 1329–39.
19. Garralda ME, Practitioner review: assessment and management of somatization in childhood and adolescence. *J Child Psychol Psychiatry* 1999; **40**: 1159–67.
20. Campo JV, Fritsch L, Somatization in children and adolescents. *J Am Acad Child Adolesc Psychiatry* 1994; **33**: 1223–34.
21. Goodman JE, McGrath PJ, The epidemiology of pain in children and adolescents: a review. *Pain* 1991; **46**: 247–64.
22. Fritz GK, Fritsch S, Hagino O, Somatoform disorders in children and adolescents: A review of the past 10 years. *J Am Acad Child Adolesc Psychiatry* 1997; **36**: 1329–38.
23. Achenbach TM, Conners CK, Quay HC, Verhulst FC, Howell CT, Replication of empirically derived syndromes as a basis for taxonomy of child/adolescent psychopathology. *J Abnorm Child Psychol* 1989; **17**: 299–323.
24. International Headache Society, Classification and diagnostic criteria for headache disorders, cranial neuralgias, and facial pain. *Cephalalgia* 1988; suppl 7: 1–96.
25. Rothner AD, Diagnosis and management of headache in children and adolescents *Neurol Clin* 1983; **1**: 511–26.
26. Barlow CF, *Headaches and Migraine in Childhood.* Philadelphia: Lippincott, 1984.

27. Egger HL, Angold A, Costello EJ, Headaches and psychopathology in children and adolescents. *J Am Acad Child Adolesc Psychiatry* 1998; **37**: 951–8.

28. Livingston R, Taylor JL, Crawford SL, A study of somatic complaints and psychiatric diagnosis in children. *J Am Acad Child Adolesc Psychiatry* 1988; **27**: 185–7.

29. Coch C, Melchior JC, Headache in childhood – a five year material from a pediatric university clinic. *Dan Med Bull* 1969; **16**: 109–14.

30. Ling W, Oftedal G, Weinberg W, Depressive illness in childhood presenting as severe headache. *Am J Dis Child* 1970; **120**: 122–4.

31. Maratos J, Wilkinson M, Migraine in children: a medical and psychiatric study. *Cephalalgia* 1982; **2**: 179–87.

32. Millichap JG, Recurrent headaches in 100 children. *Child's Brain* 1978; **4**: 95–105.

33. Kowal A, Pritchard D, Psychological characteristics of children who suffer from headache: a research note. *J Child Psychol Psychiatr* 1990; **4**: 637–49.

34. Guidetti V, Ottaviano S, Pagliarini N, Paolella A, Seri S, Psychological peculiarities in children with recurrent primary headache. *Cephalalgia* 1983; **41**(suppl 1): 215–17.

35. Guidetti V, Mazzei G, Ottaviano S, Pagliarini N, The utilization of Rorschach test in childhood migraine: a case controlled study. *Cephalalgia* 1986; **6**: 87.

36. Guidetti V, Galli F, Fabrizi P et al, Headache and psychiatric comorbidity: clinical aspects and outcome in an 8-year follow-up study. *Cephalalgia* 1998; **18**: 455–62.

37. Hockaday JM, *Migraine in Childhood*. London: Butterworths, 1988.

38. Brown JK, Migraine and migraine equivalents in children. *Dev Med Child Neurol* 1977; **19**: 683–92.

39. Rigg CA, Migraine in children and adolescents. *Acta Paediatr Scan* 1975; (suppl 256): 19–24.

40. Rothner AD, Headaches in children: a review. *Headache* 1978; **18**: 169–75.

41. Hockaday JM, Headache in children. *Br J Hosp Med* 1982; **27**: 383–92.

42. Hoelscher TJ, Lichstein KL, Behavioural assessment and treatment of child migraine: implication for clinical research and practice. *Headache* 1984; **24**: 94–103.

43. Andrasik F, Kabela E, Quinn S, Attanasio V, Blanchard AB, Rosenblum EL, Psychological functioning of children who have recurrent migraine. *Pain* 1988; **34**: 43–52.

44. Cunningham SJ, McGrath PJ, Ferguson HB et al, Personality and behavioural characteristics in pediatric migraine. *Headache* 1987; **27**: 16–20.

45. Brown LK, Fritz GK, Herzog DB, Psychosomatic Disorders. In: Wiener JM, ed. *Textbook of Child and Adolescent Psychiatry*, 2nd edn. Washington, DC: American Psychiatric Press, 1997.

46. Apley J, *The Child with Abdominal Pain*. Oxford: Blackwell, 1975.

47. Borge AIH, Nordhagen R, Development of stomach-ache and headache during middle childhood: co-occurrence and psychosocial risk factors. *Acta Paediatr* 1995; **84**: 795–802.

48. Mikkelsson M, Salminen JJ, Sourander A, Kautianen H, Contributing factors to the persistence of musculoskeletal pain in preadolescents: a prospective 1-year follow-up study. *Pain* 1998; **77**: 67–72.

49. Arav-Boger R, Spirer Z, Periodic syndromes of childhood. In: *Advances in Pediatrics*. Chicago: Mosby Year Book, 1997.

50. Karwautz A, Wöber C, Lang T et al, Psychosocial factors in children and adolescents with migraine and tension-type headache: a controlled study and review of the literature. *Cephalalgia* 1999; **19**: 32–43.

51. Del Bene E, Multiple aspects of headache risk in children. In: Cratchley M et al, eds, *Advances in Neurology*. New York: Raven Press, 1982: 187–98.

# IX

## Non-medical treatment of childhood headache

# 25

# Relaxation treatment of recurrent headaches in children and adolescents

*Bo Larsson, Frank Andrasik*

Relaxation training is a fairly old treatment method that was developed by Edmund Jacobson in Chicago during the 1920s.[1,2] He noted that increased muscular tension could be elicited by various lifestyle factors and that nervous tension could cause various types of psychosomatic reactions including headaches. Such symptoms and feelings were incompatible with a relaxed state in the body and relaxation therapy could be used to counteract or reduce increased tension in the body. Based on thorough clinic training and home practices, Jacobson developed a compressive relaxation treatment programme, which could include up to 200 hours of practice with discrimination training and differential relaxation. To accomplish this, participants engaged in a systematic series of muscle-tension and -releasing exercises, designed to help the individual discriminate various levels of muscle tension. With enhanced knowledge of muscle tension, participants could then achieve an overall state of relaxation. To facilitate generalization, participants practised these exercises in reclining and sitting positions. Jacobson also suggested that children could be excellent pupils and that teachers might be administrators or actually guide the children through treatment.

Although effective, Jacobson's procedures were quite effort intensive. In the 1960s and 1970s, researchers and clinicians began to develop and test whether radically abbreviated forms of relaxation could yield similar benefits. Such abbreviated forms of relaxation training were first developed by Wolpe and Lazarus[3] and later by Bernstein and Borkovec,[4] who have provided a very detailed description of a 10-session relaxation programme (with verbatim sample scripts). These programmes were primarily developed for adults experiencing various types of somatic or psychiatric symptoms. Cautela and Broden[5] modified these relaxation methods to be more appropriate for children: they were taught first to tighten and relax larger muscles, instructions were simplified, and tangible reinforcement was recommended to increase motivation and effort. The sessions were shorter in duration, and children received a minimum of six sessions of relaxation training.

Tensing and releasing exercises are not the only approach to relaxation. Other forms of relaxation methods, such as meditative or creative relaxation, guided imagery, and autogenic and hypnotic suggestions have been used in the treatment of various somatic symptom conditions (e.g. epilepsy, asthma, insomnia, headaches), anxiety, poor reading skills and stress reactions, but also autistic symptoms in children and adolescents.[6,7] For most of these disorders, relaxation has been taught to the children as a coping technique to be used at early signs of symptoms to reduce their frequency or intensity. As children become proficient at their relaxation skills, they may even be able to prevent symptoms from ever occurring. Various types of cognitive–behavioural methods have commonly been added to relaxation training to enhance treatment effects and generalization when working with children and adolescents. When treated with combined methods or treatment packages, children and adolescents also have greater options to use whatever technique they feel comfortable with and prefer. The availability of multiple methods might have the additional benefit of increasing treatment compliance.

## Relaxation training and recurrent headaches

Numerous studies have shown that relaxation training is an effective treatment method for adults suffering from migraine or tension-type headaches.[8,9] Typically, electromyographic (EMG) biofeedback has been used for tension-type headaches and temperature biofeedback for migraine often combined with relaxation training (more is said about biofeedback approaches in Chapter 26). For tension-type headaches, negligible differences between relaxation and biofeedback training have been found and, when these treatments have been combined, results have been comparable to those obtained for each single treatment. Similar results have also been reported for adult migraineurs by Holroyd and Penzien.[10]

In one of the first investigations of these techniques for recurrent headaches in children,

Werder and Sargent[11] evaluated the effectiveness of multiple relaxation techniques (progressive muscle relaxation, autogenic training, self-awareness and guided imagery), in addition to biofeedback training. The authors reported that this self-regulation training was very useful for migraine and tension-type headaches in children. They stated further that the relaxation response was easier to elicit in children than in adults and that such treatment was more readily accepted by children. The authors also suggested that parents and school personnel should be more aware of headache symptoms in children and adolescents and to encourage regular use of self-regulation techniques. Since Werder and Sargent's study,[11] more than 30 controlled studies have been published on the outcome of psychologically based treatment of recurrent headaches in children and adolescents.[12] Using specified criteria for evaluating the efficacy of psychological treatments in their review of the literature, Holden and colleagues[12] concluded that relaxation and self-hypnosis are a well-established and efficacious treatment for recurrent headaches in children and adolescents. Relaxation training has been included in treatment packages most commonly used for migraine headaches. It has often been combined with various biofeedback procedures, cognitive-coping strategies, problem-solving or assertiveness training as well. Although there are good clinical reasons for using such packages with children and adolescents experiencing recurrent headaches, there is minimal evidence to show that combined treatment methods are more effective than relaxation used as a treatment by itself.

Table 25.1 provides a summary of the studies in which various forms of relaxation training have been compared with other active

| Study and setting | Headache type | Treatment comparison and outcome |
|---|---|---|
| *Clinic* | | |
| Richter et al[13] | Migraine | Relaxation = cognitive coping > non-specific placebo |
| Fentress et al[14] | Migraine | Relaxation = relaxation + biofeedback > waiting-list control |
| Olness et al[15] | Migraine | Self-hypnosis > propranolol, placebo |
| McGrath et al[16] | Migraine | Relaxation = non-specific therapy = 'own best efforts' |
| Bussone et al[17] | Tension-type headache | Biofeedback-assisted relaxation > pseudo-relaxation |
| *School* *classroom based* | | |
| Setterlind[18] | Unspecified headaches | Physical teacher-administered relaxation to classes = untreated control group |
| Passchier et al[19] | Unspecified headaches | Physical teacher-administered relaxation to classes = placebo training control |
| *Individual/group-based* | | |
| Larsson and Melin[20] | Tension-type headache, migraine | Relaxation > information-contact > self-monitoring |
| Larsson et al[21] | Tension-type headache, migraine | Therapist-assisted relaxation = self-help relaxation > self-monitoring |
| Larsson et al[21] | Tension-type headache, migraine | Self-help relaxation > problem – discussion, self-monitoring |
| Larsson et al[22] | Tension-type headache | Self-help relaxation > self-monitoring; no additional improvement of a muscle relaxant drug (chlormezanone) after relaxation |
| Larsson and Carlsson[23] | Tension-type headache | School-nurse administered relaxation > self-monitoring |
| Fichtel and Larsson[24] | Migraine and tension-type headache | Therapist-assisted relaxation > self-monitoring; migraine > tension-type headache |

**Table 25.1**
*Outcomes of relaxation training for various types of recurrent headaches in children and adolescents*

treatments, attention-control conditions or self-monitoring of headaches in a daily diary. In two studies, relaxation training was administered by physical education teachers to adolescents in school classes.[18,19] However, it should be noted that many of these participants did not suffer from severe headaches, which possibly helps to explain the lack of differences between relaxation training and the control conditions. Instead, it has been suggested that relaxation training should be offered to small groups of adolescents who suffer from more severe and disabling forms of recurrent headaches.[19]

In clinical studies, relaxation training has been shown to be as effective as cognitive-coping procedures, relaxation combined with biofeedback training and prophylactic drug treatment with propranolol, and more effective than waiting-list control for migraine headaches in children.[12,25] It should be noted that in the largest outcome study published so far, McGrath and his colleagues[16] did not find any differences in headache improvement between relaxation training (six individual sessions with a therapist), placebo intervention and a single session ('own best effort') in which information regarding common headache triggers was provided.

In a theoretically interesting study, Bussone and collaborators[17] found that just sitting still in a laboratory setting with no home practice was less effective than biofeedback-assisted relaxation for adolescents with tension-type headaches. These findings suggest that active treatment components are necessary to achieve a reduction of tension-type headaches in these age groups. In a series of school-based treatment studies on primarily tension-type headaches, relaxation training has been found to be effective in particular for adolescents

(10–18 years of age) suffering from chronic tension-type headaches, i.e. daily or almost daily headaches for at least a year. Typically, relaxation training was begun in small groups of adolescents (three to four) and then the administration format was changed to individual sessions that were conducted twice per week for about 2 months (for a total of eight to ten sessions). Overall, the results showed that relaxation treatment was effective and that more than 50% of the treated participants attained at least a 50% reduction in their total headache activity (based on 3–4 weeks of systematic daily headache recordings and estimates of pre–post differences). In the school-based approach, relaxation training has also been found to be more effective than various types of attention-control approaches and self-monitoring of headaches only.[20–22,26] In line with findings for children with migraine,[13] a better improvement was obtained for those who suffered from severe recurrent headaches.[26] Adolescents with chronic tension-type headaches responded better to relaxation training than those suffering from both migraine and tension-type headaches.[26] Headache improvement among the adolescents was well maintained 3–4 years after receiving therapist-assisted relaxation.[27]

Although relaxation training has typically been provided by therapists during at least five to six sessions, various self-help formats have been used in the treatment of migraine as well as tension-type headaches in children and adolescents. Self-help treatment has been shown to provide relief, in particular for those adolescents who are highly motivated to practise at home and apply the techniques in everyday life. Such treatments have often included a few contacts or sessions with a therapist to enhance effectiveness and provide support at critical moments of the training. Outcome research has shown that self-help relaxation might be cost-effective; however, therapist-assisted training seems to be more powerful, in that a higher proportion of subjects achieve a clinically significant improvement with the assistance of a therapist (a 50% headache reduction or more).[28] Treatment administered by a school-nurse, based on audio-tapes and supervised by an experienced physiotherapist, has been shown to provide benefits to adolescents with recurrent headaches that are similar to those obtained from treatment administered by graduate psychology students.[23,26] Thus, relaxation can be effective when administered by various treatment agents, in various settings and in different formats.

## Relaxation training programme

Before training starts, the adolescents are asked to record their headaches four times a day (breakfast, lunch, afternoon, bedtime) in a diary on a 0–5 scale developed by Budzynski et al.[29] In research, participants are instructed to complete their diaries for about 3–4 weeks before treatment starts, but in clinical practice the length of headache recordings should be based on headache frequency and client motivation. Such detailed headache recordings are particularly useful in the assessment of tension-type headaches that occur in isolation or combined with migraine. It is suggested that the adolescents keep their diaries, for example, in their wallet to ease the headache recordings and increase compliance. For infrequent migraine, event-related recordings are more practical and could include various headache characteristics. Andrasik et al[30] describe the use of such an approach and how

results compare with ratings provided by parents and physicians.

In most relaxation training programmes with children and adolescents, the sequential steps have generally been the following: (1) discrimination training focusing on identification of tense and relaxed larger muscle groups; (2) differential relaxation (some muscle groups are tensed while other muscles are relaxed); (3) cued relaxation (pairing breathing to a relaxing word, such as 'calm' or 'relax'; (4) mini-relaxation focusing on a limited number of muscles in the head, neck or shoulders; and (5) application of techniques in everyday life situations when headache and stress tend to occur. In a Swedish school-based programme a CD version has been developed and complemented with a manual to be used for adolescents who would like to practise on their own. A tape and manual version has been prepared for school nurses to use in their treatment of groups of adolescents with recurrent headaches.

In the school-based programme, a treatment rationale is given to adolescents which emphasizes that treatment takes time, so they need to set aside at least half an hour per day for about 2 months for training. It is further stressed that the participants will learn a skill to be practised in everyday life situations when they notice early signs of headaches, increased muscle tension or feelings of stress. They are informed that they will learn coping skills and a mini-rapid relaxation training technique, and the more they practise the better their chances to benefit from treatment. If the participants manage to reduce their headaches they will also experience increased control over their symptoms. During the first two to three sessions, participants sit in chairs and learn to recognize feelings of tension in the body, by tensing and relaxing the various muscle groups. The participants are also asked to record in the diary everyday situations in which the headaches occur.

In the next phase, participants sit and try to relax their muscles without any previous tensing, and also to increase a relaxed state that is facilitated by deep breathing. Cue-controlled relaxation is then trained, and the participants are instructed to use a simple word that they couple with deep breathing. After this phase, differential relaxation is practised during activities, e.g. the subject may walk around in the room while still trying to keep shoulder, head and neck muscles as relaxed as possible. A rapid relaxation technique is then practised and various cues are used in everyday life situations to help prompt regular use of relaxation. As an example, a mark may be placed on the watch crystal and the subject informed: 'every time you look at your watch use this as a signal to practise rapid relaxation'. Students are also instructed to engage in practice 'when the school bell rings'.

In the last phase, participants are asked to apply rapid relaxation in as many situations as possible, in particular in those situations in which headaches and feelings of stress tend to occur. Any moments that present difficulties to the participants receive further training and are rehearsed more thoroughly during treatment. It is emphasized that rapid relaxation should be used early when headaches start to occur or when adolescents notice increased muscle tension in the body, in particular in the head, neck and shoulder muscles. The more they practise and use the technique, the better their chances of achieving a headache reduction. Participants with migraine are instructed to use the rapid relaxation technique at early

signs of an attack and not when the headache has fully developed, which will often ameliorate their headaches.

Most adolescent headache sufferers learn to apply these techniques successfully and also to differentiate between migraine and tension-type headaches.[24] Those who suffer from both headaches, which is fairly common, are instructed to use the rapid relaxation technique early in the development of both headaches. Many of the headache sufferers decrease their use of these techniques after successful treatment of their headaches, but it is not unusual for them then to use these techniques for other problems, such as difficulties falling asleep before a school test or simply to relax after a strenuous day at school. Waranch and Keenan[31] found that relaxation practices had decreased from every day during treatment to less than once a week at a 1-year follow-up. At that time most of the treated participants had mild or no headaches.

Relaxation training has been found to be a highly acceptable treatment among school adolescents who prefer this treatment to other alternatives such as medication.[32] In treatment studies, children and adolescents have also identified relaxation training as one of the most important techniques for their recurrent headaches when other components have been included in treatment packages.[14,33] At a long-term follow-up, more than 90% would also recommend relaxation to others suffering from recurrent headaches.[34] Benefits other than headache relief were reported, the chief one being better stress management, enhanced sleep and improved performance in sports.

It is recommended that individuals practise at least twice a day. However, on school days adolescents may be able to arrange only one daily practice of 20–30 min. Even though adolescents are instructed to practise every day, it has been found that they over-report both the frequency and duration of actual practice by about 50%.[35] General instructions are to perform the training in a quiet room alone with as little disturbance as possible; placing a 'please do not disturb' sign on the door is often helpful in minimizing disruptions. It is important that the adolescents are feeling fresh when starting to practise and are sitting up when they train. It is strongly advised that training should not be performed lying down on a bed with a risk of falling asleep. The strong emphasis on learning an active coping technique is an important message for the trainee, and also that relaxation is not a method to be used only to 'cool off' after a hard day's school work.

## *Causal and change mechanisms*

School stressors are commonly reported by children and adolescents to elicit both migraine or tension-type headaches[36–38] and headaches typically occur in the afternoon in school or afterwards.[36] However, it is unclear whether today's recurrent headache sufferers are exposed more often to external stressors or whether headache sufferers have developed a greater sensitivity to various stressors in everyday life as a consequence of a long-standing pain.[39]

It has been found that adults with tension-type headache respond to stress with more muscle tension than individuals with no headache.[8] Adults with chronic tension-type headache with a muscular disorder have also been shown to have lower pressure detection thresholds and tolerances than those without a disorder in various pericranial locations[40] (see

Andrasik and Passchier[41] for a review of studies addressing stress and muscle tension in tension-type headache). It has been suggested further that prolonged nociceptive stimuli from the pericranial muscles might sensitize the central nervous system, thereby leading to an increased general sensitivity to pain. Schoolchildren with frequent headaches have also shown increased sensitivity to pressure stimuli in the pericranial muscles.[41] In adults, vascular and neurogenic theories have dominated the aetiological hypotheses, but biochemical mechanisms have also been found to play an important role. The pain of migraine arises from the distension of the pial arteries and the sensitization of periarterial nociceptors.[43]

Although it is expected that theories behind recurrent headache in children and adolescents might increase our understanding of causal mechanisms, therapeutic change mechanisms might be different and therefore in need of separate research attention. In adults with tension-type headache it was found that reductions in EMG levels (increased muscle tension in the head muscles) were unrelated to headache change.[44,45] The authors therefore suggested that improvements in headache activity after treatment might be mediated by psychological changes, rather than or in addition to reduced head muscle tension itself. In a subsequent study, it was found that reductions of tension-type headache activity in young adults treated with relaxation/EMG biofeedback training correlated with increases in self-efficacy but not with changes in EMG activity.[46] Overall, these outcomes suggest that cognitive changes explain the effectiveness of relaxation and biofeedback treatments and that such mechanisms also may play an important role when using similar treatments for children and adolescents with recurrent tension-type headaches. Finally, in a study by Bussone et al,[17] in which first progressive relaxation and then EMG biofeedback was given in a laboratory clinic setting with no home practise, children with tension-type headache improved much more than participants who were exposed to the same number of pseudo-relaxation sessions without any feedback and simply asked to sit quietly. Although no differences could be seen after treatment, the first group improved continuously during a 1-year follow-up. However, it should be noted that the latter group, being a credible attention control group, also improved, suggesting that such a simple treatment method might be an easy, but still meaningful, treatment method for children with tension-type headache, e.g. in school settings such cost-effective interventions may help a larger number of children and adolescents suffering from recurrent headaches, perhaps more so for less severe cases ('take your time to rest and relax each week').

## Conclusions and recommendations

Relaxation training is a viable treatment method that has proved effective for children and adolescents suffering from frequent migraine or tension-type headaches, i.e. headaches occurring at least once a week and for an extended period of time. This treatment can be administered to smaller groups of individuals in clinics or within regular school health-care services, e.g. by a trained school nurse.[23] Highly motivated adolescents with recurrent headaches can also benefit from self-help treatment, with the emphasis on home practise or with little further support by a therapist (based on audiotapes or CD and complementing manual). It needs to be emphasized that outcomes seem to be better when treatment is delivered by experienced therapists who can provide specialized assistance to children, adolescents and their parents. Eight to ten sessions delivered twice a week (at least at the start of therapy) seem to be sufficient for most headache sufferers, but some individuals need further help to benefit from treatment. It is highly recommended that a headache diary be used some weeks before treatment and afterwards to evaluate outcome, so that both the client and the therapist can assess whether further treatment needs to be provided. Those individuals who achieve a clinically significant headache improvement can also expect these changes to be well maintained from a short-term as well as a long-term perspective.[27,34] In clinical services relaxation training for children and adolescents can preferably be integrated into a treatment package including, for example, various biofeedback, cognitive coping techniques or stress management procedures. Such packages will increase the options for the individual to use those coping techniques that they feel most comfortable with, thus increasing the compliance and likelihood that their recurrent headache complaints will be reduced.

## References

1. Jacobson E, *Progressive Relaxation*. Chicago: Chicago University Press, 1929.
2. Jacobson E, *You must relax!* New York: Whittlesey House, 1934.
3. Wolpe J, Lazarus AA, *Behavior Therapy Techniques. A guide to treatment of neuroses.* New York: Pergamon Press, 1966.
4. Bernstein DA, Borkovec TD, *Progressive Relaxation Training: A manual for the helping professions.* Champaign, IL: Research Press, 1973.

5. Cautela J, Broden J, *Relaxation*. Champaign, IL: Research Press, 1978.

6. Richter NC, The efficacy of relaxation training with children. *J Abnorm Child Psychol* 1984; **12**: 319–44.

7. Gagnon DJ, Hudnall L, Andrasik F, Biofeedback and related procedures in coping with stress. In: LaGreca AM, Siegel LJ, Wallander JL, Walker CE, eds, *Stress and Coping in Child Health. Advances in Pediatric Psychology.* New York: Guilford Press, 1992: 303–26.

8. Martin PR, *Psychological Management of Chronic Headaches.* New York: Guilford Press, 1993.

9. Holroyd KA, Penzien DB, Psychosocial interventions in the management of recurrent headache disorders 1: Overview and effectiveness. *Behav Med* 1994; **20**: 53–63.

10. Holroyd KA, Penzien DB, Pharmacological versus non-pharmacological prophylaxis of recurrent migraine headache: a meta-analytic review of clinical trials. *Pain* 1990; **42**: 1–13.

11. Werder DS, Sargent JD, A study of childhood headache using biofeedback as a treatment alternative. *Headache* 1984; **24**: 122–6.

12. Holden EW, Deichmann MM, Levy JD, Empirically supported treatments in pediatric psychology: recurrent pediatric headaches. *J Pediatr Psychol* 1999; **24**: 91–109.

13. Setterlind S, Teaching relaxation in physical education lessons. Psychological results from empirical studies in school. *Scand J Sports* 1983; **5**: 56–9.

14. Passchier J, van den Bree MBM, Emmen HH, Osterhaus S, Orlebeke JF, Relaxation in school classes does not reduce headache complaints. *Headache* 1990; **30**: 660–4.

15. Hermann C, Kim M, Blanchard EB, Behavioral and prophylactic pharmacological intervention studies of pediatric migraine: an exploratory meta-analysis. *Pain* 1995; **60**: 239–56.

16. McGrath PJ, Humphreys P, Goodman JT, Kenne D, Relaxation prophylaxis for childhood migraine: A randomized placebo-controlled trial. *Dev Med Child Neurol* 1988; **30**: 626–31.

17. Bussone G, Grazzi L, D'Amico D, Leone M, Andrasik F, Biofeedback-assisted relaxation training for young adolescents with tension-type headaches. *Cephalalgia* 1998; **18**: 463–7.

18. Larsson B, Melin L, Chronic headaches in adolescents: Treatment in a school setting with relaxation training as compared with information-contact and self-registration. *Pain* 1986; **25**: 325–36.

19. Larsson B, Daleflod B, Håkansson L, Melin L, Therapist-assisted relaxation versus self-help relaxation treatment of chronic headaches in adolescents. A school-based intervention. *J Child Psychol Psychiatry* 1987; **28**: 127–36.

20. Larsson B, Melin L, The psychological treatment of recurrent headache in adolescents: short-term outcome and its prediction. *Headache* 1988; **28**: 187–95.

21. Larsson B, Melin L, Döberl A, Recurrent tension headache in adolescents treated with self-help relaxation training and a muscle relaxant drug. *Headache* 1990; **30**: 665–71.

22. Richter IL, McGrath PJ, Humphreys PJ, Goodman JT, Cognitive and relaxation treatment of paediatric migraine. *Pain* 1986; **25**: 195–203.

23. Larsson B, Melin L, Follow-up on behavioral treatment of recurrent headache in adolescents. *Headache* 1989; **29**: 249–53.

24. Larsson B, Recurrent headaches in children and adolescents. In: McGrath PJ, Finley GA, eds, *Chronic and Recurrent Pain in Children and Adolescents, Vol. 13, Progress in Pain Research and Management.* Seattle: IASP Press, 1999: 115–40.

25. Larsson B, Carlsson J, A school-based, nurse-administered relaxation training for children with chronic tension-type headache. *J Pediatr Psychol* 1996; **21**: 603–14.

26. Budzynski TH, Stoyva JM, Adler CS, Mullaney DJ, EMG biofeedback and tension headache: a controlled outcome study. *Psychosom Med* 1973; **6**: 509–14.

27. Andrasik F, Burke EJ, Attanasio V, Rosenblum EL, Child, parent, and physician reports of a child's headache pain: Relationships prior to and following treatment. *Headache* 1985; **25**: 421–5.

28. Fichtel Å, Larsson B, Does relaxation treatment have differential effects on migraine and

tension-type headaches in adolescents? *Headache*, 2001; **41**: 290–6.

29. Waranch HR, Keenan DM, Behavioral treatment of children with recurrent headaches. *J Behav Ther Exp Psychiatry* 1985; **28**: 612–17.

30. Larsson B, Melin L, Relaxation training in the treatment of recurrent pediatric headache. The Uppsala studies. *Scand J Behav Ther* 1988; **17**: 125–37.

31. Fentress DW, Masek BJ, Mehegan JE, Bensen H, Biofeedback and relaxation-response training in the treatment of pediatric migraine. *Dev Med Child Neurol* 1986; **28**: 139–46.

32. Mehegan JE, Masek BJ, Harrison RH, Russo DC, Leviton A, A multicomponent behavioral treatment for pediatric migraine. *Clin J Pain* 1987; **2**: 191–6.

33. Engel JM, Rapoff MA, Pressman AR, Long-term follow-up of relaxation training for pediatric headache disorders. *Headache* 1992; **32**: 152–6.

34. Wiesniewski JJ, Genshaft JL, Mulick JA, Coury DL, Hammer D, Relaxation therapy and compliance in the treatment of adolescent headache. *Headache* 1988; **28**: 612–17.

35. Bille B, Migraine in schoolchildren. *Acta Paediatr Scand Suppl* 1962; **51**(136): 1–151.

36. Passchier J, Orlebeke JF, Headaches and stress in school children: an epidemiological study. *Cephalalgia* 1985; **25**: 167–76.

37. Metsähonkala L, Headache and school. *Headache Q* 1998; **9**: 233–6.

38. Holm JE, Holroyd KA, Hursey KG, Penzien DB, The role of stress in recurrent tension headache. *Headache* 1986; **26**: 160–7.

39. Jensen R, Berndtsen L, Olesen J, Muscular factors are of importance in tension-type headache. *Headache* 1998; **38**: 10–17.

40. Andrasik F, Passchier J, Psychological mechanisms of tension-type headache. In: Olesen J, Tfelt-Hansen P, Welch KMA, eds, *The Headaches*, 2nd edn. Philadelphia: Lippincott, Williams & Wilkins, 599–603.

41. Carlsson J, Tenderness in pericranial muscles in school children with headache. *Pain Clin* 1996; **9**: 49–56.

42. Olesen J, Tfelt-Hansen P, Welch KMA, eds, *The Headaches*. New York: Raven Press, 1993.

43. Andrasik F, Holroyd KA, A test of specific and nonspecific effects in the biofeedback treatment of tension headache. *J Consult Clin Psychol* 1980; **48**: 575–86.

44. Andrasik F, Holroyd KA, Specific and nonspecific effects in the biofeedback treatment of tension headache: 3-year follow-up. *J Consult Clin Psychol* 1983; **51**: 634–6.

45. Rockicki LA, Holroyd KA, France CR, Lipchik GL, France JL, Kvaal SA, Change mechanisms associated with combined relaxation/EMG biofeedback training for chronic tension headache. *Appl Psychophysiol Biofeedback* 1997; **22**: 21–41.

# 26

# Biofeedback treatment of recurrent headaches in children and adolescents

*Frank Andrasik, Bo Larsson, Licia Grazzi*

Two types of behavioural treatments predominate in the headache literature: relaxation, which was reviewed in Chapter 25, and biofeedback, which is the focus of this chapter. Relaxation and biofeedback are similar in many respects, because both have as their chief aim the reduction of physiological arousal associated with stress and headaches and both typically incorporate the same types of adjunctive approaches (diaphragmatic breathing, mental imagery, etc.) to maximize effects. As mentioned in the previous chapter, in clinical practice these two forms of treatment are often combined. Relaxation training uses what may be considered a 'shotgun' approach (seeking to effect a broad or overall state of relaxation), whereas biofeedback uses a 'rifle' or more focused approach (targeting specific response systems). The more precise focus of biofeedback has led investigators and clinicians to advocate specific approaches for distinct headache types, which is the format that we follow in this chapter.

## Biofeedback: definition

Many operational definitions have been proposed for biofeedback. Here we present the comprehensive definition of 'applied biofeedback' provided by Olson[1] which attempts to synthesize the most salient points from several different existing theoretical accounts:

> As a process, applied biofeedback is (1) a group of therapeutic procedures that (2) utilizes electronic or electromechanical instruments (3) to accurately measure, process, and 'feed back' to persons (4) information with reinforcing properties (5) about their neuromuscular and autonomic activity, both normal and abnormal, (6) in the form of analogue or binary, auditory and/or visual feedback signals. (7) Best achieved with a competent biofeedback professional, (8) the objectives are to help persons develop greater awareness and voluntary control over their physiological processes that are otherwise outside awareness and/or under less voluntary control, (9) by first controlling the external signal, (10) and then with internal psychophysiological cues. (p. 29)

The biofeedback movement in general can be traced back to the late 1960s and early 1970s, when a number of converging scientific findings and sociocultural trends fostered development of what was then viewed as a radically new approach to behaviour change.[2] At this time, empirical studies were beginning to show that both humans and animals could be conditioned to control certain autonomic nervous system functions, such as blood pressure, salivation, gastrointestinal contractions, urine formation, sweat gland activity, vasomotor response and cardiac activity.[3–11] The possibility that glandular and visceral responses, heretofore thought to function automatically and even unconsciously, could be influenced by conscious attempts of individuals opened the eyes of many medical and psychological visionaries. It was only a matter of time before clinical applications began to surface and among the first attempts were alternative ways to manage headache.

# Biofeedback training for headache: basis

## Migraine

Four distinct biofeedback approaches have been investigated for migraine headache: (1) thermal biofeedback or autogenic feedback, which is by far the most common; (2) blood volume pulse biofeedback; (3) transcranial Doppler biofeedback; and (4) contingent negative variation (CNV) biofeedback. These treatments were initially developed for adults, but subsequently they were found to be very beneficial for children and adolescents as well.

### Thermal biofeedback

Thermal biofeedback originated from a serendipitous finding at the Menninger Clinic in Topeka.[12] During a standard laboratory evaluation at this clinic, it was noted in one patient that spontaneous termination of a migraine attack was accompanied by flushing in the hands and a rapid, sizeable increase in surface hand temperature. This astute observation, combined with clinical creativity, led these researchers to pilot test whether teaching migraineurs how to increase their peripheral temperature could voluntarily afford patients some improved ability to regulate their headaches. In their early studies, highly sensitive temperature probes were attached to a patient's index finger and the middle of the forehead. The temperature differential between these two probes was displayed to the patient, who was then instructed in ways to increase hand temperature relative to forehead temperature (the goal being to shunt blood flow in the head and redirect it to the extremities, based on the prevailing view of migraine being primarily a vascular disorder). This thermal biofeedback was combined with certain components of autogenic therapy in order to augment training effects, resulting in what was termed 'autogenic feedback'.

Autogenic training has an extensive history[13] and involves having patients passively concentrate on key words and phrases selected for their ability to promote desired somatic responses. Specifically, patients were instructed to focus on feelings of warmth and heaviness in the extremities (two of the six components of autogenic therapy) to facilitate increased blood flow there. Initially, it was not known whether the temperature change occurring in patients was the result of forehead cooling, hand warming or both. Subsequent study revealed that most of the effect was essentially caused by hand warming, so most present-day biofeedback therapists monitor temperature from single peripheral sites, as depicted in Fig. 26.1.

As seen in a subsequent section, an extensive literature supports the clinical utility of this approach (with patients of all ages). However, mechanisms underlying hand warming are not fully understood at present. Current theoretical accounts speculate that

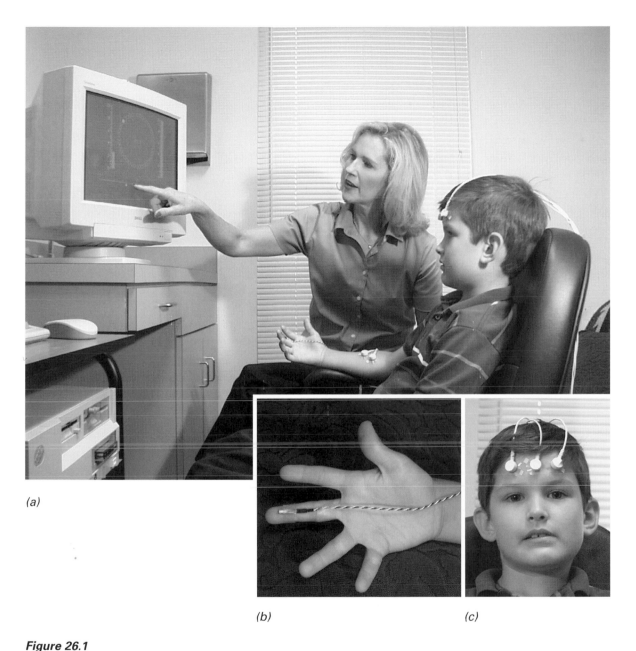

(a)

(b)                                             (c)

**Figure 26.1**
*Child receiving thermal and EMG biofeedback. (a) The therapist is explaining the feedback modalities to the child. The vertical bars on either side of the computer monitor display EMG activity from the forehead and forearm. The circle in the middle and the bar on the bottom of the monitor are providing temperature (relative) feedback. Actual temperature values are provided digitally in the middle of the circle. (b) A typical thermistor placement for monitoring surface skin temperature. (c) A typical EMG electrode array placement for treatment of tension-type headache and generalized relaxation.*

autogenic feedback (1) derives its effect *indirectly* from the decreased sympathetic nervous system arousal that must occur in order for peripheral dilatation and subsequent hand warming to take place and/or (2) serves to stabilize the vascular system and counteract vasomotor instability and perturbations, much like some prophylactic medications.[14-16] If the former account holds true, then autogenic biofeedback may well serve as yet another more generalized approach to relaxation.

### Blood volume pulse biofeedback

Hand warming biofeedback remains the predominant biofeedback approach for research into and treatment of migraine in children, adolescents and adults, but three other approaches have received some research attention. The first of these evolved from a more straightforward rationale and involves monitoring blood volume pulse (BVP) from the temporal artery to teach patients how to reduce or constrict blood flow to the temporal region. This technique for coping with migraine attacks is based on the seminal research of Wolff and colleagues,[17] who found an association between pain and both extra- and intracranial artery dilatation during migraine attacks. Thus, this procedure may be thought of as the non-drug equivalent to ergotamine therapy.

The initial effectiveness of this biofeedback treatment was evaluated by Friar and Beatty;[18] 19 adult migraineurs, 18 of whom had reported prior treatment success with ergotamine tartrate, were carefully selected from a pool of 74 potential patients. Measures of blood flow were taken from pressure-transducing plethysmographs attached at two different sites – one directly above the temporal artery or to one of its main ramifications, and the other to the ventral surface of the index finger. Participants were matched carefully and assigned randomly to receive pulse-amplitude feedback from the temporal area (experimental group) or the finger (control group), both in the direction of decreased blood flow. At the completion of eight training sessions, experimental participants were able to decrease blood flow in the temporal region by 20% during non-headache periods. (It was not possible to train patients directly during an attack, so they needed to learn the vasoconstriction strategies during non-headache intervals.) There were no significant changes in temporal blood flow in the control individuals. Experimental subjects improved by approximately 45%, versus 14% improvement for control individuals.

Friar and Beatty's procedures were very difficult to implement, because they required repeated calculations of pulse amplitude, skin temperature, pulse rate and pulse-propagation time. In addition, it was necessary simultaneously to monitor and correct for muscle-activity artefact, via visual analysis and construction of a pulse-wave template from the previous session. Although these obstacles are now more easily overcome with computers, and advanced software and sensors have been improved (reflectance plethysmography), there are still other measurement difficulties (varying reliability, inability to quantify values in an absolute sense). Consequently, research and clinical applications of BVP biofeedback lag far behind those for hand-temperature biofeedback, especially with regard to children and adolescents.

Sartory et al[19] have conducted the only controlled evaluation of the use of BVP for headache in children. Juvenile headache sufferers (migraine and non-migraine), aged between 8 and 16, were randomly assigned to receive BVP biofeedback (combined with stress-management training), relaxation training (also combined with stress-management training) or metoprolol (a β-blocker). Biofeedback resulted in significant improvements with regard to headache frequency, headache duration and mood state. Consumption of analgesics decreased considerably (by about 40%), but this change was not found to be statistically significant. Similar findings occurred for relaxation (significant improvements for frequency and intensity), with a greater proportion of patients in this condition being judged overall as clinically improved. No significant changes occurred for the β-blocker medication. These effects endured at the 8-month follow-up. Children receiving BVP feedback reduced blood flow in the temporal artery by 6–8% on average, which contrasts markedly with the reductions reported by Friar and Beatty[18] with adults (20%). Time devoted to BVP biofeedback was minimal in the study by Sartory et al.[19] Perhaps outcomes would have been improved if subjects had had increased opportunities to become more proficient in BVP regulation.

### Other biofeedback approaches

The two other biofeedback approaches for migraine are experimental and remain under development. The first involves transcranial Doppler technology in attempts to affect blood flow in the middle cerebral artery.[20] This approach is based on the observations of Friberg et al,[21] who found that migraine pain was caused by, or at least closely associated with, dilatation of the intracranial large artery. Parameters under investigation concern mean blood velocity and peripheral resistance index (systolic pressure minus diastolic pressure divided by diastolic pressure). This research

appears to be confined to adults at present. The newest biofeedback approach for migraine in children directly targets central nervous system parameters and involves self-regulation of slow cortical potentials (CNV) in the EEG.[22] This treatment, as with BVP and Doppler biofeedback, requires special therapist expertise and equipment, and will probably remain experimental for some time.

## Tension-type headache

Electromyographic (EMG) biofeedback is by far the main biofeedback treatment for tension-type headache. In this treatment, EMG electrodes are typically attached to the surface of the forehead (see Fig. 26.1), the patient is given easily processed information about the ongoing level of muscle activity in this area (via an auditory tone that is directly proportional to the electrical activity recorded), and the therapist coaches the use of strategies to facilitate relaxation and reductions in tension levels.[23] At the time this procedure was developed, it was widely believed that sustained muscular contractions were the chief cause of tension-type headache and that tension levels in the frontal area served as a good barometer for tension elsewhere in the body, especially for the head, neck and shoulder muscles. Current-day EMG biofeedback approaches to tension-type headache include more extensive, individualized assessment so that treatments can be tailored to a greater extent, e.g. varied muscles are sampled (bilateral frontal–posterior neck electrode placement, scanning of multiple sites), recordings are dynamic as well as static (taken during movement and postural changes as well as at rest) and, occasionally, readings are taken in real-life settings (via ambulatory monitoring).[24]

Research has shown that a number of cognitive and behavioural changes occur when patients undergo EMG biofeedback (e.g. confidence in coping abilities is enhanced, self-efficacy is increased, and these in turn lead the patient to attempt to cope in a more active manner), in addition to improved abilities to regulate tension levels.[25-27] These changes may well serve important mediating functions.[28] This may help explain the positive treatment effects observed for tension-type headache patients who lack evidence of pericranial muscle involvement, yet still benefit from EMG treatment.

In adult patients, brain wave and electrodermal biofeedback have been piloted, but we could find no such work with tension-type headaches in children or adolescents. Hence, we are not reviewing these approaches here.

To facilitate discussion, we have presented biofeedback as distinct treatments for distinct headache types. In practice, clinicians often employ multiple forms of biofeedback, along with related complementary behavioural approaches and medication, because a sizeable percentage of individuals with headache experience overlapping symptoms and other complicating conditions.

## Evidence base

### Migraine

Two recent articles contain extensive reviews of the literature for the major biofeedback approaches for childhood headache: thermal/autogenic feedback and EMG biofeedback. The first[29] culled all available drug and non-drug studies for childhood migraine to early 1993 and selected for analysis only those studies meeting explicit predetermined criteria,

to ensure that adequate designs and sample sizes were employed, that duplication of subjects and repetition of findings were avoided, and that samples were not specially selected. The resulting 17 behavioural treatment studies and 24 pharmacological studies were then entered into a meta-analysis, which permitted the investigators to evaluate statistically how various non-pharmacological treatments compared with each other, how various pharmacological prophylactic approaches compared with each other, and how these two forms of treatment compared with each other. The findings from this meta-analysis are presented graphically in Fig. 26.2, which lists the results in decreasing order of obtained effect sizes (for data with outliers excluded), and in Table 26.1, which reports all possible paired statistical comparisons. To illustrate how to interpret Table 26.1, first consider thermal biofeedback. By comparing down the column, it can be learned that outcomes from this treatment exceeded those obtained by progressive muscle relaxation training, multicomponent treatments (at least three or more distinct behavioural treatments combined), active medications (calcium channel blockers and serotoninergic agents), psychological and drug placebos, and no treatment controls. The addition of relaxation training (biofeedback + progressive muscle relaxation) did not add appreciably to effectiveness, although this combination exceeded all other treatment and control conditions. Of additional interest is the finding that both active medications exceeded drug placebo. Data for other medications (propranolol, dopaminergic drugs, ergotamine and clonidine) were too limited to permit meaningful analyses in the primary comparisons. Thus, thermal/autogenic feedback was shown to be highly efficacious for childhood migraine.

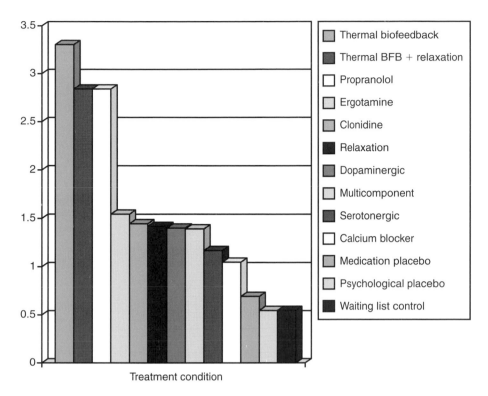

**Figure 26.2**
*Effect size values for behavioural (n = 17) and pharmacological (n = 24) treatment for childhood migraine. (Data derived from Hermann et al.[29]) BFB, biofeedback; Multicomponent, a combination of three or more behavioural treatments*

The second, and more recent, review article examined 31 behavioural studies for the extent to which they met what have become fairly standard criteria for determining efficacy of psychologically based interventions (based on seminal work by a task force for the clinical psychology division of the American Psychological Association[30]). The criteria used by Holden et al[31] are reproduced in Table 26.2. These authors came to similar conclusions about the efficacy of thermal biofeedback for childhood migraine upon examining the available evidence.

As previously mentioned, the database is too limited to permit definitive statements about efficacy of BVP, Doppler and CNV biofeedback for childhood headache.

## Tension-type headache

Investigations are far more limited for tension-type headache with children and adolescents, and only one of the two previously cited literature reviews addressed this headache type. This most recent review[31] uncovered only a small number of studies researching EMG

| | Thermal BFB | PMR | BFB + PMR | Multicomponent treatment | Psychological placebo | Waiting list | Calcium blockers | Serotoninergic drugs | Drug placebo |
|---|---|---|---|---|---|---|---|---|---|
| Thermal BFB | – | | | | | | | | |
| PMR | >** | – | | | | | | | |
| BFB + PMR | NS | <** | – | | | | | | |
| Multicomponent treatment | >** | NS | >** | – | | | | | |
| Psychological placebo | >** | >** | >** | >** | – | | | | |
| Waiting list | >** | >** | >** | >** | NS | – | | | |
| Calcium blockers | >** | NS | >** | NS | <** | <** | – | | |
| Serotoninergic drugs | >** | NS | >** | NS | <** | <** | NS | – | |
| Drug placebo | >** | >** | >** | >** | NS | NS | >* | >** | – |

(Reprinted from Table IV of Hermann et al[29] with permission.)
The inequality signs refer to the comparison between columns and rows (e.g. considering the first column, Thermal BFB was found to be superior to PMR, multicomponent, psychological placebo, waiting list, calcium blockers, serotoninergic drugs and drug placebo; the addition of PMR to biofeedback did not significantly enhance effects). The comparisons were based on the mean ES for each treatment category after removal of outliers.
*$p < 0.05$; **$p < 0.01$; NS, not significant.
BFB, biofeedback; PMR, progressive muscle relaxation.

**Table 26.1**
*Significance of the within-group effect size differences across the different behavioural and pharmacological treatments*

*Well established*
Tested in randomized group designs, wherein:
• Treatment is superior to placebo or alternative treatment
• Statistical power is adequate
Or, a large series of appropriately controlled single-case design experiments, wherein:
• Treatment is superior to placebo or alternative treatment
+ • Effects demonstrated by at least two different investigative teams
+ • Treatment must be well specified
+ • Samples must be adequately described

*Probably efficacious*
Two or more randomized group designs, wherein:
• Treatment is superior to a wait list control
Or, one study that meets the criteria for a well-established intervention

*Promising intervention*
Positive support from one well-controlled study and at least one other less well-controlled study
Or, a small number of single-case design experiments
Or, two or more well-controlled studies by the same investigative team

**Table 26.2**
*Criteria for determining efficacy of psychological treatments (Holden et al[31])*

biofeedback for tension-type headache alone (not combined with migraine features); all identified studies were published before 1991. Perhaps the strongest support for EMG biofeedback comes from a few recent studies that have been able to recruit fairly large sample sizes and collect longer-term follow-up. In the first, Bussone et al[32] randomly assigned juveniles to either EMG biofeedback (assisted by relaxation training, $n = 20$) or relaxation placebo ($n = 10$). In the placebo condition, EMG recordings were made but no feedback was provided; patients were instructed to remain calm and attempt to become more and more relaxed, by whatever means possible for them. At the completion of treatment, both conditions led to sizeable reductions (about 50%). Over time, however, children in the biofeedback condition con-

tinued to improve, whereas those assigned to placebo did not. At the 6- and 12-month follow-up, improvements shown by the biofeedback group statistically surpassed those for the placebo group (Fig. 26.3). Patients in this study were not instructed to practise biofeedback and related relaxation skills outside of therapy, and this may help explain the delayed onset to maximum symptom relief.

The efficacy of EMG biofeedback for tension-type headache in children and adolescents was replicated in a subsequent single-group outcome study ($n = 38$), with results holding over 3 years.[33] As was true for Bussone et al,[32] patients continued to improve over time. Finally, Kröner-Herwig et al[34] found EMG biofeedback to be efficacious, too, but their sample included subjects who had

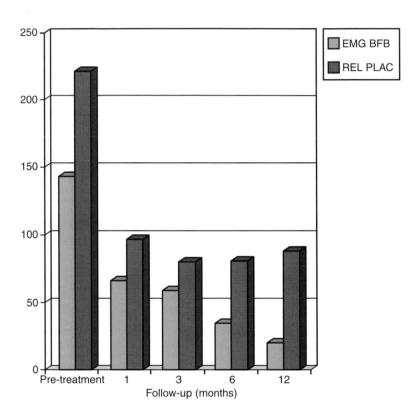

**Figure 26.3**
*Mean pain total index scores for EMG biofeedback (BFB)-assisted relaxation and relaxation placebo (REL PLAC) from pre-treatment to the 12-month follow-up*

combined headache in addition to pure tension-type headache. Thus, it is not possible to determine how each subsample fared. Taken together, however, these reports support the use of EMG biofeedback for episodic tension-type headache, although further investigation is needed before more definitive claims can be made. In future research, it will be important to separate the effects for biofeedback and relaxation alone, because most of the preceding studies combined these two components.

## Clinical considerations

Biofeedback treatments for headache were developed and field tested with adult patients.

When investigators began to turn their attention to children and adolescents, the treatments were applied with few adjustments and appeared to meet with even greater clinical success than when comparable procedures were performed with adults. To date, no direct comparisons of child and adult headache patients have been conducted within a single study. However, a recent quantitative analysis,[35] drawing upon nearly 60 existing separate child and adult studies, confirmed that children indeed have improved at a greater level when treated in a similar fashion with either temperature or EMG biofeedback (Fig. 26.4). These very encouraging findings for juveniles may need to be tempered somewhat, because it is possible that children and

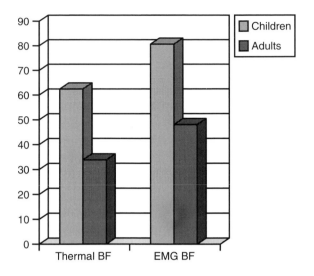

**Figure 26.4**
*Mean percentage improvement in headache
activity for children and adults treated by thermal
and EMG biofeedback. (Data from Sarafino and
Goehring.[35]) Values are subject-weighted means.
The number of subjects and the number of
studies upon which the values are based are as
follows: children's thermal BF (65/6); children's
EMG BF (19/4); adults' thermal BF (243/15); and
adults' EMG BF (238/25)*

*Advantages*
Increased enthusiasm
Quicker rate of learning
Less sceptical about self-control procedures
Greater confidence in special abilities
Increased psychophysiological lability
Fewer previous failure experiences with
  treatment
Increased enjoyment when practising
Increased reliability of symptom monitoring

*Disadvantages*
Briefer attention span
Off-task behaviours during session
Fear/apprehension about equipment
Intolerant of minor discomfort in removing
  sensors
Emotional/psychological problems
Reduced ability to comprehend
  rationale/procedures
Scheduling problems
Lack of standardized electrode placement

**Table 26.3**
*Advantages and disadvantages when treating
children by biofeedback (from Attanasio et al[36])*

adolescents may have a higher rate of spontaneous remission than adults[35] (see also Chapters 10 and 16). Few investigators have examined this aspect, but it does need consideration.

From our clinical experience, after working with 100+ children and adolescents, ranging in age from 6 to 17, we[36] identified a number of advantages in working with younger individuals, which may help account for their enhanced treatment response (Table 26.3). At the same time, certain difficulties were encountered (Table 26.3). These potential problems are easily addressed by tailoring language and

taking additional time to ensure understanding, decreasing the amount of time spent practising biofeedback within sessions (e.g. 20 min total with children versus 30–40 min for adults and inclusion of frequent rest periods if needed), and by employing contingency management strategies to help sustain performance. In trying to follow standardized protocols, which is crucial in research investigations, we found that multiple modifications were required for children aged 7 and below. The modifications were such that it became very difficult to determine with any certainty what components were being most helpful.

Green[37] presents a number of very helpful suggestions and verbatim scripts to use when teaching self-regulatory skills to very young children. Some of her specific recommendations include the following: invite the entire family to the initial session to prevent the child from being singled out as the problem or 'sick one'; have the therapist be identified as a 'biofeedback teacher', someone who teaches ideas and skills, who likes to be asked questions and who in turn likes to ask questions; demonstrate biofeedback with a response that is easily controlled or produces a quick, discernible response (EMG from the forearm, because it can be manipulated very easily; electrodermal response when playing guessing games); and incorporate adjunctive techniques, such as those discussed in Chapter 25 (belly or diaphragmatic breathing, body scanning, 'limp rag doll', imagery).

From this chapter on biofeedback and Chapter 25, it is evident that each approach is of value to child and adolescent headache patients. With adults, there is the suggestion that some patients may respond differentially to relaxation and to biofeedback.[38] Unfortunately, there are no data at all to guide therapists in selecting and sequencing which approach to apply for a given child or adolescent. Until such critical data are collected, the choice defaults to therapist and patient preference. Some therapists believe that children lacking in motivation may respond better to biofeedback because of the immediacy of feedback and its game-like, futuristic and technical qualities.

Although fairly straightforward translations of biofeedback treatment approaches have met with much success, it is possible that effects could be enhanced further by adding a developmental perspective to evaluation and treatment. Marcon and Labbé[39] discuss cogni-tive, self-regulation and psychosocial factors, and issues that arise at various stages of development. One example they discuss, illness causality, is presented here for the purposes of illustration. To the question, 'How do people get headaches?', they point out that children proceed from no to minimal comprehension ('from God'), to external causality and concrete explanations ('from running and getting hot'), to internal and physiological understanding ('from things happening to you that cause too much blood flowing to your head'), and lastly to psychophysiological explanations ('when people get nervous or do too much, this causes their body to react, with a headache'). It can readily be seen how these varied illness conceptualizations would impact treatment delivery. Other examples discussed by Macon and Labbé concern differences in language, time perception and approaches to tasks, and varied abilities to comprehend the notion of severity. They also point to the importance of considering environmental influences on headache, specifically attention from family members and teachers.

Allen and Shriver[40] recently provided a concrete illustration of this last point. Child and adolescent migraineurs, ranging in age from 7 to 18, were randomly assigned to one of two treatment conditions: standard thermal biofeedback or biofeedback combined with parent training in pain behaviour management. In the latter condition, parents were taught to (1) minimize their reactions to pain behaviour, (2) insist upon participation in normal, planned activities, and (3) praise and support biofeedback practice. Specific written guidelines were distributed to parents and reviewed at each session (Table 26.4). Thermal biofeedback, as expected, led to significant improvements, thus providing a

1.  *Encourage independent management of pain:* praise and publicly acknowledge practise of self-regulation skills during pain-free episodes. If pain is reported, issue a single prompt to practise self-regulation skills. Praise and reward normal activity when report of pain has been made.
2.  *Encourage normal activity during pain episodes:* insist upon attendance at school, maintenance of daily chores and responsibilities, participation in regular activities (lessons, practices, clubs).
3.  *Eliminate status checks:* no questions about whether there is pain or how much it hurts.
4.  *Reduce response to pain behaviour:* no effort should be made to assist the child in coping. Do not offer assistance or suggestions for coping. Do not offer medications.
5.  *Reduce pharmacological dependence:* if medication is requested, deliver only as prescribed (i.e. follow directed time table).
6.  *Recruit others to follow same guidelines:* school personnel should not send child home; child should be encouraged and permitted to practise self-regulation skills in the classroom, workload should not be modified.
7.  *Treat pain requiring a reduction in activity as illness:* if school, activities, chores or responsibilities are missed, the child should be treated as ill and sent to bed for the remainder of the day, *even if pain is resolved.* Do not permit watching television, playing games or special treatment.

**Table 26.4**
*Pain behaviour management guidelines for parents (from Allen and Shriver[40])*

further replication of the efficacy of this approach. However, the addition of parent training for pain behaviour management added a significant benefit to clinical outcome. The combined treatment group achieved greater overall reductions in headache frequency, had a larger percentage of patients displaying clinically significant improvement (reductions greater than 50%) and revealed better adaptive functioning (i.e. pain led to less interference in daily activities).

As is true for all treatments, medical and non-medical alike, no one approach benefits all patients equally. This has led to the search for variables that can predict or are associated with clinical outcome. The following have surfaced as tentative predictors of enhanced treatment response (they are labelled as 'tentative'

because they have yet to be cross-validated/replicated in varied settings and by different investigators): greater externalizing behaviour (acting out, impulse control), psychosomatic distress, home practice, unhappiness at home and/or at school and headache severity; lesser age, chronicity and maternal reinforcement of illness behaviour.[41-43]

Health-care costs continue to increase and treatments such as biofeedback can become quite expensive. In published studies, patients are typically seen in 8–12 one-hour individual sessions. In clinical practice, complicated cases may remain in treatment even longer. As a way of controlling costs, investigators working with adult headache patients have begun to explore more cost-effective and cost-competitive ways to administer treatments. The two primary approaches have been group administration[44] and home-based or minimal-contact delivery.[45,46] The typical reduced-contact treatment involves only three to five office visits, with treatment supplemented by written training manuals and audio-cassettes to use in home instruction. In addition to saving time and money, there are many theoretical and practical advantages to such an approach and few disadvantages.[47] Pilot investigations with child migraineurs suggest that autogenic feedback may work equally well when delivered in a reduced-contact mode, with either the child or the parent serving as the main treatment agent for the home instruction.[48] The therapist's skill level may become increasingly important, as time with the patient is reduced. Andrasik et al[49] review various factors that need consideration when selecting biofeedback therapists (such as training level, credentials, personal characteristics, etc.). Biofeedback therapists can be characterized as 'general practice (GP) biofeedback clinicians' or 'biofeedback specialists'.[50,51] The GP biofeedback clinician is the most common in practice settings, and this therapist is typically familiar with EMG, thermal and electrodermal approaches for reducing excess physiological arousal. This is fortunate because these are by far the most common biofeedback approaches for childhood headache. EEG and Doppler biofeedback would fall into the realm of the biofeedback specialist and such therapists are far fewer in number and much less available.

## Conclusion

Varied biofeedback approaches are available for children and adolescents who experience recurrent migraine and tension-type headaches. Biofeedback treatments receiving the greatest empirical support at present are thermal/autogenic feedback and EMG biofeedback. Other treatments show promise (BVP, Doppler and CNV biofeedback). Although comparative data are limited, meta-analysis suggests that biofeedback treatment can rival outcomes obtained for medication. Improvements appear to exceed those found when similar procedures are applied to adults. A number of variables have been tentatively identified as predictors of treatment response. However, further research, investigating patient–treatment interactions, behavioural–pharmacological interactions and sequencing effects, varied modes of administration, the role of co-morbid conditions and setting effects (clinic vs research laboratory) is clearly needed. Consideration of developmental aspects is warranted as well.

## References

1. Olson RP, Definitions of biofeedback and applied psychophysiology. In: Schwartz MS et al, eds, *Biofeedback: A practitioner's guide*, 2nd edn. New York: Guilford, 1995: 27–31.
2. Schwartz MS, Olson RP, A historical perspective on the field of biofeedback and applied psychophysiology. In: Schwartz MS et al, eds, *Biofeedback: A practitioner's guide*, 2nd edn. New York: Guilford, 1995: 3–18.
3. Engel BT, Operant conditioning of cardiac function: A status report. *Psychophysiology* 1972; **9**: 161–77.
4. Harris AH, Brady JV, Animal learning-visceral and autonomic conditioning. *Annu Rev Psychol* 1974; **25**: 107–33.
5. Kamiya J, Operant control of the EEG alpha rhythm and some of its reported effects on consciousness. In: Tart CT, ed., *Altered States of Consciousness: A book of readings*. New York: Wiley, 1969: 507–15.
6. Kimmel HO, Instrumental conditioning of autonomically mediated responses behavior. *Psychol Bull* 1967; **67**: 337–45.

7. Kristt DA, Engel BT, Learned control of blood pressure inpatients with high blood pressure. *Circulation* 1975; **51**: 370–8.

8. Miller NE, Learning of visceral and glandular responses. *Science* 1969; **163**: 434–45.

9. Miller NE, DiCara L, Instrumental learning of heart rate changes in curarized rats: Shaping and specificity to discriminative stimulus. *J Comparative Physiol Psychol* 1967; **63**: 12–19.

10. Shapiro D, Tursky B, Schwartz GE, Differentiation of heart rate and systolic blood pressure in man by operant conditioning. *Psychosom Med* 1970; **32**: 417–23.

11. Surwit RS, Shapiro E, Feld JL, Digital temperature autoregulation and associated cardiovascular changes. *Psychophysiology* 1976; **13**: 242–8.

12. Sargent JD, Green EE, Walters ED, The use of autogenic feedback training in a pilot study of migraine and tension headaches. *Headache* 1972; **12**: 120–4.

13. Schultz JH, Luthe W, *Autogenic Training*, vol. 1. New York: Grune & Stratton, 1969.

14. Dalessio DJ, Kunzel M, Sternbach R, Sovak M, Conditioned adaptation-relaxation in migraine therapy. *JAMA* 1979; **242**: 2102–4.

15. Gauthier J, Bois R, Allaire D, Drolet M, Evaluation of skin temperature biofeedback training at two different sites for migraine. *J Behav Med* 1981; **4**: 407–19.

16. Sovak M, Kunzel M, Sternbach RA, Dalessio DJ, Is volitional manipulation of hemodynamics a valid rationale for biofeedback therapy of migraine? *Headache* 1978; **18**: 197–202.

17. Tunis MM, Wolff HG, Analysis of cranial artery pulse waves in patients with vascular headache of the migraine type. *Am J Med Sci* 1952; **244**: 565–8.

18. Friar LR, Beatty I, Migraine: Management by trained control of vasoconstriction. *J Consult Clin Pyschol* 1976; **44**: 46–53.

19. Sartory G, Müller B, Metsch J, Pothmann R, A comparison of psychological and pharmacological treatment of pediatric migraine. *Behav Res Therapy* 1998; **36**: 1155–70.

20. Andrasik F, Gerber WD, Relaxation, biofeedback, and stress-coping therapies. In: Olesen J, Tfelt-Hansen P, Welch KMA, eds, *The Headaches*. New York: Raven, 1993: 833–41.

21. Friberg L, Olesen J, Iversen HK, Sperling B, Migraine pain associated with middle cerebral artery dilatation: Reversal by sumatriptan. *Lancet* 1991; **338**: 13–17.

22. Siniatchkin M, Hierundar A, Kropp P, Kuhnert R, Gerber WD, Stephani U, Self-regulation of slow cortical potentials in children with migraine: An exploratory study. *Appl Psychophysiol Biofeedback* 2000; **25**: 13–32.

23. Budzynski T, Stoyva J, Adler C, Feedback-induced relaxation: Application to tension headache. *J Behav Exp Psychiatry* 1970; **1**: 205–11.

24. Andrasik F, Assessment of patients with headaches. In: Turk DC, Melzack R, eds, *Handbook of Pain Assessment*, 2nd edn. New York: Guilford Press, 2001; 454–74.

25. Andrasik F, Holroyd KA, A test of specific and nonspecific effects in the biofeedback treatment of tension headache. *J Consult Clin Psychol* 1980; **48**: 575–86.

26. Andrasik F, Holroyd KA, Specific and non-specific effects in the biofeedback treatment of tension headache: 3-year follow-up. *J Consult Clin Psychol* 1983; **51**: 634–6.

27. Holroyd KA, Penzien DB, Hursey KG et al, Change mechanisms in EMG biofeedback training: Cognitive changes underlying improvements in tension headache. *J Consult Clin Psychol* 1984; **52**: 1039–53.

28. Bandura A, *Self-efficacy: The exercise of control*. New York: WH Freeman, 1997.

29. Hermann C, Kim M, Blanchard EB, Behavioral and prophylactic pharmacological intervention studies of pediatric migraine: An exploratory meta-analysis. *Pain* 1995; **20**: 239–56.

30. Task Force on Promotion and Dissemination of Psychological Procedures, Training in and dissemination of empirically-validated psychological treatments: Report and recommendations. *Clin Psychol* 1995; **48**: 3–23.

31. Holden EW, Deichmann MM, Levy JD, Empirically supported treatments in pediatric psychology: Recurrent pediatric headache. *J Pediatr Psychol* 1999; **24**: 91–109.

32. Bussone G, Grazzi L, D'Amico D, Leone M, Andrasik F, Biofeedback-assisted relaxation

training for young adolescents with tension-type headache: A controlled study. *Cephalalgia* 1998; **18**: 463–7.

33. Grazzi L, Andrasik F, D'Amico D, Leone M, Moschiano F, Bussone G, Electromyographic biofeedback-assisted relaxation training in juvenile episodic tension-type headache: Clinical outcome at three-year follow-up. *Cephalalgia* in press.

34. Kröner-Herwig B, Mohn U, Pothmann R, Comparison of biofeedback and relaxation in the treatment of pediatric headache and the influence of parent involvement on outcome. *Appl Psychophysiol Biofeedback* 1998; **23**: 143–57.

35. Sarafino EP, Goehring P, Age comparisons in acquiring biofeedback control and success in reducing headache pain. *Ann Behav Med* 2000; **22**: 10–16.

36. Attanasio V, Andrasik F, Burke EJ, Blake DD, Kabela E, McCarran MS, Clinical issues in utilizing biofeedback with children. *Clin Biofeedback Health* 1985; **8**: 134–41.

37. Green JA, Biofeedback therapy with children. In: Rickles WH, Sandweiss JH, Jacobs D, Grove RN, eds, *Biofeedback and Family Practice Medicine*. New York: Plenum, 1983: 121–44.

38. Blanchard EB, Andrasik F, Neff DF et al, Sequential comparisons of relaxation training and biofeedback in the treatment of three kinds of chronic headache or the machines may be necessary some of the time. *Behav Res Therapy* 1982; **20**: 469–81.

39. Marcon RA, Labbé EE, Assessment and treatment of children's headaches from a developmental perspective. *Headache* 1990; **30**: 586–92.

40. Allen KD, Shriver MD, Role of parent-mediated pain behavior management strategies in biofeedback treatment of childhood migraines. *Behavior Therapy* 1998; **29**: 477–90.

41. Andrasik F (1999, September). Biofeedback training in childhood headache. Invited presentation at the IVth International Congress on Headache in Childhood and Adolescence. Turku, Finland.

42. Hermann C, Blanchard EB, Flor H, Biofeedback treatment for pediatric migraine: Prediction of treatment outcome. *J Consult Clin Psychol* 1997; **65**: 611–16.

43. Larsson B, Recurrent headaches in children and adolescents. In: McGrath PJ, Finley GA, eds, *Chronic and Recurrent Pain in Children and Adolescents*, vol. 13. Seattle, WA: IASP Press, 1999: 115–40.

44. Napier D, Miller C, Andrasik F, Group treatment for recurrent headache. *Adv Med Psychother* 1997; **9**: 21–31.

45. Rowan AB, Andrasik F, Efficacy and cost-effectiveness of minimal therapist contact treatments of chronic headaches: A review. *Behavior Therapy* 1996; **27**: 207–34.

46. Haddock C, Rowan AB, Andrasik F, Wilson PG, Talcott GW, Stein RJ, Home-based behavioral treatments for chronic benign headache: A meta-analysis of controlled trials. *Cephalalgia* 1997; **17**: 113–18.

47. Andrasik F, Behavioral management of migraine. *Biomed Pharmacother* 1996; **50**: 52–7.

48. Burke EJ, Andrasik F, Home- vs. clinic-based biofeedback treatment for pediatric migraine: Results of treatment through one-year follow-up. *Headache* 1989; **29**: 434–40.

49. Andrasik F, Oyama ON, Packard RC, Biofeedback therapy for migraine. In: Diamond S, ed., *Migraine Headache Prevention and Management*. New York: Marcel Dekker, 1990: 213–38.

50. Andrasik F, Biofeedback. In: Mostofsky DI, Barlow DH, eds, *The Management of Stress and Anxiety in Medical Disorders*. Needham Heights, MA: Allyn & Bacon, 2000: 66–83.

51. Andrasik F, Blanchard EB, Applications of biofeedback to therapy. In: Walker CE, ed., *Handbook of Clinical Psychology: Theory, Research and Practice*. Homewood, IL: Dorsey, 1983: 1123–64.

# 27

# Psychotherapy

*Federica Galli, Vincenzo Guidetti, Antonio Pascotto, Francesca Tagliente*

All mental processes are biological, and therefore any alteration in those processes is necessarily organic.

Kandel (1998)[1]

Anatomical changes in the brain occur throughout life and are likely to shape the skills and character of an individual. The representation of body parts in the sensory and motor area of the cerebral cortex depends on their use, and, thus, the particular experience of the individual.

Does therapy work in this way? If so, where does these psychotherapeutically induced changes occur?

The mind will be to the biology of twenty-first century what gene has been to the biology of the twentieth century.

Kandel (1999)[2]

The role of psychological factors in relation to headache has been widely discussed (see Chapter 6). However, in spite of the unquestionable role of psychological factors in influencing headache crises, little is known about the aetiopathogenic relationship, the mechanisms involved, the direction of influence or the probable diverse associations according to different headache subtypes.[3,4] To date we can say that there is a relationship between psychological factors, even though much must be done in the direction of giving sound, evidence-based explanations. The role of psychological factors does not exclude the somatic point of view, in the sense that emotional factors may lead to the activation of biological–physiological pathways, triggering headache crises. Psychotherapy may be seen as working on the emotional factors, helping the patients to unwind motives of psychological distress by different channels from the body's way. Psychotherapy is clearly an indirect way to help patients cope with head pain. Obviously, we will be able to draw together all the consequences for both diagnosis and therapy only when supported by evidence-based findings. The main objective is to give each patient the most appropriate therapy, considering not only the clinical features of headache, but the mutual interplay of the co-morbid conditions, emotional triggering factors, individual pharmacogenic characteristics, etc.

These considerations substantiate the attention given to psychotherapy, starting from the developmental age.

From another point of view, non-pharmacological treatment of childhood or adolescence headache should not be seen as an alternative to the pharmacological one, and the choice of the best 'dosage' of both should be tailored according to the individual specificities.

Helping the patient to overcome the symptoms of headache, is an important part of our work.[5] Since the initial steps of the diagnostic process, attention should be dedicated to the recognition of triggering factors and the psychological ones. In a broad sense, this may represent the first step of the psychotherapeutic process, sometimes (after a complete psychodiagnostic assessment) with a proper indication for psychotherapy (individual or family). Focusing attention on psychological triggering factors may represent a valid aid in this and in the general management of headache.

From yet another point of view, the psychological work may assume different meanings. During childhood, the culture of a correct drug intake assumes preventive significance. Analgesic drug overuse may predispose to the chronicization of headache with symptomatic drug dependence and refractoriness to prophylactic medication.[6] Adult patients with chronic daily headache frequently refer the onset of headache back to their infancy or adolescence. In adults the role of analgesic overuse has been stressed in the exacerbation and maintenance of headaches over time.[6–11] However, even in childhood the occurrence of 'rebound headache' has been described.[12]

As the youngster ages, the prevention of drug overuse should be pursued as part of the general management, raising awareness in the parents and, when possible, the patient.

# Types of psychotherapy in children and adolescents

The concept of psychotherapy is a general term to indicate the psychic way of solving problems. It is an umbrella term, but additional specifications should clarify the theoretical models of reference (psychoanalysis, psychodynamic, cognitive–behavioural, systemic) and the typology of the main target (individual, couple, family, group), taking into consideration that each model may not have a unique target and may over time have enlarged it (e.g. from family focused to the individual – the systemic model). Most psychotherapies start from clinical work and observations, and the scientific basis is far from being achieved, even though there is ongoing verification of the outcome and comparative attempts between different theoretical models and techniques.[13] Epistemological questions arise from such efforts, and questions about the applicability of scientific criteria drawn from 'hard science' have been progressively brought to the attention of this field, as should the case for any method of research that ensures a scientific status. The basic equipment of any valid research should be the ability to replicate the observation, the possibility of quantification, procedures for the construction of facts (observations must be confirmable by different qualified observers), the possibility of prediction, falsifiability,[14] and unambiguous terminology.

Early forms of therapy for childhood were borrowed from adult treatment models. More recently, there has been a recognition of the need to design treatments from a child-based perspective. Consequently, several forms of psychological interventions designed specifically for children and youth have been developed and evaluated. The importance of parental involvement has also been recognized in these treatment innovations. However, a number of developmental factors have yet to be given adequate consideration in both the research and practice of childhood treatment. A number of approaches are available for childhood psychotherapy. The indication of the best treatment is mainly through personal experience, and attempts to give the best psychotherapy according to the individual characteristics is still in the embryonic stages, even though studies in this direction are advancing.

We are just at the start of understanding the biological effects of psychotherapeutic work, even though hypotheses start to arise at this level,[2] giving elements that support the scientific basis of psychotherapy.

## Psychoanalysis and the psychodynamic model

The psychoanalytical treatment of children evolved as an application of psychoanalytic therapy with adults. Forays into child treatment were attempted early in the evolution of psychoanalysis, such as Sigmund Freud's[15] own treatment of little Hans via the child's father, Ferenczi's[16] single consultation with Arpad, a 5-year-old boy who was obsessed with and phobic about chickens, and Hug-Helmuth's[17] more systematic treatment of children, using drawings and games. However, it was not until the late 1920s that child psychoanalysis became established under the guidance of two pioneers – Melanie Klein[18] and Anna Freud[19] – whose respective influences continue to dominate the field after well over half a century. Klein argued that play is the natural mode of expression for children and that the patients symbolize their inner wishes, fears and internalized relationships through this medium. Play is therefore a suitable substitute for the free association of adults. Finally, Klein[19] insisted on strict neutrality on the part of the analyst, who had to refrain from reassurance, guidance or any deviation

from supply-only interpretations. The analyst could participate in a game at the child's request, but must keep participation to the barest minimum.

Perhaps, the more pertinent characteristics of analysis of children, which reveal the disparity of Freud's system from that of Klein's, are Freud's questioning whether a child can really free associate. Freud also differs from Klein in regarding control of speech as a prerequisite for child psychoanalysis; she did not therefore recommend this form of treatment for very young children.

Psychodynamic psychotherapy is a derivative of psychoanalysis, and it is often difficult to differentiate from analytical therapy, particularly when considering the modifications in technique suggested by Freud. In psychodynamic psychotherapy, the play of a young child and the drawings of an older child are viewed as the patient's manner of revealing his or her total life situation. Children not only project their inner life into the play activity, they also reveal their reality situation. Play does not use unconscious drives or superego sanctions, but is a child's mode of communicating the totality of his or her current life. A frequently used therapeutic technique is 'the squiggle game', created by D Winnicott as a means to facilitate the child's expression of feelings or thoughts. This technique consists of exchanging drawings between the therapist and the child, with each drawing initiated by the other person's initial 'squiggle'. The therapist starts the game by drawing a straight, curved, serpentine or zig-zag line, and the child has to turn the squiggle into a drawing. He or she is then invited to comment on it. Then the roles are reversed: the child makes the squiggle and the therapist completes it. Each drawing can be used to tell a story or may stimulate questions. The game can continue as long as it is productive and enjoyable. Often, after many drawings, a child may start to feel more comfortable and spontaneously describe his or her internal psychic life. Winnicott believed that the squiggle game can facilitate the formation of a trusting relationship and shorten the initial period of therapy when a child may play in the presence of the therapist, but does not interact or exchange meaningful material.[20]

Attempts to verify and 'quantify' the effectiveness of psychoanalytical psychotherapies in scientific terms (e.g. outcome studies) are growing[21–29] with good results, even if we are far from sound evidence.

The implication of emotional factors in headache sufferers has been extensively outlined in the literature on psychodynamic orientation, paying particular attention to the conflict of aggression[30–33] (for a review see Karwautz et al[34]).

However, the lack of evidence-based findings on a cause–effect relationship and psychophysiological explanations of headache and emotional factors weakens the scientific basis of the work, in order to support the indication for a psychodynamic psychotherapy. In spite of the fact that psychoanalytical theory of pain via behaviourally oriented theories is now in decline,[34] we outline the importance of the integration of the two perspectives in the treatment of headache, searching for the likely resources that each model may give to any patient.

Probably, the patient's difficulties in modulation and recognition of his or her own emotional state and feelings, concomitant anxiety and mood disorders, and the consequent 'choice' of a body way of communicating the inner state could suggest the implementation of a psychodynamic psychotherapy.

# Behavioural model

This model consists of an approach towards treatment that emphasizes the empirical evaluation of clinical problems. When behaviour modification first emerged as a formal movement in the 1950s, the focus of treatment on overt behaviour, the absence of concern about presumed aetiology and the rejection of intrapsychic determinants were a few of the characteristics promoted.[35] Many of these characteristics were proposed as a reaction to prevailing views of intrapsychic, psychodynamic forces.

An assumption of behaviour therapy is that behaviours, when of interest in the context of therapeutic, educational, social and other settings, can be altered by providing new learning experiences. Consequently, the approach has drawn heavily on learning theories and research in psychology. Behavioural treatments essentially provide special learning experiences to alter deviant or clinically maladaptive behaviour and to increase adaptive behaviour. Treatment is conceptualized as learning new behaviours which have to be performed in everyday life. Activities in which learning needs to take place serve as the basis for developing new behaviours. The vast range of intervention techniques within behaviour therapy is the result of diverse conceptual views, and the varied clinical problems and child and adolescent populations to which they are applied.

## Distraction

Children aged less than 6 years respond well to distraction techniques such as blowing bubbles and video games, whereas those aged over 6 years engage well in external or abstract interventions, such as guided imagery, and counting and breathing techniques.

## Suggestion

Children are susceptible to the power of suggestion, which makes the 'magic glove' technique especially effective. An imaginary glove is placed on a child's hand, finger by finger, where a procedure is to be performed. The basic principles of these cognitive strategies include willingness to be involved, trust in the coach, and the ability to have enough strength and energy to participate.[36]

## Breathing techniques

Two types of breathing can be used. Rhythmic, deep-chest breathing is performed by taking in slow breaths through the nose and exhaling through the mouth. Patterned, shallow breathing consists of shallow breaths in through the nose and out through the mouth. Younger children benefit from patterned, shallow breathing using their own images to think about, such as a train. They are instructed to take two shallow nose inhalations and mouth exhalations and, on the second one, to say 'toot' like a train while breathing out. The pattern and noise require the concentration and attention of the children, thereby taking their minds away from pain. Older children may like to use the rhythmic, deep-chest breathing while they are reminded to relax and 'push the tenseness out'.

## Guided imagery

Guided imagery is a form of relaxed, focused concentration that can be used as a coping mechanism for pain problems. Guided imagery tapes, such as a mix of new age music, meditative exercises and positive thinking, are being used with good results in adult patients. Children can be encouraged, often by nurses, psychologists or child-life specialists trained in imagery, to imagine being in their favourite places and imagine doing their favourite activity.

## Progressive muscle relaxation

Progressive muscle relaxation is designed to help children to recognize and reduce body tension associated with pain and to decrease anxiety and discomfort. Learning to decrease body tension is an acquired skill, and relaxation training requires frequent practice to be successful. This skill is often taught by psychologists and physiotherapists or occupational therapists. Rules for practice require that it be done in a quiet, relaxing place. Children can be taught to tense and relax different muscle groups, starting with the hands and feet, and moving centrally from the arms and legs to the shoulders, neck, chest, abdomen, etc.[37]

## Biofeedback

Biofeedback uses instruments to detect and amplify specific physical states in the body, which usually we do not notice and help bring them under our voluntary control.

# Family therapy

Family theory focuses on human behaviour and psychiatric disturbances in the context of interpersonal relationships.[36] This theory forms the basis of family therapy, which is an umbrella term for a number of clinical practices that treat psychopathology within the family system rather than in individuals. Interventions are designed to effect change in family relationships rather than in an individual.[39-42]

Family theory considers the family as an interpersonal system with cybernetic qualities.

The relationships among the components of the system are non-linear (or circular) and the interactions are cyclical rather than causative.

A person's problems cannot be evaluated or treated apart from the context in which they occur and the functions that they serve. It is assumed, therefore, that an individual cannot be expected to change unless the family system changes.[43]

For a more detailed theoretical and clinical analysis of the issues related to the family therapy see Chapter 35.

# Group therapy

Children and adolescents live, play, study and work with peers in numerous group settings. Group treatment offers unique opportunities and challenges to use these everyday group processes to therapeutic advantage. A large variety of group treatment approaches is available for work with children. Group therapy simulates aspects of the family and school environment and closely approximates a child's daily experiences and challenges. Groups for children may be classified by various dimensions, such as theoretical framework and technique, group composition, goals, physical setting or treatment duration.

Activity group therapy is a psychoanalytically oriented, non-directive, non-interpretative, small-group treatment in which four to eight latency-age children are seen for 2 years or more.[44] To be eligible for this type of group therapy, children must have the potential to relate to others and the ability to change attitudes and conduct through corrective experiences. The types of problems treated with activity group therapy include withdrawal, constriction, anxiety, social fears, overprotection and mildly disordered behaviours.

Interpretative group psychotherapy involves facilitating conflicts, defences and fantasies via play and verbalization. An interpretative model is appropriate for latency-age children with psychosomatic symptoms, anxiety, intense sibling rivalry or behavioural disturbances.[45]

Short-term treatment emphasizes patient strengths and avoids excessive dependence. Diagnostic groups were an early form of short-term therapy conceived by Redl.[46] A series of group diagnostic contacts may be useful to observe in-group behaviour, provide intrinsic therapeutic value and avoid the artificiality of the dyadic interview. Whereas heterogeneous groups may be preferred for long-term intensive therapy, homogeneous groups are advantageous when the goal is specifically short-term support or symptomatic relief. Homogeneous groups attain cohesion more rapidly, have less conflict and offer more immediate support.

# Hypnosis

The history of psychotherapy preceding the use of hypnosis abounds with dramatic reports of healing disabling symptoms by ceremonies that change the state of consciousness in the patient. This healing was believed in past centuries to result from a spiritual leader invoking divine intervention. Efforts to conceptualize these phenomena in more secular, scientific terms led to a variety of formulations during the eighteenth and nineteenth centuries and to the emergence of the term 'hypnosis' to describe them.[47]

Hypnosis is a state in which the individual is able to respond to appropriate suggestions by experiencing changes of perception, memory or mood. It is implicit that overt behaviour (as in a hypnotic induction procedure) may be one useful indicator of the trance state, but this indicator requires associated enquiry into the subjective experience of the patient to document the existence of a trance state.

Furthermore, when hypnosis is applied in a clinical setting, transference is of relevance. This refers to the patient's tendency to elaborate subjectively on the therapy transaction, based on life experiences as well as hopes and expectations about the therapy relationship. In contrast to the psychoanalytical approach, hypnosis actively, and by detracting, exploits the therapeutic leverage inherent in the transference with a view to expediting therapeutic change.[48–50]

Hypnosis, in the hand of enthusiastic proponents, has been used to treat a wide array of psychiatric and medical disorders in children and adolescents, as documented by Olness and Kohen.[51]

## Psychological treatments and headache

A wide range of behavioural and cognitive techniques has been found to be efficacious for helping children to cope with acute pain. The methods typically involve the use of many areas of expertise to manage pain. The integration of different forms of pain management, including education, relaxation techniques and biofeedback to the standard methods, may improve the management of children with acute pain. New directions in the non-drug treatment of childhood headache are related to new insight in the field.

An initial study draws therapeutic implications about the role of sleep in migraine sufferers (see Chapter 32), showing that indications for correct sleep hygiene bring a high improvement in headache crises.[52]

An exploratory study[53] on the probable therapeutic implications of increased amplitudes of slow cortical potentials in migrainous children[54,55] gives preliminary evidence of clinical efficacy, meriting further investigations.

Studies on psychological stress-management treatments have been shown to be efficacious and are often preferred because of the reluctance on the part of adolescents and parents to use daily prophylactic medication. Psychological treatments most often involve stress reduction by teaching coping strategies with muscle relaxation or hypnosis and other behavioural and cognitive strategies.[56,57] Labbe and Williamson[58] compared the effects of autogenic feedback in a waiting-list control group and in 28 children with migraine aged between 7 and 16 years. Using a criterion of 50% reduction in headaches as clinical improvement, 93% of the autogenic group had improved at the end of treatment and the 1-month follow-up.

Fentress et al[59] randomly assigned 18 children with migraine between the ages of 8 and 12 years to one of three groups: relaxation–response, relaxation–response plus biofeedback, and waiting-list control. The result for the two active treatment groups were superior to those for the control group.

A randomized controlled trial was undertaken to evaluate the efficacy and efficiency of a predominantly self-administered treatment: 87 adolescents ranging in age from 11 to 18 years were randomly assigned to receive a self-administered treatment, the same treatment delivered by a therapist or a control treatment. The self-administered treatment was substantially more efficient.[60]

Biofeedback has been especially useful in

children and adolescents with migraine and in patients wishing to avoid the use of medication. Both muscle relaxation training using electromyographic (EMG) feedback and thermal regulation using hand warming have been successful.

When family stress is a contributing factor, family counselling has been shown to be useful.[61,62]

Work carried out in school settings and in paediatric outpatient clinics for children and adolescents with migraine and functional headaches has shown that tension-type headaches can be improved by relaxation training. In a number (not all) of studies of adolescents, this has been shown to be superior to the placebo and effective if administered both at the clinic and as a home-based self-administered treatment.[63,64]

Hermann et al[65] located 38 behavioural treatment trials with a group design, which they included in their meta-analysis of effective size. After eliminating outliers, they found that thermal biofeedback had the greatest effect size, which was similar to that of combined thermal biofeedback and relaxation training, but significantly greater than that of relaxation training alone. In a study of 43 children migraine sufferers, relaxation and stress-management training reduced the headache index (frequency × intensity of headache episodes) more effectively than metoprolol with biofeedback and stress-management training in between.[66]

In another study of 30 children with headache, clinical improvement was greatest in the biofeedback group (80%), followed by the relaxation group (50%), with no relief in the group with no therapy. Migraine and tension-type headache improved with relaxation and biofeedback; these benefits are long lasting and are still present 10 years after completion of the training.[67]

Bussone et al[68] reported that combined EMG biofeedback/relaxation training was more effective than relaxation placebo in reducing episodic tension-type headaches in patients aged 11–15 years; notably, the relative benefits of biofeedback training were most evident at 6-month and 12-follow-up evaluations.[67]

In another study, McGrath et al[64] evaluated the effectiveness of relaxation training in the treatment of childhood migraine, in a total of 99 children and adolescents. Relaxation training was compared with two control groups: placebo and 'own best effort'. Relaxation training consisted of a series of six individual, 1-hour, weekly sessions with a therapist. The children were taught sequential tensing and relaxation of large muscle groups and the use of deep breathing to achieve total body relaxation. They were then taught sequential relaxation without tensing.

Placebo treatment consisted of six individual, 1-hour, weekly sessions with a therapist, in which children were taught to recognize and label their emotions, to relate them to their life situation and to discuss their feelings daily with a friend or a parent. 'Own best effort' treatment consisted of a single session to discuss the use of the headache diary to determine what was triggering the migraine attacks. In all three treatment groups, patients showed a significant reduction in headaches, but relaxation training was not found to be superior in reducing headache compared with the other two forms of treatment.

The above findings suggest the general efficacy of non-drug therapy for headache sufferers from a young age, even though scientific trials must necessarily deal with several obstacles. First, changing the clinical characteristics and the tendency to spontaneous remission of childhood headache (both migraine and tension-type) have been well documented,[67,69,70] and we should consider analysing the long-term efficacy of any intervention. Second, the probable implication of placebo effect in the short and medium term should always be considered, before drawing conclusions. Third, the fact that patients attending specialty centres are 'self-selected patients' (the so-called Berkson's bias), with peculiar personality characteristics and/or environmental (familial, social) factors leading or predisposing to headache improvement, should also be taken into consideration.

## Conclusion

Why, when, which psychotherapy for headache patients? These three key questions have led our discussion on psychotherapy for headache sufferers. However, it is difficult to draw clear-cut conclusions, inasmuch as the same psychotherapy is in search of answers for similar questions within its field to avoid problems of auto-reference (Which are the cross factors explaining the efficacy of different psychotherapy? Which is the best psychotherapy for different problems? How to verify the outcomes in scientific terms?, etc.).

Probably, such environmental factors may modulate or even alter the gene expression (phenotype), because the psychological intervention by psychotherapy may produce effects in biological terms (producing changes in gene expression?), giving elements of analysis and explanation beyond simply speculative points of view (for a review see Kandel[2]). Psychoanalysis (or other psychotherapy approaches) may be seen as successful, bringing significant and persistent changes in personal attitudes, conscious and unconscious behaviours, habits, etc. Biological, structural modifications in the brain probably correspond with these changes. Challenges for the immediate future will be finding the matched changes, and monitoring them by imaging techniques (as Kandel hypothesizes[2]).

In the headache field, there is general agreement that psychological factors are important, even if there are few carefully controlled trials to demonstrate the effectiveness of psychological management in general and the comparative merits of the various forms of treatment employed. However, many areas need further investigations to provide evidence that therapies work well. What is known now suggests that the use of these adjunctive methods of pain management may complement pharmacological pain management, bringing physicians closer to the optimal care of children with pain.[72,73]

Our knowledge about the management of children with headache is based largely on clinical reports, but a number of open trials and methodologically stronger studies are progressively showing that headache can respond to psychological treatments. However, further studies on this issue are essential, mainly during the developmental age, inasmuch as fewer treatment trials have been carried out in children compared with adults with migraine. However, the studies of the long-term efficacy of non-drug treatment must deal with the tendency towards spontaneous remission of headache with onset in childhood.[67,69,70]

There are no sound evidence-based data in the literature about other forms of psychological interventions (in particular psychotherapy) in children and adolescents with migraine or tension-type headache. In particular, we stress the lack of controlled studies on psychodynamic and family therapy for headache sufferers, considering particularly their anecdotal and experiential use.

Our clinical experience shows that psychodynamic-oriented or family therapy can be useful in improving headache, even more so if used in association with a pharmacological approach. It depends on the specificity of the case. Only after a complete psychological assessment are we able to decode the likely meanings of 'that headache' in 'that patient' within his or her familial and social context, and so decide on the best therapy, e.g. we can say that the occurrence of headache and psychiatric co-morbidity, problems in school achievement and peer relationship, sleep problems, somatization and psychopathology in siblings and the whole family of the patient should push for psychotherapy, although there is still a lot of experiential and clinical intuition involved. The challenge will be to find scientific criteria for tailoring the best psychotherapy for each patient, according to age, type and history of headache, psychiatric co-morbidity, psychosocial characteristics, etc.

# References

1. Kandel ER, A new intellectual framework for psychiatry. *Am J Psychiatry* 1998; **155**: 457–69.
2. Kandel ER, Biology and the future of psychoanalysis: A new intellectual framework for psychiatry – revisited. *Am J Psychiatry* 1999; **156**: 505–24.
3. Galli F, Guidetti V, Psychiatric comorbidity. *Semin Headache Manage* 1997; **2**: 4.
4. Guidetti V, Galli F, Fabrizi P et al, Headache and psychiatric comorbidity: clinical aspects and outcome in an 8-year follow-up study. *Cephalalgia* 1998; **18**: 455–62.
5. Lance JW, Goadsby PJ, Migraine: Treatment. In: Lance JW, Goadsb PJ, eds, *Mechanism and Management of Headache*, 6th edn. Oxford: Butterworth-Heinemann, 1998: 117–18.
6. Solomon S, Lipton RB, Newman LC, Clinical features of chronic daily headache. *Headache* 1992; **32**: 325–9.
7. Mathew NT, Stubits E, Nigam MR, Transformation of episodic migraine into daily headache: analysis of factors. *Headache* 1982; **22**: 66–8.
8. Mathew NT, Kurman R, Perez F, Drug induced refractory headache – clinical features and management. *Headache* 1990; **30**: 634–8.
9. Mathew NT, Chronic daily headache: clinical features and natural history. In: Nappi G, Bono G, Sandrini G, Martignoni E, Miceli G, eds, *Headache and Depression*. New York: Raven Press, 1991: 49–58.
10. Silberstein SD, Appropriate use of abortive medication in headache treatment. *Pain Manage* 1991; **4**: 22–8.
11. Silberstein SD, Tension-type and chronic daily headache. *Neurology* 1993; **43**: 1644–9.
12. Vasconcellos E, Piña-Garza JE, Millan EJ, Warner JS, Analgesic rebound headache in children and adolescence. *J Child Neurol* 1998; **13**: 443–7.
13. Fonagy P, The future of an empirical psychoanalysis. *Br J Psychother* 1996; **13**: 106.
14. Popper K, *The Logic of Scientific Discovery*. London: Routledge & Kegan Paul, 1959.
15. Freud S, Analysis of a phobia in a five-year-old boy (1909). In: Strachey J, ed., *The Standard Edition of the Complete Psychological Works of Sigmund Freud*. London: Hogarth Press, 1955: 1–149.
16. Ferenczi S, A little chanticleer (1913). In: Brunner R, ed., *Sex and Psychoanalysis*. New York, 1950: 240–52.
17. Hug-Helmuth H, On the technique of the analysis of children. *Int J Psychoanal* 1920; **1**: 361–2.
18. Klein M, *Psychoanalysis of Children*. London: Hogarth Press, 1932.
19. Freud A, *Normality and Pathology in Childhood: Assessments of Development*. New

York: International Universities Press, 1965.

20. Winnicott DW, *Therapeutic Consultation in Child Psychiatry*. New York: Basic Books, 1971.

21. DeWitt K, Wallerstein R, Scales of psychological capacities: measure of structural change. *Psychoanal Contemp Thought* 1999; **22**: 453–80.

22. Doidge N, Empirical evidence for the efficacy of psychoanalysis. *Psychoanal Inquiry* 1997; **17**(suppl): 102–50.

23. Gedo PM, Single case studies in psychotherapy research. *Psychoanal Psychol* 1999; **16**: 274–80.

24. Lepper G, Between science and hermeneutics: Towards a contemporary empirical approach to the study of interpretation in analytic psychotherapy. *Br J Psychother* 1996; **13**: 219.

25. Luborsky L, Luborsky E, The era of measures of transference: the CCRT and other measures. *J Am Psychoanal Assoc* 1993; **41**(suppl): 329–52.

26. Schachter J, Luborsky L, Who's afraid of psychoanalytic research? Analysts' attitudes. *Int J Psychoanal* 1998; **79**: 965–70.

27. Waldron S, How can we study the efficacy of psychoanalysis. *Psychoanal Q* 1997; **66**: 283–322.

28. Wallerstein R, The relation of theory to therapy: an alternative vision. *Psychoanal Inquiry* 1996; **16**: 491–507.

29. Wallerstein R, Fonagy P, Psychoanalysis research and IPA: history, present status, future potential. *Int J Psychoanal* 1999, **80**: 91–110.

30. Fromm-Reichmann F, Contribution to the psychogenesis of migraine. *Psychoanal Rev* 1937; **24**: 26–33.

31. Weber H, The psychological factors in migraine. *Br J Med Psychol* 1932; **12**: 151–73.

32. Sperling M, *Psychosomatic Disorders in Childhood*. New York: Jason Aronson, 1978.

33. Alexander F, *Psychosomatic Medicine*. New York: Norton, 1950.

34. Karwautz A, Wöber-Bingöl C, Wöber C, Freud and migraine: the beginning of psychodynamically oriented view of headache a hundred years ago. *Cephalalgia* 1996; **16**: 22–6.

35. Kazdin AE, *History of Behavior Modification: Experimental Foundations of Contemporary Research*. Baltimore: University Park Press, MD, 1978.

36. Kachoyeanos MK, Freidhoff M, Cognitive and behavioral strategies to reduce children's pain. *Maternal Child Nursing* 1993; **18**: 14–19.

37. Schecter NL, Berde CB, Yaster M, *Pain in Infants, Children and Adolescents*. Baltimore: Williams & Wilkins, 1993.

38. Lansky MR, Family therapy. In: Kaplan HI, Sadock BJ, eds, *Comprehensive Textbook of Psychiatry/V*, 5th edn, Vol 2. Baltimore: Williams & Wilkins, 1989: 1535–41.

39. Bell JE, *Family Therapy*. New York: Jason Aronson, 1975.

40. Minuchin S, *Families and Family Therapy*. Cambridge: Harvard University Press, 1974.

41. Olson DH, Marital and family therapy: integrative review and critique. *J Marriage Family* 1970; **32**: 501–38.

42. Shapiro R, Psychodynamic family therapy with children and adolescents. In: Sholevar GP, ed., *Treatment of Emotional Disorders in Children and Adolescents*. Jamaica: SP Medical and Scientific Books, 1986: 135–59.

43. Haley J, *Strategies of Psychotherapy*. New York: Grune & Stratton, 1963.

44. Slavson SR, Schiffer M, *Group Psychotherapies for Children: A Textbook*. New York: International Universities Press, 1975.

45. Schammess G, Differential diagnosis and group structure in the outpatient treatment of latency age children. In: Riester AE, Kraft IA, eds, Child *Group Therapy: Future tense*. Madison, CT: International Universities Press, 1986: 29–68.

46. Redl F, Diagnostic group work. *Am J Orthopsychiatry* 1944; **14**: 53–67.

47. Ellenberger HI, *The Discovery of the Unconscious*. New York: Basic Book, 1970.

48. Spiegel D, Hypnosis. In: Talbott J, Hales R, Yudofsky S, eds, *The American Psychiatric Press Textbook of Psychiatry*, 2nd edn. Washington: American Psychiatric Press, 1994: 1115–42.

49. Orne M, Dinges D, Bloom P, Hypnosis. In: Kaplan HI, Sadock B, eds, *Comprehensive Textbook of Psychiatry/VI*, 6th edn, Vol 2.

Baltimore: Williams & Wilkins, 1995: 1501–16.

50. Williams DT, Hypnosis. In: Kestenbaum CJ, Williams DT, eds, *Handbook of Clinical Assessment of Children and Adolescent*, Vol 2. New York: New York University Press, 1988: 1129–46.

51. Olness K, Kohen D, *Hypnosis and Hypnotherapy with Children*, 3rd edn. New York: Guilford Press, 1996.

52. Bruni O, Galli F, Guidetti V, Sleep hygiene and migraine in children and adolescents. *Cephalalgia* 1999; **19**(suppl 25): 57–9.

53. Siniatchkin M, Hierundar A, Kropp P et al, Self-regulation of slow cortical potentials in children with migraine: An exploratory study. *Appl Psychophysiol Biofeedback* 2000; **25**: 15–34.

54. Kropp P, Kirbach U, Detlefsen JO et al, Slow cortical potentials in migraine: a comparison of adults and children. *Cephalalgia* 1999; **19**(suppl 25): 60–4.

55. Siniatchkin M, Kropp P, Gerber WD, Stephani U, Migraine in childhood – are periodically occurring migraine attacks related to dynamic changes of cortical information processing? *Neurosci Lett* 2000; **279**(1): 1–4.

56. Richter IL, McGrath PJ Goodman JT, Firestone P, Keene D, Cognitive and relaxation treatment of pediatric migraine. *Pain* 1986; **25**: 195–203.

57. Olness K, MacDonald JT, Uden DL, Comparison of self hypnosis and propranolol in the treatment of juvenile classic migraine. *Pediatrics* 1987; **79**: 593–7.

58. Labbe EL, Williamson DA, Treatment of childhood migraine using autogenic feedback training, *J Consult Clin Psychol* 1984; **52**: 968–76.

59. Fentress DW, Masek BJ, Mehegan JE, Benson H, Biofeedback and relaxation-response training in the treatment of pediatric migraine. *Dev Med Child Neurol* 1986; **28**: 139–46.

60. MacGrath PJ, Humphreys P, Keene D et al, The efficacy and efficiency of a self-administered treatment for adolescent migraine. *Pain* 1992; **49**: 321–4.

61. Jensen VK, Rothner AD, Chronic nonprogressive headaches in children and adolescents. *Semin Pediatr Neurol* 1995; **2**: 151–8.

62. McGrath PJ, Reid GJ, Behavioral treatment of pediatric headache. *Pediatr Ann* 1995; **24**: 486–91.

63. Larsson B, Mellin L, The psychological treatment of recurrent headache in adolescents – short-term outcome and its prediction. *Headache* 1988; **28**: 187–95.

64. MacGrath PJ, Humphreys P, Goodman JT, Keene D, Fireston P, Jacob P, Cunningham SJ, Relaxation prophylaxis for childhood migraine: a randomized placebo-controlled trial. *Dev Med Child Neurol* 1988; **30**: 626–31.

65. Hermann C, Kim M, Blanchard EB, Behavioral and prophylactic pharmacological intervention studies of pediatric migraine: an exploratory meta-analysis. *Pain* 1995; **60**: 239–56.

66. Sartory G, Muller B, Metsch J, Pothmann, A comparison of psychological and pharmacological treatment of pediatric migraine. *Behav Res Ther* 1998; **36**: 1155–70.

67. Dooley J, Bagnell A, Prognosis and treatment of headache in children: a ten years follow-up. *Can J Neurol Sci* 1995; **22**: 47–9.

68. Bussone G, Grazzi L, D'Amico D, Leone M, Andrasik F, Biofeedback-assisted relaxation training for pediatric tension-type headache: a controlled study. *Cephalalgia* 1998; **18**: 463–7.

69. Prensky AL, Sommer D, Diagnosis and treatment of migraine in children. *Neurology* 1979; **29**: 506–10.

70. Guidetti V and Galli F, Evolution of headache in childhood and adolescence: an 8-year follow-up. *Cephalalgia* 1998; **18**: 452–4.

71. Rusy LM, Weisman SJ, Complementary therapies for acute pediatric pain. *Pediatr Clin North Am* 2000; **47**: 589–99.

72. Chen E, Joseph MH, Zeltzer LK, Behavioral and cognitive interventions in the treatment of pain in children. *Pediatr Clin North Am* 2000; **47**: 513–25.

# X

## Symptomatic headaches

# 28

## Symptomatic headaches
*George Russell (unless otherwise noted)*

Confronted by a child with headache, every paediatrician and primary care physician is aware that the differential diagnosis includes a wide variety of underlying conditions, many of potentially grave importance. In practice, such anxieties are for the most part unfounded. The great majority of chronic or recurrent headaches fall into one of the categories of primary headache, and most acute headaches, perhaps a greater source of anxiety, are related to minor though not necessarily easily diagnosed conditions.

Headache is a common symptom in otherwise healthy children. In a study of 1754 Aberdeen schoolchildren,[1] we found that two-thirds had had one or more headaches over the past year, a figure almost identical to that of 64% reported in a recent study from Finland.[2] In only one-third of these cases was the headache severe enough to interfere with normal activities, a borrowed but simple criterion for severity,[3] giving an overall incidence of severe headache over the past year of 22%. Primary headaches did not figure largely in the parental explanations offered for these headaches, migraine being the explanation in only 15% (although this figure increased once the children were interviewed and examined).

Intercurrent infection was thought to be the cause of one-third of these severe headaches, and trauma accounted for 5%. In almost half, the parents had no explanation to offer, or explained the headache on the basis of tiredness, hot weather, menstruation, lack of sleep, food intolerance or constipation. Clinical interview and examination of the children with severe headaches failed to uncover a single serious underlying disorder which might otherwise have been missed.

Nevertheless, headaches can on occasion reflect serious underlying pathology such as brain tumour, subdural haematoma or hypertension, and all children who present with otherwise unexplained headache must be carefully evaluated. Even in the presence of an apparently obvious diagnosis, a full examination will sometimes uncover unexpected pathology (see Case 1).

In a recent review of 288 children presenting to a paediatric emergency room with a main complaint of headache,[4] the principal diagnoses were as shown in Table 28.1. An important finding was that no case of brain tumour or bacterial meningitis was identified in children in whom headache was the presenting complaint. Nevertheless, in some children headache was associated with significant pathology – in particular, 15 cases (5.2%) had viral meningitis, and there were occasional cases of other intracranial pathologies.

In contrast, in an older study of 200 patients of all ages presenting to a primary care practice

| Diagnosis | % |
|---|---|
| Viral illness | 39.2 |
| Sinusitis | 16.0 |
| Migraine | 15.6 |
| Post-traumatic headache | 6.6 |
| Streptococcal pharyngitis | 4.9 |
| Tension headache | 4.5 |

**Table 28.1**
*Diagnosis in children presenting to an emergency department with headache as the primary complaint[4]*

with headache, Jerrett[5] found two children with brain tumours, a reminder that headache is by no means always a benign symptom.

From a practical point of view, it is helpful to divide headaches into two categories, those with and those without fever. Headache without fever may be due to trauma, vascular disorders, brain tumour and a variety of extracranial disorders such as temporo-mandibular joint dysfunction and cervicogenic headache. In contrast, headache with fever is almost always associated with infection, either intracranial or extracranial.

# Head injuries and intracranial haemorrhage

In the accident and emergency series already discussed in the Introduction to this section,[4] post-traumatic headache was the most common cause of secondary acute headache without fever. Although diagnoses made in hospital attendees do not necessarily reflect the prevalence of disease in the population from which they are drawn, in our own population-based study the most common cause of non-febrile secondary

headache was also trauma,[1] with an incidence during the previous year of 1.1%, similar to the figure of 2% reported from Finland.[2]

Head injuries are common in children, arising as the result of a wide variety of accidents and, occasionally, from non-accidental injury. In most cases, it is obvious that the child has been injured and, if there is a complaint of headache, that its origin is traumatic. However, this is not always the case, and even older children may give incomplete histories unless searching questions are asked (see Case 2). In some, failure to provide an accurate history reflects retrograde amnesia after injury.

## Post-traumatic headache

The term 'post-traumatic headache' is used to describe headaches that follow trauma, and are not otherwise classifiable. Minor head injuries frequently trigger pre-existing headache syndromes, particularly migraine (e.g. 'footballer's migraine' from heading the ball). Such cases should be classified according to the pre-existing headache type,[3] and trauma should be regarded as a triggering factor rather than the primary cause of the headache. Similarly, more severe head trauma may precipitate headache caused by subdural or epidural haematoma, in which headache is clearly symptomatic of the haematoma, and should be classified as such.

Head injuries are easily remembered, rather frightening occurrences, and it is likely that in many cases the relationship between the injury and the headache is more apparent than real. The term 'post-concussional headache' is frequently used to describe headaches that follow significant trauma from headaches after minor injury, and this appears to have been the thinking behind the International Headache Society (IHS)[3] classification presented in Table 28.2.

**1.** ***Acute post-traumatic headache***
*1.1  With significant head trauma and/or confirmatory signs*
*Diagnostic criteria:*
A.    Significance of head trauma documented by at least one of the following:
    1.  Loss of consciousness
    2.  Post-traumatic amnesia lasting more than 10 min
    3.  At least two of the following exhibit relevant abnormality: clinical neurological examination, radiograph of skull, neuroimaging, evoked potentials, spinal fluid examination, vestibular function test, neuropsychological testing
B.    Headache occurs less than 14 days after regaining consciousness (or after trauma, if there has been no loss of consciousness)
C.    Headache disappears within 8 weeks after regaining consciousness (or after trauma, if there has been no loss of consciousness)

*1.2  With minor head trauma and no confirmatory signs*
*Diagnostic criteria:*
A.    Head trauma that does not satisfy 1.1A
B.    Headache occurs less than 14 days after injury
C.    Headache disappears within 8 weeks after injury

**2.**  ***Chronic post-traumatic headache***
*2.1  With significant head trauma and/or confirmatory signs*
*Diagnostic criteria:*
B.    Significance of head trauma documented by at least one of the following:
    1.  Loss of consciousness
    2.  Post-traumatic amnesia lasting more than 10 min
    3.  At least two of the following exhibit relevant abnormality: clinical neurological examination, radiograph of skull, neuroimaging, evoked potentials, spinal fluid examination, vestibular function test, neuropsychological testing
C.    Headache occurs less than 14 days after regaining consciousness (or after trauma, if there has been no loss of consciousness)
D.    Headache continues more than 8 weeks after regaining consciousness (or after trauma, if there has been no loss of consciousness)

*2.2  With minor head trauma and no confirmatory signs*
*Diagnostic criteria:*
A.    Head trauma that does not satisfy 2.1A
B.    Headache occurs less than 14 days after injury
C.    Headache continues more than 8 weeks after injury

**Table 28.2**
*International Headache Society[3] classification of post-traumatic headache*

### Acute post-traumatic headache

Not surprisingly, trauma to the head is often followed by head pain. In most instances it is obvious that the trauma is responsible for the pain, which settles rapidly with recovery from the injury (Table 28.2, Category 1.2). More worrying is the headache that follows more severe head injury (as defined in Table 28.2, Category 1.1) in which the essential differential diagnosis is from intracranial haematoma. In the complete absence of neurological signs, it is probably unnecessary to undertake neurological investigation and imaging but the child must be observed carefully, and the parents warned of the need to seek medical advice at the earliest sign of neurological compromise. The presence of neurological signs is, of course, an absolute indication for neuroimaging (see Chapter 2).

### Chronic post-traumatic headache

There are various alternative terms to describe chronic post-traumatic headache, including post-concussional syndrome. It is widely believed that chronic post-traumatic headache is mainly a problem in adults, in whom it is often attributed to a desire for financial compensation following the injury. However, children also suffer from chronic headache, and indeed other symptoms, after head injury.[6] In a series of patients whose ages ranged from 4 to 69 years, de Beneditiis[7] found that the age of the patient and the apparent severity of the injury were unrelated to the occurrence of chronic post-traumatic headache. Several other studies have suggested that chronic headache is more likely to follow mild than severe head injury.[8,9] In a 2-year follow-up of 44 children who had had either a mild head injury or a fractured bone, Overweg-Plandsoen et al[10] found a significantly greater incidence of headache, dizziness, fatigue and memory problems in the mildly head-injured children. Symptomatic children have frequently had no evidence of intracranial injury or cerebral oedema at the time of the injury, and the reasons for the subsequent development of symptoms are obscure. The lack of a satisfactory explanation for such symptoms frequently leads to the suggestion that they are psychogenic in origin. However, although the symptoms are often of a psychological nature (memory loss, irritability, personality change), it is clear that their origin is physical and it is important that both the child and the parents should appreciate this. For a more in depth discussion of post-traumatic headache, see Chapter 29.

## Intracranial haemorrhage

Serious lesions associated with head injury include subdural haematoma, epidural haematoma, and intracerebral bleed.

### Subdural haematoma

Subdural haemorrhage results from venous haemorrhage into the subdural space. In the neonate, it may follow birth trauma, and in children under the age of about 2 years it is often associated with non-accidental injuries sustained by shaking. However, in the age group old enough to complain of headache, subdural haematoma may follow any type of injury associated with rapid acceleration–deceleration of the head, the injury itself sometimes appearing so trivial as to have been forgotten by the time the child presents. Typical injuries include falling (especially from a height), automobile accidents and sporting injuries.

The clinical picture is determined by the

underlying brain damage (if any) and by the rate at which the haematoma enlarges. With a rapidly enlarging haematoma, extensive neurological signs may develop rapidly as a result of brain herniation, constituting an acute neurosurgical emergency and requiring immediate neuroimaging and drainage.

In patients with slower accumulation of haematoma, including the osmotic enlargement that occurs in chronic subdural haematoma, headache is often the predominant and sometimes the only symptom. However, raised intracranial pressure may result in vomiting, visual disturbance, ataxia and mental confusion (often manifest as irritability), accompanied by papilloedema, cranial nerve palsies and long tract signs. On occasion, especially in younger children, separation of the cranial sutures may result in a 'cracked pot' note on percussing the skull. However, headache may be the only feature and the absence of neurological signs is common in subdural haematoma.

In a series of 260 patients, van Havenbergh et al[11] found that the only useful prognostic indicator in chronic subdural haematoma was the neurological condition of the patient at the time of treatment. Computed tomography (CT) findings such as haematoma volume, midline shift and residual subdural collections had no influence on the outcome. It is important therefore that surgical aspiration should not be delayed until the onset of neurological impairment.

### Epidural haematoma

Here the haematoma is in the extradural space, the result of damage to the middle cerebral artery or the dural veins. Epidural haematoma usually results from direct trauma to the overlying temporal bone, so the injury tends to be remembered. The rapidity of onset of neurological involvement after the injury varies widely. With oozing from the dural veins, there may be a silent interval of several days, during which there may be chronic headache but no other findings. Neurological dysfunction then accompanies the headache, including vomiting, papilloedema, ipsilateral pupillary and third nerve palsy, and contralateral hemiparesis. In contrast, with a brisk bleed from the middle meningeal artery, the haematoma may enlarge rapidly, with a silent interval of only a few minutes between the injury and the onset of neurological disturbance, which can include convulsions, coma and death.

A skull radiograph frequently shows a temporal fracture, but neuroimaging is required to demonstrate the haematoma, which should be evacuated without delay.

### Traumatic intracerebral haemorrhage

Severe head injury is associated with cerebral contusion and oedema. The neurological features overshadow complaints such as headache.

## Non-traumatic causes of intracranial haemorrhage

Intracranial haemorrhage is a life-threatening emergency in children. There is usually an underlying vascular abnormality, either an arteriovenous malformation or a berry aneurysm.

### Arteriovenous malformation

Arteriovenous malformations are congenital lesions in which there is maldevelopment of the normal capillary bed linking the cerebral arteries and veins. Many of these lesions remain asymptomatic throughout life, but in others the dilated vessels raise intracranial pressure to produce headaches that may mimic migraine, although the affected side tends to be constant. At this stage, the astute clinician may make the diagnosis based on the finding of an intracranial bruit on auscultation over the skull or eyeball.

These lesions may rupture at any time, usually without warning or predisposing factor. Although the clinical picture depends on the site of the malformation and the extent of the bleeding, most patients have some sub-arachnoid haemorrhage resulting in extremely severe headache, often occipital, with vomiting and neck stiffness. Cerebral damage is almost invariable, with altered consciousness, hemi-paresis and convulsions.

Cerebral imaging to delineate the lesion is urgently required; modern neurosurgical tech-niques, including stereotactic radiosurgery, have resulted in great improvements in the prognosis for arteriovenous aneurysms, including those identified both before and after rupture.[12]

### Cerebral aneurysm

In children, cerebral aneurysms (berry aneurysms) are responsible for intracranial bleeding much less frequently than arteriove-nous malformations. In some cases, the under-lying vascular weakness may also be associated with coarctation of the aorta and polycystic kidney disease.[13] The lesions tend to be located on the larger arteries rather than the circle of Willis, and sometimes reach a considerable size ('giant aneurysms') to produce mass effects such as cranial nerve palsies. When aneurysms rupture, they produce the classic picture of acute subarach-noid haemorrhage. However, there may be a

'warning leak'[14] resulting in much less devas-tating effects, justifying an aggressive diagnos-tic approach in children with acute headache with neck stiffness, even if it proves transient.

Cerebral aneurysm is sometimes familial, and a recent study showing a 9.5% prevalence of unruptured aneurysms among the first-degree relatives of patients with cerebral aneurysm concluded that magnetic resonance (MR) angiography screening of first-degree relatives was cost-effective.[15] However, figures for the heritability of cerebral aneurysms vary widely, and screening remains the subject of considerable controversy. It is reasonable to recommend screening in any child with unusual (particularly unilateral) headaches who is a first-degree relative of a patient with an aneurysm.

## Hypertension

Numerically, hypertension accounts for an extremely small proportion of childhood headaches. However, because such headaches are easily confused with primary headaches, and because hypertension is an important and dangerous condition, measuring the blood pressure is an integral component of the initial assessment of any child presenting with headache. Careful attention should be paid to measurement technique; in particular, the use of an inappropriately sized cuff can result in major inaccuracies. Once made, the measure-ment must be compared with normal values for the child's age.[16]

In childhood, hypertension is most often secondary to renal disease, but can result from a variety of other underlying conditions. These include endocrine disorders such as phaeochromocytoma[17] and hyperadrenalism, congenital cardiovascular disease such as coarctation of the aorta and, of relevance to the investigation of headache, from raised intracranial pressure. It should also be remembered that a number of drugs, including 'recreational' drugs such as 'Ecstasy' and 'Herbal Ecstasy'[18] can raise the blood pressure. Essential hypertension is rarely diagnosed before adolescence, although the use of appropriate blood pressure standards for children may result in this diagnosis being made more often in future.

As a result of simple hydrostatic mechanisms, the headache associated with hypertension tends to be worse first thing in the morning (matutinal headache), and to improve during the course of the day. However, this is by no means invariable (see Case 2). Often throbbing, its bilateral location is said to be useful in distinguishing it from migraine but, because so many children with migraine have generalized headache, this feature is of little practical value. In adults, the development of hypertension can exacerbate pre-existing migraine, and the blood pressure may rise during migraine attacks.[19] It is not known if these comments are equally applicable to children.

Making the diagnosis of hypertension relies not on the details of the history, but on ensuring the routine measurement of blood pressure in every child presenting with headache.

## Cerebral tumour and pseudotumour

Brain tumours are the most common solid tumours encountered in children, and a common reason for consultation with headache is to exclude this possibility.

Although brain tumour is an unusual cause of headache, the implications of delayed diagnosis are such that this diagnosis must be constantly in the mind of the clinician dealing with headaches. Headache is the first symptom in about one-third of children with cerebral tumour, and is sometimes the only symptom of raised intracranial pressure, although there continue to be unacceptable delays in diagnosing brain tumours.[20]

Brain tumour may present as an acute emergency when there is haemorrhage into the lesion or when there is rapid obstruction to the flow of cerebrospinal fluid (CSF). Most, however, present with a more gradually evolving picture, with symptoms reflecting raised intracranial pressure, focal neurological disturbance or both.

Raised intracranial pressure results in headaches that tend to be worse in the mornings, are exacerbated by coughing, straining or lying down, and are often accompanied by vomiting. In most the pain is intermittent and, although usually dull and steady, may be throbbing, leading to confusion with migraine. Strabismus is common as a result of third or sixth nerve palsy, but children seldom complain of diplopia or, if a complaint is made, it is of something vague such as 'things looking funny' which may cause confusion with the visual aura of migraine.

Over half the tumours are located in the posterior fossa, and dizziness is a common complaint. The inability of many children to give an accurate account of their symptoms compounds the diagnostic problem, and it is all too easy to accept these symptoms as migrainous manifestations.

Enquiry must also be made about psychological changes that may antedate by weeks or even months the onset of headache or neurological features. These changes include behavioural problems, an appearance of depression, apathy or irritability, inattentiveness or other problems at school, and slowing or even regression of intellectual development.

Careful neurological examination is therefore a mandatory part of the initial assessment of the child with headache. In particular, examination must include visualization of the optic fundi, careful evaluation of eye movements, examination of the other cranial nerves, and examination of the motor system with particular emphasis on coordination. It must also be remembered that raised intracranial pressure may result in bradycardia and/or hypertension.

The consequences of missing a cerebral tumour are dire, and it is better to err on the side of caution by over-investigating. The principal indication for neuroimaging in headache is the presence of neurological signs; this issue is discussed in Chapter 2.

## Pseudotumour cerebri (benign intracranial hypertension)

As the interchangeable names imply, this is a condition in which raised intracranial pressure mimics brain tumour, but in which there is no evidence of tumour, and the ventricular anatomy and cerebrospinal fluid are normal. As the course is by no means always benign, the term 'idiopathic intracranial hypertension' is preferred by some.

### Aetiology
Although most cases are indeed unexplained, pseudotumour can be associated with a wide variety of conditions, some of which are listed in Table 28.3. Perhaps the most common association is with obesity,[21] particularly when weight gain has been rapid, as in re-feeding after maternal deprivation or after cystic fibro-

sis has been diagnosed,[22] or after the initiation of growth hormone treatment.[23] An additional factor in some of these cases may be hypervitaminosis A resulting from over-enthusiastic use of vitamin supplements during the re-feeding process.[24]

A small number of familial case have been reported, showing both autosomal dominant and autosomal recessive inheritance.[25] It should also be noted that in many cases, although no underlying pathology can be identified initially, with the passage of time a variety of conditions including brain tumour can be unmasked, and a cautious prognosis should always be offered.

### Epidemiology
The prevalence of pseudotumour is uncertain. In Nova Scotia, Gordon[26] found an annual incidence of symptomatic disease of 0.9 per 100 000 children, with a 2.7-fold female preponderance. In Iowa, Babikian et al[27] reported that they saw only about one affected child per year in a large referral hospital. Pseudotumour is therefore an uncommon condition even in a highly specialized paediatric practice, and much of the literature on the subject is of necessity anecdotal.

### Clinical features
The usually accepted diagnostic criteria include the clinical features of raised intracranial pressure in an alert, conscious patient without truly localized clinical signs, normal neuroradiology, normal CSF cytology and biochemistry, but raised CSF pressure.[28] Sixth nerve palsy, which can reasonably be regarded as non-localizing, is common in pseudotumour, but some children have other cranial nerve palsies.[29]

The single most common symptom of

| Group | Examples |
|---|---|
| Infection | Roseola infantum |
| | Lyme disease (neuroborreliosis) |
| | Ear and sinus infections |
| | Guillain–Barré syndrome |
| Endocrine disorders | Growth hormone treatment |
| | Addison's disease |
| | Hyperadrenalism, including prolonged corticosteroid treatment |
| | Hypoparathyroidism and pseudohypoparathyroidism |
| | Menstrual disorders, including use of contraceptive pill |
| Metabolic disorders | Severe obesity |
| | Hypervitaminosis A |
| | Galactosaemia |
| | Hypophosphatasia |
| Drugs | Nalidixic acid |
| | Tetracyclines |
| | Chemotherapeutic agents |
| Haematological disorders | Anaemias |
| | Polycythaemia |
| Immune disorders | Systemic lupus erythematosus |
| | Wiscott–Aldrich syndrome |

**Table 28.3**
*Conditions associated with pseudotumour cerebri*

pseudotumour is headache, although this is not invariably present.[30] The pain occurs on a daily basis, is frequently throbbing in character and, as might be expected in the presence of raised intracranial pressure, is frequently present first thing in the morning. Other common symptoms include blurred or double vision,[30–32] visual loss,[32,33] neck stiffness[32] and nausea and vomiting.[30,34] On occasion, there may be a wide variety of other neurological disturbances, including flashing lights, vertigo and photophobia, suggesting migraine, dizziness, unsteady gait and tinnitus (sometimes pulsatile), suggesting posterior fossa tumour, and non-specific complaints such as change in personality, paraesthesiae and weakness. It should also be borne in mind that pseudotumour may coexist with other causes of headache such as migraine[35] and sinusitis.[36]

On examination, the most consistent feature is bilateral papilloedema, but even this is not invariable.[30,32,33,37] In some, there may be retinal haemorrhages and exudates. The retinal findings are reflected in decreased visual acuity,[30,33,38] visual field loss[39] and scotomata, although of course these may be difficult or impossible to assess in younger children. Visual evoked responses are impaired early in the course of pseudotumour, often before any clinical abnormality of vision is apparent, a finding that has been suggested as a useful means of assessing progress and response to treatment in pseudotumour.[40] Other visual features include disturbed colour vision and decreased contrast sensitivity, although these are difficult to assess in younger children, and are in any case less sensitive than visual field assessment in the diagnosis of pseudotumour.[39] In infants, pseudotumour results in bulging of the fontanelle.

### Investigations

Neuroimaging is mandatory in any child with headache and papilloedema (see Chapter 8). Whether this is by radiology or magnetic resonance imaging (MRI) will depend on locally available facilities. Until this has been performed, and a normal result obtained, the diagnosis of pseudotumour must remain provisional. The role of further investigations such as cerebral angiography and single photon emission computed tomography (SPECT) scanning remains uncertain, but ultrasonography of the optic nerve is a non-hazardous, non-invasive technique that promises to be useful in assessing intracranial pressure in pseudotumour.[41]

Once intracranial pathology has been ruled out, lumbar puncture must be performed. This will almost invariably show a CSF pressure in excess of 150 mmH$_2$O, and usually in excess of 200 mmH$_2$O. Normally contraindicated in the presence of raised intracranial pressure, the safety of lumbar puncture in the presence of cerebral pseudotumour is well established, perhaps because of increased brain stiffness.[42] Occasionally, the pressure rise that characterizes pseudotumour is intermittent,[31] and is detectable only on continuous CSF pressure monitoring.

The detection of possible underlying disorders may involve other investigations, such as the assessment of vitamin A status, endocrine function, etc.

### Management

As a result of the rarity of pseudotumour, there have been no randomized controlled trials of its management. Management is therefore based on empirical observations,[38] the reliability of which is confounded by the variability of the natural history of the condition.

The therapeutic options have been summarized by Salman[43] (Table 28.4). Initial treatment is usually with acetazolamide, a carbonic anhydrase diuretic which can produce clinically significant hypokalaemia and metabolic acidosis. Careful monitoring of electrolytes and acid–base status is therefore recommended. Alternative diuretics have also been used.[44] The use of corticosteroids is more controversial. Although it has been pointed out that they are of unproven benefit, or even unnecessary,[44] most authors recommend their use for eye involvement.[32] The sudden withdrawal[38,45] of corticosteroids may precipitate pseudotumour.

Children with pseudotumour should be monitored carefully, paying particular attention to ophthalmological features. If there is any evidence of deterioration on medical treatment, surgical intervention should be considered. The main alternatives are optic nerve fenestration[46] and lumboperitoneal shunt,[47] although subtemporal decompression,[48] formerly in vogue, has been shown on prolonged follow-up to produce good results. In the absence of randomized controlled trials, the choice of surgery will continue to be determined by local expertise and prejudice.[49]

| Treatment | Example |
|-----------|---------|
| Management of underlying condition | Dietary, endocrine, etc. |
| Supportive | Analgesia, education, social support, etc. |
| No other treatment | As indicated in text, many cases run a benign course with rapid spontaneous recovery |
| Repeated lumbar punctures | Seldom if ever employed in children |
| Osmotic agents | Glycerol |
| | Isosorbide |
| Diuretics | Acetazolamide |
| | Furosemide/frusemide |
| Corticosteroids | Prednisolone |
| | Dexamethasone |
| Surgical | Lumboperitoneal shunt |
| | Optic nerve fenestration |

**Table 28.4**
*Therapeutic options in pseudotumour cerebri (based on Salmon[43])*

Attention must of course be paid to any underlying condition that is found, the management of which will vary from case to case.

### Prognosis

Pseudotumour runs a variable course. Some patients recover spontaneously after a period that may be as short as a few days, sometimes after a single diagnostic lumbar puncture, whereas others continue to have symptoms for many years. Although in general the long-term prognosis is good, it must be remembered that a proportion of children will develop visual impairment,[32,39,46] and, despite the lack of objective proof of the efficacy of treatment, it is wise to adopt an aggressive approach to management when there is evidence of visual involvement.

## Extracranial infections

Headache is a common feature of febrile illnesses, particularly influenza,[50] and in most cases is of no particular significance. In infants, febrile illness is often accompanied by a bulging fontanelle, suggesting that fever is accompanied by a rise in intracranial pressure.

## Sinusitis

Sinusitis is a common problem in children. In the series by Burton et al,[4] sinusitis accounted for 16% of headaches presenting to an accident emergency department. In the early years of life, the frontal sinuses have not yet developed, and inflammation is confined mainly to the maxillary antra and ethmoids. Sinusitis is an integral part of most upper respiratory tract infections, and may well explain associated headaches, but such inflammation does not usually persist. However, in some instances bacterial superinfection occurs, sometimes a few days after the original cold has gone. In many such cases there are underlying drainage problems associated with respiratory tract allergy. The symptoms may include purulent nasal discharge, headache that is often poorly localized (seldom facial in children) and low-grade fever. The diagnosis may be obvious when there is redness and swelling of the overlying skin, but more often in children the picture is vague, leading to diagnostic difficulty. It is increasingly appreciated that, in cases of diagnostic difficulty, investigation should include direct endoscopy and tomography as well as standard radiographs.[51] Sphenoidal sinusitis enjoys a particular reputation for presenting with intractable headache, often peri- or retro-orbital, with few diagnostic clues.[52] It is all too often detected as an incidental finding when cerebral imaging is performed for intractable headache (see Case 2).

The mainstay of management is antibiotic therapy – account should be taken of the propensity of local organisms to produce β-lactamase. The efficacy of topical and systemic decongestants remains in doubt. In persistent cases, consideration should be given to surgical lavage and drainage of the sinuses.

Occasionally sinusitis is associated with intracranial spread, resulting in abscess formation and meningitis.[53] Such cases require expert and aggressive management.

## Middle-ear infection

Middle-ear infection results in pain which, in some young children, is poorly localized and may be described as headache. As paediatricians include otoscopic examination in their diagnostic routine, such cases are seldom missed, and most older children are able to localize the pain to the ear.

## Acute virus infections

Headache is one of the principal symptoms of influenza[50] and other virus infections, and during epidemics the diagnosis is usually obvious. However, headache may occur in the course of any febrile illness, when the main concern will be to exclude meningitis. Recent media interest in meningitis had led to the presentation of many such children with a provisional but erroneous diagnosis of meningitis. In many instances, it is impossible to make a precise aetiological diagnosis in fever-associated headache, and it is important not to traumatize the child with excessive investigations. A normal blood count or lymphocytosis, and a normal or only modestly elevated C-reactive protein (CRP) offer reassurance that the infection is unlikely to be serious. In most cases no further investigation is necessary, although it is important to ensure that the headache does settle when the fever resolves.

## Serious systemic infections associated with headache

Headache occurs in the course of numerous serious systemic infections, many of which have encephalitic or meningitic as well as systemic components. It is impossible within the scope of this chapter to deal with these in any detail, and in these conditions headache is usually only one of a constellation of symptoms. Some examples are given in Table 28.5,[54–67] but this list is by no means exhaustive.

## Dental abscess

Young children are well known for their diffi-

| Group | Example |
|---|---|
| Helminthic infections | Cestodiasis (neuroysticercosis)[54] |
| | Echinococcosis (hydatid disease)[55] |
| | Filariasis |
| Protozoan infections | Malaria, especially cerebral[56] |
| | Amoebic meningoencephalitis |
| | Toxoplasmosis, especially in immunocompromised individuals |
| | African trypanosomiasis |
| Fungal infections | Cryptococcosis[57] |
| Bacterial infections | Tuberculous meningitis[58,59] |
| | Lyme disease,[60,61] |
| | Brucellosis[62,63] |
| Rickettsial infections | Typhus[64] |
| | Erlichiosis[65] |
| | Rocky Mountain spotted fever |
| | Q fever |
| Virus infections | Arbovirus encephalitides[66] |
| | Epstein–Barr virus.[67] |

**Table 28.5**
*Some infections that may present with headache as a major feature*

culty in localizing the site of pain. It is therefore not uncommon for the chronic pain of a dental abscess to be described as headache, and there may be considerable delay (and expenditure on investigation) before the correct diagnosis is made.

# Substances or their withdrawal

## Analgesic misuse headache

### David NK Symon

Analgesic misuse headache occurs when drugs given for the treatment of headache aggravate symptoms. The condition has been described as headache occurring during daily intake of medication for symptomatic headache. The headache occurs daily or almost daily but disappears within a few weeks of withdrawal of medication.[68,69] Analgesic misuse headache has been recognized in adults for many years[70] but has only recently been described in children.[69,71,72] It should be suspected in any child with a history of headache on 4 or more days per week.[72]

Analgesic misuse headache may be caused by a wide range of drugs. Most patients with analgesic misuse headache have been using combination preparations of a simple analgesic such as paracetamol with caffeine, codeine, benzodiazepines or barbiturates.[73] In some of these cases the headache may be caused by excessive use of the 'non-analgesic' drug in the compound, particularly caffeine.[74] In adults abuse of single preparations of aspirin, phenacetin or paracetamol is rare, but this probably reflects the pattern of drug use in adults[75] rather than being a necessary part of the syndrome. In children, analgesic abuse headache may be induced by mild analgesics such as paracetamol or ibuprofen used alone.[69,71,72] Many children and their parents do not consider the use of mild analgesics, available without prescription, to be drug therapy, and will deny any drug therapy when the initial clinical history is taken.[72] It is often necessary to use direct leading questions to obtain a history of the use of non-prescription drugs.

Typically children with analgesic misuse headache will give a history of infrequent headaches, which may be either migraine or tension-type headaches, starting months or even years before they present to medical attention. The headaches then become increasingly frequent until they are occurring on most days. Many of the children will say that they feel that the drugs are not of benefit in relieving symptoms, but continue to take them anyway.[72] Despite lack of benefit, others are given analgesic drugs by their parents who feel that they do not wish their child to suffer pain without treatment being given. We have seen children who take analgesic drugs on a regular daily basis in an attempt to *prevent* attacks of headache, with further doses being given when the headache occurs. Perhaps surprisingly, analgesic misuse headache has not been reported in patients taking regular analgesic drugs for other (non-headache) chronic painful conditions.

There is no information on the prevalence of analgesic misuse headache in children. The condition is probably uncommon, but is important because the frequency of symptoms results in considerable disability for those affected.

The treatment of analgesic misuse headache is the complete withdrawal of all analgesic drugs.[76] This may be done abruptly on an outpatient basis[72,77] and no alternative drug therapy is required although some clinicians will give a short course of amitriptyline.[69,77] Many parents will be reluctant to follow this advice and they must be persuaded that this is necessary as the drug treatment is causing an increased frequency of headaches. After withdrawal of analgesics the headaches do not resolve immediately, but after several weeks most patients will see a reduction in headache frequency and many will become symptom free. Some patients may continue to have intermittent episodic migraine headaches after their daily headache has resolved and this may then be treated with specific therapy. Some patients who do not respond to drug withdrawal or who only partially respond may benefit from psychiatric or psychological therapy.[72]

## Caffeine-related headaches

Headaches resulting from caffeine withdrawal are well recognized in adults, but it is sometimes forgotten that, although children may not consume caffeine as tea or coffee, they frequently consume large amounts in the form of cola drinks. Withdrawal from these may occur for instance at weekends, resulting in yet another cause of weekend headache.[78]

Excessive consumption of caffeine on a regular basis, often in the form of cola drinks, may cause a chronic tension-type headache. This may resolve when the cola drinks are gradually withdrawn.[79]

## Solvent abuse

Organic solvent abuse, commonly known as glue-sniffing, involves the inhalation of fumes from a wide variety of sources, including adhesives, typewriter correction fluids,[80] dry cleaning fluids, butane cigarette lighter refills, spray paints and thinners,[81] aerosol propellants and gasoline. The individuals involved tend to be adolescents from deprived backgrounds, although younger children may also indulge, and no social group is immune. When the desired psychological effects of inhaling these substances wears off, there may be symptoms similar to those of a post-alcoholic hangover, including headache. There is likely to be reluctance on the part of the teenager to admit to the origin of these symptoms, which may include vomiting and malaise as well as headache. The youngster may then come to medical attention with suspected intracranial pathology. Suspicious features include skin lesions around the mouth and nose, unusual odours on the breath or skin, drunken behaviour, unexplained listlessness, anorexia and moodiness.[82] There may be otherwise unexplained perturbations of blood chemistry including abnormal liver function tests. Flanagan and Ives[82] point out that the paraphernalia for sniffing, including empty adhesive tubes or other containers, potato crisp (American – chip) bags, cigarette lighter refills and aerosol spray cans, are often found in the child's bedroom or elsewhere. It is important to detect and, if possible, put a stop to solvent abuse, because it can lead to permanent neurological dysfunction[83] and death.[84]

## Headache as a side effect of prescribed medication

Many frequently used drugs are capable of inducing headache in children, and can cause considerable diagnostic confusion, e.g. children with asthma have an increased tendency to have headaches,[85] but this association is complicated by the fact that theophylline, β-agonists and leukotriene antagonists, all commonly used anti-asthma drugs, include headache among their side effects. A list of drugs frequently used in paediatric practice that can cause headache is given in Table 28.6. this list is by no means comprehensive; drug history is particularly important in children with headache and, when a child is found to be on medication, reference should be made to the manufacturer's data-sheet. It should also be remembered that adolescents may well be taking non-prescribed medications containing, for instance, amphetamines.

## Metabolic disorders

Headache occurs during episodes of metabolic decompensation in a wide variety of metabolic disorders, including inborn errors of metabolism such as the hyperammonaemias and organic acidaemias, and secondary metabolic disorders such as renal and hepatic failure. In most cases the other features of the illness predominate, and it is obvious that headache is but one of a constellation of clinical features. These cases are unlikely to be confused with any of the primary headache syndromes, but may be confused with cyclic vomiting syndrome, discussed in Chapter 17.

| Group of drugs | Example(s) |
|---|---|
| Analgesics | Codeine |
| Anti-asthma | β-Agonists, especially long acting |
| | Theophylline |
| | Montelukast |
| Antibiotics | Quinolone derivatives |
| | β-Lactams |
| | Fusidic acid |
| Anticonvulsants | Vigabatrin |
| | Lamotrigine |
| Anti-emetics | Ondansetron |
| Antifungal agents | Fluconazole, ketoconazole, etc. |
| Anti-neoplastic agents | Aromatase inhibitors |
| Anti-platelet agents | Dipyridamole |
| Antiviral agents | Ganciclovir |
| | Lamivudine |
| Calcium blockers | Nifedipine |
| Cold 'cures' | Ephedrine |
| Hormone preparations | Oral contraceptives |
| | Corticosteroids |
| Immunosuppressants | Tacrolimus |
| Proton pump inhibitors | Omeprazole |
| Vaccines | Hepatitis B |
| Vasodilators | Glyceryl trinitrate |

**Table 28.6**
Commonly used drugs that can produce headaches as a side effect

# Other headaches originating in the head and neck

Pain can be referred to the head from a number of extracranial structures, and can cause a great deal of confusion by presenting with symptoms suggestive of one of the primary headaches, particularly migraine or tension headache. The inability of younger children to give a detailed account of their symptoms, and perhaps also the failure of adults to listen carefully to them, encourage erroneous diagnoses and hence inappropriate treatment. Cervicogenic headache with retro-orbital pain is a particular source of confusion in children.

## Ocular headaches

It is widely believed by the general population that headaches commonly result from ocular causes. In practice, this is seldom the case,[86,87] although on occasion there may be a convincing relationship between refractive error and headache.[88] Untreated strabismus, astigmatism and occasionally simple refractive errors may all on occasion be associated with headache, and in a recent study refractive errors were thought to account for headache in 2% of children.[2] However, by the time most children with headaches reach the paediatric or neurology clinic, the eyes have been examined by an optometrist and, in general, no abnormality has been found. In the author's experience, eye problems seldom result in headaches, and even when refractive errors are uncovered, their correction has no therapeutic effect on the headache.

## Temporomandibular joint disorders

Temporomandibular joint (TMJ) dysfunction is a common cause of headache and facial pain in adolescents and young adults, but is relatively uncommon in children. Rarely, it may result from primary joint disease such as juvenile chronic arthritis or after trauma, but more often it reflects underlying dental malocclusion or bruxism. In many cases no underlying abnormality can be found, but studies have shown a low pain threshold in some sufferers.[89] At all ages it is more common in females than in males.

Usually, the pain comes on gradually, but it can evolve rapidly. Typically, it is felt on chewing, but it is seldom localized to the joint. More often it radiates all over the head, to the temporal region or to the ear.[90] The patient may hear a variety of clicks and other noises on jaw movement, and these may also be heard through a stethoscope placed over the TMJ. Recently developed techniques to quantify the vibratory energy underlying these sounds may prove useful in confirming the diagnosis.[91] Jaw movement is usually limited, and various indices exist to quantify this restriction.[92]

TMJ dysfunction causes diagnostic difficulty when the patient fails to relate the pain to chewing or jaw movement, especially if the pain is intermittent and confined to one side, when it may mimic migraine, or if it is referred to an ear that is already the site of pathology such as 'glue ear'.

Management is by orthodontic correction and is beyond the scope of this chapter. A typical case history is presented in Case 4.

## Cervicogenic headaches

Pathology in the neck has for many years been classified as a potential cause of headache.[93-96] However, there has never been agreement on the precise mechanism by which such headaches are caused, and even today many neurologists and neurosurgeons are reluctant to make the diagnosis.

One difficulty arises from the apparent discrepancy between the distribution of dermatomes as mapped by classic techniques, and the distribution of pain of cervical origin. Thus, Poletti[97] mapped the C2 and C3 pain dermatomes in humans, and described the C2 dermatome as an occipital parietal area 6–8 cm wide in adults, ascending paramedially form the subocciput to the vertex. The C3 pain dermatome comprised a craniofacial area including the scalp around the ear, the pinna

363

itself, the lateral cheek over the angle of the jaw, the submental region, and the lateral and anterior aspects of the upper neck. Although these areas are involved in headaches of cervical origin, it is also common for the painful area to extend frontally well beyond these distributions, with retro-orbital and periorbital pain being particularly frequent.[98]

Sjaastad and his colleagues[99] have provided useful criteria for the diagnosis of cervicogenic headache (Table 28.7) and, although these have not been validated in paediatric practice, they provide a useful guideline.

In children, headache of cervical origin is seen in four main situations:

(1) Post-traumatic, sometimes after whiplash injury in motor vehicle accidents, but more often as a result of injury sustained in collision sports.
(2) In association with cervical spine involvement in juvenile chronic polyarthritis.
(3) In association with rubella and other virus infections that cause occipital lymphadenitis.
(4) With congenital malformations such as atlantoaxial dislocation, occipitalization of the atlas and Chiari malformation.[100–102]

In most instances the diagnosis is immediately apparent, but, on occasion, particularly in post-traumatic cases, the presence of head pain may wrongly be interpreted as the result of head rather than neck injury.

The management of cervicogenic headache will depend on the cause.

In post-traumatic cases, it is usual to begin with some sort of physical therapy. Various approaches have their advocates; in the absence of controlled trials, it is impossible to make firm recommendations. Simple traction may give instant relief, although it is often only temporary. Cervical spine manipulation may give more prolonged relief,[103,104] although it is not without danger.[105] Di Fabio[106] found 177 reports of adverse events in the course of cervical spinal manipulation in a literature review covering 72 years. Most of the injuries involved damage to either the vertebral arteries or the brain stem. Interestingly, injuries at the hand of physical therapists were rare. Other simple therapies to be considered at this stage include adjustment of dental occlusion[107] and the use of a simple roll-shaped pillow,[108] although neither of these approaches has been formally investigated in children. Various more invasive approaches have been used in adults, but experience of their use in children is limited. These include the epidural injection of corticosteroids[109] and blocade with local anaesthetic of the greater occipital nerve[110,111] or cervical nerve roots,[112] which may be useful in localizing the lesion. Radiofrequency neurotomy shows promise in the treatment of adults,[110,112] but information on its use in children is scant.

In headaches associated with juvenile chronic polyarthritis of the spine, manipulation is generally best avoided, and reliance should be placed on the suppression of the disease with anti-inflammatory and immunosuppressive agents.

Cervicogenic headaches associated with infections are usually transient, and no specific treatment is required. Simple analgesics, including non-steroidal anti-inflammatory agents, may be required briefly.

In cervicogenic headaches associated with congenital malformations, the management is directed at the relevant lesion, and will usually be surgical.

Major symptoms and signs

I.    Unilaterality of the head pain, without side shift
II.   Symptoms and signs of neck involvement:
      (a)  Provocation of attacks:
           (1)  Pain, seemingly of a similar nature, triggered by neck movement and/or sustained
                awkward head positioning
           (2)  Pain similar in distribution and character to the spontaneously occurring pain
                elicited by external pressure over the ipsilateral upper, posterior neck region or
                occipital region
      (b)  Ipsilateral neck, shoulder, and arm pain of a rather vague, non-radicular nature
      (c)  Reduced range of motion in the cervical spine

Pain characteristics

III.  Non-clustering pain episodes
IV.   Pain episodes of varying duration or fluctuating continuous pain
V.    Moderate, non-excruciating pain, usually of a non-throbbing nature
VI.   Pain starting in the neck, eventually spreading to oculo-frontotemporal areas, where the
      maximum pain often is located

Other important criteria

VII.  Anaesthetic blockades of the major occipital nerve and/or of the C2 root on the symptomatic
      side abolish the pain transiently, provided complete anaesthesia is obtained
VIII. Female sex
IX.   Head and/or neck trauma (whiplash) by history

Minor, more rarely occurring, non-obligatory symptoms and signs

Various attack-related phenomena:
X.    Autonomic symptoms and signs:
      (a)  Nausea
      (b)  Vomiting
      (c)  Ipsilateral oedema, and, less frequently, flushing, mostly in the periocular area
XI.   Dizziness
XII.  Phono- and photopobia
XIII. 'Blurred vision' in the eye ipsilateral to the pain
XIV.  Difficulties in swallowing

**Table 28.7**
*Diagnostic criteria for cervicogenic headache[99]*

## Other causes

Most of the other causes of headache arising in the head and neck are infective in nature, and are dealt with in the chapters on intracranial and extracranial infections.

# Other causes of headache

Headache occurs in a wide variety of circumstances, in response to all manner of stimuli, many of which are specific to the affected individual. Most such headaches are likely to remain unexplained, but in some instances the features occur sufficiently frequently for them to be recognised as a distinct syndrome. Some of these are discussed in this chapter, although this list is by no means exhaustive.

## Headache produced by external cold stimulus

Headache may follow the exposure of the head to a cold environment. The aetiology is usually obvious from the history, but in children the phenomenon may give rise to unnecessary parental anxiety. Management is by protecting the head in sub-zero temperatures and parental reassurance.

## Headache produced by ingestion of cold material (ice-cream headache)

The ingestion of cold drinks and foods such as ice cream can result in headaches which although often severe are of brief duration, generally less than 5 minutes. The area of stimulus is usually the palate or posterior pharyngeal wall, and the pain is generally frontal or retro-orbital, although in migraineurs it may occur in the area normally affected by migraine. The parent is usually relieved to find that the child has a well-recognized complaint. The only further management required is the avoidance of cold stimuli.

## External compression headache (goggle migraine)

Neuralgic head pains have been reported following nerve compression by swimming goggles.[113] Other forms of external compression, such as wearing tight hats, headbands and baseball caps, have the same effect. Usually the cause and the remedy are obvious, but on occasion prolonged pressure may precipitate a full-blown migraine attack, which continues after the compression has been removed.

## Headache following lumbar puncture

Headache following lumbar puncture is usually attributed to cerebral hypotension resulting from leakage of CSF at the site of the puncture,[114] although the precise mechanism by which this produces pain is uncertain. The incidence of such headaches is greater in patients with a prior history of headache,[115,116] and it has been suggested that there may be a psychogenic element in the causation of these headaches.[117] However, it has been shown that the incidence is unrelated to the expectation of headache,[118] and sufferers appear to have no significant personality traits when compared with controls.[119]

Various techniques for spinal puncture have been suggested to reduce the incidence of headache, including the use of atraumatic pencil-point (Whitacre) needles rather than cutting-point (Quincke) needles, the insertion of cutting-point needles with the bevel parallel to the longitudinal axis (to coincide with the direction of dural fibres[120]), and bed rest after the procedure. Although it seems sensible to use the finest possible needle, there is evidence that the choice of needle design has no effect on the incidence of postspinal puncture headache in children,[121] and the routine imposition of bed rest has been shown to be of no prophylactic benefit.[118,122–124]

Headache following spinal puncture is common, and usually settles after a few days of bed rest. If the headache persists for more than a few days, the injection of autologous blood into the epidural space around the site of the original puncture ('blood patch') is almost invariably successful in plugging the leak and abolishing the headache. This technique is probably ineffective as a prophylactic,[125] although it has its advocates.

## Idiopathic stabbing headache

Sudden, severe, stabbing, unilateral headaches have, over the years, been described as ice-pick headaches and cephalgia fugax. The IHS Classification Committee[3] recommends the term 'idiopathic stabbing headache' to describe such headaches, which occur spontaneously and in the absence of organic disease of the underlying structures or the cranial nerves. The pain is usually confined to the distribution of the first division of the fifth cranial nerve, although similar pains with an occipital distribution may be encountered. The pain is recurrent, attacks occurring at widely varying intervals. The sharpness and severity of the pain are such that the child may accuse a bystander of having hit or even stabbed him or her. Treatment is generally unnecessary, and most parents are relieved to find that their

child has a well-recognized syndrome that poses no serious threat. In children with frequent attacks, low-dose indomethacin[126] should be tried.

## Benign cough headache

This term is applied to headache precipitated by coughing in the absence of any intracranial disorder.[3] The pain is usually bilateral but brief, lasting for only a few minutes, and the relationship to coughing is obvious. Although it is seldom a problem in children, it can cause distress to children with whooping cough, cystic fibrosis or asthma. Whereas the cause is self-apparent, the management may be difficult, because coughing in these conditions is involuntary and difficult to suppress, even if that were desirabe. Indomethacin is probably the most effective analgesic for these children.

Benign cough headache must be distinguished from symptomatic cough headache in which coughing exacerbates already raised intracranial pressure. Ophthalmoscopy is therefore a mandatory component of the initial assessment of a child with cough-related headache, particularly if the symptom is persistent.

## Exercise-related headache

The IHS Classification[3] defines benign exertional headache as headache precipitated by any form of exercise, and fulfilling the following criteria:

- The headache is specifically brought on by physical exercise
- It is bilateral, throbbing in nature at onset, and may develop migrainous features in those patients susceptible to migraine

- It lasts from 5 min to 24 h
- It is prevented by avoiding excessive exertion, particularly in hot weather or at high altitude
- It is not associated with any systemic or intracranial disorder.

In children in whom exercise tends to be a spontaneous, everyday occurrence, the association between exercise and headache is easily overlooked. Moreover, management by the avoidance of exercise is difficult and not necessarily desirable. Some children respond to migraine prophylactics such as propranolol, or to indomethacin taken before planned exercise such as formal athletic activity.

## Post-coital and post-masturbatory headache

Headache associated with sexual activity may cause considerable anxiety to adolescents, who may attribute the headache to extraneous factors ranging from intracranial tumour to divine retribution. In practice, most such headaches are benign,[127,128] and may even be familial,[129] but intracranial haemorrhage is not unknown during sexual activity, and should be considered if the headaches are of recent onset or if the pain is persistent.[128]

Most teenagers are satisfied with an explanation for their headaches, and reassurance that there is no serious underlying abnormality. Various forms of medication have been tried, including β-blockers, calcium channel blockers and indomethacin, but have never been subjected to controlled trials; there is no information on their use during adolescence.

## Headache associated with hypoxia

### Obstructive sleep apnoea

Sleep deprivation from any cause is a well-known precipitant of headache syndromes, particularly migraine. In sleep apnoea syndromes, the effects of lack of sleep are compounded by those of nocturnal hypoxia, and morning headaches are common. Obstructive sleep apnoea is particularly common in various craniofacial syndromes,[130] including Down's syndrome,[131] although children with Down's syndrome also have disturbed sleep for reasons unrelated to respiratory obstruction.[132]

The management of OSA is physical, improving the nasal airway either by the application of continuous positive airway pressure, or by removing redundant tissue from the nose or pharynx.[133–135] These options are reviewed by Marcus.[136,137] For further discussion, see Chapter 32.

### Central sleep apnoea (Ondine's curse)

Central sleep apnoea may occur as an isolated developmental anomaly in otherwise normal children, when it is commonly known as Ondine's curse. It also occurs as part of more complex congenital syndromes,[138] and in association with congestive heart failure, nervous system disorders,[139–141] Hirschsprung's disease (Haddad's syndrome[142]) and obesity. In some cases, it appears to be familial. In very young children, central apnoeas are of course an integral feature of prematurity.

Following an apnoeic episode sufficient to induce hypoxia, headache is common.

### Headache in mountain sickness

Children are more liable than adults to develop medical problems at altitudes over

2750 m, and headache is an integral if not quite universal feature of the syndrome of mountain sickness. Usually, the cardiorespiratory features predominate, but headache can be an important warning sign that the child is having problems, and should be taken seriously. Management is by immediate cessation of activity, the administration of oxygen if available and evacuation to a lower altitude as soon as is practicable.

## Headache associated with constipation

### David NK Symon

Many paediatricians who treat children with constipation are aware that some of these children will complain of recurrent headaches. Constipation is not listed as a cause of headache in the IHS classification.

There appears to be an association between constipation and tension-type headaches, which may be recurrent episodic headaches or may become chronic tension-type headache. Constipation should be suspected particularly where the headache is associated with abdominal symptoms such as abdominal pain or nausea.

The diagnosis of constipation is often not immediately apparent in patients presenting with a history of tension-type headaches. Many children and adolescents will deny constipation and some even complain of diarrhoea, which is a symptom of constipation with overflow. Most parents of school age children are not aware of their child's bowel habit. Constipation may be found on clinical examination by the finding of palpable rocks of faeces on abdominal examination, or by observing loaded bowel on a plain abdominal radiograph.

In many patients the headaches will resolve if the constipation is treated with laxatives. Treatment may have to be continued for several months until a normal bowel habit is restored, and laxatives should then be gradually withdrawn and not abruptly stopped.

## Headaches associated with depression and/or anxiety

This is dealt with in Chapter 24.

## Symptomatic headache: cases

### Case 1

A 7-year-old boy presented with a 6-month history of throbbing headaches, gradually increasing in severity and frequency. Recently he had been having headaches three or four ties a week but was apparently well between attacks. The headaches came on at any time of day, and during them he would lie down in a quiet darkened room. He often suffered accompanying nausea, vomiting and periumbilical pain. His mother suffered from migraine, and felt that her son's attacks were similar to her own. A diagnosis of migraine was made, and he was started on pizotifen. A few days later he was admitted to hospital with an unusually severe headache, and was found to be severely hypertensive. Investigation uncovered unilateral renal artery stenosis.

This boy broke all the rules! His headaches were intermittent (unlike his hypertension), he was well between attacks, there was no suggestion of matutinal onset and the periumbilical pain gave no hint of underlying renal disease. However, his hypertension was continuous, and the cardinal error was failure to check his blood pressure when he was first seen.

## Case 2

A 12-year-old boy returned from school one evening complaining of a headache of gradually increasing severity. It had been sports afternoon, and he had been playing rugby football, but he denied any injury to his head. He sat down and watched television before eating his evening meal, and his parents were not unduly concerned. However, as the evening wore on his complaints became more vociferous, and medical advice was sought. When the history was taken, he was unable to localize the pain except to say that it was all over his head. However, there was marked tenderness and spasm of the posterior nuchal muscles, and flexion of his neck reproduced his headache. He then revealed that, although he had not injured his head, he had several times tackled boys bigger than himself. Gentle traction relieved his pain. A cervical spine radiograph showed no bony injury, and he was issued with a cervical collar. By the time he saw an orthopaedic surgeon 2 days later, his symptoms had gone.

This boy answered the questions about head injury quite accurately, but did not see the need to volunteer the additional information about tackling. As the pain of cervicogenic headache is commonly referred all over the head and behind the eyes, this diagnosis continues to be missed, particularly in the acute setting, and may lead to unnecessary and inappropriate investigation.

## Case 3

A 12-year-old girl presented with a 3-week history of severe unrelenting headaches which, she said, were 'getting on top' of her. The pain was 'all over' her head, had no special

characteristics and was simply described as being extremely painful. Physical examination revealed no abnormality, but she was clearly miserable and depressed. A psychogenic aetiology was suspected, but careful evaluation by a clinical psychologist failed to uncover any problems, and it was concluded that the problem was organic. At this point she was admitted to hospital, where it was found that she was running a low-grade fever – her temperature had not been measured in the outpatient department. An elevated C-reactive protein prompted a CT scan, which showed bilateral sphenoidal opacity. Recovery began within a few hours of starting antibiotics.

## Case 4

An 8-year-old boy presented at a headache clinic with a 6-month history of right-sided headache, present almost every morning on waking, and gradually improving as the day wore on. He had difficulty in describing the pain, but he was able to attend school. Physical examination revealed normal optic discs, cranial nerves, peripheral nervous system and blood pressure, and he was asked to keep a pain diary and return in a few weeks. He did so, at which point his mother volunteered the information that the pain had started when he was fitted with an orthodontic brace. Re-examination revealed tenderness over the right TMJ, and further enquiry revealed nocturnal bruxism. Some simple adjustments to his brace cured the bruxism, and with it the headaches.

Although physical examination is seldom revealing in children with headache, this does not mean that it need not be done. TMJ dysfunction was considered only when the mother commented on the temporal association with the orthodontic treatment, but tenderness over the joint was almost certainly present at the time of the initial consultation.

# References

1. Abu-Arefeh I, Russell G, Prevalence of headache and migraine in schoolchildren. *BMJ* 1994; **309**: 765–9.

2. Anttila P, Epidemiology of headaches and other pains in schoolchildren. *Annales Universitatis Turkuensis* 2000; **D400**: 1–78.

3. Headache Classification Committee of the International Headache Society, Classification and diagnostic criteria for headache disorders, cranial neuralgias and facial pain. *Cephalalgia* 1988; 8(suppl 7): 1–96.

4. Burton LJ, Quinn B, Pratt-Cheney JL, Pourani M, Headache etiology in a pediatric emergency department. *Pediatr Emerg Care* 1997; **13**: 1–4.

5. Jerrett WA, Headaches in general practice. *Practitioner* 1979; **222**: 549–55.

6. Lundar T, Nestvold K, Pediatric head injuries caused by traffic accidents. A prospective study with 5-year follow-up. *Childs Nerv Syst* 1985; **1**: 24–8.

7. De Benedittis G, De Santis A, Chronic post-traumatic headache: clinical, psychopathological features and outcome determinants. *J Neurosurg Sci* 1983; **27**: 177–86.

8. Wilkinson M, Gilchrist E, Post-traumatic headache. *Ups J Med Sci Suppl* 1980; **31**: 48–51.

9. Yamaguchi M, Incidence of headache and severity of head injury. *Headache* 1992; **32**: 427–31.

10. Overweg-Plandsoen WC, Kodde A, van Straaten M et al, Mild closed head injury in children compared to traumatic fractured bone; neurobehavioural sequelae in daily life 2 years after the accident. *Eur J Pediatr* 1999; **158**: 249–52.

11. van Havenbergh T, van Calenbergh F, Goffin J, Plets C, Outcome of chronic subdural haematoma: analysis of prognostic factors. *Br J Neurosurg* 1996; **10**: 35–9.

12. Humphreys RP, Hoffman HJ, Drake JM, Rutka JT, Choices in the 1990s for the management of pediatric cerebral arteriovenous malformations. *Pediatr Neurosurg* 1996; **25**: 277–85.

13. Chester AC, Harris JP, Schreiner GE, Polycystic kidney disease. *Am Fam Physician* 1977; **16**: 94–101.

14. Jakobsson KE, Saveland H, Hillman J et al, Warning leak and management outcome in aneurysmal subarachnoid hemorrhage. *J Neurosurg* 1996; **85**: 995–9.

15. Brown BM, Soldevilla F, MR angiography and surgery for unruptured familial intracranial aneurysms in persons with a family history of cerebral aneurysms. *Am J Roentgenol* 1999; **173**: 133–8.

16. Harshfield GA, Alpert BS, Pulliam DA, Somes GW, Wilson DK, Ambulatory blood pressure recordings in children and adolescents. *Pediatrics* 1994; **94**: 180–4.

17. Ciftci AO, Tanyel FC, Senocak ME, Buyukpamu-Kau N, Phaechromocytoma in children. *J Pediatr Surg* 2001; **36**: 447–52.

18. Yates KM, O'Connor A, Horsley CA, 'Herbal Ecstasy': a case series of adverse reactions. *N Z Med J* 2000; **113**: 315–17.

19. Mathew NT, Migraine and hypertension. *Cephalalgia* 1999; **19**(suppl 25): 17–19.

20. Edgeworth J, Bullock P, Bailey A, Gallagher A, Crouchman M, Why are brain tumours still being missed? *Arch Dis Child* 1996; **74**: 148–51.

21. Scott IU, Siatkowski RM, Eneyni M, Brodsky MC, Lam BL, Idiopathic intracranial hypertension in children and adolescents. *Am J Ophthalmol* 1997; **124**: 253–5.

22. Couch R, Camfield PR, Tibbles JA, The changing picture of pseudotumor cerebri in children. *Can J Neurol Sci* 1985; **12**: 48–50.

23. Malozowski S, Tanner LA, Wysowski DK, Fleming GA, Stadel BV, Benign intracranial hypertension in children with growth hormone deficiency treated with growth hormone. *J Pediatr* 1995; **126**: 996–9.

24. Lucidi V, Di Capua M, Rosati P, Papadatou B, Castro M, Benign intracranial hypertension in an older child with cystic fibrosis. *Pediatr Neurol* 1993; **9**: 494–5.

25. Kharode C, McAbee G, Sherman J, Kaufman M, Familial intracranial hypertension: report of a case and review of the literature. *J Child Neurol* 1992; **7**: 196–8.

26. Gordon K, Pediatric pseudotumor cerebri: descriptive epidemiology. *Can J Neurol Sci* 1997; **24**: 219–21.

27. Babikian P, Corbett J, Bell W, Idiopathic intracranial hypertension in children: the Iowa experience. *J Child Neurol* 1994; **9**: 144–9.

28. Smith JL, Whence pseudotumor cerebri? *J Clin Neuroophthalmol* 1985; **5**: 55–6.

29. Capobianco DJ, Brazis PW, Cheshire WP, Idiopathic intracranial hypertension and seventh nerve palsy. *Headache* 1997; **37**: 286–8.

30. Dhiravibulya K, Ouvrier R, Johnston I, Procopis P, Antony J, Benign intracranial hypertension in childhood: a review of 23 patients. *J Pediatr Child Health* 1991; **27**: 304–7.

31. Soler D, Cox T, Bullock P, Calver DM, Robinson RO, Diagnosis and management of benign intracranial hypertension. *Arch Dis Child* 1998; **78**: 89–94.

32. Cinciripini GS, Donahue S, Borchert MS, Idiopathic intracranial hypertension in prepubertal pediatric patients: characteristics, treatment, and outcome. *Am J Ophthalmol* 1999; **127**: 178–82.

33. Amacher AL, Spence JD, Spectrum of benign intracranial hypertension in children and adolescents. *Child Nerv Syst* 1985; **1**: 81–6.

34. Grant DN, Benign intracranial hypertension. A review of 79 cases in infancy and childhood. *Arch Dis Child* 1971; **46**: 651–5.

35. Mathew NT, Ravishankar K, Sanin LC, Coexistence of migraine and idiopathic intracranial hypertension without papilledema. *Neurology* 1996; **46**: 1226–30.

36. Keren T, Lahat E, Pseudotumor cerebri as a presenting symptom of acute sinusitis in a child. *Pediatr Neurol* 1998; **19**: 153–4.

37. Marcelis J, Silberstein SD, Idiopathic intracranial hypertension without papilledema. *Arch Neurol* 1991; **48**: 392–9.

38. Baker RS, Baumann RJ, Buncic JR, Idiopathic intracranial hypertension (pseudotumor cerebri) in pediatric patients. *Pediatr. Neurol* 1989; **5**: 5–11.

39. Rowe FJ, Sarkies NJ, Assessment of visual function in idiopathic intracranial hypertension: a prospective study. *Eye* 1998; **12**: 111–18.

40. Sorensen PS, Trojaborg W, Gjerris F, Krogsaa B, Visual evoked potentials in pseudotumor cerebri. *Arch Neurol* 1985; **42**: 150–3.

41. Shuper A, Snir M, Barash D, Yassur Y, Mimouni M, Ultrasonography of the optic nerves: clinical application in children with pseudotumor cerebri. *J Pediatr* 1997; **131**: 734–40.

42. Salman M, Why does tonsillar herniation not occur in idiopathic intracranial hypertension? *Med Hypotheses* 1999; **53**: 270–1.

43. Salman MS, Idiopathic 'benign' intracranial hypertension in childhood: an update and review. *Pediatr Today* 1999; **7**: 63–9.

44. Jefferson A, Clark J, Treatment of benign intracranial hypertension by dehydrating agents with particular reference to the measurement of the blind spot area as a means of recording improvement. *J Neurol Neurosurg Psychiatry* 1976; **39**: 627–39.

45. Neville BG, Wilson J, Benign intracranial hypertension following corticosteroid withdrawal in childhood. *BMJ* 1970; **3**: 554–6.

46. Goh KY, Schatz NJ, Glaser JS, Optic nerve sheath fenestration for pseudotumor cerebri. *J Neuroophthalmol* 1997; **17**: 86–91.

47. Burgett RA, Purvin VA, Kawasaki A, Lumboperitoneal shunting for pseudotumor cerebri. *Neurology* 1997; **49**: 734–9.

48. Kessler LA, Novelli PM, Reigel DH, Surgical treatment of benign intracranial hypertension – subtemporal decompression revisited. *Surg Neurol* 1998; **50**: 73–6.

49. Brazis PW, Lee AG, Elevated intracranial pressure and pseudotumor cerebri. *Curr Opin Ophthalmol* 1998; **9**: 27–32.

50. Nicholson KG, Clinical features of influenza. *Semin Respir Infect* 1992; **7**: 26–37.

51. Clerico DM, Sinus headaches reconsidered: referred cephalgia of rhinologic origin masquerading as refractory primary headaches. *Headache* 1995; **35**: 185–92.

52. Haimi-Cohen Y, Amir J, Zeharia A, Danziger Y, Ziv N, Mimouni M, Isolated sphenoidal sinusitis in children. *Eur J Pediatr* 1999; **158**: 298–301.

53. Giannoni C, Sulek M, Friedman EM, Intracranial complications of sinusitis: a pediatric series. *Am J Rhinol* 1998; **12**: 173–8.

54. Weisse ME, Raszka WV, Jr, Cestode infection in children. *Adv Pediatr Infect Dis* 1996; **12**: 109–53.

55. Ersahin Y, Mutluer S, Dermirtas E, Yurtseven T, A case of thalamic hydatid cyst. *Clin Neurol Neurosurg* 1995; **97**: 321–3.

56. Steele RW, Baffoe-Bonnie B, Cerebral malaria in children. *Pediatr Infect Dis J* 1995; **14**: 281–5.

57. Chan KH, Mann KS, Yue CP, Neurosurgical aspects of cerebral cryptococcosis. *Neurosurgery* 1989; **25**: 44–7.

58. Alsoub H, Tuberculous meningitis: a clinical and laboratory study of 20 patients in Qatar. *Int J Clin Pract* 1998; **52**: 300–4.

59. Kumar R, Singh SN, Kohli N, A diagnostic rule for tuberculous meningitis. *Arch Dis Child* 1999; **81**: 221–4.

60. Eppes SC, Nelson DK, Lewis LL, Klein JD, Characterization of Lyme meningitis and comparison with viral meningitis in children. *Pediatrics* 1999; **103**: 957–60.

61. Kan L, Sood SK, Maytal J, Pseudotumor cerebri in Lyme disease: a case report and literature review. *Pediatr Neurol* 1998; **18**: 439–41.

62. Estevao MH, Barosa LM, Matos LM, Barroso AA, da Mota HC, Neurobrucellosis in children. *Eur J Pediatr* 1995; **154**: 120–2.

63. Hendricks MK, Perez EM, Burger PJ, Mouton PA, Brucellosis in childhood in the Western Cape. *S Afr Med J* 1995; **85**: 176–8.

64. Masalha R, Merkin-Zaborsky H, Matar M, Zirkin HJ, Wirguin I, Herishanu YO, Murine typhus presenting as subacute meningoencephalitis. *J Neurol* 1998; **245**: 665–8.

65. Wallace BJ, Brady G, Ackman DM et al, Human granulocytic ehrlichiosis in New York. *Arch Intern Med* 1998; **158**: 769–73.

66. Steele MT, Update on emerging infections from the Centers for Disease Control and Prevention. Arboviral infections of the central nervous system – United States, 1996–1997. *Ann Emerg Med* 1999; **33**: 365–7.

67. Domachowske JB, Cunningham CK, Cummings DL, Crosley CJ, Hannan WP, Weiner LB, Acute manifestations and neurologic sequelae of Epstein-Barr virus encephalitis in children. *Pediatr Infect Dis J* 1996; **15**: 871–5.

68. Diener HC, Tfelt-Hansen P, Headache associated with chronic use of substances. In: Olesen J, Tfelt-Hansen P, Welch KMA, eds, *The Headaches*, New York: Raven Press, 1993: 721–7.

69. Vasconcellos E, Pina-Garza JE, Millan EJ, Warner JS, Analgesic rebound headache in children and adolescents. *J Child Neurol* 1998; **13**: 443–7.

70. Kudrow L, Paradoxical effects of frequent analgesic use. *Adv Neurol* 1982; **33**: 335–41.

71. Symon DNK, Analgesic headache in children. *Cephalalgia* 1997; **17**: 292–3.

72. Symon DNK, Twelve cases of analgesic headache. *Arch Dis Child* 1998; **78**: 555–6.

73. Wallasch TM, Medikamentös induzierter Kopfschmerz. *Fortschr Neurol Psychiatr* 1992; **60**: 114–18.

74. Mathew NT, Stubits E, Nigam MP, Transformation of episodic migraine into daily headache: analysis of factors. *Headache* 1982; **22**: 66–8.

75. Pfaffenrath V, Niederberger U, What kind of drugs are taken by patients with primary headaches? In Diener HC, Wilkinson M, eds, *Drug-induced Headache*, Berlin: Springer-Verlag, 1988: 44–62.

76. Olesen J, Analgesic headache. *BMJ* 1995; **310**: 479–80.

77. Hering R, Steiner TJ, Abrupt outpatient withdrawal of medication in analgesic-abusing migraineurs. *Lancet* 1991; **337**: 1442–3.

78. Couturier EG, Hering R, Steiner TJ, Weekend attacks in migraine patients: caused by caffeine withdrawal? *Cephalalgia* 1992; **12**: 99–100.

79. Hering-Hanit R, Gadoth N, Caffeine-induced headache in childhood and adolescents. *IVth International Congress on Headache in*

*Childhood and Adolescence*, Turku, Finland 1999.

80. Pointer J, Typewriter correction fluid inhalation: a new substance of abuse. *J Toxicol Clin Toxicol* 1982; **19**: 493–9.

81. Komiyama M, Yamanaka K, Chronic misuse of paint thinners. *J Neurol Neurosurg Psychiatry* 1999; **67**: 247.

82. Flanagan RJ, Ives RJ, Volatile substance abuse. *Bull Narc* 1994; **46**: 49–78.

83. Byrne A, Kirby B, Zibin T, Ensminger S, Psychiatric and neurological effects of chronic solvent abuse. *Can J Psychiatry* 1991; **36**: 735–8.

84. Johns A, Volatile solvent abuse and 963 deaths. *Br J Addict* 1991; **86**: 1053–6.

85. Wilkinson IA, Halliday JA, Henry RL, Hankin RG, Hensley MJ, Headache and asthma. *J Paediatr Child Health* 1994; **30**: 253–6.

86. Cameron ME, Headaches in relation to the eyes. *Med J Aust* 1976; **1**: 292–4.

87. Romano PE, Pediatric ophthalmic mythology. *Postgrad Med* 1975; **58**: 146–50.

88. Hutter RF, Rouse MW, Visually related headache in a preschooler. *Am J Optom, Physiol Opt* 1984; **61**: 711–13.

89. Maixner W, Fillingim R, Booker D, Sigurdsson A, Sensitivity of patients with painful temporomandibular disorders to experimentally evoked pain. *Pain* 1995; **63**: 341–51.

90. List T, Wahlund K, Wenneberg B, Dworkin SF, TMD in children and adolescents: prevalence of pain, gender differences, and perceived treatment need. *J Orofac Pain* 1999; **13**: 9–20.

91. Olivieri KA, Garcia AR, Paiva G, Stevens C, Joint vibrations analysis in asympotmatic volunteers and symptomatic patients. *Cranio* 1999; **17**: 176–83.

92. Miller VJ, Bookhan V, Brummer D, Singh JC, A mouth opening index for patients with temporomandibular disorders. *J Oral Rehabil* 1999; **26**: 534–7.

93. Telling WH, Nodular fibromyositis, an everyday affection, and its identity with so-called muscular rheumatism. *Lancet* 1911; **i**: 154.

94. Hartsock CL, Headache from arthritis of the cervical spine. *Med Clin North Am* 1940; 329–333.

95. Barré M, Sur un syndrome sympathique cervical posterieur et sa cause frequente: l'arthrite cervicale. *Rev Neurol (Paris)* 1926; **33**: 1246–8.

96. Friedman AP, Finley KH, Graham JR, Classification of headache. *JAMA* 1962; **179**: 717–18.

97. Poletti CF, C2 and C3 pain dermatomes in man. *Cephalalgia* 1991; **11**: 155–9.

98. Fredriksen TA, Hovdal H, Sjaastad O, 'Cervicogenic headache': clinical manifestation. *Cephalalgia* 1987; **7**: 147–60.

99. Sjaastad O, Fredriksen TA, Pfaffenrath V, Cervicogenic headache: diagnostic criteria. *Headache* 1990; **30**: 725–6.

100. Milhorat TH, Chou MW, Trinidad EM et al, Chiari I malformation redefined: clinical and radiographic findings for 364 symptomatic patients. *Neurosurgery* 1999; **44**: 1005–17.

101. Park JK, Gleason PL, Madsen JR, Goumnerova LC, Scott RM, Presentation and management of Chiari I malformation in children. *Pediatr Neurosurg* 1997; **26**: 190–6.

102. Weinberg JS, Freed DL, Sadock J, Handler M, Wisoff JH, Epstein FJ, Headache and Chiari I malformation in the pediatric population. *Pediatr Neurosurg* 1998; **29**: 14–18.

103. Nilsson N, Christensen HW, Hartvigsen J, The effect of spinal manipulation in the treatment of cervicogenic headache. *J Manipulative Physiol Ther* 1997; **20**: 326–30.

104. Shekelle PG, Coulter I, Cervical spine manipulation: summary report of a systematic review of the literature and a multidisciplinary expert panel. *J Spinal Disord* 1997; **10**: 223–8.

105. Hurwitz EL, Aker PD, Adams AH, Meeker WC, Shekelle PG, Manipulation and mobilization of the cervical spine. A systematic review of the literature. *Spine* 1996; **21**: 1746–59.

106. Di Fabio RP, Manipulation of the cervical spine: risks and benefits. *Phys Ther* 1999; **79**: 50–65.

107. Karppinen K, Eklund S, Suoninen E, Eskelin M, Kirveskari P, Adjustment of dental occlusion in treatment of chronic cervicobrachial pain and

headache. *J Oral Rehabil* 1999; **26**: 715–21.

108. Hagino C, Boscariol J, Dover L, Letendre R, Wicks M, Before/after study to determine the effectiveness of the align-right cylindrical cervical pillow in reducing chronic neck pain severity. *J Manipulative Physiol Ther* 1998; **21**: 89–93.

109. Martelletti P, Di Sabato F, Granata M et al, Epidural steroid-based technique for cervicogenic headache diagnosis. *Funct Neurol* 1998; **13**: 84–7.

110. Bovim G, Sand T, Cervicogenic headache, migraine without aura and tension-type headache. Diagnostic blockade of greater occipital and supra-orbital nerves. *Pain* 1992; **51**: 43–8.

111. Vincent M, Greater occipital nerve blockades in cervicogenic headache. *Funct Neurol* 1998; **13**: 78–9.

112. van Suijlekom HA, van Kleef M, Barendse GA, Sluijter ME, Sjaastad O, Weber WE, Radiofrequency cervical zygapophyseal joint neurotomy for cervicogenic headache: a prospective study of 15 patients. *Funct Neurol* 1998; **13**: 297–303.

113. Pestronk A, Pestronk S, Goggle migraine. *N Engl J Med* 1983; **308**: 226–7.

114. Wang LP, Schmidt JF, Central nervous side effects after lumbar puncture. A review of the possible pathogenesis of the syndrome of postdural puncture headache and associated symptoms. *Dan Med Bull* 1997; **44**: 79–81.

115. Ramamoorthy C, Geiduschek JM, Bratton SL, Miser AW, Miser JS, Postdural puncture headache in pediatric oncology patients. *Clin Pediatr (Phila)* 1998; **37**: 247–51.

116. Kuntz KM, Kokmen E, Stevens JC, Miller P, Offord KP, Ho MM, Post-lumbar puncture headaches: experience in 501 consecutive procedures. *Neurology* 1992; **42**: 1884–7.

117. Kaplan G, The psychogenic etiology of headache post lumbar puncture. *Psychosom Med* 1967; **29**: 376–9.

118. Hilton-Jones D, Harrad RA, Gill MW, Warlow CP, Failure of postural manoeuvres to prevent lumbar puncture headache. *J Neurol Neurosurg Psychiatry* 1982; **45**: 743–6.

119. Vilming ST, Ellertsen B, Troland K, Schrader H, Monstad I, MMPI profiles in post-lumbar puncture headache. *Acta Neurol Scand* 1997; **95**: 184–8.

120. Fink BR, Walker S, Orientation of fibers in human dorsal lumbar dura mater in relation to lumbar puncture. *Anesth Analg* 1989; **69**: 768–72.

121. Kokki H, Heikkinen M, Turunen M, Vanamo K, Hendolin H, Needle design does not affect the success rate of spinal anaesthesia or the incidence of postpuncture complications in children. *Acta Anaesthesiol Scand* 2000; **44**: 210–13.

122. Handler CE, Smith FR, Perkin GD, Rose FC, Posture and lumbar puncture headache: a controlled trial in 50 patients. *J R Soc Med* 1982; **75**: 404–7.

123. Dieterich M, Brandt T, Is obligatory bed rest after lumbar puncture obsolete? *Eur Arch Psychiatry Neurol Sci* 1985; **235**: 71–5.

124. Spriggs DA, Burn DJ, French J, Cartlidge NE, Bates D, Is bed rest useful after diagnostic lumbar puncture? *Postgrad Med J* 1992; **68**: 581–3.

125. Palahniuk RJ, Cumming M, Prophylactic blood patch does not prevent post lumbar puncture headache. *Can Anaesth Soc J* 1979; **26**: 132–3.

126. Rothner AD, Miscellaneous headache syndromes in children and adolescents. *Semin Pediatr Neurol* 1995; **2**: 159–64.

127. Lance JW, Headaches related to sexual activity. *J Neurol Neurosurg Psychiatry* 1976; **39**: 1226–30.

128. Kumar KL, Reuler JB, Uncommon headaches: diagnosis and treatment. *J Gen Intern Med* 1993; **8**: 333–41.

129. Johns DR, Benign sexual headache within a family. *Arch Neurol* 1986; **43**: 1158–60.

130. Hoeve HL, Joosten KF, van den BS, Management of obstructive sleep apnea syndrome in children with craniofacial malformation. *Int J Pediatr Otorhinolaryngol* 1999; **49**(suppl 1): S59–61.

131. Jacobs IN, Gary RF, Todd NW, Upper airway obstruction in children with Down syndrome. *Arch Otolaryngol Head Neck Surg* 1996; **122**: 945–50.

132. Levanon A, Tarasiuk A, Tal A, Sleep characteristics in children with Down syndrome. *J Pediatr* 1999; **134**: 755–60.

133. Coleman SC, Smith TL, Midline radiofrequency tissue reduction of the palate for bothersome snoring and sleep-disordered breathing: A clinical trial. *Otolaryngol Head Neck Surg* 2000; **122**: 387–94.

134. Troell RJ, Powell NB, Riley RW, Li KK, Guilleminault C, Comparison of postoperative pain between laser-assisted uvulopalatoplasty, uvulopalatopharyngoplasty, and radiofrequency volumetric tissue reduction of the palate. *Otolaryngol Head Neck Surg* 2000; **122**: 402–9.

135. Elsherif I, Kareemullah C, Tonsil and adenoid surgery for upper airway obstruction in children. *Ear Nose Throat J* 1999; **78**: 617–20.

136. Marcus CL, Advances in management of sleep apnea syndromes in infants and children. *Pediatr Pulmonol Suppl* 1999; **18**: 188–9.

137. Marcus CL, Management of obstructive sleep apnea in childhood. *Curr Opin Pulm Med* 1997; **3**: 464–9.

138. Gurewitz R, Blum I, Lavie P et al, Recurrent hypothermia, hypersomnolence, central sleep apnea, hypodipsia, hypernatremia, hypothyroidism, hyperprolactinemia and growth hormone deficiency in a boy – treatment with clomipramine. *Acta Endocrinol Suppl (Copenh)* 1986; **279**: 468–72.

139. Keefover R, Sam M, Bodensteiner J, Nicholson A, Hypersomnolence and pure central sleep apnea associated with the Chiari I malformation. *J Child Neurol* 1995; **10**: 65–7.

140. Guilleminault C, Briskin JG, Greenfield MS, Silvestri R, The impact of autonomic nervous system dysfunction on breathing during sleep. *Sleep* 1981; **4**: 263–78.

141. Frank Y, Kravath RE, Inoue K et al, Sleep apnea and hypoventilation syndrome associated with acquired nonprogressive dysautonomia: clinical and pathological studies in a child. *Ann Neurol* 1981; **10**: 18–27.

142. Haddad GG, Mazza NM, Defendini R et al, Congenital failure of automatic control of ventilation, gastrointestinal motility and heart rate. *Medicine (Baltimore)* 1978; **57**: 517–26.

# 29

# Post-traumatic headache
*Paul Winner*

Head injury in children is extremely common. Children and adolescents involved in motor vehicle accidents, bicycle accidents, sports-related injuries or child abuse may develop headache symptoms within the first 24 hours to 2 weeks, even after what would seem to be a trivial head injury. Most children admitted after head injury have a Glasgow Coma Scale (GCS) ranging from 13 to 15 (Table 29.1). For children and adolescents who develop headache after a minor head injury, it often clears within 2–3 months of the injury. In some individuals, this headache and the collection of symptoms are sometimes referred to as post-traumatic syndrome or postconcussion syndrome. The symptoms include vertigo, dizziness, difficulty concentrating, memory disorders, depression, altered school performance, behavioural disorders and sleep alteration.[1–3]

The pathophysiology associated with post-traumatic headache and postconcussion syndrome in minor head injuries is not as well understood as that after severe head injury. The severity of the symptoms is not clearly dictated by the severity of the head injury. Severe headaches, impaired memory and difficulty in concentrating have been reported with traumatic or relatively minor head injury.[4] The headaches associated with the postconcussion syndrome can present either as a migraine-like

| Eye opening (E) | |
|---|---|
| Spontaneous | 4 |
| To sound | 3 |
| To pain | 2 |
| None | 1 |
| *Verbal response (V)* | |
| Oriented | 5 |
| Confused | 4 |
| Inappropriate | 3 |
| Incomprehensible | 2 |
| None | 1 |
| *Best motor response (M)* | |
| Obeys | 6 |
| Localizes | 5 |
| Withdraws | 4 |
| Abnormal flexion | 3 |
| Extends | 2 |
| None | 1 |

**Table 29.1**
Glasgow Coma Scale (GCS).

headache, or seemingly as a tension-type headache, or a combination of migraine-like and tension-type headaches often referred to as chronic daily headache; even cluster-type headaches have been reported after head injury.[5] Children with no reported concussion symptoms as a result of mild head injury, plus a GCS of 13–15 may have no detectable structural abnormality, focal perangular brain lesions or dural haemorrhages.

The clinical and neurobehavioural abnormalities after mild head injury have been fairly well established using a monkey model for a minor acceleration/deceleration non-impact head injury in the saggital plain, in which the animal sustained a brief loss of consciousness, but no neurological deficits were reported. Degenerating axons in the pons and dorsal midbrain were noted 7 days after injury.[6] Observations of injury in experimental animals and humans suggest that trauma causes a disorganization of the neurofilament cytoskeleton and axolemma, resulting in axonal disconnection.[7] Minor acceleration/deceleration injury involving rotational forces may result in axonal sheering or tearing, especially in areas of the midbrain, superior cerebellar peduncles, corpus callosum and the central white matter of the brain.[8] Acceleration/deceleration of the brain may also damage the labyrinth and mechanoreceptor in the neck and central vestibular connections, resulting in the symptoms of dizziness and vertigo that are often reported in patients with postconcussion syndrome. Blood vessels may be stretched or injured during head injury, impairing the vascular contractility in an autoregulation that may result from direct vascular damage or residual tissue injury. Acceleration/deceleration forces may also result in stretching and straining of the cervical ligaments, muscle and supporting bony structures of the neck and back.[9]

Postconcussion syndrome symptoms appear to occur more commonly after a mild-to-moderate head injury than after a severe head injury. Direct impact is not necessary to cause postconcussion syndrome. The unsynchronized rotational forces that may develop

| |
|---|
| • Begins within days to weeks |
| • Migraine-like quality |
| • Cognitive difficulties |
| • Symptoms may not equal injury |
| • Subsides spontaneously? |

**Table 29.2**
*Post-traumatic headache.*

between the cerebral hemisphere, the cerebellum and axons in the upper brain stem are more vulnerable to diffuse axonal injury, which may have a role in the above symptom complex developing after head injury. The persistence of the headache and the associated symptoms may not correlate with the duration of unconsciousness, post-traumatic amnesia or skull fracture. Clearly, further work is necessary to further understand the pathophysiology and clinical relationship. Concussion produced by rotational forces to a semi-solid brain within a skull can result in, and give rise to, shearing and diffuse axonal injury.[7] This correlation needs to be addressed further.

## Diagnosis

As we develop greater understanding of neurophysiology, further observations and clinical understanding of the pathophysiology of head pain and its associated symptom complex will be forthcoming. The criteria of the International Headache Society (IHS) have attempted to set initial guidelines for diagnosis, including the requirement that the onset of headache occurs within 2 weeks of head injury or 2 weeks from the time that the patient regains consciousness. This is a reasonable guide, although clinically patients may report the onset of their headaches as late as 1 month after the injury. The clinical report may be complicated by the patient's attention to the other injuries sustained or the more notable issues of other associated symptoms. Patients may report the onset of their initial migraine symptoms after they have reported the head injury, although some patients report migraine-like headache after injury, and then often do not respond as well to standard migraine medications.[11-13] The neurological sequelae of mild head injuries in children and adolescents who report headache may also have even more prominent associated symptoms: hyperactivity, difficulty concentrating, memory disorders, vertigo, dizziness, depression, altered personality affecting altered school performance and behavioural disorders[14,15] (Table 29.3). It is important to review the symptoms with both the patient and the family, and to explain that the associated symptoms are common, may include mild irritability as well as fatigue, but may have a high likelihood of resolving over the course of the next several weeks to months. The vast majority of children will be symptom free within a few months of a mild head injury. With regard to sports-related injuries, a severe brain injury is relatively rare, especially under the age of 12.[16] The potential for long-term sequelae after minor head injury in young athletes is unknown. Concern arises with second impact syndrome. In each situation an athlete with minor head injury can recover uneventfully and some time within the next week another minor head injury can occur, resulting in rapid cerebral oedema and death.[17] The concern is that effects of sequential minor injuries to the brain may be compounded, resulting in cerebral swelling and diminished

| |
|---|
| • Headache |
| • Hyperactivity |
| • Decreased attention span |
| • Sleep disturbances |
| • Behavioural disorders |
| • Dizziness |

**Table 29.3**
*Postconcussion syndrome after minor head injury.*

intracranial compliance. An athlete may return to athletics after a mild concussion if he or she is asymptomatic (experiences no dizziness, headaches, or impaired concentration, orientation or memory) for 1 week. The issue of when an athlete returns after a second or third minor head injury or a severe first or second head injury is more complicated.[18]

There are reports that idiopathic intracranial hypertension, pseudotumour cerebri with or without papilloedema after minor head injury, as well as carotid sheath injuries, temporomandibular joint injuries and temporomandibular joint dysfunction may be headache triggers.[19] Some children report sleep disturbances, including insomnia, daytime drowsiness, non-specific staring episodes, periodic loss of consciousness, neurocognitive deficits and the inability to process information.[20]

## Diagnostic evaluations

Currently, most patients who are hospitalized for a mild-to-moderate head injury will undergo computed tomography (CT). Unfortunately, the absence of an abnormality on a CT scan or on magnetic resonance imaging

(MRI) does not predict whether a patient will develop post-traumatic headaches or post-concussion syndrome. For those patients who report a mild behavioural abnormality with a GCS of <15, but for whom neuroimaging has not been done, we suggest MRI of the brain to rule out any potential chronic subdural haematoma, hydrocephalus or possible structural lesion unrelated to trauma.[21] If a patient has associated cervical symptoms, it is recommended to do MRI of the cervical region as well. In the future SPECT (single photon emission CT) may prove to be very beneficial. Some initial studies suggest that this form of imaging may be helpful in predicting central nervous system (CNS) outcome.[22–24] From these early assessments the SPECT may be more sensitive as a long term outcome predictor than more traditional neuroimaging.[25]

Brain-stem auditory evolved potentials have been found to be abnormal in 10–20% of individuals with postconcussion syndrome associated with head injury.[21] This relationship and the predictors for postconcussion sequelae still need further assessment about clinical correlation.

## Neuropsychological testing

In patients with postconcussion syndrome, abnormalities may be found in information processing, auditory vigilance, reaction time, attention, visual and verbal memory and analytical capability.[26] A hierarchy of functional recovery after mild head injury seems to exist in those who are fortunate enough to recover; in children and adolescents, this is the vast majority of individuals. Deficits in attention and concentration tend to resolve within 6 weeks. Visual memory, imagination and analytical capability also resolve in the subsequent 6-week pattern. Verbal memory abstraction, cognitive selectivity and speed of information, processing may take over 12 weeks to recover.[26]

As noted previously patterns of migraine, and tension-type, cluster and chronic daily cluster headaches have all been reported in patients with minor head injury.[27–28] It has been noted that patients who reported post-traumatic headache more commonly had a prior history of headache.[29,30] Although most children show clinical improvement in their headache sequelae within several weeks, and most within several months, some patients still do not have complete recovery of the headache and associated symptoms of postconcussion syndrome. In adults, there are reports of patients whose symptoms do not abate over 3–5 years, even when financial compensation is not involved.[31–33] The formal diagnosis of post-traumatic headaches and postconcussion syndrome requires the symptoms of the syndrome, with an onset that is related to the trauma, in addition to exclusion of the differential diagnosis of subdural haemorrhage, cerebral vein thrombosis, cavernous sinus thrombosis, carotid artery dissection, epilepsy, cerebral haemorrhage, CNS neoplasm or hydrocephalus.[21] Head injury accounts for the largest number of children coming to the accident and emergency department.[34]

## Treatment

Children and adolescents with head injury need rapid clinical assessment, as well as anticipation of the potential development of intracranial complications. The treatment of post-traumatic headaches is currently symptomatic. Often patients with post-traumatic headaches are misdiagnosed or go undiagnosed; in the case of children and adolescents, they may not receive the necessary attention of their parents or guardian because it is only a headache. If other associated symptoms of postconcussion syndrome are present, as described earlier, this may also further complicate issues when these symptoms are not diagnosed or related to recent head injury. Thus, a comprehensive approach to the education of both the parents and the patient about what could happen is the most beneficial approach. It may even be therapeutic simply to discuss what post-traumatic headache and postconcussion syndrome are and what could happen over the course of the next few weeks and months.

The initial headache symptoms and soft-tissue injuries may be treated quite effectively with mild analgesics and non-steroidal anti-inflammatory drugs (NSAIDs) over the first few weeks. Depending on the clinical situation, a short course of physical therapy for the cervical region might also prove quite efficacious, if there are associated cervical soft-tissue symptoms, depending on the patient's age and circumstances. If there is a more prominent headache symptomatology or associated symptoms of anxiety, depression or cognitive difficulties, more intervention may be necessary.

Post-traumatic headache symptomatology will usually respond to medications used for chronic daily and chronic tension-type headache therapies, although, to date, no specific medication or treatment profile has been found to alter the underlying disturbance of the CNS and there is no clearly defined treatment protocol. The tricyclic antidepressants, such as amitriptyline and nortriptyline, are often the medication of choice. In children,

specific cardiac side effects may need to be addressed. β Blockers may also prove potentially helpful, although they may potentiate fatigue or produce depression; this should be monitored closely. Cyproheptadine may also prove helpful, especially in patients with sleep disorders, because it can be given as a single night-time dose. Cyproheptadine often produces sedation, which is the reason for its use in the evening. For those patients who have frequent headaches, it is important to review the concerns of medication overuse in relation to the potential development of rebound headache; currently it is recommended to limit the dose of analgesics to no more than twice a week. The potential development of rebound headaches from NSAID use is still not fully understood; it is recommended that they should also be limited to two to three times a week. The potential gastrointestinal and renal side-effect profile of NSAIDs must also be addressed in this population if the drugs are to be used long term.

For those patients with migraine-like post-traumatic headaches, triptans with or without an antiemetic may prove beneficial. Some patients respond to dihydroergotamine, especially if there is a persistent headache pattern. For those who wish to consider non-pharmacological profiles, use of biofeedback and stress management can be quite effective, even in children as young as 9 years.[14] As part of the non-pharmacological comprehensive programme, it is important to address other family members as well as teachers, particularly for children who are having difficulty in school after a minor headache injury – about postconcussion syndrome and some of the potential associated sequelae. The addition of a psychologist may also prove helpful for both older children and adolescents in order to teach a coping mechanism for pain. In most patients whose symptoms do not resolve over the course of several weeks or a few months, it may be necessary to consider more physiological testing and reassessment of pharmacological treatment for both acute and preventive regimens.

In the past it has been felt that young children are less vulnerable to long-term sequelae of brain injury than older children or adults. More recent research on animals and humans has not supported this concept that younger brains recover better or more comprehensively after injury.[36] Differences based on focal lesions are not consistently seen, and younger brains do not appear to recover any better than the brains that have undergone severe diffuse injury in older children or adults.[37–39] The relationship between age and outcome of CNS injury appears to be quite complex, and depends on a variety of factors involving the nature and timing of the injury and the environmental contacts.[40] It is felt that the skills that are in a state of development are more vulnerable to CNS injury or cerebral injury than well-formulated skills.[41] Present evidence suggests that the outcome of minor head injuries is similar in adults and children.[42,43]

With the present studies using different study designs and definitions for head injury, it is difficult to ascertain the prognosis of posttraumatic headache in available studies. One month after mild head injury, up to 90% of patients in the adult population have reported headaches;[44] 2–3 months after injury up to 78% report headaches;[15] 1 year after head injury 35–54% of patients report headache symptoms;[45] 2–4 years after injury, 20–24% of patients have been noted to have persistent headache symptomatology. Approximately one-third of adults are unable to return to work after a head injury.[46]

The criteria for predicting the clinical outcome for children and adolescents after a head injury still need to be developed. After injury most headaches in children and adolescents gradually taper off over a period of 3–6 months; those children who experienced persistent symptoms, which did not abate over the course of months to years, have probably sustained a diffuse injury resulting from acceleration/deceleration forces, which plays a significant role in the lack of full recovery. Children and adolescents may benefit from a combination of pharmacological and non-pharmacological therapies for symptomatic relief. Children who do not recover fully within a few months to 6 months after injury may benefit from neurophysiological testing carried out 6 months after injury, to help formulate recommendations for future intervention; earlier assessments may, however, also prove beneficial for those children who have more significant difficulties.

# References

1. Evans RW, The postconcussion syndrome and the sequelae of mild headache injury. *Neurol Clin* 1992; **10**: 815–47.
2. Rizzo M, Tranel D, *Pediatric Trauma*. Eichelberge: Mosby, 1993: 352–61.
3. Goldstein B, Powers KS, Head trauma in children. *Pediatr Rev* 1994; **15**: 213–19.
4. Rizzo M, Tranel D, *Head Injury and Post Concussive Syndrome*. Edinburgh: Churchill Livingstone, 1996: 51–2.
5. Reik L, Cluster headache after head injury. *Headache* 1987; **27**: 509–10.
6. Jane JA, Steward O, Gennarelli T, Axonal degeneration induced by experimental non-invasive minor head injury. *J Neurosurg* 1985; **62**: 96–100.

7. Christman CW, Grady MS, Walker SA et al, Ultrastructural studies of diffuse axonal injury in humans. *J Neurotrauma* 1994; **11**: 173–86.

8. Rizzo M, Tranel D, *Head Injury and Post Concussive Syndrome.* Edinburgh: Churchill Livingstone, 1996: 55.

9. Gordon B, Postconcussional syndrome. In: Johnson RT ed., *Current Therapy in Neurologic Disease.* Philadelphia: BC Decker, 1990: 208–13.

10. Gennarelli TA, Mechanisms of brain injury. *J Emerg Med* 1993; **1**: 511.

11. Evans RW, The postconcussion syndrome and the sequelae of mild head injury.

12. Mandel S, Minor head injury may not be 'minor'. *Postgrad Med* 1989; **85**: 213–15.

13. Brenner C, Friendman AP, Merritt HH et al, Post-traumatic headache. *J Neurosurg* 1944; **1**: 317–91.

14. Winner P, *Current Management in Child Neurology.* Decker, Inc, London 1999: 57–8.

15. Rimel RW, Giordani B, Barth JT, Boll TJ, Jane JA, Disability caused by minor head injury. *Neurosurgery* 1981; **9**: 221–8.

16. Bruce DA, Schut L, Sutton LN, Brain and cervical spine injuries occurring during organized sports activities in children and adolescents. *Clin Sports Med* 1982; **1**: 495–514.

17. Saudners RL, Harbaugh RE, The second impact in catastrophic contract-sports head trauma. *JAMA* 1984; **252**: 538–9.

18. Rizzo M, Tranel D, *Head Injury and Post Concussive Syndrome.* Edinburgh: Churchill Livingstone, 1996: 449.

19. Silberstein S, Marceils J, Pseudotumor cerebri without papilledema. *Headache* 1990; **30**: 304.

20. Gronwall D, Wrightston P, Delayed recovery of intellectual function after minor head injury. *Lancet* 1974; **ii**: 605–9.

21. Silberstein S, Lipton R, Goadsby P, *Headache in Clinical Practice.* Oxford: Isis Medical Media, 1998: 139.

22. Abdel-Dayem HM, Sadek SA, Kouris K et al, Changes in cerebral perfusion after acute head injury: comparison of CT with Tc: 99m – PAO SPECT. *Radiology* 1987; **165**: 221–6.

23. Reid, RH, Gulenchn K, Ballinger JR, Ventureyra EC, Cerebral perfusion imaging with technetium-99m HMPAO following cerebral trauma. Initial experience. *Clin Nucl Med* 1990; **15**(6): 383–8.

24. Abdel-Dayem H, Masdeu J, O'Connel R et al, Brain perfusion abnormalities following minor/moderate closed head injury: comparison between early and late imaging in two groups of patients. *Eur J Nucl Med* 1994; **21**: 750.

25. Gray BG, Ichise M, Chung D et al, Technetium 99-m HMPAO SPECT in the evaluation of patient with a remote history of traumatic brain injury: a comparison with X-ray computed tomography. *J Nucl Med* 1992; **33**: 52–8.

26. Silberstein S, Lipton R, Goadsby P, *Headache in Clinical Practice.* Oxford: Isis Medical Media, 1998: 140.

27. Weiss HD, Sterm BJ, Goldbert J, Post traumatic migraine: chronic migraine precipitated by minor head or neck trauma. *Headache* 1991; **31**: 451–6.

28. Haas DC, Laurie H, Trauma-triggered migraine: an explanation for common neurologic attacks after mild head injury. *J Neurosurg* 1988; **68**: 181–8.

29. Jensen OK, Nielsen FF, The influence of sex and pretraumatic headache on the incidence and severity of headache after head injury. *Cephalalgia* 1990; **10**: 285–93.

30. Russell MB, Olesen J, Migraine associated with head trauma and its relation to migraine. *Eur J Neurol* 1996; **3**: 424–8.

31. Medina JL, Efficacy of an individualized outpatient program in the treatment of chronic post-traumatic headache. *Headache* 1992; **32**: 180–3.

32. Packard RC, Ham LP, Post-traumatic headache: determining chronicity. *Headache* 1993; **33**: 133–4.

33. Packard RC, Post-traumatic headache: permanency and relationship to legal settlement. *Headache* 1992; **32**: 496–50.

34. Kraus JF, Fife D, Cox P et al, Incidence, severity and external causes of pediatric brain injury. *Am J Dis Child* 1986; **140**: 687–93.

35. Silberstein S, Lipton R, Goadsby P, *Headache in Clinical Practice.* Oxford: Isis Medical Media, 1998: 137.

36. Goldman PS, An alternative to development plasticity: hererology of CNS structures in infants and adults. In: Stein DG, Rosen JJ, Butters N, eds, *Plasticity and Recovery from Brain Damage*. Orlando, FL: Academic Press, 1974: 149–74.

37. Mahoney WJ, D'Souza BJ, Haller JA et al, Long-term outcome of children with sever head trauma and prolonged coma. *Pediatrics* 1983; **71**: 756–62.

38. Kriel RL, Krach LE, Panser LA, Closed head injury: comparison of children younger and older than 6 years of age. *Pediatr Neurol* 1989; **5**: 296–300.

39. Filley CM, Cranberg ID, Alexander MP, Hart EJ, Neurobehavioral outcome after closed head injury in childhood and adolescence. *Arch Neurol* 1987; **44**: 194–8.

40. Kolb B, Brain development, plasticity, and behavior. *Am Psychol* 1989; **44**: 1203–12.

41. Ewing-Cobbs L, Levin HS, Eisenberg HM, Fletcher JM, Language functions following closed-head injury in children and adolescents. *J Clin Exp Neuropsychol* 1987; **9**: 575–92.

42. Dikman S, McLean A, Temkin N, Neuropsychological and psychosocial consequences of minor head injury. *J Neurol Neurosurg Psychiatry* 1986; **49**: 1227–32.

43. Fay GC, Jaffe KM, Polissar NL et al, Mild pediatric traumatic brain injury: a cohort study. *Arch Phys Med Rehabil* 1993; **74**: 895–901.

44. Denker PG, The postconcussion syndrome: prognosis and evaluation of the organic factors. *NY State J Med* 1944; **44**: 379–84.

45. Dencker SJ, Lofving BA, A psychometric study of identical twins discordant for closed head injury. *Acta Psychiatr Neurol Scand* 1968; (suppl 33): 1958.

46. Rutherford WH, Merrett JD, McDonald JR, Sequelae of concussion caused by minor head injuries. *Lancet* 1977; **i**: 14.

# 30

# Intracranial infections
*Antonio La Vitola and Francesco Peltrone*

In infectious diseases with systemic involvement, headache is generally present. A headache of moderate severity and sensitive to analgesic drugs characterizes the more frequent viral infections. It appears, generally, at the onset of the infection and lasts for a short time. In contrast, a headache of greater intensity and duration which does not respond to analgesic drugs suggests potential central nervous system (CNS) involvement.[1] Assessment of the clinical characteristics of the headache is therefore crucial for timely aetiological diagnosis and therapy.[2–4] Keeping these concepts in mind, we will focus on the more frequent CNS infectious diseases underlying severe headache in children and adolescents. Furthermore, we present some case reports in which the multiparametric evaluation of headache provided a clue for correct diagnosis.

## Meningitis

The annual incidence of meningitis in developed countries,[5–8] ranges between 15 and 20 cases per $10^5$ patients under 14 years of age, increasing to around 100 cases per $10^5$ children in underdeveloped countries.[9] Despite diagnostic and therapeutic progress, the disease continues to have a significant mortality rate, ranging from 3% to 30%, the range

reflecting socio-economic differences. Similarly, the incidence of late complications is higher in underdeveloped countries (50%) compared to developed countries (10%).[10] Common to all these diseases is an inflammatory involvement of leptomeninges caused by bacterial, viral, mycotic and protozoan agents.

## Purulent meningitis

### Aetiology
Agents causing bacterial meningitis vary with the age of the child, e.g. in the newborn Gram-negative enterobacteria, group B streptococcus, *Listeria monocytogenes* and more rarely *Haemophilus influenzae* type b are the usual infecting organisms. The pattern of infectious agents changes substantially after the second month of life when *Haemophilus influenzae* type b, *Streptococcus pneumoniae* and *Neisseria meningitidis* account for more than 90% of all cases of meningitis (Table 30.1).[11,12]

### Risk factors and pathogenesis
Infections of the upper respiratory tract are frequent in normal children. They are caused by the same pathogenic agents potentially responsible for meningitis, but only occasionally is there invasion of the bloodstream. The risk factors for such an event reflect poor

| Age | Aetiological agents |
|---|---|
| <1 month | *Escherichia coli*, group B streptococci, *Listeria monocytogenes*, *Klebsiella pneumoniae* |
| >1–3 months | Gram-negative enterobacteria, *Haemophilus influenzae*, group B streptococci, *L. monocytogenes* |
| >3 months–16 years | *H. influenzae*, *Neisseria meningitidis*, *Streptococcus pneumoniae*, *Tuberculosis mycobacterium* |

**Table 30.1**
*Aetiological agents of bacterial encephalitis at various ages.*

socio-economic conditions, such as malnutrition and reduced immunological response. In some cases, once bacteraemia is produced, micro-organisms are removed from the reticulo-endothelial system. In other cases the infections are blocked, at this stage, by the establishment of antibiotic therapy. In rare cases infections cannot be stopped and therefore, after crossing the blood brain barrier (BBB), they reach the meninges, causing inflammation.[13]

Less frequently, pathogenic agents reach the meninges through surrounding tissues, for example in meningitis complicating sinusitis, purulent otitis and mastoiditis.[14] Other less frequent causes are infections of a pilonidal sinus or dermoid cyst, traumatic fractures of the cribriform plate and infections complicating neurosurgery.[10] What is not clear is why children exposed to the same risk factors do not all contract the disease. There are various studies that support the existence of genetic predisposition to meningitis: certain human leukocyte antigen (HLA) configurations have been observed in children suffering from *Haemophilus influenzae*. Recurrence of meningitis has been observed in the relatives of these

children, as well as a modest antibody response after the administration of the polysaccharide-ribitolo-phosphated (PRP) antigen capsular of *Haemophilus influenzae*.[15] Furthermore, in patients suffering from meningococcal meningitis, a reduction in some complement factors, in particular C5 and C8, was found. The organisms penetrate the cerebrospinal fluid (CSF) through the choroid plexus, which is the weakest area of the BBB. At this level micro-organisms replicate quickly because antibody activity is insufficient, and they activate an inflammatory response with a concentration of polymorphonuclear leukocytes. The polysaccharide of the bacterial capsular in the Gram-negative bacteria (endotoxin), and the teicoico acid and peptidoglycan present on the cellular part of the Gram-positive bacteria stimulate the release of cytokines and other pro-inflammatory mediators (IL-1, IL-6, TNF, prostaglandin E, etc.). The presence of such mediators causes an increase of vascular permeability, further neutrophilic infiltration, BBB alterations and vascular thrombosis.[16,17] Many studies have shown that, even after CSF sterilization induced by antibiotic therapy, the inflammation caused by the cytokines can continue, causing persistence of the acute symptomatology and possibly contributing to its sequelae. In the initial phase of treatment, the use of corticosteroids has been advised to hinder such events.[18]

*Symptomatology*

The pathognomonic clinical signs of meningitis are common to all forms. They are the expression of CNS involvement due both to intracranial hypertension and the inflammatory process on the spinal and cranial root nerves and on the corticoencephalic areas. Symptoms arise suddenly and rapidly become serious. Headache, hyperpyrexia and nuchal rigidity are present in 85% of cases of meningitis. Headache can, in the initial phase, represent the most alarming and, on occasion, the only symptom, although this is more typical of tuberculous meningitis (*qv*). Generally, headache is intense and continuous; initially frontally located, it then spreads to the whole head. Projectile vomiting, photophobia, and sometimes hyperacusis, and restlessness with rapid impairment of the general state generally accompany the headache.[1] Sometimes the evolution is tumultuous as a consequence of severe cerebral oedema leading, in some instances, to transtentorial herniation with trunk compression. This course, which is possible in purulent meningitis caused by all three common pathogenic agents (*Haemophilus influenzae*, *Neisseria meningitidis* and *Streptococcus pneumoniae*), is more frequent in the meningococcal forms. Sometimes a macular rash is observed in meningococcal meningitis, but the most characteristic rash is purpuric, occurring in 50% of cases and associated with meningococcal septicaemia. Purpura and petechiae, which are rarely seen in the other two forms, are often accompanied by a severe clinical picture characterized by cardiovascular shock and disseminated intravascular coagulation. Generalized seizures can occur early in the course of the illness; these do not necessarily carry a serious prognosis. In contrast, focal seizures are generally associated with neurological sequelae, and late seizures with complications such as purulent subdural collections and cerebral or spinal thrombophlebitis.

In newborns and infants the clinical symptoms are less specific; fever or nuchal rigidity may be lacking, and in one third of cases the fontanel is tense and bulging. Non-specific signs include irritability, mood swing with apathy, lethargy, hypotonia, anorexia, vomiting, diarrhoea, respiratory insufficiency and icterus. Seizures are more frequent (40% infants) (Table 30.2).[11]

*Diagnosis*

A lumbar puncture should be performed promptly if there is any suspicion of meningitis. In most cases such a procedure carries no particular risks. However, lumbar puncture should be avoided when signs of intracranial hypertension are detected. Caution should also be used in the case of cardiorespiratory distress, or infection of the area where the needle

Headache
Fever
Nausea and vomiting
Lack of interest
Irritability and torpidity
Meningeal irritation signs

**Table 30.2**
*Clinical symptoms related to meningitis in children.*

is to be inserted. The final diagnosis depends on examination of the CSF. Measurements of interest include pressure, macroscopic characteristics such as colour and cloudiness, concentration of glucose and proteins, immunoglobulin specificity, and qualitative and quantitative characteristics of cellular elements when present. In meningitis the CSF pressure is generally increased and its appearance ranges from opalescent to clearly purulent; glucose is decreased below 2/3 of the blood value; protein is increased >40 mg/dl; immunoglobulin concentration is increased; cells are up to $10^3$–$10^4$, mainly polymorphonuclears. The pathogenic agent can be shown by gram staining (which is positive in over 90% of cases) and with the bacterioscope. A CSF culture should always be performed, although difficulties in culturing the organism and/or previous antibiotic therapy may lead to a negative result in 10–20% of cases.[19] There are also rapid tests that allow the identification of the infectious agent through indirect assays, based on the presence of bacterial antigens in the CSF. The methodology most commonly used is latex agglutination and counterimmuno-electrophoresis.[20]

The responsible organism may also be found on blood culture, and both urine and blood may contain bacterial antigens. In meningococcal septicaemia, the organism may also be identified in scrapings from the purpuric lesions.

Neutrophilic leukocytosis is generally present. Leukopenia is rarely found, and tends to carry an adverse prognosis. In cases with a longer course, a platelet disorder or coagulation time alternation may occur, with an increase in the prothrombin and partial thromboplastin times. Blood electrolytes must be determined due to the possibility in verifying hyponatremia due to inappropriate secretion of antidiuretic hormone (SIADH).

Electroencephalography (EEG),[10] computed tomography (CT) or a nuclear magnetic resonance (NMR),[21,22] although not included in the routine procedures, should be performed in those cases presenting with coma, seizures, especially focal or late, persistence of neurological signs and persisting fever, 5 days after the start of therapy (Table 30.3)[11–19]

## Therapy

Treatment of meningitis should be started immediately after carrying out lumbar puncture, if the macroscopic evaluation of CSF suggests this diagnosis. Antibiotics are used initially on an empirical basis.[3] Ceftriaxone, a third-generation cephalosporin, is the frontline therapy for bacterial meningitis in patients, aged less than 1 month. This antibiotic is given intravenously (80 mg/kg per day) in twice-daily doses for the first 2 days, then once a day.[23] The patient with allergy to β-lactams can be treated with chloramphenicol. Once the result of the CSF examination is obtained, specific treatment based on aetiology can be administered. It has been traditional to

Lumbar puncture: chemical examination, culture and bacterial antigen research
Cultures: nose and throat, intratympanal exudate
Blood culture
Complete blood count
C-reactive protein (CRP)
Electrolyte and blood gas analysis
Creatinine, azotaemia, glycaemia

**Table 30.3**
*Investigations for diagnosing meningitis.*

continue treatment for 10 days, but recently there has been a trend to reduce treatment to 7 days in early responders with sterilization of CSF in the first 24–48 hours. In the case of *Strep. pneumoniae* strains that are resistant to third-generation cephalosporins, vancomycin may be used in a dose of 15 mg/kg every 6 hours.[24] In infants ampicillin should be given with ceftriaxone. The use of steroids is a controversial issue and they are clearly indicated only in cases with intracranial hypertension. There are many studies supporting the effectiveness of dexamethasone in reducing oedema and the inflammatory response, thus limiting the production of cytokines primed by bacterial endotoxin. Dexamethasone is given intravenously for 4 days, in a daily dose of 0.6 mg/kg, divided into 4 doses. This treatment should begin half an hour before antibiotic treatment.[18,26] In various studies the use of steroids has led to a reduction of fever, headache, CSF changes and particularly of secondary sensorineural hearing loss and neurological deficiency.[27]

## Complications

Patients with meningitis should be observed closely in order to ensure the early identification of neurological complications. Cerebral oedema may arise within the first 48 hours and must be treated rapidly because it can be life-threatening. Brain abscess may occur at any time during the course of disease and needs timely neuro-imaging. Subdural effusion is the most frequent complication; it is often asymptomatic and can usually be treated successfully with prolonged antibiotic therapy. Generalized seizures arising after the third day of therapy, or focal seizures arising at any time, are possible signs of neurological damage or alternation of CSF circulation.

These require immediate neuroradiological study. Persistent fever lasting more than 5 days from the beginning of therapy is consistent with previously mentioned complications, or others such as osteomyelitis, arthritis or endocarditis.[10]

## Development and prognosis

In the last few years mortality resulting from bacterial meningitis has been reduced to around 5% thanks to prompt and appropriate treatment. Most deaths result from the accompanying septicaemia rather than the meningitis itself. In the past there was considerable morbidity following meningitis, affecting about 30% of cases. Modern antibiotic therapy together with the appropriate use of dexamethasone has ensured that neurological complications occur in only 5–20% of cases.[27–29] Neurological sequelae include hearing loss, visual impairment, hydrocephaly, semi- or partial paralysis, secondary epilepsy, cognitive disturbance and delay in acquisition of language.

# Tuberculous meningitis

In comparison to the other forms of meningitis tuberculous meningitis is relatively rare. It has been estimated that, for every 300 lung infections, there is one case of tuberculous meningitis. The highest incidence is in the first 5 years of life. It is a complication of primary tuberculosis with or without miliary spread.[30] In most instances the onset is insidious and symptoms are quite non-specific. The earliest symptoms are moderate fever, general malaise, anorexia and irritability. Later, persistent headache and signs of meningeal irritation may appear. On occasion, headache is the only significant symptom, perhaps accompanied by slight mood swing. After one or two weeks seizures, paralysis of cranial nerves and coma may appear. The diagnosis is based on a positive intradermal test to tuberculin, radiological signs of the tubercular disease and CSF modifications (appearance clear aspect to frosted glass, slight pleocytosis between 30/500 white blood cells per mm³, protein between 100/1500 mg/dl, glucose less than 40 mg/dl). Isolation of tuberculous mycobacterium is difficult with both bacterioscopical and cultural tests. Recently new methodologies have been introduced, such as ELISA or latex agglutination to determine the soluble antigen in the CSF micro-bacteria. However, these tests still need further validation. Therapy is based on the combination of three drugs: isoniazid (15–20 mg/kg per day); rifampicin (15–20 mg/kg per day), and streptomycin (20 mg/kg per day) or ethambutol (15–25 mg/kg per day) for the first two months. These are followed by isoniazid and rifampicin for an additional ten months. The use of steroids (prednisone 1–3 mg/kg per day to be reduced gradually after the first or second week) is advised in the initial phase in patients with increased intracranial pressure to prevent transtentorial herniation and in patients with high CSF protein levels to prevent a medullar block. An early diagnosis of tuberculous meningitis reduces mortality to 10–15%. Sequelae are observed in 20% of cases, and consist of convulsions, delayed cognitive developments, motor deficiency and intracranial calcification, especially in the sellar area.[31–33]

## Aseptic meningitis

Most cases of aseptic meningitis are of viral aetiology, most frequently enteroviruses (ECHO virus and coxsackie virus) and the parotitis virus. The symptoms of the disease are heterogeneous; in some cases they are indistinguishable from signs of the infection (fever, mild headache, vomiting, irritability and drowsiness) and they can regress in 3 or 4 days. In other cases, specific signs of meningeal irritation accompanied by intense headache can be so evident as to require a lumbar puncture which shows clear CSF and slightly elevated glucose levels. In the presence of parotitis, lumbar puncture can be avoided because the meningeal syndrome is frequently found in mumps (in some forms it is found in 50% of the cases), is benign, with spontaneous resolution without complications. Therapy of aseptic meningitis is symptomatic with antipyretics, analgesics, and antiemetic drugs. Anti-oedema drugs are rarely used. Symptoms regress in a few days without sequelae.[34,35]

# Encephalitis

## Definition and epidemiological aspects

Encephalitis is an inflammatory process of the cerebral parenchyma of infectious aetiology. Today it is still considered one of the most life-threatening diseases in children and adolescents. Viruses are frequently involved as causal agents, and usually involve the meninges as well as the brain parenchyma (meningoencephalitis). The illness occurs in 3–5 cases per year in $10^5$ individuals during developmental age, and 10% of the cases occur in the first year of life.[36]

## Aetiology

Encephalitis can be caused by various infectious agents, but viruses are the most common, bacteria, protozoa and mycetes

| Viruses | Bacteria | Protozoa | Mycetes |
|---|---|---|---|
| Enteroviruses (Coxsackie, echovirus, polio) | Rickettsiae | *Plasmodium* sp. | *Candida* sp. |
| Parotitis virus | *Tuberculosis mycobacterium* | *Toxoplasma* sp. | *Cryptococcus* sp. |
| Herpes simplex types 1 and 2 | *Mycoplasma* sp. | Free-living A | *Coccidioides* sp. |
| HIV | *Borrelia* sp. (Lyme disease) | *Trypanosoma* sp. | *Aspergillus* sp. |
| Adenovirus | *Listeria* sp. | | |
| Varicella-zoster virus | | | |
| Measles | | | |
| Cytomegalovirus | | | |
| Arbovirus | | | |
| Rubella | | | |
| Rabies | | | |
| Influenza A and B | | | |
| Epstein–Barr virus | | | |
| Parainfluenza virus 1–3 | | | |
| Respiratory syncytial virus | | | |
| Parvovirus | | | |

**Table 30.4**
*Most common agents responsible for encephalitis in order of incidence.*[39,40]

being rarer aetiological agents. Often agents causing such illness cannot be identified even after sophisticated laboratory tests. In Table 30.4 aetiological agents are shown by order of incidence.

## Pathogenesis

Under the pathogenic profile, three different types of encephalitis can be considered: acute viral encephalitis, post-infectious viral encephalitis and slow encephalitis.

In acute encephalitis, after a systemic and proliferation phase, the virus reaches the CNS. The virus enters the host, invading the endothelium capillary cell or spreading via neurons, finally passing the BBB. Enteroviruses, Herpesviruses and Togaviruses produce a direct cytoclastic effect on the cells of the grey matter, which are killed.

Post-infectious viral encephalitis suggests an autoimmune mechanism, characterized by a host reaction to the viral antigens that produce demyelination phenomena (immune T-cell response against myelin basic proteins), lymphocytosis and perivascular oedema. Symptoms arise after 1–2 weeks after infection.

Slow encephalitis, is characterized by symptoms which appear some years after the virus has entered the host, via a slow and progressive evolution, after the viral antigen has been in contact with the encephalic cells for a long time (typical examples are subacute sclerosing encephalitis after measles, and progressive rubella panencephalitis).[37]

## Clinical manifestations

Clinical symptomatology is heterogeneous, ranging from abortive forms with mild manifestations and complete recovery within a few days (5–10), to fulminant forms with convulsions, paresis, sensorial modification, intracranial hypertension, coma and death. Parotitis (mumps) virus encephalitis represents an example of a benign form, whereas a serious form is Herpes simplex encephalitis. After a prodromic phase lasting 4–5 days, characterized by fever, myalgia, arthralgia and malaise, often exanthematous and rhino-conjunctival manifestations, a typical symptomatology arises with intense headache, nausea, vomiting and awareness alternations. General or focal seizures, nuchal rigidity, focal neurological signs (hemiparesis, cranial nerve paralysis), behavioural changes and language problems are likely to be associated with these symptoms. The clinical picture is related to various factors, from the degree to which the CNS is involved, to the virulence of the pathogenic agent and the host's immunological response.[38–41]

## Laboratory tests and investigations

Lumbar puncture and CSF examination are mandatory for correct diagnosis. Before CSF sampling, a few necessary precautions should be taken if intracranial hypertension or cardio-respiratory depression is present. CSF generally flows out under normal or slightly increased pressure, and it is generally clear though rarely xanthochromatic. Slight pleiocytosis is present, which varies from 10 to 1000/mm$^3$ with increased mononuclear cells during illness although initially a transient increase of polymorphonuclear cells may occur. Glucose level is normal, or may be increased by up to 50% of normal. This is important for the differential diagnosis and the viral aetiological diagnosis. Also of great importance for the identification of the virus are the new methodologies, which are based on polymerase chain reaction (PCR).[42] In post-infectious encephalitis with methodological radioimmunity the research for basic protein myelin can be positive. Blood, rhinopharynx, urine and faeces sampling should be collected to have confirmation of the disease. Over 50% of cases of acute infectious encephalitis cases are not aetiologically diagnosed due to difficulty in obtaining CSF and in performing the necessary laboratory tests.

Before contemplating lumbar puncture and CSF examination, it is essential that the optic discs be examined for evidence of raised intracranial pressure. The clinician should proceed to lumbar puncture only if completely satisfied that there is no intracranial hypertension. However, lumbar puncture and CSF examination are mandatory. Other examinations that may be helpful are:

- EEG which can show the presence of various abnormalities, slowed rhythm, of theta type, locally or spread, and paroxysmal phenomena
- CT or MRI is able to show signs of cerebral oedema and focal inflammation of the brain or adjacent areas.[22]

## Diagnosis

A careful anamnesis is essential for a correct diagnosis. Anamnestic and epidemiological data such as the local community, possible exposures to the illness during the past 2–3 weeks and exanthematous illnesses in the area along with viral infections prevalent in the geographical area and the season, possible stays in areas considered at risk, and tick or insect punctures should be analyzed to give a specific aetiological agent. It is also useful to enquire about recent immunizations or if there is a possibility of exposure to heavy metals (encephalopathy) or of accidental ingestion of drugs. The differential diagnosis is wide, and includes other illnesses from which recovery is possible, as well as the various encephalitides. The evaluation of clinical and laboratory results requires great care (Table 30.5).[36]

## Therapy and prevention

For herpes simplex encephalitis a specific treatment consisting of aciclovir is available: three intravenous doses of 30 mg/kg per day for 15 days. For other viral forms, available treatment is not specific, so only supportive therapy can be given. Until a bacterial cause has been ruled out, parenteral antibiotic therapy should be given. All patients with

fever, seizures, inadequate electrolyte balance, cardio-respiratory inadequacy, cerebral oedema and coma should be monitored in an intensive care unit. Use of osmotic diuresis (mannitol) should be used to reduce cerebral oedema. Use of steroids (dexamethasone) is not advised in viral replication encephalitis. However, it is useful in 'allergic' encephalitis. The widespread use of viral vaccines for measles, rubella and mumps has drastically reduced the incidence of CNS complications from these diseases. Control of insect and animal vectors is necessary to reduce incidence of encephalitis due to arboviruses.[40]

## Prognosis

In the first phase of the disease, clinical outcome of viral encephalitis is unpredictable. This is true for either life-expectancy or late complications. However, when patients are stratified according to their age, a more favourable outcome characterizes the adult patient.[43]

## Brain abscess

Typically, brain abscess presents with the triad of headache, fever and neurological deficit, commonly in the presence of some predisposing factor (Table 30.6). Not all cases are typical, and the clinical features, especially in the early stages of the infection, may be non-specific with no clear indication of intracranial pathology. Acute phase reactants may suggest bacterial infection, and oral antibiotic therapy may result in some improvement. However, evidence of intracranial pathology eventually appears with symptoms such as headache, vomiting, convulsions and altered consciousness, accompanied by clinical signs such as

Meningitis
Toxic and drug encephalopathy
Brain abscess
Subarachnoid haemorrhage resulting from aneurysm breakage, vascular malformation or trauma
Intracranial expansive process
Reye's syndrome
Metabolic disease
Collagen disease
Epilepsy
Guillain–Barré syndrome
Acute cerebellar ataxia

**Table 30.5**
*Illnesses to be differentiated from encephalitis.*

| Group | Examples |
|---|---|
| Congenital heart disease with right-to-left shunting[45] | Tetralogy of Fallot |
| Intracranial infections | Meningitis |
| | Venous sinus thrombosis |
| Cranial infections | Sinusitis[46] |
| | Otitis media |
| | Mastoiditis |
| Soft tissue infections | Orbital cellulitis |
| | Face and scalp infection |
| Injuries | Dental extractions, scalp wounds |
| | Ventricular drainage tubes |
| Pulmonary suppuration | Cystic fibrosis[47] |
| Immunodeficiency states | AIDS |
| | Chronic granulomatous disease |

**Table 30.6**
Conditions predisposing to brain abscess.

papilloedema and neurological deficits including cranial nerve or long tract signs. In cerebellar abscess, the unilateral signs may be particularly dramatic.

Investigations usually show an acute phase reaction suggestive of bacterial infection, but blood culture is seldom positive. The CSF findings are variable and cannot be relied upon to point to the diagnosis; in any case, lumbar puncture carries the danger of 'coning' in the presence of any space-occupying lesion, especially an abscess that may be expanding rapidly. The diagnosis of brain abscess should be based on neuro-imaging, which should be performed as soon as the diagnosis is suspected.

The management of brain abscess is a combined medical and surgical effort. Initial treatment is with intravenous antibiotics, the choice depending on the likely source of the organism, the progress of the lesion being closely monitored by regular scanning. Surgi-

cal excision has largely given way to aspiration, and is reserved for large abscesses causing mass effects, and for chronic encapsulated abscesses; the use of stereotactic frames allows accurate placement of aspiration needles.[44]

The published prognosis for brain abscess varies widely, but in most western countries a mortality of less than 10% can be expected, although the damage to cerebral tissue which is inherent to abscess formation results in neurological sequelae at least half the survivors.

## Conclusion

This chapter provides an appraisal of natural history of intracranial infectious in children. As previously discussed headache is a key symptom of these diseases. In acute infections the rapid increase of endocranial pressure, together with a pain-producing vascular involvement, leads to a sudden onset of headache. Headache is generally diffuse and very intense, accompanied by vomiting, photophobia and fever. These symptoms are followed by antalgic hypertonic features and impairment of general conditions. In less acute forms, e.g. in tuberculous meningitis, the headache at the beginning is less intense and signs of meningeal irritation are absent or few. These symptoms increase gradually within a few days. In chronic forms, e.g. in meningeal infections caused by mycetes, which occur mostly in immunodepressed individuals, headache is the only symptom for a long time. Initially the headache is of moderate intensity, later becoming persistent, intense and diffuse.

In conclusion, headache in acute forms is often the first symptom of intracranial infection. Its correct evaluation facilitates early diagnosis and prompt treatment. The earlier the treatment, the better the outcome. In subacute and chronic forms, headache can be the only evocative symptom during the first days or even during the first weeks, which could persuade physicians to suspect an intracranial infection.

## Case 1: Pneumococcal meningitis with otorrhoea and maxillary sinusitis

Daniele M, aged 7 years and 7 months, with negative anamnesis, was hospitalized in our paediatric department because of a high fever that had started 7 days earlier. Two days later, repeated vomiting episodes and right otorrhoea with strong headache appeared. This last symptom led Daniele's parents to bring him to hospital. Before admission to hospital, a paracetamol-based therapy was given.

On initial clinical observation, Daniele

complained of intense headache. He was in a poor clinical condition, pale, with hyperthermia (40 °C). It was possible to reveal the presence of purulent material in his right acoustic canal as well as features of meningeal irritation (nuchal rigidity, Brudzinski and Lasegue positive). Such symptoms persuaded us to formulate a possible diagnosis of meningitis. A prompt lumbar puncture resulted in a CSF with high pressure. CSF examination displayed: albumin 166 mg/dl; glucose 45 mg/dl, Pandy reaction ++−, Nonne Appelt ++++, $1.0 \times 10^3$ cells, mainly neutrophils. On culture assay, Strep. pneumoniae was found in the material from the acoustic canal. Other examinations performed showed: neutrophilic leukocytosis (white blood cells [WBCs] 21 920, neutrophils 88%), erythrocyte sedimentation rate (ESR) at hour 1 = 66, C-reactive protein (CRP) 208 mg/l, haemopoietic tests within normal values (PT, PTT, fibrinogen, platelets). On day 2 a brain CT scan was performed. Only right maxillary sinus opacification was found. Therapy including ceftriaxone for 10 days and dexamethasone for 3 days was given. On day 3 there was a reduction in temperature and remission of headache, along with disappearance of the meningeal irritation. Daniele was discharged 7 days later. At that time, the biological indices of inflammation were normal. The final diagnosis was a purulent meningitis as a result of otogenic dissemination. At clinical follow-up no further complications were observed.

## Case 2: Headache with tuberculous meningitis

Two-year-old Rosarina G was hospitalized in our department because of symptoms that had arisen 2 months earlier. Such symptomatology was characterized by fever, initially sporadic and later continuous, during the last 3 weeks accompanied by mood swing, irritability and especially intense headache – intense to the point where the child would grasp her head between her hands and slam it on various objects (pillows, walls, beds and mother's breast). Upon arrival, the child was crying and showed great suffering during the physical examination, with slight resistance to flexing of her head. Routine laboratory examinations showed: ESR at hour 1 = 32, neutrophilic leukocytosis, negative blood culture and negative viral markers. A Mantoux intradermic test was performed which revealed positivity in both the child and her parents. A chest radiograph showed reinforcement of the hilar design. Chest radiographs of her parents were negative. A family history led to the discovery that Rosarina's grand-father had tuberculosis in an acute phase. A lumber puncture was therefore performed revealing xanthochromic CSF with thick fibrin reticulum, alumbin level in the CSF of 330 mg/dl, glucose level of 75 mg/dl in the CSF, positive Pandy reaction and None Appelt, and 55 cells made up of lymphoid elements negative to culture examination and BK research. Such CSF findings, not usual in tuberculous meningitis, are described in long-standing tuberculosis and spinal caseous TB. A CT scan was performed giving negative results. Specific therapy was started (streptomycin, rifampicin, isoniazid, and prednisone and vitamin $B_6$). In the next few days, her temperature fell and there was a progressive resolution of clinical symptomatology and headache. Clinical examinations and CSF findings began to normalize without persistent neurological deficiency. Clinical observation over the time demonstrated a favourable outcome.

## Case 3: Headache during epidemic parotitis

Seven-year-old Giuseppe S with epidemic parotitis was sent to our department from an outlying hospital. After a brief stage of improvement, he began to exhibit a fever, intense headache, with phono- and photophobia and repeated vomiting. Symptomatology alerted his parents to the point that they asked that their child could be transferred to a 'better-equipped' hospital.

Upon arrival at our hospital, clinical examination showed swelling of the parotid gland, signs of meningeal irritation (nuchal rigidity, Lasegue and Brudzinski II positive) and hyperpyrexia.

The general conditions of the boy did not cause a great deal of concern, so a lumbar puncture was not performed as it would probably have revealed clear CSF, which usually occurs during parotitis. Such an examination would have given insufficient information and unnecessary pain. Routine examinations were negative except for the serum amylase level (non-pancreatic) which was increased to 659 IU/ml.

The child was treated with an antidiuretic (intravenous glycerol) and an antipyretic (paracetamol).

Rapid clinical remission was achieved and within 2 days the fever had disappeared; the child was discharged on the third day.

## Case 4: Encephalitis during varicella (chickenpox)

Elena V, age 5 years and 7 months, had for 10 days had moderate fever, malaise and anorexia. Two days after this her red spots became rapidly papular and blister like. The paediatrician diagnosed varicella and treated it with paracetamol and an antihistamine (loratadine) for the itching.

Between days 8 and 9, during the regression phase of symptomatology, Elena had a fever spike accompanied by diffuse cephalalgia not sensitive to paracetamol. Such symptoms caused her parents to seek paediatric advice once more.

During the visit the child had convulsions characterized by general tonic–clonic contractions, fixed gaze and loss of awareness. Diazepam given rectally stopped the convulsions within 30 min and the child was immediately admitted at our hospital.

On initial observation, Elena appeared to be ailing and had agitated psychosomatic phases that alternated with phases of torpidity.

The physical examination showed hyperreflexia at her lower extremities with slight nuchal rigidity. An EEG revealed the presence of slow waves coming mostly from the left and complex slow-wave points coming mostly from the right. Lumbar puncture was performed (clear CSF at increased pressure) culture examination and negative chemical physical of 2 cells/mm$^3$. Treatment immediately began with aciclovir, an antidiuretic (mannitol), cortisone (prednisone) and phenobarbital. On the second day of treatment, the child had a convulsive seizure with the same characteristics as the first, but lasting 10 min this time. A CT scan gave a negative result. On the third day, the fever disappeared and the clinical picture regressed; the sensory picture was normal and the child showed more interaction with her environment. Upon discharge, physical examination gave negative results, phenobarbital was prescribed and a regular follow-up programmed.

# Case 5: Meningoencephalitis with clear CSF and status epilepticus

Salvatore M, age 5 years and 11 months, was brought to our hospital with a fever that had begun 2 days earlier, at first very low grade and then high grade, along with an increasing headache. The child did not stop crying and kept grasping his head. Such a state alerted his parents who sought immediate medical advice. He arrived at the emergency room with hyperpyrexia (39.8 °C). During the visit, a convulsion crisis, characterized by clonic–tonic contractions, on the right hemisphere, drooling and loss of awareness, was observed. Diazepam was administered rectally, stopping the seizure within 10 min. Transient Todd's paralysis of the right hemisphere, slight nuchal rigidity, and Lasegue and Babinski positive signs on the left were noticed. An eye examination and CT scan gave negative results. The emergency room doctors then hospitalized the child in our department.

Lumbar puncture resulted in clear CSF with increased pressure and hyperglycaemia (glycaemia of 136 mg/dl, glucose level 88 mg/dl), but the culture examination was negative. The following day, more convulsive seizures occurred, so an antidiuretic (mannitol) along with aciclovir via intravenous therapy was initiated. After 24 hours, another seizure occurred located on the left clonic–tonic hemisphere, and was successfully treated with diazepam. Therapy with phenobarbital was started. An EEG showed the presence of asymmetrical slow waves, without showing where they were coming from. The situation became more critical and required transfer into an intensive care unit, where Salvatore was put on to assisted ventilation and treated with intravenous phenobarbital. After 24 hours, the seizures ceased and he was moved back to our department. Examinations showed a slight increase in ESR, CRP and GPT. A search for neurotropic viruses in the serum and CSF resulted in negative values, particularly insignificant for cytomegalovirus (CMV) and herpes simplex. The child had no more seizures, and on physical examination showed recovery. Upon discharge, physical examination was negative, the barbiturate level was at 23 mg/dl and home therapy with phenobarbital was prescribed. Regular follow-up was carried out.

## Case 6: Acute encephalitis caused by herpes virus simplex type 1

Six-year-old GC, with negative anamnesis, presented symptomatology for 3 days characterized by epistaxis and repeated vomiting with blood and mucous clots, for which he was hospitalized in our surgical department and discharged after resolution of these symptoms. After 24 hours of being in a good condition, intense headache developed along with double vision, fixed gaze (inability to move eyes towards the sides), motor impairment, speech difficulty and unusual drowsiness alternating with irritability. For all these symptoms he was admitted to our paediatric department. Physical examination showed torpidity, bilateral lid ptosis, conjugated paresis of lateral gaze, diplopia, dysarthria and ataxia. Both tone and muscular strength were normal. Meningeal irritation findings were absent and the same applied to Babinsky's findings. An eye examination gave a normal result. Evalu-

ation by an ophthalmologist confirmed lateral external ophthalmoplegia. Lumbar puncture resulted in a clear CSF, with 8 lymphoid cells/mm$^3$, and no reaction to Nonne Appelt and Pandy. Culture and bacterial tests were negative. Inflammation indices (WBCs, ESR and CRP) were within normal values. Tests carried out for possible metabolic or intoxication pathologies (blood gas analysis, ammonaemia and liver enzymes) gave normal or negative results. Considering the signs and symptoms described and the test results, the most logical diagnostic hypothesis was encephalitis. Diagnosis was completed with an encephalo-MRI (Fig. 30.1a,c) which showed the presence in various areas of altered signal intensity, especially in the bilateral frontotemporal insula. The clinical picture was consistent with herpes encephalitis. The EEG picture (diffused slowing down of brain activity) was compatible with the above-mentioned pathology. Diagnostic confirmation was based on the detection of IgM and IgG antibodies against herpes simplex in either CSF or serum. Aciclovir treatment was given for 15 days. Initially, a cerebral antidiuretic (mannitol) was also given. The child's general state rapidly improved while the neurological symptomatology gradually regressed. Clinical course was complicated by the presence of SIADH, which was appropriately treated. On discharge, a horizontal nystagmus on forced lateral ocular movements was discovered. During follow-up 1 month later, MRI (Fig. 30.1b,d) showed sensible reduction of the areas of altered density, seen in the last radiological evaluation, and almost complete regression of the nystagmus.

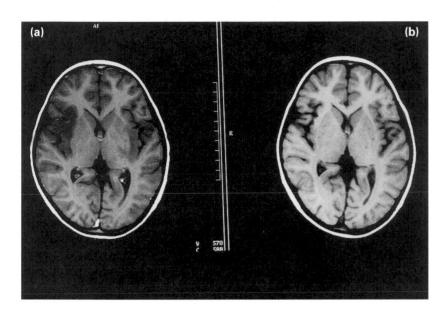

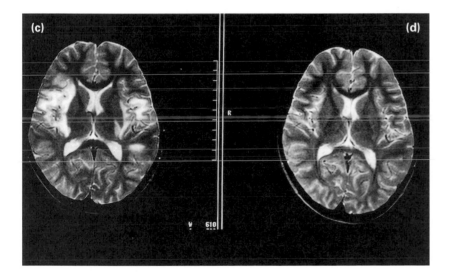

**Figure 30.1**
Patient's MRI scan affected by encephalitis caused by herpes virus simplex type 1. SE sequence dependent on T1 (a, b) and T2 (c, d). (a, d) Onset, cellular oedema swelling and interstitial on medial temporal lobe and insula, bilaterally expressed by hypodensity in TI-weighted and hyperintensity in T2-weighted image (c). During check-up after 30 days (b, d) and after antiviral therapy with aciclovir, a clear regression is seen. (Courtesy of Dr S Vero.)

# References

1. Passali D, Guidetti V, Cefalee infettive da farmaci e da tossici. In: Calvani M, ed., *Cefalee in eta Evolutiva*, pp. 190–201. Rome: CIC Edizioni Internazionali, 1987.

2. Sztajnkrycer M, Jauch EC, Unusual headaches. *Emerg Med Clin North Am* 1998; **16**: 741–61, 6th.

3. Nemer JA, Tallick SA, O'Connor RE, Reese CL, Emergency medical services transport of patients with headache: mode of arrival may indicate serious etiology. *Prehosp Emerg Care* 1998; **2**: 304–7.

4. Gutierrez A, Ramoz MA, Sanz JC, Bernal A, Agirrezabal J, Casado Y et al, Meningitis purulenta en urgencias. Factores asociados al retraso del tratamiento antibiotico. *Enferm Infecc Microbiol Clin* 1998; **16**: 302–6.

5. Progress toward eliminating Haemophilus influenzae type b disease among infants and children – United States, 1987–1997. *MMWR Morb Mortal Wkly Rep* 1998; **47**: 993–8.

6. Peltola H. Haemophilus influenzae type b disease and vaccination in Europe: lessons learned. *Pediatr Infect Dis J* 1998; **17**: S126–32.

7. Herf C, Nichols J, Fruh S, Holloway B, Anderson CU, Meningococcal disease: recognition, treatment, and prevention. *Nurse Pract* 1998; **23**: 30, 33–0, 40.

8. Diomina AA, Spirikhina LV, Koroliova IS, Volkova MO, Childhood Haemophilus influenzae type b meningitis in Russia. *Eur J Pediatr* 1999; **158**: 85.

9. Shembesh NM, el Bargathy SM, Rao BN, Kashbur IM, A prospective study of bacterial meningitis in children from north-eastern Libya. *Ann Trop Paediatr* 1998; **18**: 203–7.

10. Cernibori A, Tamburlini G, Neuropsichiatria per il Pediatra. Rome: Nuova Edizione Italiana, 1992.

11. Tunkel AR, Scheld WM, Acute bacterial encephalitis. *Lancet* 1995; **346**: 1675–80.

12. Fernandez-Jaen A, Borque AC, del Castillo MF, Pena GP, Vidal Lopez ML, Meningitis bacteriana en la edad pediatrica. Estudio de 166 casos. *An Esp Pediatr* 1998; **48**: 495–8.

13. Quagliarello V, Scheld WM, Bacterial meningitis: pathogenesis, pathophysiology, and progress. *N Engl J Med* 1992; **327**: 864–72.

14. Gallagher RM, Gross CW, Phillips CD, Suppurative intracranial complications of sinusitis. *Laryngoscope* 1998; **108**: 1635–42.

15. Kearns AM, Ingham HR, Cant AJ, Spickett GP, Breathnach AS, Abnormal phagocytic function in children under one year of age. *J Infect* 1996; **32**: 103–7.

16. Angstwurm K, Freyer D, Dirnagl U, Hanisch UK, Schumann RR, Einhaupl KM et al, Tumour necrosis factor alpha induces only minor inflammatory changes in the central nervous system, but augments experimental meningitis. *Neuroscience* 1998; **86**: 627–34.

17. Tuomanem E, Bacterial infections and the hemo-encephalic barrier. *Le Scienze (Italian Edition)* 1993; **269**.

18. Schaad UB, Lips U, Gnehm HE, Blumberg A, Heinzer I, Wedgwood J, Dexamethasone therapy for bacterial meningitis in children. Swiss Meningitis Study Group. *Lancet* 1993; **342**: 457–61.

19. Feigin RD, McCracken GH, Klein JO, Diagnosis and management of meningitis. *Pediatr Infect Dis J* 1992; **11**: 785–814.

20. Cherian T, Lalitha MK, Manoharan A, Thomas K, Yolken RH, Steinhoff MC, PCR-Enzyme immunoassay for detection of Streptococcus pneumoniae DNA in cerebrospinal fluid samples from patients with culture-negative meningitis. *J Clin Microbiol* 1998; **36**: 3605–8.

21. Daoud AS, Omari H, al Sheyyab M, Abeukteish F, Indications and benefits of computed tomography in childhood bacterial meningitis. *J Trop Pediatr* 1998; **44**: 167–9.

22. Smith RR, Caldemeyer KS, Neuroradiologic review of intracranial infection. *Curr Probl Diagn Radiol* 1999; **28**: 1–26.

23. Marshall WF, Blair JE, The cephalosporins. *Mayo Clin Proc* 1999; **74**: 187–95.

24. Infection and Immunisation Committee NZPS. Penicillin- and cephalosporin-resistant pneumococcal meningitis: the future is now. *NZ Med J* 1999; **112**: 14–15.

25. Arditi M, Mason EO, Bradley JS et al, Three-

year multicenter surveillance of pneumococcal meningitis in children: clinical characteristics, and outcome related to penicillin susceptibility and dexamethasone use. *Pediatrics* 1998; **102:** 1087–97.

26. Quagliarello VJ, Scheld WM, Treatment of bacterial meningitis. *N Engl J Med* 1997; **336:** 708–16.

27. Axon PR, Temple RH, Saeed SR, Ramsden RT, Cochlear ossification after meningitis. *Am J Otol* 1998; **19:** 724–9.

28. Richardson MP, Williamson TJ, Reid A et al, Otoacoustic emissions as a screening test for hearing impairment in children recovering from acute bacterial meningitis. *Pediatrics* 1998; **102:** 1364–8.

29. Taylor HG, Schatschneider C, Watters GV et al, Acute-phase neurologic complications of Haemophilus influenzae type b meningitis: association with developmental problems at school age. *J Child Neurol* 1998; **13:** 113–19.

30. Abernathy RS, Tuberculosis: an update. *Pediatr Rev* 1997; **18:** 50–8.

31. Nozaki H, Tanaka K, Central nervous system tuberculosis: diagnosis and therapy (Japanese). *Nippon Rinsho* 1998; **56:** 3100–3.

32. Donald PR, Schoeman JF, Van Zyl LE et al, Intensive short course chemotherapy in the management of tuberculous meningitis. *Int J Tuberc Lung Dis* 1998; **2:** 704–11.

33. Yaramis A, Gurkan F, Elevli M et al, Central nervous system tuberculosis in children: a review of 214 cases. *Pediatrics* 1998; **102:** E49.

34. Cherry JD, Enteroviruses: Polioviruses (poliomyelitis), coxsackieviruses, echoviruses and enteroviruses. In: Feigin RD, Cherry JD, eds, *Textbook of Pediatric Infectious Diseases*, pp 1705–53. Philadelphia: WB Saunders, 1992.

35. Rorabaugh ML, Berlin LE, Heldrich F et al, Aseptic meningitis in infants younger than 2 years of age: acute illness and neurologic complications. *Pediatrics* 1993; **92:** 206–11.

36. O'Meara M, Ouvrier R, Viral encephalitis in children. *Curr Opin Pediatr* 1996; **8:** 11–15.

37. Whitley RJ, Viral encephalitis. *N Engl J Med* 1990; **323:** 242–50.

38. Bourguerra L, Encephalites aigues de l'enfant. *Arch Pediatr* 1996; **3:** 267–73.

39. Arboviral infections of the central nervous system – United States, 1996–1997. *Can Commun Dis Rep* 1998; **24:** 156–9.

40. Whitley RJ, Gnann JW, Acyclovir: a decade later. *N Engl J Med* 1992; **327:** 782–9.

41. Turkulov V, Madle-Samardzija N, Ilic A et al, Virusi herpesa simpleks i limfocitarnog horiomeningitisa u infekcijama centralnog nervnog sistema-klinicke i likvorske karakteristike. *Med Pregl* 1998; **51:** 436–40.

42. Ito Y, Ando Y, Kimura H et al, Polymerase chain reaction-proved herpes simplex encephalitis in children. *Pediatr Infect Dis J* 1998; **17:** 29–32.

43. Bartolozzi G, Guglielmi M, Infezioni del sistema nervoso centrale. In: Bartolozzi G, ed., *Pediatria*, pp 926–33. Milan: Masson, 1998.

44. Barlas O, Sencer A, Erkan K et al, Stereotactic surgery in the management of brain abscess. *Surg Neurol* 1999; **52:** 404–10.

45. Strong WB, Cerebral abscess and congenital heart disease. *Pediatr Rev* 1995; **16:** 277.

46. Giannoni C, Sulek M, Friedman EM, Intracranial complications of sinusitis: a pediatric series. *Am J Rhinol* 1998; **12:** 173–8.

47. Cooper DM, Russell LE, Henry RL, Cerebral abscess as a complication of cystic fibrosis. *Pediatr Pulmonol* 1994; **17:** 390–2.

# 31

## Tropical infections: neurocysticercosis

*Deusvenir de Souza Carvalho*

Symptomatic or secondary headaches, classified in groups 5–11 of the International Headache Society (IHS) system,[1] elicit the intriguing question about how they fit into the headache process and can sometimes mimic the primary headaches (groups 1–4). Studies of secondary headaches can help in the understanding of the pathophysiology and pathogenesis of primary headaches.

Tropical infections are a large group of diseases invariably accompanied by headache symptoms. Systemic infectious diseases frequently presenting severe headache include the rickettsial group, dengue fever, influenza, mycobacterial infection, malaria, opportunistic infections caused by *Toxoplasma gondii*, *Cryptococcus neoformans* and *Candida albicans*, and infectious diseases of the central nervous system such as secondary forms of untreated syphilis and viral, parasitic, bacterial or fungal meningitis or encephalitis. Several other tropical infections are also accompanied by the headache symptom but are outside of the scope of this chapter.

Neurocysticercosis can be considered to be typical of the situations that frequently bring together knowledge in the fields of neurology, infection and headache. *Taenia solium* is a tapeworm first recognized by Hippocrates, and 'mealy' pork containing cysticerci has been recognized for centuries.[2] To some extent, therefore, it is obligatory to present neurocysticercosis in a book about headache.

## Human neurocysticercosis

### Epidemiology

Neurocysticercosis is an important public health problem in South and Central America and in south Asia, where it is widely prevalent. On account of the characteristic life cycle of cestodes, cysticercosis is common in developing countries, where sanitation is poor and there are large numbers of stray pigs that ingest human faeces. Negligent care by adults and the play behaviour of children, can make this even worse in childhood.

Although cysticercosis was common in mediaeval Europe, it has been eradicated from developed countries apart from a few exceptions.[3,4] It is also being recognized with increasing frequency in the south-western USA, because of large-scale Hispanic immigration.[4] Several large series of neurocysticercosis have been reported from India and some countries in South and Central America.[5,6] In Latin America it is most frequent in Mexico, Brazil, Peru and Chile.[7] About 2.92–8.5%[7,8] of neurological inpatient cases in Brazil are caused by neurocysticercosis. Patients' ages range from 8 months to 88 years and 1.76% are under 13 years old.[8]

## Aetiology

Human neurocysticercosis is caused by the presence of cysticercus cellulosae, the larval form of *Taenia solium*, in the central nervous system (CNS) and by the biological parasite–host interactions, leading to severe symptoms and high morbidity and lethality.[9] Humans are the definitive host of taeniasis and harbour the adult tapeworm in their intestines as a result of ingesting insufficiently cooked pork that contains viable larvae of *Taenia solium* or cysticerci.

After the ingestion of a living cysticercus, the larva develops in the small intestine into a tapeworm 1–8 m in length.[2,8] The tapeworm causes few clinical symptoms but can release terminal proglottids, bearing up to 50 000 eggs per proglottid. Terminal proglottids are passed into the stool, liberating viable ova.[10] If these ova contaminate food or water that is eaten by pigs, the life cycle of the tapeworm continues.

The pig is the intermediate host for the larvae that develop from taenia eggs. When ova are ingested by pigs, the gastric juices within the stomach dissolve the thick outer shell of the ova to release the oncosphere. The oncosphere, or immature larva, then penetrates the mucosa of the pig's stomach and intestine to be carried by the bloodstream to lodge in diverse body organs, especially the muscles. Within 60–70 days, the oncosphere is transformed into a mature cyst with a bladder wall containing a single invaginated scolex nodule or protoscolex. The mature cyst, cysticercus cellulosae, is a transparent cyst and measures 5–15 mm in diameter, and forms the larval stage of *Taenia solium*.

The life cycle continues when humans eat undercooked pork that contains the viable cysticercus.[10] Human cysticercosis occurs when people become an intermediate host because of autoinfection or food contamination by taenia eggs. Human cysticercosis is acquired via the faecal–oral route, by autoinfection in a patient with an intestinal tapeworm, from a family member or from communal contact with a tapeworm. Ingested ova develop into larva and lodge in soft tissues, primarily the brain, eyes, muscles, and skin (Fig. 31.1). In about 95% of cases this infection occurs when the individual ingests food or water that is contaminated with *Taenia solium* ova. These patients do not or will not develop an intestinal tapeworm. In the remaining 5%, the patients have an intestinal tapeworm.[10]

The mechanism is very well described by Davis.[2] When humans ingest *Taenia solium* ova, they are partially digested in the stomach, releasing oncospheres that penetrate the stomach and intestinal mucosa to reach the bloodstream. These oncospheres may lodge in any body tissue in humans but show a predilection for the brain. Less common sites include the retina, heart, skeletal muscle and subcutaneous tissue.

In the brain, the oncospheres commonly lodge in small cerebral blood vessels located between the grey and white matter. The oncospheres then appear to burrow through the vessel walls into the adjacent brain or into the leptomeninges, often deep within the sulci, possibly even expanding within the occluded blood vessel.[11] Oncospheres may also lodge in the meninges, ependyma and choroid plexus of the ventricles. Cysts involving the spinal cord are somewhat unusual.[12,13]

About 10% of cysticerci lodge in the meninges or ventricular spaces. In the subarachnoid space, some cysticerci grow to over 5 cm in diameter. These giant cysticerci often

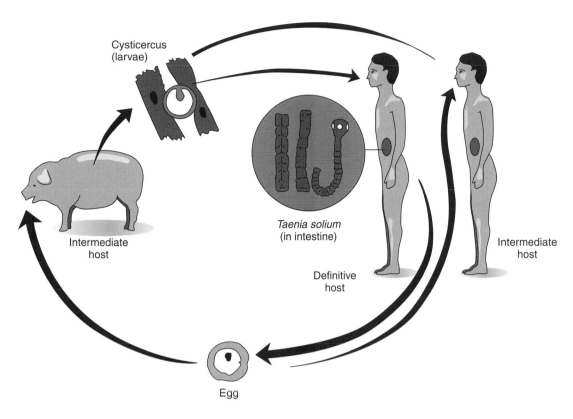

Cysticercus
(larvae)

*Taenia solium*
(in intestine)

Intermediate
host

Definitive
host

Intermediate
host

Egg

**Figure 31.1**
*Biological cycle of teniasis–cysticercosis.*

produce focal neurological signs and increased intracranial pressure with headaches and papilloedema.[14] Other cysticerci in the subarachnoid space or ventricles never develop a protoscolex and produce a grape-like or racemose structure.[15] These non-viable cysts frequently leak foreign antigens into cerebrospinal fluid (CSF), producing ventriculitis, chronic meningitis or arachnoiditis. Over time, the arachnoiditis may obstruct CSF pathways, particularly at the level of the basal cisterns. Occasional lateral ventricular cysts may dislodge and travel until they reach the

aqueduct of Sylvius, where they obstruct the CSF pathway, producing acute obstructive hydrocephalus.[16] In addition, the chronic meningeal inflammation can cause vasculites in traversing arteries sufficient to cause vessel thrombosis and brain-stem or basal ganglia infarctions.

The immune system does not react to live organisms and intraparenchymal larva may live for months or even years with no symptoms in the definitive host unless many cysts are present. When the organism dies, an immune response is generated and the cyst is surrounded by inflammation. In the brain, marked oedema may occur. The dead organism is absorbed, sometimes leaving a calcified granuloma.[3] The disease can be resolved when a small number of parasites infect the tissue and die after maturation.

## Clinical aspects

The clinical picture of neurocysticercosis in humans can vary enormously, from asymptomatic to severe forms. It depends on the number of cysts, their CNS location and the state of health presented by the cyst. The diagnostic difficulties demand knowledge about its clinical aspects. Patients with one or two cysts never develop clinical symptoms.

In general, cysticerci do not produce clinical symptomatology until the cysts begin to degenerate. Cyst degeneration begins from 2 to more than 10 years after the original infestation. As the cyst degenerates, cysticercus antigens leak into the adjacent brain or meninges and produce an intense inflammatory reaction. It is not known how long it takes for the degenerating cyst to die and involute, but it is in a range from months up to a few years. The inflammatory reaction produces clinical symptoms, such as seizures, headaches, altered mental status and focal neurological signs, e.g. hemiparesis, visual loss and paraparesis.[2] The clinical manifestations of neurocysticercosis can be classified into two major groups: benign forms and malignant forms (Table 31.1).

Data collected in the Neuropaediatrics Section of Hospital das Clinicas, University of São Paulo reflect some important aspects of the clinical picture of neurocysticercosis in childhood.[8] During a period of 35 years (1945–80), there were 100 inpatients suffering from neurocysticercosis, of whom 62 were boys and 38 girls; 54% were between the ages of 6 and 9, 27% between 1 and 5 and 19% between 10 and 13; 89% were white. The diagnosis based on symptoms and signs is presented in Fig. 31.2. Although absent from this sample, other rare syndromes have been described, such as pyramidal, extrapyramidal and cerebellar syndromes.[17] A preponderance of females has been observed[18] and the preponderance of whites over other races is noticeable in Brazilian populations. There were positive family antecedents of neurocysticercosis in 27% of this sample, although this in itself is not enough to suggest that autoinfection and contaminated food ingestion can occur predominantly in childhood.

| Benign syndromes | Malignant syndromes |
|---|---|
| Psychological symptoms | Elevated intracranial pressure |
| Headache | Meningitis |
| Epilepsy | Meningoencephalitis |
| Cranial nerve palsy | |

**Table 31.1**
*The main clinical presentations of neurocysticercosis.*

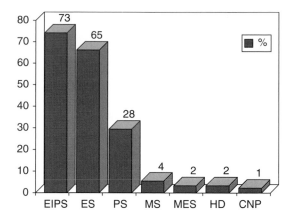

**Figure 31.2**
*Frequency (%) of clinical syndromes in 100 patients with neurocysticercosis. EIPS, elevated intracranial pressure syndrome; ES, epileptic syndrome; PS, psychic syndrome; MS, meningitis syndrome; MES, meningoencephalitic syndrome; HD, headache; CNP, cranial nerve palsy. (Translated from Manreza[8] with author's permission.)*

Headache symptoms are present in most neurocysticercosis syndromes, both in isolation and in association with elevated intracranial pressure, meningitis and meningoencephalitis. Migraine or tension-type characteristics are common, and sometimes patients complain of intractable headaches.[19] Progressive or paroxysmal elevated intracranial pressure syndrome (EIPS), in isolation or associated with other symptoms or syndromes, especially epilepsy, is the more frequent clinical picture for neurocysticercosis. Motor deficits are rare.[20] Paroxysmal EIPS suggests obstruction of the CSF pathway by a racemoso cysticercus (Brun's sign[21]). Occasionally it is followed by remission periods or, more frequently in childhood, it becomes severe, with psychic and visual disturbances, and

seizures caused by oedematous lesions in the brain, resulting in death.

Epileptic syndromes have become more frequently seen since the advent of computed tomography studies.[2,14] Generalized, partial or mixed seizures have been observed, which are clinically easy to treat and well controlled. Benign febrile convulsion and Wests syndrome have also been described.[22,23]

Psychic syndromes are variable, often associated with other syndromes and described as dementia, mental involution, agitation, confused status, hallucination, and other altered psychic and mental statuses. These disturbances disappear after control of EIPS, seizures, inflammation, etc.

Other syndromes observed in the sample presented in Fig. 31.2 are rare. Meningitis and meningoencephalitis occasionally occur and sometimes their reoccurrence suggests neurocysticercosis.[8] Cranial nerve palsy involving the optical, abducens and acoustic–vestibular nerves has been observed.[8] Degenerated colloid cysts may cause severe perivascular inflammation after months or years or vasculitis, leading to thrombosis and stroke.[2]

## Diagnosis

As a result of the variable clinical symptomatology in endemic countries, neurocysticercosis should be considered in young adults and children who present unexplained seizures, subacute meningitis, obstructive hydrocephalus, strokes or signs of a CNS mass. The clinical diagnosis is established if computed tomography (CT) scan, magnetic resonance imaging or the CSF demonstrates the typical cysticercus cellulosae interaction with the host. The CSF from someone with neurocysticercosis can show slight pleocytosis and the presence of

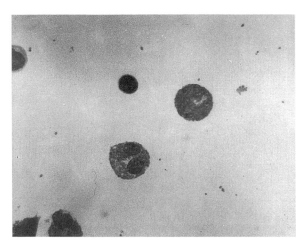

**Figure 31.3**
*Eosinophilic granulocytes in the CSF of a child with neurocysticercosis. (Haematoxylin and eosin staining, ×800.) (Courtesy of Reis CSF Laboratory.)*

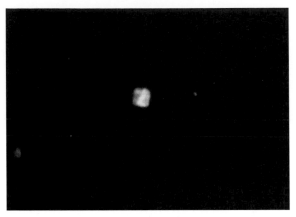

**Figure 31.4**
*Positive immunofluorescence assay for neurocysticercosis (×800). (Courtesy of Reis CSF Laboratory.)*

eosinophils (Fig. 31.3), although serological tests are more important in the study of immunodiagnosis and therapeutic trials to differentiate active from inactive forms of the disease.[24,25] Weimberg's complement fixation test is usually positive in more than 70%.[26] Improved tests in the CSF include immuno-fluorescence assay (Fig. 31.4) and ELISA (enzyme-linked immunosorbent assay) for cysticercosis with sensitivity of more than 80% and specificity of 90%.[27]

Enzyme-linked immunoelectrotransfer blot assay in serum, using the metacestode glyco-protein antigens of *Taenia solium* affinity purified on lentil lectin, is even more sensitive.[2] The serum test has high specificity[28] and is quite sensitive for patients with multiple cysts; false-negative tests occur most often in patients with few cysts. Tests are variable in patients with only calcified cysts. In endemic countries, however, positive serological tests have limited value.[29]

Neuroimaging using CT scans defines the illness and stage (Fig. 31.5). Early in the infection CT shows up homogenous contrast-enhancing lesions with an evolution towards non-enhanced lesions after maturation, ending in calcified nodules. MRI using gadolinium is more sensitive to early stages, showing ring enhancement on T1-weighted images which can sometimes even suggest scolex-shaped lesions (Fig. 31.6). Identification of cysts within the ventricles or meninges is often difficult. The cyst fluid is usually isodense with CSF and can be detected on the basis of distortion or enlargement of third or fourth ventricles outlined by non-ionic contrast CT ventriculography or MRI.[30]

## Differential diagnosis

The differential diagnosis of neurocysticercosis depends on the type of clinical presentation. If

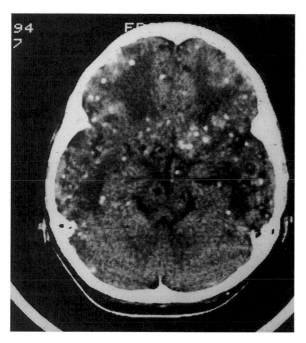

**Figure 31.5**
*Non-contrasting CT (axial view) of 4-year-old child with neurocysticercosis, showing numerous intraparenchymal calcified nodules and some cysts. The concomitant cysts and calcified nodules indicate multiple infestations. (Courtesy of Neuropaediatrics Section, UNIFESP.)*

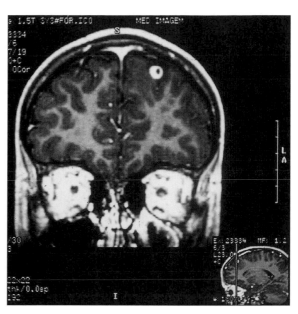

**Figure 31.6**
*MRI (coronal view) of 11-year-old child with neurocysticercosis showing a giant cyst with ring-contrast enhancement over the cortical sulcus. (Courtesy of Neuropaediatrics Section, UNIFESP.)*

cysts are identified on CT and/or MRI, major diagnoses to be considered include tuberculoma, brain abscess, syphilitic gumma, arteriovenous malformation, metastatic tumour, small primary tumour or other parasitic cysts, such as schistosomas or amoebas. Tuberculomas tend to be larger than 20 mm in diameter, have an irregular outline, cause more mass effect and have a progressive focal neurological deficit, whereas cysticercus cellulosae cysts tend to be less than 20 mm in diameter, have a smooth regular outline and seldom cause progressive focal neurological deficits. If the patient presents subacute or chronic meningitis or obstructive hydrocephalus, then tuberculous meningitis, fungal meningitis, cerebrovascular syphilis, neurosarcoidosis, meningeal carcinomatosis and CNS vasculitis need to be considered. The presence of CSF eosinophils increases the probability of meningeal cysticercosis.[2,31]

## Treatment

The treatment of cysticercosis includes medication and surgical intervention. Most symptomatic patients are clinically treated with praziquantel or albendazole. Both drugs are capable of killing cysticerci and *Taenia solium* tapeworms by mechanisms that are poorly understood. Praziquantel appears to kill the scolex, whereas albendazole appears to interfere with cyst metabolism.[2] As both drugs act by killing the cysticercus, the drugs are not useful in the treatment of patients with dead calcified cysts.[2] In addition, occasional patients with multiple cysts may develop increased CNS symptoms, especially headaches, lethargy and seizures, shortly after the start of drug treatment.[31]

Increased symptomatology appears to be the result of rapid death of cysticerci, with a sudden release of cysticercus antigen into the surrounding brain and stimulation of an intense reactive inflammation. Dexamethasone 12–24 mg/day is often added to lessen the intensity of the inflammation.[32] Praziquantel is well tolerated orally and has minimal side effects. The adverse effects usually include gastrointestinal upsets, dizziness, fever, headaches and occasionally a diminished sense of well-being.[31] The drug is well absorbed through the gastrointestinal tract and has a plasma half-life of $1–1\frac{1}{2}$ hours.

There appears to be a wide variation in plasma levels of praziquantel after a standard oral dose. Some of this variation appears to result from the extensive primary hepatic metabolism of praziquantel during its first passage through the liver. Praziquantel is bound by albumin, but free praziquantel readily crosses the blood–brain barrier to achieve therapeutic concentrations in the CSF and even within the cyst fluid.[33] Concomitant administration of cimetidine often increases praziquantel blood levels, whereas corticosteroids, phenytoin or carbamazepine may lower blood levels.[34–36] The usual dosage of praziquantel is 50 mg/kg per day, divided into three oral doses, for about 15 days.[31] Further studies should evaluate the efficacy of a new

regimen of single-day 100 mg/kg dosage, divided into three doses at 2-hourly intervals, for therapy of parenchymal brain cysticercosis.[37] In most studies, praziquantel treatment reduces the cyst burden by 50–80% over 3–6 months.[31]

Albendazole is available in many endemic countries, although not approved in the USA.[2] According to Albendazole Drug Monographs,[38] it is moderately absorbed by oral administration and is rapidly metabolized by the liver to an active sulphoxide metabolite. This metabolite is about 70% protein bound and is eliminated in urine with an elimination half-life of 8.5 hours. The CSF serum ratios of albendazole (mean 43%) are considerably higher than for praziquantel (mean 24%), suggesting that albendazole may be better for treatment of subarachnoid and ventricular cysts.[39] In a study of 63 children, albendazole proved to be beneficial in 31, with focal seizures and single, small, CT-enhanced lesions, compared with 32 who received placebo.[40] The drug is well tolerated with minimal side effects such as dizziness, gastrointestinal distress, leukopenic rashes or elevated serum liver enzymes. Albendazole is less expensive than praziquantel, and some studies find it to be slightly more efficacious.[41] Albendazole is usually given at an oral dose of 15 mg/kg per day divided into two or three doses for 14–30 days.

Rare patients with hundreds of intra-parenchymal cysts present a therapeutic dilemma because treatment with either of these anticysticercal drugs may result in overwhelming cerebral oedema and brain hernia, even if high doses of corticosteroids are given.[42,43] Unfortunately, these patients also do poorly in the absence of treatment.[2]

As many patients have a benign natural

history, questions have been raised about whether all patients with neurocysticercosis require treatment.[44,45] Patients who are asymptomatic and have only a few intraparenchymal cysts may not require treatment. The argument in favour of treatment stems from the observation that anticysticercus drugs rapidly kill cysticerci with collapse of the cysts within weeks instead of months, and this rapid death reduces the incidence of neurological sequelae.[2] Patients who develop seizures should be treated with anticonvulsant medication. Patients who develop obstructive hydrocephalus from a chronic arachnoiditis or blockade of intraventricular CSF pathways require placement of a ventriculoperitoneal shunt. Intraventricular cysts usually require surgical removal.[16] Death may occur from shunt malfunction or from vasculitis of brainstem blood vessels, resulting in brain-stem or thalamic infarction.[2] The multiple infection or miliary form with a huge number of cysticerci in brain parenchyma, meninges or ventricular spaces causes a severe prognosis and is more common in childhood neurocysticercosis.[8]

## Prevention

To prevent development of the intestinal tapeworm, all pork should be thoroughly cooked before eating.[46] Freezing pork to −20°C for several days will also inactivate cysticerci.[47] Prevention of neurocysticercosis is accomplished by avoiding ovacontaminated food and water. In endemic regions, the dimunition of the frequency of the disease relies on prevention through health education campaigns, pending the achievement of an efficient vaccine.[48] Also, in endemic areas, consumption of raw vegetables should be avoided because they may be contaminated with human fertil-

izer. Heating food above 60°C or freezing below −30°C is usually sufficient to kill ova.[10] Restaurant workers from endemic areas should have their stools routinely checked for the presence of tapeworm ova.[2]

## Prognosis and complications

Most patients with neurocysticercosis have an excellent prognosis.[2] Many remain asymptomatic throughout the entire infection. However, those with intraparenchymal cysts often develop transient acute symptoms during cyst degeneration, but these often resolve within a period of between a few months and 2 years.

Some patients develop epilepsy with either focal or generalized seizures. Usually these seizures respond well to anticonvulsant therapy. The rare patients with large numbers of CNS cysts do poorly and may die from the overwhelming CNS infection. Patients who develop a chronic meningitis may also fair poorly. About 5% will develop obstructive hydrocephalus. These patients, if untreated, may suffer brain hernia and death.[49] The occasional patient with a cyst in the spinal cord may be left with paraparesis or quadriparesis.[13] Patients who develop intraocular cysts may lose vision in the affected eye.[2] During pregnancy, oncospheres that reach the blood could potentially lodge in the placenta but will not cross the placenta. Therefore, the fetus should not be infected, and most pregnancies proceed normally. No experience with praziquantel usage during pregnancy has been published, but animal studies have not found teratogenic effects.[2] Albendazole has been shown to cause teratogenic effects in animals and therefore should be avoided during pregnancy.[38]

# Acknowledgments

We are very grateful to Professor Vincenzo Guidetti for kindly inviting us to write about this subject using material from our country, Professor Dr João Baptista dos Reis Filho, Head of Reis CSF Laboratory, for Figs 31.3 and 31.4 and Professor Dr Luiz Celso Pereira Vilanova, Head of Neuropaediatrics Section at UNIFESP for Figs 31.5 and 31.6.

# References

1. International Headache Society, Classification and diagnostic criteria for headache disorders, cranial neuralgias, and facial pain. *Cephalalgia* 1988; 8(suppl 7): 1–96.
2. Davis LE, Neurocysticercosis. In: Gilman S, Goldstein GW, Waxman SG, eds, *Neurobase – The information resource for clinical neurology.* CD-ROM, 4th edn. San Diego: Arbor Publishing Corp, 1999.
3. Mitchell WG, Crawford TC, Intraparenchymal cysticercosis in children: diagnosis and treatment. *Pediatrics* 1988; 82: 76–82.
4. Richards FO Jr, Schantz PM, Ruiz-Tiben E, Sorvillo FJ, Cysticercosis in Los Angeles county. *JAMA* 1985; 254: 3444–8.
5. Singh G, Neurocysticercosis in south-central America and the Indian subcontinent: a comparative evaluation. *Arq Neuropsiquiatr* 1997; 55: 349–56.
6. Schenone H, Ramirez R, Rojas A, Aspectos epidemiológicos de la neurocisticercosis en América Latina. *Bol Chile Parasit* 1973; 28: 61.
7. Takayanaghi O, Jardim E, Aspectos clínicos da Neurocisticercose: análise de 500 casos. *Arq Neuropsiquiatr* 1983; 41: 50–63.
8. Manreza MLG, Neurocisticercose. In: Diament A, Cypel S, eds, *Neurologia Infantil Lefrève,* 2nd edn. Rio de Janeiro: Livraria Atheneu, 1989: 921–35.
9. Spina-França A, Patogenia das infecções do SNC e LCR: análise crítica da contribuição diagnóstica. *Rev Paul Med* 1989; 107: 169–74.
10. Lawson JR, Gemmell MA, Hydatidosis and cysticercosis: the dynamics of transmission. *Adv Parasitol* 1983; 22: 261–308.
11. Thomas JA, Knoth R, Volk B, Disseminated human neurocysticercosis. *Acta Neuropathol* 1989; 78: 594–604.
12. McCormick GF, Zee C-S, Heiden J, Cysticercosis cerebri: review of 127 cases. *Arch Neurol* 1982; 39: 534–9.
13. Dantas FLR, Pereyra WJF, Souza CTS et al, Cisticercose intramedular: relato de caso. *Arq Neuropsiquiatr* 1999; 57: 301–5.
14. Del Brutto OH, Santibanez R, Noboa CA et al, Epilepsy due to neurocysticercosis: analysis of 203 patients. *Neurology* 1992; 42: 389–92.
15. Bickerstaff ER, Cloake PCP, Hughes B et al, The racemose form of cerebral cysticercosis. *Brain* 1952; 75: 1–18.
16. Apuzzo MLJ, Dobkin WR, Zee C-S et al, Surgical considerations in treatment of intraventricular cysticercosis. An analysis of 45 cases. *J Neurosurg* 1984; 60: 400–7.
17. Canelas HM, Cruz OR, Neurocisticercose: formas clínicas pouco frequentes. Formas hemiplégicas. *Arq Neuropsiquiatr* 1962; 20: 89.
18. Lima JGC, Cisticercose encefálica. Aspectos clínicos. Postdoctoral thesis. São Paulo: Escola Paulista de Medicina, 1966.
19. Cruz ME, Cruz MD, Preux P-M et al, Headache and cysticercosis in Ecuador, South America. *Headache* 1995; 35: 93–7.
22. Lefèvre AB, Estudo clínico dos tumores intracranianos em crianças. Considerações a propósito de 127 casos. *Rev Hosp Clin Fac Med São Paulo* 1966; 21: 1–32.
21. Bruns L, Neuropathie demonstration. *Neurol Z* 1906; 61: 25–540.
22. Tasker WG, Plotkin AS, Cerebral cysticercosis. *Pediatrics* 1979; 63: 761–8.
23. Frochtengarten ML, Scarante O, Sindrome de West evoluindo para sindrome de Lennox–Gastaut em paciente com cisticercose cerebral. *Arq Neuropsiquiatr* 1973; 31: 319.
24. Sotelo J, Guerrero V, Rubio F, Neurocysticercosis: a new classification based on active and inactive forms. A study of 753 cases. *Arch Intern Med* 1985; 145: 442–5.

25. Bruck I, Antoniuk SA, Wittig E et al, Neurocysticercosis in childhood. I. Clinical and laboratory diagnosis. *Arq Neuropsiquiatr* 1991; **49**: 43–6.

26. Reis JB, Bei A, Reis Filho JB et al, *Líquido cefalorraquiano*. São Paulo: Sarvier, 1980: 1–250.

27. Rosas N, Sotela J, Nieto D, ELISA in the diagnosis of neurocysticercosis. *Arch Neurol* 1986; **43**: 353–6.

28. Gabbai AA, Contribuição ao estudo da reação de fixação de complemento para cisticercose no soro sanguíneo. Thesis. São Paulo: Escola Paulista de Medicina, 1981.

29. Garcia HH, Herrera G, Gilman RH et al, Discrepancies between cerebral computed tomography and western blot in the diagnosis of neurocysticercosis. *Am J Trop Med* 1994; **50**: 152–7.

30. Woody RC, Rutledge JC, Sklar F, Intraventricular neurocysticercosis. *Pediatr Infect Dis* 1984; **3**: 328–33.

31. Sotelo J, Escobedo F, Rodriguez-Carbajal J et al, Therapy of parenchymal brain cysticercosis with praziquantel. *N Engl J Med* 1984; **310**: 1001–7.

32. de Ghetaldi LD, Norman RM, Douglas AW, Cerebral cysticercosis treated biphasically with dexamethasone and praziquantel. *Ann Intern Med* 1983; **99**: 179–81.

33. Overbosch D, van der Nes JCM, Groll E et al, Penetration of praziquantel into cerebrospinal fluid and cysticerci in human cysticercosis. *Eur J Clin Pharmacol* 1987; **33**: 287–92.

34. Drachman WD, Adubofour KO, Bikin DS et al, Cimetidine-induced rise in praziquantel levels in a patient with neurocysticercosis being treated with anticonvulsants. *J Infect Dis* 1994; **169**: 689–91.

35. Vasquez ML, Jung H, Sotelo J, Plasma levels of praziquantel decrease when dexamethasone is given simultaneously. *Neurology* 1987; **37**: 1561–2.

36. Bittencourt PRM, Carcia CM, Martins R et al, Phenytoin and carbamazepine decrease oral bioavailability of praziquantel. *Neurology* 1992; **42**: 492–6.

37. Del Brutto OH, Campos X, Sánchez J et al, Single-day praziquantel versus 1-week albendazole for neurocysticercosis. *Neurology* 1999; **52**: 1079–81.

38. *Albendazole Drug Monographs*. In: Gelman CR, Rumack BH, eds, *Drugdex Information System*, CD-ROM. (Micromedex, Denver, May 1993 edition.)

39. Jung H, Hurtado M, Sanchez M, Medina MT et al, Plasma and CSF levels of albendazole and praziquantel in patients with neurocysticercosis. *Clin Neuropharmacol* 1990; **13**: 559–64.

40. Baranwal AK, Singhi PD, Khandelwal M, Singhi SC, Albendazole therapy in children with focal seizures and single small enhancing computerized tomographic lesions: a randomized, placebo-controlled, double blind trial. *Pediatr Infect Dis J* 1998; **17**: 696–700.

41. Takayanagui OM, Jardim E, Therapy for neurocysticercosis. Comparison between albendazole and praziquantel. *Arch Neurol* 1992; **49**: 290–4.

42. Wadia N, Sesai S, Bhatt M, Disseminated cysticercosis. *Brain* 1988; **111**: 597–614.

43. Thomaz JÁ, Knoth R, Volk B, Disseminated human neurocysticercosis. *Acta Neuropathol* 1989; **78**: 594–604.

44. Kramer LD, Medical treatment of cysticercosis – ineffective. *Arch Neurol* 1995; **52**: 101–2.

45. Del Brutto OH, Sotelo J, Roman CG, Therapy for neurocysticercosis: a reappraisal. *Clin Infect Dis* 1993; **17**: 730–5.

46. Biagi F, Velez G, Gutierrez ML, Destruction de los cisticercos en la carne de cerdo prensa. *Med Mex* 1963; **28**: 253–7.

47. Sotelo J, Rosas N, Palencia G, Freezing of infested pork muscle kills cysticerci. *JAMA* 1986; **256**: 893–4.

48. Grill J, Pillet P, Rakotomalala W et al, Neurocysticercosis: pediatric aspects. *Arch Pediatr* 1996; **3**: 360–8.

49. Keane JR. Death from cysticercosis: seven patients with unrecognized obstructive hydrocephalus. *West J Med* 1984; **140**: 787–9.

# XI

## Special issues

# 32

# Sleep and headaches

*Oliviero Bruni, Vincenzo Guidetti*

Clinical observations supported by experimental data suggest that sleep and headache share common anatomical, physiological and biochemical substrates.

> The stupid-looking lazy child frequently suffers from headaches at school, breathes through his mouth instead of his nose, snores and is restless at night, and wakes up with a dry mouth in the morning, is well worthy of the solicitous attention of the school medical officer.[1]

This note highlighted the association between headache and sleep-disordered breathing; since then, several aspects of co-morbidity between sleep and headache have been confirmed, showing an involvement of the whole sleep–wake cycle, which contributed to worsening of the quality of life in people with headaches.

Sleep represents the only well-documented behavioural state related to the occurrence of some headache syndromes, whereas headache may cause various degrees of sleep disruption and seems to be associated with several sleep disturbances either in adults or in children. Headaches are known to occur during sleep, after sleep and in relationship to various sleep stages. An excess or lack of sleep or a bad quality or inadequate duration of sleep could cause headache. Many chronic headache patients, whatever the type of headache or migraine may be, complain of insufficient sleep, lack of restoration in the morning, severe snoring, etc.[2]

One of the first medical reports on the relationship between sleep problems and headache in children was that of Hill:[1]

Different studies proposed a model of interaction between headache and sleep.[2,3] Table 32.1 showed a model combining clinical data and experimental evidence.

Clinic-based studies demonstrated that sleep, either spontaneous or induced by hypnotics, was efficacious in relieving the head pain or even terminating the attacks in those who have headache.[4,5] The intrinsic mechanism that leads to head pain relief is still unknown and insufficiently studied; the hypothesis that sleep could trigger an autonomic reset seems to be the most reasonable.[6] However, the power of sleep in terminating the attack is counterbalanced by the ability to precipitate the attack. Although sleep was more commonly referred to as a relieving factor for migraine (70%), migraine attack was also precipitated by sleep deprivation in 24% and by sleep excess in 6% of cases.[7] Sleep is a precipitating factor for either nocturnal headache (awakening during a usual sleep period with a headache) or morning arousal with headache (headache present at arousal at the end of a behaviourally defined

- Sleep as trigger factor for headache (excessive, reduced or disrupted, increased deep sleep)
- Sleep as relieving factor for headache
- Sleep disturbance as cause of headache (especially sleep apnoea)
- Headache as cause of sleep disturbance (especially attacks occurring during sleep)
- Sleep disorders in headache patients (parasomnias, somnambulism)
- Sleep-related headache
  (a)  Temporal relationship (during or after sleep)
  (b)  Sleep stage relationship[1]
      (1)  REM sleep (migraine, cluster, chronic paroxysmal hemicrania)
      (2)  Slow-wave sleep (migraine)
- Headache/sleep association:
  (a)  Intrinsic origin (modulation through the same neurotransmitters)
  (b)  Extrinsic origin (i.e. fibromyalgia syndrome)
  (c)  Reinforcement (bad sleep hygiene)

**Table 32.1**
*Models of relationships between sleep and headache*

sleep period). It has been hypothesized that depth of sleep could be responsible for the migraine attack. The use of a technique called 'sleep rationing', which consists of the reduction of total sleep time and of relaxed sleep and almost leading to a reduction of rapid eye movement (REM) sleep and slow wave sleep, was successful in reducing both the intensity and the severity of the migraine attacks.[8]

## Adult epidemiological studies

Some epidemiological studies in adults showed that one of the most common factors reported to provoke headache, together with emotional stress, physical strain and particular foods, was lack of sleep; further, migraine sufferers reported bad sleep more frequently than controls.[9] Another questionnaire study[10] evaluating fatigue and sleep in chronic headache sufferers showed that, with regard to sleep, the

headache sufferers slept significantly less (6.7 hours) than the controls (7.0 h); it also took them longer to fall asleep (31.4 vs 21.1 min) and longer to fall back asleep after waking up at night (28.5 vs 14.6 min).

A large epidemiological study on 385 migraineurs and 313 non-migraine headache sufferers demonstrated that the most frequent precipitating factors (reported at least once by more than 10% of subjects [range 18–80%] in both groups) were fatigue, sleep, stress, food and/or drinks, menstruation, heat/cold/ weather and infections in both groups. Mean intensity of headache related to these factors, but sleep problems, rather than provoking migraine, can be a premonitory symptom similar to mood changes, food cravings or surges of energy, and can occur many hours before the migraine attack.[11]

With regard to the prevalence of sleep disorders in headache patients, a Portuguese research group, studying a group of 75 adult chronic headache patients compared with 50 healthy controls, found, in the former, more difficulty at sleep onset, more awakenings, more nocturnal symptoms (hypnagogic startles, restless leg syndrome, pain, respiratory problems, sweating, bruxism), and more awakening symptoms such as non-refreshing sleep, fatigue, paralysis and daytime somnolence.[12] Comparing the headache entities, significant differences have been found in only a few items: headache linked to chronic substance abuse had a significantly lower sleep duration, more restless legs and hypnagogic startles and a higher incidence of snoring; tension headaches had more nocturnal disturbances. In this sample, childhood sleep disturbances were more frequent in patients with migraine, supporting the evidence of a more disturbed sleep in children with migraine. Half of the patients had nocturnal headaches during either the second half of the night or at awakening; in addition, lack of sleep was a frequent trigger for headache. From this study, it becomes evident that there is a broader connection between headache and sleep; this suggests that we are not dealing with a 'psychological insomnia' and that there is a need for polysomnographic studies to uncover the links between these two disorders.

## Clinical studies in childhood and adolescence

Even though several studies demonstrated a high prevalence of sleep disorders in headache subjects, sleep disorders are not seen as a co-morbid or causative factor for headache. Although patients complain about their sleep disorders, these manifestations are usually considered to be 'common insomnia' of psychological origin and tend to be considered irrelevant by doctors. The head pain could be the consequence of a subtle sleep disorder that has not been diagnosed or of bad sleep habits, which are difficult to evaluate in adults. In children, this estimation could be even more difficult because the perception of disturbed sleep is missed or underestimated, and it is easier for a child to refer to headache than to poor sleep quality. Therefore the symptom 'headache' in children has to be evaluated from different points of view, including an accurate evaluation of sleep behaviours and disturbances.

## Early sleep problems and other manifestations as migraine variants

In childhood there are different symptoms that can be viewed as migraine variants and their diagnosis can be difficult because the symptoms frequently do not include headache. Migraine variants in early childhood include paroxysmal vertigo, paroxysmal torticollis, paroxysmal ataxia and benign sixth nerve palsy. A recent report showed that migraine in early childhood should also be suspected in the presence of colic associated with irritability, slapping of the head with the hands and upper eyelid retraction, and a family history of migraine.[13] It is known that colicky infants are also candidates for sleep disorders when growing up, and the pathogenesis of colic has been linked to the maturation of the sleep–wake control mechanism.[14]

Another association reported is between migraine and hyperreactivity syndrome during infancy;[15] typical of this syndrome are night awakenings and difficulties falling asleep. The symptoms of periodic syndromes (recurrent vomiting and abdominal pain, migrating limb pain, vertigo, recurrent hyperthermia with no visible cause, sleep disturbances and eating disorders) could be viewed as precursors or the equivalent of migraine in children[16] and they might be considered as risk and predisposing factors.[17,18]

A retrospective evaluation of six children aged under 3 years showed that the classic symptoms may not be present in young children with migraine; from a list of presenting signs, sleep disorders were in fourth place after irritability, head pain and emesis.[19]

It is therefore possible that the same pathogenic mechanism underlying headache or migraine and sleep could have been acting since early life, and that migraine variants are the presenting symptoms of a later developing headache, supporting the hypothesis of a common intrinsic origin.

Early sleep disorders have been also related to psychiatric co-morbidity and involved in the endurance of headache in children and adolescents. In an 8-year follow-up study, it has been found that the most frequent co-morbid disorders at the onset of the headache were sleep disorders (12%), followed by anxiety (11%); of the nine patients with sleep disorders as a co-morbid factor at the onset of headache, at follow-up six had enduring headache and three were headache free.[20]

## Headache and parasomnias

Several reports have described the association between headache and parasomnias in children. One of the first studies correlating these two disorders was that of Barabas et al:[21] they analysed four groups of patients (60 with migraine, 42 with non-migraine headache, 60 with epilepsy and 60 with learning disabilities/neurological impairment) and found a history of at least two episodes of somnambulism in 30% of migraineurs versus 4.8% of those with non-migraine headaches, 5% of those with learning disabilities/neurological impairment and 6.6% of children with epilepsy. Other studies confirmed these data. Pradalier et al[22] found an incidence of somnambulism in 21.9% of migraine subjects versus 6.6% of controls. Giroud et al[23] found a history of somnambulism in 29.4% of migraine subjects versus 5.4% of non-migraine headache subjects; the analysis of different types of migraine showed that the highest prevalence was found in ophthalmic migraine (70%), common migraine (24%) and classic migraine (20%). As somnambulism appeared before migraine, the authors hypothesized that this sleep disorder and migraine could be a different age-related expression of the same neurotransmitter imbalance, probably of the serotoninergic axis.

It seems, however, that the association between migraine and parasomnias is not limited to somnambulism, but also includes pavor nocturnus (nightmares) and enuresis: Dexter,[24] when asking parents of 100 migrainous patients about the occurrence of these three disorders in the first two decades of life, compared with a control group of patients with non-headache pain problems, found an incidence of 71% of pavor nocturnus (vs 11% of controls), 55% of somnambulism (vs 16% of controls) and 41% of enuresis (vs 16% of controls).

## Headache and sleep disorders

Few systematic studies about the wide spectrum of sleep disorders in children with headache syndromes have been carried out. The first survey on a wide paediatric population confirmed the strong association between headache and different sleep disorders, not only parasomnias.[25] This questionnaire-based study involved a sample of 283 children with headache (144 boys/139 girls) aged 5.0–14.3 years: 164 with migraine (M) headache (141 migraine without aura and 23 migraine with aura), 119 with tension-type (T) headache (84 episodic tension-type headache and 35 chronic tension-type headache), compared with an age-matched healthy control (C) group. Significant differences between headache patients and controls have been found in several areas as follows.

## Sleep duration and sleep latency

Migraine and tension-type headache children had a shorter sleep duration – duration < 8 hours in about 18% of headache children (M = 17.68%; T = 17.65%) vs 9.6% of controls – and a longer sleep latency than controls (sleep latency > 30 min in 13.4% [M = 12.2%; T = 15.1%] vs 6.6%).

## Bedtime problems

Headache children showed a higher prevalence of difficulty getting to sleep (M = 20.1%; T = 17.6%; C = 8.9%) and of fears or anxiety when falling asleep (M = 30.5%; T = 22.7%; C = 8.2%).

## Night awakenings

Headache children showed a more interrupted sleep, with more than two awakenings per night in 12.8% of the M group and 12.6% of the T group vs 6.83% of the controls.

## Parasomnias

Sleeptalking, bruxism and reports of frightening dreams were the items in which the migraine children were significantly different from controls, although no differences were found for the prevalence of somnambulism,

bed-wetting and sleep terrors (Table 32.2). These findings were in agreement with those of another survey on migraine subjects[26] which did not find a higher incidence of somnambulism. As there were different reports of a higher prevalence of somnambulism during childhood in adults with migraine,[21–24] the authors analysed the migraine subgroups and found a higher frequency of somnambulism in migraine with aura (13.04%) vs migraine without aura (2.84%; $p < 0.05$) and vs controls (3.14%; $p < 0.005$). This result is in accord with the only report that attempted to differentiate between subgroups[23] which found a higher occurrence of somnambulism in ophthalmic migraine and a lower one in common migraine and classic migraine.

## Sleep breathing disorders

Sleep breathing problems were more frequent in children with migraine vs controls, whereas tension-type headache failed to show a difference (Table 32.2), confirming data already reported in children and adults.[27,28]

## Morning symptoms and daytime sleepiness

Both children with migraine (35.37%) and those with tension-type headache (30.25%) reported more restless sleep than controls (19.71%); daytime sleepiness affected both headache groups in a higher percentage with respect to controls (12.20% in migraine, 10.92% in tension type, 4.48% in controls).

Although no statistical differences have been found for the prevalence of sleep disturbances between migraine and tension-type headache children, the migraine group seemed to be the one with the more 'disturbed sleep', with increased prevalence of nocturnal symptoms such as sleep breathing disorders and certain parasomnias. Of 283 participants,

| | Controls (%) | Migraine (%) | Tension type (%) | Significant comparisons vs controls[a] |
|---|---|---|---|---|
| *Parasomnias* | | | | |
| Hypnic jerks | 5.0 | 16.5** | 14.3** | M and T |
| Rhythmic movements while falling asleep | 2.7 | 6.1* | 5.0 | M |
| Hypnagogic hallucinations | 1.5 | 4.3* | 4.2* | M and T |
| Somnambulism | 3.1 | 4.3 | 4.2 | NS |
| Sleeptalking | 14.4 | 28.7* | 19.3 | M |
| Bedwetting | 2.3 | 3.7 | 3.4 | NS |
| Bruxism | 7.4 | 12.2* | 7.6 | M |
| Sleep terrors | 1.3 | 3.0 | 1.7 | NS |
| Nightmares | 2.5 | 8.5** | 6.7** | M and T |
| Report of frightening dream | 10.6 | 18.9* | 12.6 | M |
| *Sleep breathing disorders* | | | | |
| Sleep breathing difficulties | 6.8 | 16.5** | 10.1 | M |
| Sleep apnoea | 1.0 | 6.1** | 3.4 | M |
| Snoring | 14.7 | 21.9* | 15.9 | M |

M, migraine; T, tension-type headache.
*$p < 0.05$; **$p < 0.005$; NS, not significant.
[a]No differences have been found between the two headache entities M and T.

**Table 32.2**
*Prevalence of parasomnias and sleep breathing disorders (presence more than 1/week)*

20 (7.77%) presented recurrent nocturnal headache attacks and showed more sleep disorders than patients with diurnal attacks – particularly bedtime struggles, night wakings, parasomnias and daytime sleepiness. The occurrence of nocturnal headache attacks deeply modifies the sleep pattern and affects the occurrence of night symptoms, confirming the involvement of common pathways in the pathogenesis of both conditions.

In the same study, a higher prevalence of sleep disturbances in parents, sleep disturbances in infancy and from colic, as well as an increased level of familial headache, were found in migraine sufferers, showing that a genetic link could subsist between migraine and sleep and indicate that the common neurobiological substrate might have acted since the start of life and/or that there is a co-morbidity between the two disorders. This hereditary connection was not sufficiently supported in our participants with tension-type headache.

Other studies confirmed this survey. A report on 48 elementary and junior high school students with primary headache highlighted the association with sleep disorders: night wakings (41.7%) and difficulty falling asleep (20.8%) were the most prevalent disorders; parasomnias were also represented: pavor nocturnus and nightmares (14.6%), enuresis (8.3%) and somnambulism (6.3%).[29] Treatment with L-5-hydroxytryptophan (5HTP) in these subjects determined the improvement of both conditions – headache and sleep disorders – in particular, frequent awakenings and some parasomnias.[29] An Hispanic study, carried out on 97 children aged 3–15 years with primary chronic headache and compared with 127 age-matched control children showed a decreased duration of sleep at night, and an increased frequency of poor sleep hygiene (insomnia and night wakings), some parasomnias (somnambulism, sleeptalking, enuresis) and nocturnal snoring.[30]

## Headache, circadian rhythms and sleep hygiene

Headache has been described as related to biological cycles and there is evidence of the relationship of different headache syndromes to a variety of cyclic phenomena; however, few studies focused on the sleep–wake cycle and the circadian aspects.

The involvement of the suprachiasmatic nucleus in the pathogenesis of migraine attacks,[31] and the reduction of the nocturnal peak of melatonin in cluster headache and migraine without aura, provide evidence of the links between the biological clock and migraine.[32] Migraine attacks showed different periodicities:

(1) A circadian periodicity of migraine attacks with an over-representation during the hours of waking (between 4am and 9am)

(2) A menstrual periodicity with a peak after the onset of menses

(3) A weak seasonal periodicity with a mild over-representation during summer months.[33]

In childhood, the precursors of the migraine called 'migraine variants' such as colic and periodic syndromes showed a recurrent circadian pattern. Another indirect demonstration of the involvement of the circadian rhythms is the report of five patients with different kinds of headache (migraine without aura, cluster headache and chronic tension-type headache) associated with delayed sleep phase syndrome who were successfully treated with melatonin.[34] As the melatonin levels were normal and did not differ from those of the patients with delayed sleep phase syndrome who did not have headaches, the authors explain the results by the chronological action of melatonin, which synchronizes the patients' biological clock with their lifestyle.[34] From another point of view, we can say that in these patients melatonin has had a 'sleep hygiene effect', which is in agreement with the results of migraine improvement in childhood and adolescence after the application of sleep hygiene guidelines.[35] Sleep hygiene has been defined as the conditions and practices that promote continuous and effective sleep: these include regularity of bedtime and rising time; conformity of time spent in bed to the time necessary for sustained and individually adequate sleep (i.e. a total sleep time sufficient to avoid sleepiness when awake); restriction of beverages, foods and compounds (that tend to disrupt sleep) before bedtime; and use of exercise, nutrition and environmental factors so that they enhance, rather than disturb, restful sleep.

In the aforementioned study, 70 migraineur children with poor sleep hygiene were randomly assigned to two groups: group A were instructed to follow directions to improve sleep hygiene; group B had no instructions on improvement of sleep hygiene. After the application of the sleep hygiene guidelines, the mean duration of migraine attacks was significantly reduced in the A group (from 234 to 65 min at 6-month follow-up), whereas the B group showed an initial but insignificant reduction. The frequency of migraine attacks also showed a reduction from 35% to 11% in the A group only. The severity of the attacks did not change, and seemed to be independent of bad sleep habits and related more to the presence of sleep disorders such as hypnic (sleep) jerks, nightmares or restless sleep. The frequency and duration of migraine attacks were therefore sensitive to the modification of the sleep habits, whereas the severity was related more to the alteration of the sleep structure.[35]

A further report on the association between headache and sleep deprivation showed that, in three children, the head pain complaints resolved after a modification of bad sleeping habits, notably problems with falling asleep, confirming that awareness of this connection can provide a clue to the successful treatment of headache.[36] The application of sleep hygiene guidelines could represent an alternative approach to the treatment of migraine by correcting inappropriate sleep behaviour, without resorting to pharmacological treatment.

Few studies in children focused on the whole sleep–wake cycle and the circadian aspects for assessing the relationships with migraine. A recent preliminary report evaluated the sleep–wake cycle in 10 participants with migraine on a long-term basis (2 weeks), using the actigraph, which allows an activity-based assessment of the sleep–wake cycle. A total of 155 days for migraine and 66 days for control children were recorded. The mean activity during the night was globally reduced in migraine vs control children and there was

an increase in wakenings after sleep onset and number of wakenings, and a reduction in sleep efficiency and average duration of each sleep episode, indicating an alteration in sleep continuity. Correlating the actigraphic data with the temporal occurrence of migraine attacks, it has been found that there was reduced activity during the night after the migraine attack; however, the observation that the activity index (percentage of periods with activity > 0) is higher led to the hypothesis that children with migraine move less intensively but more continuously during the night. These results supported the hypothesis of a dopaminergic imbalance in migraine children.[37]

## Polysomnographic studies in adults

Several polysomnographic studies analysed sleep organization in headache and did not find any peculiar characteristics of sleep architecture in the adult population, except for the strict relationship of some particular subgroups with specific sleep stages:

(1) Migraine attacks seem to be linked to REM stages and associated with a large amount of deep sleep[38,39]
(2) Cluster headache is triggered by REM[40] and non-REM (NREM) sleep, particularly stage 2[41]
(3) Chronic paroxysmal hemicrania is associated with a reduction of total sleep time and REM phase, and an increase in awakenings during REM.[42]

The evaluation of sleep architecture in chronic headache patients through ambulatory recording showed, compared with published norms, an increased number of awakenings and being awake during sleep and a slight reduction of NREM stage 2, with minor differences among the three headache groups analysed: slow-wave sleep was slightly increased in migraine patients and markedly reduced in tension-type headache; and REM latency was markedly diminished in mixed vascular headache.[43]

Headache is the presenting symptom of several sleep disorders that could therefore be misdiagnosed; Paiva et al[3] demonstrated that, in several cases of adult migraine, after a polysomnographic study, the diagnosis has been changed in half the patients and the treatment of the underlying clinical condition improved the symptomatic headache greatly. Among the 25 patients, 13 were misdiagnosed as headache: after the polysomnographic study the diagnosis was changed to periodic limb movement of sleep in four cases, to fibromyalgia syndrome in six cases and to obstructive sleep apnoea syndrome in three cases.

## Migraine headache

The first polysomnographic study of patients with sleep-related headache showed that awakening-related migraine attacks were associated with REM sleep in all patients: six awakenings from REM sleep; one within 3 min of the completion of a REM period; one on awakening 9 min after the termination of a REM period.[39] The prevalence of REM-related attacks could be linked to the chronobiology of migraine because the peak time of attack onset (4am to 9am) is during the hours of REM maximal representation.[33] However, even in a different sleep schedule (7-h sleep shift), the attacks continued to occur during REM sleep (even if during the day), demonstrating that migraine was related to sleep rather than to circadian rhythms.[44]

Some relationships with NREM sleep have also been found: headache-related awakening occurred from non-REM sleep in two or three patients with nocturnal headache.[45]

As the reduction of total sleep time and depth of sleep through sleep rationing was effective in preventing migraine attacks,[8] it could be expected that migraine is somewhat related to NREM slow-wave sleep: Dexter[38] confirmed this hypothesis, showing that the morning arousals with headache were associated with sleep periods that had large amounts of NREM slow-wave sleep and REM sleep.

## Cluster headache and chronic paroxysmal hemicrania

The description by Wolfe[46] of cluster headache (CH) attacks during sleep, in which patients jump out of bed before fully awake, suggested that there was a concurrent presence of a disorder of arousal that preceded or was the consequence of the pain attack. Some authors found that nocturnal attacks in cluster headache occurred mainly from REM sleep[39] whereas others found that they occurred from NREM sleep.[41] Recently, it has been found that symptoms of sleep-disordered breathing (SBD) predicted reported occurrence of CH in the first half of the night, which suggested that CH could be triggered in some cases by unrecognized SBD.[47] In most cases of CH, the treatment of the sleep apnoea either with surgical interventions or with continuous positive airway pressure solved or greatly improved the head pain.[48]

Chronic paroxysmal hemicrania is characterized by frequent nocturnal arousals with pain which occurred mainly from REM sleep and by marked fragmentation of sleep with an excessive number of sleep-stage shifts, and a reduction of total sleep time and of REM.[42] This fragmentation of sleep is similar to what is seen in chronic cluster headache.

## Hypnic headache syndrome

First described by Raskin in 1988,[49] this is a rare, recurrent, benign, headache disorder occurring exclusively during sleep and in older people. The common symptom is regular awakening from nocturnal sleep caused by headache attacks lasting 30–60 min. Since the first description, about 45 patients have been described. Recent polysomnographic studies of this syndrome showed conflicting results with a more consistent association with REM sleep in three cases[50] and with stage III NREM in one case.[51]

## Headache and sleep apnoea

It is well known that headache could be a sign of sleep-disordered breathing and the presenting complaint of sleep apnoea, a subtle and often undiagnosed symptom in several headache patients. Guilleminault et al[52] reported a 36% incidence of morning headaches in 50 patients with sleep apnoea. Dexter[53] reported 11 patients with chronic recurring headaches who had a history suggestive of sleep apnoea, which was confirmed polysomnographically: 10 of these patients had sleep apnoea and one had mixed sleep apnoea. Mathew et al[27] have also reported headache in patients with sleep apnoea: three out of eighteen patients with chronic headaches and one of four patients with cluster headache had sleep apnoea. Kudrow et al[40] found a 60% prevalence of sleep apnoea among ten patients with cluster headaches: four of these patients had central apnoeas, and two obstructive apnoeas.

An association, therefore, seems to exist between sleep apnoea and different types of headache syndrome. To clarify this relationship, Boutros[54] showed that, although the incidence of headache in general did not differ between sleep apnoea patients and controls, those with sleep apnoea had a significantly higher incidence of morning headache and a higher severity of pain. It has been also demonstrated that, although early morning headache takes place more often in patients with sleep apnoea than in people with normal sleep, it occurs even more frequently in patients who underwent sleep studies for other reasons.[55] It seems, therefore, that headache attacks could be secondary to the sleep disruption rather than to the sleep apnoea itself.

In migraine patients, either obstructive or central sleep apnoea has been found. In the study by Paiva et al[3] the authors found 3 patients with obstructive sleep apnoea syndrome among 13 migrainous patients, whereas Kudrow's study[40] showed evidence of sleep apnoea in 6 of 10 cluster headache patients: 4 of these patients had central apnoea, and 2 obstructive apnoea.

Several mechanisms have been proposed to explain the increased incidence of headaches in sleep apnoea patients: hypercapnia, hypoxaemia, altered cerebral blood flow, increased intracranial pressure, alterations in sympathetic nerve activity and increases in blood pressure secondary to multiple arousals.[27] Another hypothesis is that a brain-stem dysfunction could be the cause of the three disorders: migraine, sleep disruption and sleep apnoea. A brain-stem activation occurs during spontaneous migraine attacks and the same anatomical structures are involved in the control of vigilance state and arousals, and of respiratory drive.[56]

| | Migraine Mean (SD) | Controls Mean (SD) | p |
|---|---|---|---|
| Time in bed | 524.83 (32.62) | 532.50 (64.53) | NS |
| Total sleep time | 473.50 (41.39) | 489.45 (54.81) | NS |
| Sleep period total | 513.39 (30.35) | 520.40 (63.91) | NS |
| Sleep efficiency | 90.18 (4.26) | 92.16 (4.89) | NS |
| Sleep latency | 10.78 (6.76) | 12.60 (9.69) | NS |
| No. of awakenings | 2.89 (3.41) | 1.40 (1.51) | NS |
| No. of stage shifts | 89.33 (42.42) | 34.20 (23.56) | < 0.005 |
| Movement time (%) | 4.63 (1.92) | 2.59 (2.02) | < 0.05 |
| Wake after sleep onset (%) | 3.20 (3.35) | 1.77 (2.15) | NS |
| Time spent in stage I NREM (%) | 10.78 (4.75) | 8.41 (4.58) | NS |
| Time spent in stage II NREM (%) | 47.47 (6.72) | 43.41 (4.96) | NS |
| Time spent in slow-wave sleep (%) | 19.13 (6.88) | 24.57 (7.87) | NS |
| Time spent in stage REM (%) | 14.77 (3.91) | 19.42 (5.18) | < 0.05 |
| REM latency | 134.72 (50.81) | 73.85 (19.46) | < 0.005 |
| No. of REM periods | 4.78 (0.83) | 5.00 (1.25) | NS |

NS, not significant.

**Table 32.3**
Comparison of polysomnographic data

# Polysomnographic studies in children

In children, there is a real paucity of polysomnographic studies. In a preliminary study, our group analysed the sleep structure in 10 migraine children compared with 10 age-matched controls. These subjects underwent a polysomnographic recording for two consecutive nights in our sleep laboratory. Table 32.3 summarizes the polysomnographic data; we found differences in number of stage shifts (55.7 vs 20.8; $p < 0.005$), in movement time (5.16% vs 2.7%; $p < 0.05$) and in time spent in stage I NREM sleep (11.7% vs 6.9%; $p < 0.05$), whereas no differences have been found for time in bed, total sleep time, sleep period total, sleep latency, time in stage II NREM and stage III–IV NREM sleep and REM latency.[57] Therefore, the main feature of sleep organization in migraine children was represented by a highest degree of sleep instability, as demonstrated by increased number of stage shifts, movement time and percentage of stage I NREM sleep.

The description of a changing diagnosis in several headache adults, after a polysomnographic study (periodic limb movements of sleep, fibromyalgia syndrome and obstructive sleep apnoea syndrome), raised the possibility of similar conditions in children. As periodic limb movements and fibromyalgia syndrome are uncommon in childhood and adolescence, it could be expected that sleep-disordered breathing is involved in childhood migraine. The first report of sleep apnoea in eight children[58] highlighted the importance of daytime symptoms such as excessive daytime sleepiness, decrease in school performance, abnormal daytime behaviour, recent enuresis, morning headache, abnormal weight and progressive development of hypertension. These symptoms, when associated with loud snoring and interrupted by pauses during sleep, could be suggestive of childhood sleep apnoea syndrome. As stated, morning headache could also be one of the major signs of sleep apnoea in children. As, in a previous study,[24] we found a high prevalence of sleep-disordered breathing in migraine children vs controls – snoring (21.9% vs 14.7%), sleep breathing difficulties (16.5% vs 6.8%) and sleep apnoea (6.1% vs 1.0%) – we decided to analyse the respiratory pattern in ten migraine subjects in order to evaluate the presence of sleep apnoea.[59] Of the ten patients, three had normal sleep architecture, two showed an insomnia pattern (increased awakenings and being awake after sleep onset), three had a decrease in slow-wave sleep, two showed a diminution of REM sleep including absence of the first REM period and increased REM latency. Respiratory analysis revealed that two out of ten patients had obstructive apnoeas.

The two patients with sleep apnoea reported habitual snoring and associated sleep disturbances such as restless sleep and hypnic jerks. In adults, Dexter[53] showed that the symptoms associated with sleep apnoea were snoring in 72% of cases, severe-to-moderate obesity in 54%, excessive daytime sleepiness (EDS) in 36%, enuresis in 18% and restless sleep in 100%. Accordingly, in all of our sleep apnoea patients, we found an association with restless sleep and snoring; EDS was not a com-plaint in our sample because, in children, the symptom EDS was often represented by hyperactivity or attention deficit.[60] Although parents could not be aware of this symptom in their children, the report of habitual snoring associated with restless sleep could be a reliable marker of sleep apnoea in migraine children.[59]

# Conclusion: linking the studies' results

We can hypothesize a model that could explain the relationship between sleep and headache, linking the clinical findings with biochemical and anatomical aspects. We can imagine a structural co-alteration of serotoninergic and dopaminergic pathways that affect migraine and sleep.

The involvement of the serotoninergic system is reflected by an unsteadiness of serotonin levels, which may result in a derangement in the smooth transition through various sleep states. This could account for the abnormalities of sleep architecture and mainly for problems in sleep continuity, reflected by increased number of stage shifts and movement time. Also the higher prevalence of sleep disorders, either night wakings or sleep–wake transition disorders, could be related to this serotonin abnormality.

Dopamine has also been involved in migraine and sleep. Drugs such as amphetamine and cocaine, which enhance the release or synaptic concentrations of the catecholamines, dramatically enhance and prolong wakefulness; conversely, drugs that deplete or decrease the catecholamines produce a decrease in activity and cortical activation, and in certain cases appear to increase sleep. Prodromal symptoms, such as yawning, drowsiness, irritability, mood changes, hyperactivity and sleep disturbances, support a direct role for the dopaminergic system in migraine pathogenesis.[61]

A dopaminergic receptor hypersensitivity or a dopaminergic imbalance with a temporary elevation could account for increased awakening and being awake during sleep, whereas a temporary diminution could lead to a decrease in activity and cortical activation. Therefore, the dopaminergic involvement could explain either the increase of movement time during sleep or the actigraphic evidence of reduced mean activity, with a negative peak during the night after the attack and increased awakening during sleep. These two neurotransmitter systems are interconnected: the dopaminergic system is modulated by the serotoninergic system; a reduced release of serotonin between attacks could lower dopamine release, which would lead to receptor hypersensitivity.[62]

The hypothesized dysfunction of the serotoninergic and dopaminergic system could act since the early period of life in migraineurs, leading to disorders of the sleep–wake rhythm in infancy that tend to persist during childhood and adolescence.

The common anatomical substrate could be represented by the suprachiasmatic nucleus (SCN). This is an organ for the control and organization of circadian and circannual biorhythms, which has also been involved in the pathogenesis of migraine: the prodromal phase of a migraine attack could be a syndrome of SCN functional insufficiency.[31] SCN insufficiency entails reactive functional denervation hypersensitivity and a spreading depression which, via the genicolo-hypothalamic tract and optic radiation, leads to visual phenomena of the aura, whereas the affection of raphe nuclei (serotoninergic) and locus ceruleus (catecholaminergic) – which represents an integral part of central anti-nociceptive network – determines pain and intracranial and extracranial vasomotor phenomena in the pain phase.

The activation of the raphe nuclei, implicated in the generation of NREM sleep and in inhibitory control of REM phasic activity, could explain the influence of sleep in terminating or triggering the attacks.

The involvement of the locus ceruleus, implicated in the generation of REM sleep, could account for the occurrence of migraine attacks during REM sleep.

The high co-morbidity between headache and sleep could, therefore, be linked to the sharing of common anatomical structures and to the involvement of the same neurotransmitters.

# References

1. Hill W, On some causes of backwardness and stupidity in children. *BMJ* 1889; **ii**: 711–12.
2. Sahota PK, Dexter JD, Sleep and headache syndromes: A clinical review. *Headache* 1990; **30**: 80–4.
3. Paiva T, Batista A, Martins P, Martins A, The relationship between headaches and sleep disturbances. *Headache* 1995; **35**: 590–6.
4. Wilkinson M, Williams K, Leyton M, Observations on the treatment of an acute attack of migraine. *Res Clin Stud Headache* 1978; **6**: 141–6.
5. Blau JN, Resolution of migraine attacks: Sleep and the recovery phase. *J Neurol Neurosurg Psychiatry* 1982; **45**: 223–6.
6. Dexter JD, Relationship between sleep and headache syndromes. In: Thorpy MJ, ed., *Handbook of Sleep Disorders*. New York: Marcel Dekker, 1990: 663–71.
7. Inamorato E, Minatti Hannuch SN, Zukerman E, The role of sleep in migraine attacks. *Arq Neuropsiquiatr* 1993; **51**: 429–32.
8. Gans M, Treating migraine by sleep rationing. *J Nerv Ment Dis* 1951; **113**: 405–29.
9. D'Alessandro R, Benassi G, Lenzi PL et al, Epidemiology of headache in the Republic of San

Marino. *J Neurol Neurosurg Psychiatry* 1988; **51**: 21–7.

10. Spierings EL, van Hoof MJ, Fatigue and sleep in chronic headache sufferers: an age- and sex-controlled questionnaire study. *Headache* 1997; **37**: 549–52.

11. Chabriat H, Danchot J, Michel P, Joire JE, Henry P, Precipitating factors of headache. Prospective study in a national control-matched survey in migraineurs and nonmigraineurs. *Headache* 1999; **39**: 335–8.

12. Paiva T, Martins P, Batista A, Esperanca P, Martins I, Sleep disturbances in chronic headache patients: a comparison with healthy controls. *Headache Q* 1994; **5**: 135–41.

13. Katerji MA, Painter MJ, Infantile migraine presenting as colic. *J Child Neurol* 1994; **9**: 336–7.

14. Weissbluth M, Colic. In: Ferber R, Kryger M, eds, *Principles and Practice of Sleep Medicine in the Child*. Philadelphia: WB Saunders, 1995: 75–8.

15. Guidetti V, Ottaviano S, Pagliarini M, Childhood headache risk: warning signs and symptoms present during the first six months of life. *Cephalalgia* 1984; **4**: 237–42.

16. Lanzi G, Zambrino CA, Balottin U, Tagliasacchi M, Vercelli P, Termine C, Periodic syndrome and migraine in children and adolescents. *Ital J Neurol Sci* 1997; **18**: 283–8.

17. Del Bene E, Multiple aspects of headache risk in children. *Adv Neurol* 1982; **33**: 187–98.

18. Carvalho D de S, Zukerman E, Hanuch SN, Levyman C, Lima JG, Risk factors in headache in children from 7 to 15. *Arq Neuropsiquiatr* 1987; **45**: 371–8.

19. Elser JM, Woody RC, Migraine headache in the infant and young child. *Headache* 1990; **30**: 366–8.

20. Guidetti V, Galli F, Fabrizi P et al, Headache and psychiatric comorbidity: clinical aspects and outcome in an 8th years follow-up study. *Cephalalgia* 1998; **18**: 455–62.

21. Barabas G, Ferrari M, Matthews WS, Childhood migraine and somnambulism. *Neurology* 1986; **33**: 948–1048.

22. Pradalier A, Guittard M, Dry J, Somnambulism, migraine and propranolol. *Headache* 1987; **27**: 143–5.

23. Giroud M, D'Athis P, Guard O, Dumas R, Migraine et somnambulisme. Une enquete portant sur 122 migraineux. *Rev Neurol* 1986; **142**: 42–6.

24. Dexter JD, The relationship between disorders of arousal from sleep and migraine. *Headache* 1986; **26**: 322.

25. Bruni O, Fabrizi P, Ottaviano S, Cortesi F, Giannotti F, Guidetti V, Prevalence of sleep disorders in childhood and adolescence headache: a case–control study. *Cephalalgia* 1997; **17**: 492–8.

26. Bille B, Migraine in school children. *Acta Paediatr Scand* 1962; **51**: 3–151.

27. Mathew NT, Glaze D, Frost J Jr, Sleep apnea and other sleep abnormalities in primary headache disorders. In: Rose C, ed., *Migraine, Proceedings of the Fifth International Migraine Symposium*. London: Karger, 1985: 40–9.

28. Palayew MD, Kryger MH, Sleep apnea and headache. *Headache Q* 1994; **5**: 227–30.

29. De Giorgis G, Miletto R, Iannuccelli M, Camuffo M, Scerni S, Headache in association with sleep disorders in children: a psychodiagnostic evaluation and controlled clinical study – L-5-HTP versus placebo. *Drugs Exp Clin Res* 1987; **13**: 425–33.

30. Smeyers P, Headaches in childhood: association with sleep disorders and psychological implications. *Rev Neurol* 1999; **28**: S150–5.

31. Zurak N, Role of the suprachiasmatic nucleus in the pathogenesis of migraine attacks. *Cephalalgia* 1997; **17**: 223–8.

32. Leone M, Lucini V, D'Amico D, Twenty-four hour melatonin and cortisol plasma levels in relation to timing of cluster headache. *Cephalalgia* 1995; **15**: 224–9.

33. Fox AW, Davis RL, Migraine chronobiology. *Headache* 1998; **38**: 436–41.

34. Nagtegaal JE, Smits MG, Stuart ACW, Kerkhof GA, van der Meer YG, Melatonin-responsive headache in delayed sleep phase syndrome: preliminary observations. *Headache* 1998; **38**: 303–7.

35. Bruni O, Galli F, Guidetti V, Sleep hygiene and migraine in children and adolescents. *Cephalalgia* 1999; **19**(suppl 25): 58–60.

36. Feikema WJ, Headache and chronic sleep deprivation: an often missed relationship in children and also in adults. *Ned Tijdschr Geneeskd* 1999; **143**: 1897–900.

37. Guidetti V, Bruni O, Violani C, Casiello B, Devoto A, Galli F, Sleep wake cycle variations in migrainous children. *Cephalalgia* 1999; **19**: 278 (abstract).

38. Dexter J, The relationship between stage 3 + 4 + REM sleep and arousals with migraine. *Headache* 1970; **19**: 364–9.

39. Dexter J, Weitzman ED, The relationship of nocturnal headaches to sleep stage patterns. *Neurology* 1970; **20**: 513–18.

40. Kudrow L, McGinty D, Phillips E, Stevenson M, Steep apnea in cluster headache. *Cephalalgia* 1984; **4**: 33–8.

41. Pfaffenrath V, Pöllmann W, Rüther E, Lund R, Hajak G, Onset of nocturnal attacks of chronic cluster headache in relation to sleep stages. *Acta Neurol Scand* 1986; **73**: 403–7.

42. Kayed K, Godtlibsen O, Sjaastad O, Chronic paroxysmal hemicrania IV: 'REM sleep locked'? nocturnal attacks. *Sleep* 1978; **1**: 91–5.

43. Drake ME, Pakalnis A, Andrews JM, Bogner JE, Nocturnal sleep recording with cassette EEG in chronic headaches. *Headache* 1990; **30**: 600–3.

44. Dexter JD, Riley TL, Studies in nocturnal migraine. *Headache* 1975; **15**: 51–62.

45. Cirignotta F, Coccagna T, Sacquegna E et al, Nocturnal headache: systemic arterial pressure and heart rate during sleep. *Cephalalgia* 1983; **1**(suppl): 54–7.

46. Wolfe H, *Headache and Other Head Pain*, 2nd edn. New York: Oxford University Press, 1963.

47. Chervin RD, Nath Zallek S et al, Sleep disordered breathing in patients with cluster headache. *Neurology* 2000; **54**: 2302–6.

48. Zalleck SN, Chervin RD, Improvement in cluster headache after treatment for obstructive sleep apnea. *Sleep Med* 2000; **1**: 135–8.

49. Raskin NH, The hypnic headache syndrome. *Headache* 1988; **28**: 534–6.

50. Dodick DW, Polysomnography in hypnic headache syndrome. *Headache* 2000; **40**: 748–52.

51. Molino Arjona JA, Jimenez-Jimenez FJ, Vela-Bueno A, Tallon-Baranco A, Hypnic headache associated with stage 3 Slow Wave Sleep. *Headache* 2000; **40**: 753–4.

52. Guilleminault C, Clinical overview of the sleep apnea syndromes. In: Guilleminault C, Dement W, eds, *Sleep Apnea Syndromes*. New York: Alan R. Liss, 1978: 1–12.

53. Dexter J, Headache as a presenting complaint of the sleep apnea syndrome. *Headache* 1984; **24**: 171.

54. Boutros N, Headache in sleep apnea. *Tex Med* 1989; **85**: 34–5.

55. Aldrich M, Chauncey J, Are morning headaches part of obstructive sleep apnea syndrome? *Arch Intern Med* 1990; **150**: 1265–7.

56. Diener HC, May A, New aspects of migraine pathophysiology: lessons learned from positron emission tomography [editorial]. *Curr Opin Neurol* 1996; **9**: 199–201.

57. Guidetti V, Bruni O, Canitano R, Romoli M, Napoli L, Migraine and headache in childhood: sleep disorders and sleep organization. *Cephalalgia* 1995; **S16**: 10–12 (abstract).

58. Guilleminault C, Eldridge FL, Simmons FB, Dement WC, Sleep apnea in eight children. *Pediatrics* 1976; **58**: 23–30.

59. Bruni O, Miano S, Galli F, Verrillo E, Guidetti V, Sleep apnea in childhood migraine. *J Headache Pain* 2000; **1**(3): 169–72.

60. Chervin RD, Dillon JE, Bassetti C, Ganoczy DA, Pituch KJ, Symptoms of sleep disorders, inattention, and hyperactivity in children. *Sleep* 1997; **20**: 1185–92.

61. Peroutka SJ, Dopamine and migraine. *Neurology* 1997; **49**: 650–6.

62. Mascia A, Afra J, Schoenen J, Dopamine and migraine: a review of pharmaceutical, biochemical, neurophysiological and therapeutic data. *Cephalalgia* 1998; **18**: 174–82.

# 33

## Stress and quality of life in juvenile headache sufferers
*J Passchier*

This chapter discusses two major and related concepts in the area of headache research: 'stress' and 'quality of life'. Stress has mainly been studied as a provoking factor of migraine attacks, and quality of life as a consequence of chronic headache (tension-type or migraine). Most studies so far have been performed on adult patients; because their outcome may also have implications for younger patients, these results are also taken into consideration here.

## Stress

Human life is demanding. Whereas in older times these demands were mainly of a physical nature, such as defence against predators, the exertions of hunting, tribal fights, and a great deal of walking and carrying of goods, in modern society *psychosocial* stress is predominant. Children are obliged to go to school, are pestered by their schoolmates, compete for popularity, do examinations and are controlled or neglected by parents.

Stress can be defined as a physiological state, often one that reflects the sympathetic activation needed for energy expenditure, but sometimes a parasympathetic state, as in the freezing reaction of an animal cornered by its predator and not in control of the situation.[1] Stress can also be defined as a situation that requires adaptation – a minor daily hassle, e.g.

leaving for work and the car breaks down, to a major life event, such as the loss of a parent by sudden death. Alternatively, stress can be conceived of as an internal mental state of unrest when the person realizes that he or she may lack the coping possibilities to solve the problem comfortably. This last definition considers stress as an interaction between the person's perceived capabilities and the demands of the situation.

Each of these three stress concepts are discussed below. Stress produces both psychological and physical symptoms. It can elicit pain. Incidental pain caused by stress is not a reason for concern, although stress becomes a problem when:

- the stress is chronic
- the symptoms are easily and frequently elicited by an underlying physical pathology
- the symptoms occur with high intensity.

Patients suffering from chronic headache, both youngsters and adults, have these problems.

## The concept of physiological stress and chronic headache

In Selye's conception,[1] stress was considered as a physiological reaction pattern to demanding situations. His work was carried out mainly on animals that underwent a variety of unusual and unpleasant situations, such as being encaged in a too hot or too cold environment, having to swim without possibilities of escape or being handled repeatedly. He found that these different situations elicited a similar physiological reaction pattern, characterized by successive phases: an *alarm phase* in which increased cortisol excretion is paralleled by heart acceleration, increase in blood pressure and muscle tension, and other changes that are mediated by activity of the sympathetic nervous system; a *resistance phase* during which the organs resume their original baseline activity but the cortisol levels are still increased; and an *exhaustion phase* in which the cortisol level cannot be maintained and drops dramatically, while the heart rate, blood pressure and other physiological systems increase their activity again. It is in this last phase that the animal has a decreased immunological resistance and a higher susceptibility to disease. When the stressful situation continues, the animal dies.

This non-specific physiological reaction pattern that unfolds itself during successive phases, was named the 'general adaptation syndrome' by Selye. The syndrome was related to the view that being continuously or repeatedly subjected to stressful stimuli causes wear and tear of the body. This idea has inspired many researchers in their explorations for the origin and maintenance of somatic diseases with an unclear physical cause. Studies were often based on the theoretical concept that the increased physiological response to stress would, in the long term, afflict those physiological systems that, as a result of congenital weakness or sensitivity, showed the highest degree of response.[2] Later research[3,4] has challenged the idea of a non-specific response pattern. Which system was most vulnerable and responsive differed between individuals, so this concept was known as 'individual response specificity'.

Later investigators emphasized that it was not the magnitude of the reaction to stress that was maladaptive, but the incapability of recovering and resuming baseline activity.[5]

As stress provokes headaches, the idea of individual specificity inspired many researchers to investigate the hypothesis that migraine patients show abnormal extracranial responses to stress. The interest in this physiological system was based on the vascular abnormalities during a migraine attack.[6] Experimental studies were carried out in which the extracranial and peripheral responses of migraine patients were compared with those of healthy controls. A whole array of stressful stimuli was applied, such as mental arithmetic, stressful imagery, putting the hand in ice water, IQ tests and real-life stressors such as an examination. So far, the outcome of these studies has been inconsistent.[7] Some studies found more extracranial dilatation,[8] others extracranial constriction,[9] or no differences between patients and controls.[10]

Many studies had methodological flaws, e.g. the absence of any check of whether stress had actually occurred and whether it was followed by a headache. The disappointing findings are reflected in a waning interest in such studies.[11]

Adult patients with tension-type headache who have been submitted to these stress experiments showed, however, according to recent meta-analytical studies, an increased response of head muscles compared with control patients.[7]

Given that the physiological systems are

relatively uncompromised by drug use in children, it can be recommended that these experimental studies be replicated in the young age group.

## Stress as a demanding situation and chronic headache

A different scientific approach concerned mainly questioning which type of external stimuli lead to physiological and psychological dysregulations in humans. At first, the focus was on severe intrusions in life, which required a lot of adaptive recovery on the part of the person – the so-called 'life events'. Major life events were, for example, the loss of a partner or child, and a marital separation. The investigators made lists of such events, ordered according to the amount of adaptation that was required. One of the first questionnaires is the Social Readjustment Rating Scale (SRRS) of Holmes and Rahe.[12] It has been shown that individuals in the normal population who experience more major life events have a higher risk ratio for headache than those who do not.[13] Similar instruments have been designed for children.[14]

Later researchers found that less intense but more frequent stressful moments were associated with more physical complaints than the highly intrusive but less frequent life events. They designed a questionnaire for these minor stressors – the so-called 'daily hassles and uplifts list'.[15] Daily stress has clearly been found to be a provoking factor for headache attacks in adult patients. Retrospective studies, in which patients with chronic headache were asked which factors were most likely to elicit headaches, showed 'mental stress' as the most commonly mentioned factor. Prospective diary studies were less consistent.[16] A recent study

using a computer device for registration revealed that migraine patients experienced more hassles and psychological arousal in the days before an attack.[17]

## Stress as an interaction between person and environment

According to Cox,[18] stress arises when there is an imbalance between a perceived demand and a person's perception of his or her capability of meeting that demand. This approach regards the organism as an active being, in contrast to the rather mechanistic previous views. Both cognitive appraisal and problem-solving abilities are relevant for the experience of stress. Personality variables also come into play, because these may determine the perception of demands as a challenge or a problem, and one's own capabilities as being sufficient or lacking.

The interactional approach has led to the studies into *coping* with stress. Its emphasis on the possibilities of the individual inspired the application of stress management programmes for those suffering from stress and its consequences.

## Stress and juvenile headache

From all reported causes of headache, stress is mentioned most frequently, by both elementary and secondary school students,[19,20] followed by physical fatigue and sleep problems.[21,22] Within the stress domain, in particular, school problems appear to be important; it was found that these account for a significant part of the variance in headache complaints.[20]

A salient finding by Sillanpää[23] is that of a threefold increased prevalence of headache when comparing children who started school in 1974 with those who started in 1992, using the same design and a similar child population. As this was found to a larger extent in the urban districts with the highest social instability, the authors assume that underlying stress factors might be causally related to this headache trend.

In one study,[24] juvenile migraine and non-migrainous headache patients were asked to describe their stressful events in a headache diary. Most of these events appeared to be related to school. Migraine patients noted more stressful events than non-migrainous headache patients. Across the groups, the association between the number of stressful events and the amount of headache (summarized as a headache index and derived from a 4-week diary report) was not significant.

A (quasi)-experimental test of the hypothesis that stress elicits headaches can be found in the effect studies of programmes that aim to prevent the headaches by teaching the patients how to relax and how to cope with their stress in an adaptive way (evaluation of these programmes is discussed in Chapter 25). The overwhelming majority of these studies find positive clinical effects from cognitive–behavioural techniques and relaxation, in particular on headache frequency.[25–29] This outcome strongly supports the hypothesis that stress provokes headaches.

A psychological mechanism that can act as a mediator between stress and pain is the disposition of some people to experience events as more stressful and physical sensations as more painful than is common. This trait, known as 'negative affectivity', is derived from the theory of Pennebaker.[30] Related traits, such as anxiety and depression, have been found in juvenile headache patients, in particular those with migraine, to a higher degree than in their healthy counterparts.[31,32]

The positive outcome of the forementioned treatment programmes of headache, in which the juvenile patient learns by cognitive interventions how to interpret unfavourable events in a less stressful way, indicates the importance of specific ways of *stress coping* for the provocation and prevention of headaches. Generally, ways of stress coping that are passive, such as worrying, appear in school students from the general population to be associated with higher headache intensity and duration.[33] In a review of stress coping and quality of life in school-aged children, Bandell et al[34] conclude that children with recurrent headaches report a variety of active and passive coping strategies for their headaches, but the effectiveness of each of these on their headaches and quality of life is still unknown.

Psychophysiological studies on stress in juvenile patients have seldom been carried out. Hermann and Blanchard[35] assessed the pulse amplitudes of the temporalis and supraorbitalis arteries of the finger, as well as the finger temperature, in 30 migraine patients aged 8–16 years. A subtraction task and parent–child conflict served as stressors. They found no differences in these physiological responses to stress between the patients and a control group.

## Conclusion

Although not yet demonstrated in longitudinal studies, much evidence strongly suggests that stress elicits headaches in children and adolescents. So far, the underlying physiological pathways of this relationship are unknown. Active coping of the patient with the stress seems more beneficial than passive ways of coping.

# *Quality of life*

A child with chronic headache suffers not only from pain, but can also feel depressed, anxious and unmotivated. Pleasant activities, such as playing, doing sport or watching television, are sometimes stopped or carried out at a reduced level. During severe headaches the young patient stays away from school or performs school tasks less well.

It was not until the end of the twentieth century that these life-encompassing problems could be assessed in children and adolescents in a standardized valid way. For the first time, we can give an overview of the problems that these patients meet in different life areas and compare these with those of other patient groups. Now, we can measure the benefit of the treatment of juvenile headache in terms of both headache relief and quality of life.

## *Definition and measurement of quality of life in general*

After the first use of the term 'quality of life' in medicine by Elkinton in 1967,[36] and an application in patients who suffered from a life-threatening disease, such as renal failure and cancer, the first decades were mainly used for a delineation of the concept. Currently, three approaches to a definition can be differentiated, all of which have in common that the patient's judgement is what counts. So the instruments that are made to measure quality of life, mostly questionnaires, rely on the responses of the patients. The multidimensional approach considers quality of life as a construct that consists of several interrelated dimensions. There is a consensus that quality of life encompasses physical, psychological and social dimensions. Many investigators include daily functioning as well, and some recommend the inclusion of separate dimensions for cognitive functioning, sleep and pain. This leads to the construction of multidimensional instruments in which each of these domains is represented by a separate, mostly short, subscale. These so-called 'generic' quality of life (or 'health status') measures can be applied in patients with different types of diseases, and also in healthy people.

A second approach considers quality of life as a concept that can be evaluated only in the context of a specific disease, e.g. McKenna[37] defines quality of life as the possibility of the patient satisfying his or her needs in life. A patient's quality of life is therefore determined by the extent to which the disease forms an obstruction to achievement of this satisfaction. These problems are specific for particular diseases, e.g. whereas in a patient with acne the problem is the shame resulting from an afflicted face, a typical problem in a migraine patient is the anxiety about bad performance because of an unexpected migraine attack. An instrument for the measurement of this disease-specific quality of life is useful only for the patient group for which it was designed.

A third approach considers quality of life undimensionally as an overall impression of the life satisfaction of the patient. It can be quantified on the basis of just one rating, with or without the use of a description of different health states (such as the EuroQol[38] or a Visual Analogue Scale [VAS]). This produces one score that can be compared between patient groups and healthy people, and has found its way into economic evaluations of treatment.

A fourth approach considers quality of life as an individual determined concept.[39] Here, the *individual* patient determines the goals that he or she values most in his or her life and, in the next step, indicates to what extent the disease interferes with achieving these goals. The semi-structured interview is the optimal method for measurement in this approach. So far, this method has seldom been applied because of its time-consuming nature and lack of generalization across patients.

At present, most studies have used a combination of multidimensional, disease-specific and global measures in the evaluation of quality of life in adult patients with chronic headache.

## Why is it important to measure quality of life?

Measurement of quality of life can serve several purposes and each purpose has its own preferred way of measurement. First, politicians might be interested in the quality of life of different populations, healthy or sick, in order to know which groups deserve priority in the allocation of resources. Often a global and short, standardized questionnaire is used, which can easily be compared between groups and gives a high response rate because of the low time demands. This global method can also be applied to compare patients who differ in disease category, in order to determine the most urgent groups in health care. Sometimes a generic questionnaire is used to see which life dimensions are most affected in which patients. Osterhaus and Townsend,[40] for example, found that on the Nottingham Health Profile (NHP) migraine patients have lower scores for social functioning than patients with hypertension. Second, quality-of-life measures are used as secondary end-points in clinical trials to evaluate the positive and

negative effects of treatments on the life of the patients. Often a generic measure and a disease-specific questionnaire are simultaneously used in these investigations. For instance, studies showed that sumatriptan not only had a positive clinical effect on the migraine, but also on the quality of life of the migraine patient.[41,42] Finally, the individual patient might benefit from the individual approach with a semi-structured quality-of-life interview. Its outcome can be applied in tailor-made care for the patient. So far, this individual approach has not been applied in the field of chronic headache.

The number of studies on quality of life in children in pain, although few, is increasing. To date, these studies have mainly been restricted to the evaluation of the quality of life in young patients with headache in relation to their pain parameters. Hunfeld et al,[43] for instance, compared the quality of life of juvenile headache patients with that of youngsters who had chronic pain at other locations, such as abdominal and back pain. It can be expected, however, that in a few years the number of investigations that use quality of life as an outcome measure in trials on youngsters with migraine will be multiplied.

A conceptual and practical problem in measuring quality of life is the result of the level of cognitive development of the children under study. Most questionnaires refer to a timeframe of the past week, 2 weeks or even the past month. Young children (aged <7 years), are, however, not capable of answering written questions about the past, and those below 3 years of age are unable to communicate clearly about their quality of life at a sufficiently verbal level. Therefore, we have to resort to a proxy judgement, often from the mother. Inevitably this introduces some error, because the perception of the mother is determined by the behaviour that she observes and her interpretation. From research in juvenile adolescents with headache, we know that the evaluation by parents can differ considerably from that of the children.[44] One can, however, expect that these differences are less in a younger group that spends more time in the environment of the parent than that of peers.

## Findings on quality of life

### Adult

An increasing number of studies demonstrate an impaired health status in adult migraine patients. Osterhaus et al[40] showed that these patients report physical functioning and health status scores comparable with those of patients suffering from arthritis, gastrointestinal disorders, myocardial infarction and diabetes, but lower scores for role functioning, social functioning, pain and mental health. Essink-Bot et al[45] found, in the general population, that migraine patients had problems with role functioning, household work, social functioning and home life. In addition, they felt less energetic and healthy than a normal control group. In these studies, the differences could not be explained by the patient's higher tendency towards depression. The impairment they showed was, however, small in comparison with that of other groups, such as patients who have to undergo a liver transplantation. The discrepant findings of the studies about the severity of the impact of chronic headache can be attributed to the type of (sub)populations under study. Passchier et al[46,47] found that the quality of life was more reduced in patients who belong to the subgroup of those who consult the physician for their headaches or those who belong to the society of migraine

patients, than in patients who belong to a random sample of the general population. Patients with chronic tension-type headache appeared to be impaired to a comparable degree[46,47] or even more impaired than those with migraine.[48]

Quality-of-life measures have also been demonstrated to reflect the positive effects of medication, which shorten the migraine attack.[41]

### Children and adolescents

Most studies in children and youngsters did not focus on the measurement of quality of life in a multidimensional way, but were limited to one or a few of its constituent domains. In particular, the psychological domain was investigated. Engström[49] found that juvenile patients from 9 to 18 years with recurrent headache had more anxiety and depression than healthy subjects. Andrasik et al[50,51] also observed that children with migraine or recurrent headache scored higher on scales for depression, somatic complaints and anxiety than controls who were matched for age, sex and social class. Also Larsson [52] found more psychological distress and somatic symptoms in patients with recurrent headache than in their headache-free counterparts. Although fear of failure was higher in school students with frequent headaches,[20] it is salient that the cognitive and intellectual functioning of the pupils, as reflected in their school marks, do not seem to be affected.[53] The average annual number of days of school absence as a result of frequent or severe headache, as determined by the National Health Survey in the USA in 1988, was 3.3.[54] Although this figure seems relatively low, according to a recent diary study in the Netherlands,[43] adolescents with chronic headache in the age range 12–18 years reported a school absence of 2 days per month, which was about four times the school absence in juvenile patients with other chronic pain types (i.e. abdominal, limb or back pain).

It seems plausible that a child who complains often about pain, and demonstrates its suffering by a lack of interest in playing, no appetite and school absence, also forms a source of stress for the family. The pain intensity and frequency for the child with chronic pain were recently found to be associated with a diminished health status of the mother and more strain in the family.[55]

The recent development of a reliable and valid quality-of-life questionnaire enables the researcher to make an overall evaluation of the quality of life of the adolescent with chronic headache.[44] In this self-report questionnaire, the life domains 'physical', 'social' and 'psychological functioning', and 'functional status' are assessed, as well as the general satisfaction with life and health. In a prospective follow-up study, Langeveld et al[24] asked adolescents with chronic headache to keep a diary over 4 weeks and to complete this quality-of-life questionnaire (the 'Quality-of-life-headache – Youth questionnaire – QLH-Y') at the end of each week. A negative relationship was found between the spontaneous fluctuations of the diary-registered headaches and the functional status, psychological functioning, satisfaction with life and satisfaction with health. Of specific interest is the finding that the headache severity was related to a reduced psychological functioning and satisfaction with health only in patients who had experienced a lot of stress in the previous weeks. This suggests that the impact of headache on the patient's life is intensified by other stress experiences.

Lanzi et al[56] applied the QLH-Y in young migraine patients and other chronic headache patients who attended secondary school. They found that migraine patients reported more impact of the headache on daily activities and leisure activities than patients with other types of headache. Stress and other somatic symptoms also occurred more often in the migraine group. The patients with chronic headache were also less satisfied with their life in general.

An interesting question is whether the quality of life in children with chronic headache complaints is more impaired than in children with chronic pain at other locations. Recently, it was found that juvenile patients with headache and back pain had comparable quality-of-life scores. However, the *amount* of pain as measured in a 3-week diary was more strongly related to a reduction in quality of life in the headache patients than in juvenile patients with abdominal or back pain. From the pain parameters, intensity and frequency, it was the pain intensity that showed the clearest association with a reduction in quality of life, which was found on each life domain with the exception of social functioning.

## Conclusion

Overall, the quality of life in young patients with chronic headache seems to be afflicted by their disease in many life domains. That their social functioning seems to be at a normal level looks reassuring: the headaches might not impede their contacts with friends and relatives. As all studies on quality of life in juvenile patients are cross-sectional, we do not know whether the impairments found are in fact a *consequence* of the headaches. Studies on the effect of headache treatment on quality of life may give a definite answer to this causal question. Considering the fact that adult patients mention the negative impact on their life as the largest problem, evaluation studies of behavioural and medical interventions should include at least a quality-of-life measure as a major outcome variable.

# References

1. Selye H, A syndrome produced by diverse nocuous agents. *Nature* 1936; **138**: 32.
2. Malmo RB, Shagass C, Physiologic study of symptom mechanism in psychiatric patients under stress. *Psychosom Med* 1949; **11**: 25–9.
3. Lacey JI, Individual differences in somatic response patterns. *J Comp Physiol Psychol* 1950; **43**: 338–50.
4. Lacey JI, Bateman DE, Vanlehn R, Autonomic response specificity; an experimental study. *Psychosom Med* 1953; **15**: 8–21.
5. Dienstbier RA, Arousal and physiological toughness: Implications for mental and physical health. *Psychol Rev* 1989; **96**: 84–100.
6. Dalessio DJ, *Wolff's Headache and Other Head Pain*. New York: Oxford University Press, 1980.
7. Flor H, Turk DC, Psychophysiology of chronic pain: do chronic pain patients exhibit symptom-specific psychophysiological responses? *Psychol Bull* 1989; **105**: 215–59.
8. Drummond PD, Extracranial and cardiovascular reactivity in migrainous subjects. *J Psychosom Res* 1982; **26**: 317–31.
9. Passchier J, Goudswaard P, Orlebeke JF, Verhage F, Migraine and defense mechanisms: psychophysiological relationships in young females. *Soc Sci Med* 1988; **26**: 343–50.
10. Stronks DL, Tulen JH, Verheij R et al, Serotonergic, catecholaminergic, and cardiovascular reactions to mental stress in female migraine patients. A controlled study. *Headache* 1998; **38**: 270–80.
11. Passchier J, A critical note on psychophysiological stress research into migraine patients. *Cephalalgia* 1994; **14**: 194–8.
12. Holmes TH, Rahe RH, The Social Readjustment Rating Scale. *J Psychosom Res* 1967; **11**: 213–18.
13. Passchier J, Schouten J, van der Donk J, van Romunde LK, The association of frequent headaches with personality and life events. *Headache* 1991; **31**: 116–21.
14. Berden GFMG, Althaus M, Verhulst FC, The relation between major life events and changes in the emotional/behavioural functioning of children. *J Child Psychol Psychiatry* 1990; **31**: 949–59.
15. Kanner AD, Feldman SS, Control over uplifts and hassles and its relationship to adaptational outcomes. *J Behav Med* 1991; **14**: 187–201.
16. Passchier J, Andrasik F, Migraine. Psychological factors. In: Olesen J, Tfelt-Hansen P, Welch MA, eds, *The Headaches*. New York: Raven Press, 1993: 233–40.
17. Sorbi MJ, Maassen GH, Spierings EL, A time series analysis of daily hassles and mood changes in the 3 days before the migraine attack. *Behav Med* 1996; **22**: 103–13.
18. Cox T, *Stress*. Hong Kong: MacMillan Press, 1978: 1–25.
19. Maratos J, Wilkinson M, Migraine in children: a medical and psychiatric study. *Cephalalgia* 1982; **2**: 179–87.
20. Passchier J, Orlebeke JF, Headaches and stress in schoolchildren: an epidemiological study. *Cephalalgia* 1985; **5**: 167–76.
21. Chu ML, Shinnar S, Headaches in children younger than 7 years of age. *Arch Neurol* 1992; **49**: 79–82.
22. Bruni O, Fabrizi P, Ottaviano S, Cortesi F, Giannotti F, Guidetti V, Prevalence of sleep disorders in childhood and adolescence with headache: a case–control study. *Cephalalgia* 1997; **17**: 492–8.
23. Sillanpää M, Anttila P, Increasing prevalence of headache in 7-year-old schoolchildren. *Headache* 1996; **36**: 466–70.
24. Langeveld JH, Koot HM, Passchier J, Headache intensity and quality of life in adolescents. How are changes in headache intensity in adolescents related to changes in experienced quality of life? *Headache* 1997; **37**: 37–42.
25. Larsson B, Melin L, Doeberl A, Recurrent tension headache in adolescents treated with self-help relaxation training and a muscle relaxant drug. *Headache* 1990; **30**: 665–71.

26. Larsson B, Melin L, The psychological treatment of recurrent headache in adolescents – short-term outcome and its prediction. *Headache* 1998; **4**: 187–95.

27. Reid GJ, McGrath PJ, Psychological treatments for migraine. *Biomed Pharmacother* 1996; **50**: 58–63.

28. Osterhaus SO, Passchier J, Van der Helm-Hylkema H et al, Effects of behavioral psychophysiological treatment on schoolchildren with migraine in a nonclinical setting: Predictors and process variables. *J Pediatr Psychol* 1993; **18**: 697–715.

29. Osterhaus SO, Passchier J, Van der Helm-Hylkema H et al, The behavioral treatment of juvenile patients with migraine in a nonclinical setting: Effects and observations. *Gedragstherapie* 1994; **27**: 3–18.

30. Watson D, Pennebaker JW, Health complaints, stress, and distress: exploring the central role of negative affectivity. *Psychol Rev* 1989; **96**: 234–54.

31. Cooper PJ, Bawden HN, Camfield PR, Camfield CS, Anxiety and life events in childhood migraine. *Pediatrics* 1987; **79**: 999–1004.

32. Cunningham SJ, McGrath PJ, Ferguson HB et al, Personality and behavioural characteristics in pediatric migraine. *Headache* 1987; **27**: 16–20.

33. Bree MBMvd, Passchier J, Emmen HH, Influence of quality of life and stress coping behaviour on headaches in adolescent male students: an explorative study. *Headache* 1990; **30**: 165–8.

34. Bandell-Hoekstra I, Abu-Saad HH, Passchier J, Knipschild P, Recurrent headache, coping and quality of life in children: a review. *Headache* 2000; **40**(5): 357–70.

35. Hermann C, Blanchard EB, Psychophysiological reactivity in pediatric migraine patients and healthy controls. *J Psychosom Res* 1998; **44**: 229–40.

36. Elkinton JR, Medicine and the quality of life. *Ann Intern Med* 1966; **64**: 711–14.

37. McKenna SP, Quality of life assessment in the conduct of economic evaluations of medicines. *Br J Med Economics* 1995; **8**: 33–8.

38. EuroQol Group, EuroQol* – a new facility for the measurement of health-related quality of life. *Health Policy* 1990; **16**: 199–208.

39. O'Boyle CA, McGee H, Hickey A, O'Malley K, Joyce CR, Individual quality of life in patients undergoing hip replacement. *Lancet* 1992; **339**: 1088–91.

40. Osterhaus JT, Townsend RJ, The quality of life of migraineurs: A cross sectional profile. *Cephalalgia* 1991; **11**(11): 103–4.

41. Jhingran P, Osterhaus JT, Miller DW, Lee JT, Kirchdoerfer L, Development and validation of the Migraine-Specific Quality of Life Questionnaire. *Headache* 1998; **38**: 295–302.

42. Perry CM, Markham A, Sumatriptan. An updated review of its use in migraine. *Drugs* 1998; **55**: 889–922.

43. Hunfeld et al *Cephalalgia*, in press.

44. Langeveld JH, Koot HM, Loonen MC, Hazebroek-Kampschreur AA, Passchier J, A quality of life instrument for adolescents with chronic headache. *Cephalalgia* 1996; **16**: 183–96.

45. Essink-Bot ML, van Royen L, Krabbe P, Bonsel GJ, Rutten FFH, The impact of migraine on health status. *Headache* 1995; **35**: 200–6.

46. Passchier J, de Boo M, Quaak HZ, Brienen JA, Health-related quality of life of chronic headache patients is predicted by the emotional component of their pain. *Headache* 1996; **36**: 556–60.

47. Passchier J, Mourik J, Brienen JA, Hunfeld JA, Cognitions, emotions, and behavior of patients with migraine when taking medication during an attack. *Headache* 1998; **38**: 458–64.

48. Solomon GD, Skobieranda FG, Gragg LA, Does quality of life differ among headache diagnoses? Analysis using the medical outcomes study instrument. *Headache* 1994; **34**: 143–7.

49. Engstrom I, Mental health and psychological functioning in children and adolescents with inflammatory bowel disease: a comparison with children having other chronic illnesses and with healthy children. *J Child Psychiatry* 1992; **33**: 563–82.

50. Andrasik F, Burke EJ, Attanasio V, Rosenblum EL, Child, parent, and physician reports of a child's headache pain: relationships prior to

and following treatment. *Headache* 1985; **25:** 421–5.

51. Andrasik F, Psychologic and behavioral aspects of chronic headache. *Neurol Clin* 1990; **8:** 961–76.

52. Larsson B, The role of psychological, health-behaviour and medical factors in adolescent headache. *Dev Med Child Neurol* 1988; **30:** 616–25.

53. Bille B, Migraine in school children. *Acta Paediatr Scand* 1962; **51**(136): 1–151.

54. Newacheck PW, Taylor WR, Childhood chronic illness: prevalence, severity, and impact. *Am J Public Health* 1992; **82:** 364–71.

55. Hunfeld JAM, Perquin CW, Duivenvoorden HJ et al, Chronic pain and its impact on quality of life in adolescents and their families. *J Pediatr Psychol* 2001; **26:** 145–53.

56. Lanzi G, Balotti U, Zambrino CA, Quality of life in the adolescent. *IVth International Congress on Headache in Childhood and Adolescence*, Turku, Finland, 1999.

# 34

# Developmental age psychology: elements for general framing of headaches

*Federica Galli, Vincenzo Guidetti*

The evaluation of a patient during developmental ages has to take into account the multiplicity of factors that are strictly embedded in the child's development. To treat a child or adolescent who has headaches requires a good knowledge of developmental tasks.

In clinical practice, dealing with a preschooler, a school-age child, or a young or older adolescent is very different. The ways of communicating problems, the kind of assessment and diagnosis, the implementation of therapy and the adherence to treatment will differ significantly in relation to age. The wide range of problems and diseases brought to attention by a headache compels us to have a sound knowledge of the normal developmental framework, in addition to the clinical view.

The development of a child has always been analysed using different theoretical views (genetic, biomedical, psychoanalytical, behavioural, cognitive, sociological, etc.). Each perspective has often focused attention on single aspects of development (e.g. genes, sexuality or behaviour), often ignoring other aspects and giving few categories for framing and understanding diseases. However, we need a theoretically comprehensive framework to help to decode the complex psychology of a child, which takes into consideration the implications of genetic, biological, familial and social influences in modulating the relations, emotions and cognitions of the child.

Drawing on personal clinical experiences, we give preference to an *eclectic* approach, built on the basis of insights of the most important models of the child's development. The clinical framing of headache and the diagnostic and therapeutic intervention need to take account of the *individual* (e.g. cognitive and sexual development) and the *wider* (e.g. family life phase, schooling matters) psychological background. Developmental tasks may be differently experienced even within a normal range, and several factors may influence their expression and modulation. Headache is 'a symptom' and should always be framed by its biological and psychological background.

We look particularly at the stages of cognitive development (conceptualization of pain and illness, coping strategies), sexuality, attachment system and family relations, considering their importance in the lives of the children and adolescents.

Space does not allow us to analyse each model in detail. We look at the gist of each model, focusing on specific aspects according to their relevance to clinical practice. References to research in the headache field are made, often leading to further analyses.

# Cognitive development

Piaget's theory on cognitive development[1] has been widely used as a conceptual basis in most of the research into children's cognitive processing. The basic assumption of Piaget's theory is that development is the expression of a child's active, progressive construction of reality.[2] Cognitive development, as conceptualized by Piaget, provided an increasing ability to engage logical thought and to separate internal realities from the outside world, an increasing ability to distinguish other people's points of view from those of the child's.

The role of action is essential in a process made up of successive adaptations, resulting in four qualitatively different stages of reality construction. The process is a function of the complementary process of assimilation (the environmental stimuli are modified to conform to the existing cognitive structures) and accommodation (changing of cognitive structures after the encounter with the environment). The schema represents a basic element in Piaget's theory, consisting of a pattern of behaviour in response to a particular stimulus from the environment. The four stages may vary in rate, not in sequence of emergence, because of a genetically fixed process that regulates the progression ('genetic epistemology').

## Sensorimotor stage (from birth to 2 years)

The infant progressively acquires schemata related to the body – the object ('permanence of object') – begins to explore, actively produces changes in the environment, searches for novel events and, finally, shows evidence of some reasoning. Actions are employed only to achieve concrete goals.

## Preoperational stage (from 2 to 7 years)

Symbolic thought and representation develop, together with decentration. The child becomes gradually able to realize actions, at first symbolically rather than only by motor skills. Language becomes increasingly important. The child is egocentric, namely, he or she is unable to view the difference between self and the world, his or her own perspective and that of others. The concept of time is not available. The prevalent logic is 'transducive', namely, the events may be viewed as related simply on the basis of spatial or temporal contiguity.

## Concrete operational stage (from 7 years to adolescence)

The child progressively decentres his or her point of view. Social interactions and involvement increase. The child begins to discover the viewpoints of others and is no longer bound to the immediate perceptions. Being able to take into account two variables at the same time, he or she is capable of reasoning according to basic logical principles. The child is readily capable of distinguishing between fantasy and reality.

## Formal operational stage (from adolescence)

Logical thought processes become more complex and integrated. The adolescent is able to use hypotheses, experiment, make deductions and reason from particular to general, without concrete stimuli and independently by specific contents.

## Conceptualization of pain and illness: coping strategies in children and adolescents

Piaget's theory represents a rich framework to understand how the child conceptualizes physical pain and illness, which are the developmental steps and the ways of communicating it. The cognitive–developmental level influences the child's appraisals of pain and medical procedures.

Children's understanding of illness is primarily determined by cognitive maturation. Children have their own conceptions of what has happened to them. Less mature cognitive development may place limitations on children's memory of previous medical stressors, their capacity to define the parameters of procedures (e.g. intensity and duration), and their ability to understand the complex functions of pain and procedures.[3]

Not explaining to the child what happens in a medical setting may increase anxiety and fears. However, each explanation has to be tailored individually, according to the age, familial context and content of the diagnosis. For this reason, it is crucial to have basic information about children's understanding of illness causality and to present our findings, trying to involve the patient even at the youngest ages.

Children's understanding of pain can show some conceptual deficiencies, which are correlated with their level of cognitive develop-

ment.[4] Using a piagetian framework to study developmental changes, researchers have found that definitions of pain shift with age from concrete, perceptually bound descriptions to increasingly abstract, generalized descriptions.[5]

The possibility of documenting a developmental pattern in children's understanding of pain is supported by the findings of age-related patterns in children's understanding of illness.[6,7] Researchers studying children's perspectives on pain[8,9] suggested that most children are familiar with the word pain, have had painful experiences and can communicate about them if asked in terms that they understand. However, younger children are less able to communicate their views than older children.[10] The simpler communications of younger children could reflect different cognitive processing. On this basis, it is essential to stress the importance of tailoring questions according to age, using concrete examples to address questions with the youngest, and shifting to more abstract, generalized approach with adolescents.

Pre-school children's understanding of illness causality is influenced by 'magical' qualities or observable events that are temporally or spatially related to the illness. In this age, the reason for treatment is not understood, because it does not appear to be related to the illness,[11] and appears to be the consequence of a punishment.[12,13] Probably an adequate explanation of the reason for treatment or diagnostic invasive procedures may be helpful to avoid misconceptions, and to prevent the risk that treatment may be interpreted as punishment. When 'magical' thinking about the illness is overcome, children may acquire a greater sense of responsibility for their health and engage in self-control strategies that may facilitate treatment.[14] At early developmental levels children tend to be more likely to view medical procedures as physical attacks and less likely to understand the beneficial aspects of the procedures.[15]

Schoolchildren tend to be 'concrete' in their thoughts, lacking abstract causal understanding. Explanations of this type may be useful, in order to involve the child in the treatment. Making the child aware of his or her role in preventing illness may improve compliance and help in avoiding headache attacks by triggers.

Older children are more likely to recognize the usefulness of treatment and the empathy of the medical staff, and are better able to comprehend the long-term benefit of the procedures.[15] Children with a cognitive–developmental level characterized by beliefs of finalism, imminent justice and syncretism may believe that illness is caused by personal wrong-doing and, consequently, that treatment is a punishment.[9]

In adolescence, the emergence of logical, conceptual, formal thought leads to the understanding of physiological mechanisms that cause illness, and of interventions and biological mechanisms by which illness may be diagnosed and treated.[16] Adolescents and more developmentally advanced children may understand the role of psychological factors in illness causation and exacerbation.[17]

Spirito et al[18] found that adolescents were more likely to focus on the implications of the disease, whereas children were more likely to focus on symptoms. Rudolph et al[4] defined the child developmental level as a moderator, influencing coping and coping outcome.

The attention paid to children's cognitive developmental level may allow medical staff to understand the way in which children can assimilate the information given about medical procedures, resulting in the children understanding and cooperating with treatment.[6]

Children's levels of response to questions about the causes of their illness, intent of medical procedures and role of medical staff fell into three stages:[6]

(1) Children at the preoperational stage (aged < 7 years) conceptualized disease as resulting from human actions: according to the final reasoning, the illness was the outcome of wrongdoing. Children stated that medical procedures were carried out to punish them for being bad.

(2) Children in the concrete operational stage (aged 7–10 years) were capable of separating the cause of illness from direct human actions. Children believed in a single physical cause for their illness, usually answering that illness is caused by germs, and denying any personal responsibility for illness. Children knew that medical procedures were addressed to help them get well, but their ability to infer empathy is limited, because they believed that the empathy of the staff depends on their own expressed pain.

(3) Children at the formal operational level (aged > 9 years) knew that illness can have multiple causes, so that they offered multiple explanations for the cause of the disease, including their own actions.

Bibace and Walsh[20] observed developmental changes in children's concept of illness, coherent with the three stages of Piaget's cognitive development:

(1) Preoperational stage (aged 2–6): there are two types of prelogical explanation of

illness – phenomenism (the cause of illness is perceived to be an external concrete phenomenon that co-occurs with the illness) and contagion (objects or people that affect the child through proximity or magic).

(2) Concrete operational stage (aged 7–10): the children mentioned contamination (through physical contact and/or internalization) as a cause of illness.

(3) Formal operational stage (10–14 years): physiological and psychophysiological explanations.

In addition, children at the highest cognitive–developmental stage can hold on to egocentric or magical concepts in stressful situations. In this case, the children's belief that the illness was caused by something wrong may serve as an important defence mechanism against feelings of helplessness.[6] In fact, adults also prefer to blame themselves rather than admit that illness may be caused by chance and that nothing can be done to control it.[19] Children at the highest cognitive level can infer intention of treatment and medical staff's empathy, because they say that doctors and nurses can put themselves in the children's place in order to know how they feel.

Comprehension of the characteristics of coping strategies could give us additional and important elements to clarify the ways in which headache sufferers react and modulate stressing experiences, focusing the implication of cognitive variables within the general framing of headaches.

Lazarus and Folkman[21] defined the coping response as an intentional physical or mental action, initiated in response to a perceived stressor, and directed towards external circumstances or an internal state. Coping is viewed as a mediator between a stressor and the outcome of exposure to that stressor.[3] Strategies for coping with pain are cognitive and behavioural responses emitted by patients to manage painful episodes; the effectiveness of pain-coping strategies depends on their outcome in terms of pain relief, emotional adjustment or functional status.[22] Many children are able to identify techniques for coping with pain.[23]

Studies on children's coping strategies found different coping styles, depending on the authors' framework:

- Behavioural (support seeking, direct efforts to maintain control) vs cognitive (attempts to divert one's thoughts away from the stressors, cognitive restructuring) coping[24]
- Problem-focused (directed at altering the situation) vs emotion-focused (directed at regulating the emotional consequences of an event) coping[25]
- Primary (efforts to influence the objective event) vs secondary (effort to maximize one's fit to the event) coping[26]
- Approach (active efforts to confront the stressor) vs avoidance (attempts to avoid the event) coping.[27]

Varni et al[22] designed the questionnaire called the Waldron/Varni Pediatric Pain Coping Inventory (PPCI) to assess children's and parents' perceptions of the mechanisms that the child uses to cope with pain. The administration of the PPCI to a sample of children aged 5–16 years, with musculoskeletal pain associated with rheumatological diseases, has revealed the co-presence of five factors in patients' coping responses (Cognitive Self-Instruction, Seek Social Support, Strive to Rest and Be Alone, Cognitive Refocusing, Problem-Solving Self-Efficacy).[22]

A developmental trend in the use of the coping strategies has been outlined: the younger the child, the more he or she was likely to use the coping strategies of Seek Social Support or Cognitive Refocusing, whereas the oldest children were more likely to manage pain with Strive to Rest or Be Alone.

Older children are more likely to invoke some type of coping strategy and use more cognitive or secondary control coping strategies[23] vs behavioural or primary control strategies. In the oldest children, the use of cognitive or secondary strategies is more likely during uncontrollable medical procedures.[24]

Weiz[30] has hypothesized that cognitive or secondary control coping in older children may reflect either enhanced awareness of the ineffectiveness of behavioural or primary control strategies within uncontrollable medical situations or increased access to intrapsychic mechanisms of control.

Problem-focused or primary control coping in uncontrollable circumstances is viewed as maladaptive, because active attempts to alter conditions are ineffective and likely to lead to frustration. Likewise, the use of emotion-focused or secondary control coping in controllable circumstances may interfere with the application of more active techniques to alter the objective situation.[31]

To assess the adjustment outcomes of the children's pain-coping strategies, Varni et al[22] made a correlation between coping strategies and scores assessing the disease's severity, depressive symptoms, state and trait anxiety, general self-esteem and internalizing–externalizing behaviour problems. The results let the authors construct a hypothesis about the adaptiveness of the pain-coping strategies in a sample of children aged 5–16: greater use of Cognitive Refocusing coping was associated with lower worst pain and depressive symptoms reported by the patient, and lower internalizing emotional problems rated by the parents. The authors concluded that the active cognitive concentration away from pain perception may result in lower perceived pain intensity and lower emotional distress. The coping strategy of Problem-Solving Self-Efficacy was also adaptive.

On the contrary, coping by Strive to Rest and Be Alone, Seek Social Support and Cognitive Self-Instruction appeared to be maladaptive coping strategies, with regard to their relationship to pain and adjustment.[22] Previous stressful experiences in younger children could increase their likelihood of engaging in automatic, conditioned responses to fear the stressor without conscious cognitive mediation, whereas older children are more likely to use memories of past experience to cope with the stressor.[4] The influence of prior exposure may be markedly different, depending on children's cognitive constructions of their experiences; the psychological impact of previous stressors may depend on the stage at which the original stressor was experienced, or the maturity of the children's central nervous system.[4]

Research into person-specific moderators[4] has presupposed the presence of coping styles with a stable tract. Temperamental characteristics may exert a direct effect on children's adjustment to medical stressors or may moderate children's preferences for certain styles of coping. Temperamental difficulties have been found to predict poorer behavioural and emotional adjustment in chronically ill children,[33] e.g. children with high reactivity, low adaptability and low threshold for responsiveness to stimuli may demonstrate high levels of distress with a medical stressor and may prefer coping strategies that decrease their perception of the stressor (e.g. information avoiding and distraction). The same child may be less likely to use coping responses that involve direct confrontation with the stressor (e.g. information seeking and sensory focusing).[4] The individual differences in pain-coping strategies can explain the differences in patient responses to cognitive–behavioural and other treatments of childhood pain and, finally, in the variability of treatment outcome.[22]

The dispositional vs the situational nature of coping could be evaluated by examining the degree of consistency in children's coping responses across stressors that differ in type, severity and duration. Wrong cognitive beliefs that are responsible for maintenance of the pain in adult chronically ill patients have been hypothesized.[34]

The influences of coping strategies in childhood and adolescence headache have not been studied. Holm et al[35] found different coping strategies between sufferers of adult tension-type headache and a control group in similar stressing conditions. Headache sufferers showed autocritical and avoidant coping strategies, compared with the preference by controls for social support.

## Psychoanalytical view

Freudian theory represents the traditional framework for analysing psychosexual development in children. Although several revisions, adaptations and criticisms have occurred, the psychoanalytical perspective represents an indispensable load of knowledge and language for clinical work with the developmental ages.

The central assumption of the psychosexual model is that a child's development reflects a continual effort to gratify needs, obtain pleasure and relieve discomfort, from infancy to adolescence.

Id (the biological, instinctual, unconscious components), Ego (the conscious part, with a mediating role between the pressure of Id and the need of reality) and Superego (the moral sense, overall expression of reality and social rules) represent the three main structures that indicate the innate tendency towards psychological organization.

Early experiences represent the main organizer of a child's development. The mother is the primary source of stimulation for the infant. The child's maturation goes across phases related to age, need and ways of gratification. In the oral phase, self-stimulating body activities (such as mouthing and sucking) represent the means for achieving pleasure. In the anal phase, the anal mucosa is said to become erotogenized, and the bowel movements of holding in and letting go of faeces represent the means of gratification, explaining the ambivalence characterizing this period (2- and 3-year-old children). The phallic–oedipal phase occurs between the ages of 3 and 6 years. The child at this phase is said to experience sexual desires towards the parent of the opposite sex, and hostility and rivalry towards the parent of the same sex. The resolution of the tasks of each phase carry through to the emergence of the Superego and the entrance of the latency phase. Between the ages of 6 and 12 years, defence mechanisms take control of unacceptable impulses and fantasies experienced in the previous phases. Only with adolescence is a mature primacy of the genital zone established.

According to this view, psychopathology is sustained by the mechanisms of fixation (persistence of behaviour beyond the appropriate age) and regression (resumption of pre-existing behaviour). Important extensions of psychoanalytical view have been realized by Anna Freud and Melanie Klein. A Freud proposed the concept of 'developmental lines',[36] defined as graduated steps in the emergence of a child's personality. Incongruence or age inappropriateness of the process leads to imbalances of developmental lines, with clinical implications sustained by defence mechanisms. Klein's theory[37] is another extension of Freud's original formulation. Differing from Freud's perspective, the child is more active in regulating his or her own development by innate and unconscious fantasies that are internally produced. A central point is related to the presence since early infancy of a self-destructive and self-preserving instinct, and defence mechanisms such as projection, introjection and splitting for dealing with anxieties and conflicts. Abnormal development is seen as the failure of the Ego to develop adequately in terms of its conscious and unconscious parts.

Avoiding too speculative issues, outwith our main interests, we can draw important elements from the psychoanalytical perspective and subsequent developments, helping to create the framing of headache sufferers in childhood and adolescence. The importance of the first mother–infant experiences in modulating the psychological development of the child, the role of sexuality and aggressiveness, and the description of unconscious mechanisms may give us elements of analysis that aid the diagnostic process.

# Development of an attachment system

Currently, the theory of attachment[38] is one of the most fertile approaches to the analysis of children's developmental patterns of relationships. It provides a theory for child development: ethological, cognitive, psychoanalytical principles represent the main factors.

In contrast to the psychoanalytical view, the child develops the first relationship with the mother not to achieve gratification of the oral libido, but to protect him- or herself from the dangers of the environment in biological terms, developing a 'secure base'. Through the primary relations with caregivers, 'internal working models' are created which reproduce original relations and situations in different ones. The key concept is the kind of attachment built on the earliest experiences, the main distinction being between secure and insecure attachment. The former is related to constant and appropriate caregiving, which allows the child to explore away from the caregiver, providing a 'secure base' to return to.[39] The latter displays several clinical types (avoidant, anxious resistant and disorganized/disoriented), consequent on a nursing environment that is not optimal.[40,41]

The avoidant style is characterized by rejecting the expectations of the caregiver. It represents an obstacle towards new experiences and asking for help in situations of pain or suffering. The child is closed in in a sort of emotive self-sufficiency. The basis of this kind of attachment is said to be repeated refusal of the child's needs. The anxious-resistant insecure style is related to doubtful and unpredictable answers from caregivers about the child's requests for help and grief. The child lacks a secure base to move away and to come back from 'exploration of the world'.

The disorganized/disoriented model is a mixture of the avoidant and anxious–resistant patterns of attachment.

'The strange situation'[41] and the 'adult

attachment interview'[42] represent the scientific procedure that addresses the systematic evaluation of patterns of attachment. There are no scientific studies about the likelihood of links between headache and the attachment models, even when considering the role of separation anxiety (from caregivers) in the creation of a psychological framing of headache, and particularly when elements related to school phobia co-occur. Problems with schooling are probably related not only to problems in the achievement of good results but also to conflicts with teachers or schoolmates.

The school-age period represents a moment of greater demand for independence and autonomy, and the extent to which the child emerges successfully from this stage depends on many factors. The parents may facilitate or hinder the child's progress, or the child may be anxious and reluctant to leave home to go to school, for instance, when he or she feels that there are uncontrollable or unexplained changes in the daily environment (e.g. conjugal conflicts). Headache may represent a way of obtaining the closeness of the caregivers of 'controlling' the situation – it is a sign and/or a probable result of a stressful and difficult period.

# The family system

## Edited by Mimma Tafa

Throughout the life history of the family, events occur that make the functioning of ordinary family life ineffective. In such situations, deep changes should take place, entailing a consistently rapid rebuilding of the family organization, the roles played by the family members and, finally, their relationships and expectations.

The 'family life cycle' approach is highly relevant to an appropriate study of these changes. This approach, addressed differently by researchers and reviewed critically by Breunlin,[43] has proved to be a useful conceptual tool when approaching the family dimension. It considers the difficulties of a family in the light of its past, the current developmental tasks confronting it, and the future towards which it is inevitably moving. The symptoms and the problems may be understood in relation to the actual family functioning over time.[44]

In particular, this approach highlights the different stages of family life from its very beginning. Through these stages, the family has to face and solve specific developmental tasks, the positive solution of which allows progression to the next phase.[44–47]

With 'uncommon therapy', the family therapist Haley[48] entered the family life cycle concept into the psychotherapeutic domain,[49] broadening its initial definition which primarily referred to ordinary family life functioning. In his opinion, family distress is more intense when it coincides with transition from one stage of the developmental process to another, when the pathological symptoms are frequently manifest during the breaking off or disorganization of the life cycle progression.

These symptoms stand for the presence of a stalemate or difficulty in the transition to the next stage. For careful analysis of the symptom of one of the family members in a therapeutic context, it is crucial to take into account the development of the family process, along with its salient stages.

Bowen,[50] another family therapist, argued that at least three generations have to be considered with respect to each life cycle phase. In his opinion, it is of no use doing without a broader family context for a comprehensive evaluation of the individual, because each phase is defined by a complex role that differentiates every single member from the others, and that determines the intersubjective features of the interpersonal relationships.

Within the 'family developmental orientation' approach to the family processes, McGoldrick and Carter[44] made an important contribution to understanding family functioning through the concept of the life cycle. In their opinion, the family system encompasses the whole emotional system of at least three generations. The family bounds are identified by their double features of tie and resource. The authors described the tie as the role played in relation to a particular event, and the resource (coping) as the family organizational ability – core of the family functioning – to cope with the change demands springing from inside and outside the family.

Attachment, looking after and loyalty are other core characteristics of the family bounds. The first two are obviously prominent in the mother–child relationship. In particular, attachment is a relational phenomenon that in many ways will affect the individual's social relationships throughout his or her life.[51] Loyalty is particularly referred to as a sort of silent intergenerational commitment. Every member is trustee of its own perception of a present, past and future double-entry bookkeeping, which is invisibly written into family duties.[52]

The normal model of family functioning described by the authors is built on a horizontal and a vertical axis. The horizontal axis includes the relationship and functioning structures that are handed down along the generations, through the emotional triangulation process that Bowen[50] described (attitudes, taboos, expectations, beliefs and preconceptions that influence the individual upbringing).

The vertical axis describes the effects on the family in terms of anxiety caused by distress resulting from the developmentally crucial life cycle changes and transitions. In the authors' opinion, the difficulties inherent to the 'here and now' dimension (social context) have to be added to the difficulties inherited from the previous generations (vertical axis) and to what is experienced in the life cycle (horizontal axis).

The normative and paranormative events invariably represent family crisis risk factors, because both the ordinary system functioning is no longer adequate and the events are highly likely to result in a change in family life. The critical event does not directly imply a passage to the next stage, but it outlines a process by which an initial crisis is followed by a reorganization/disorganization of the family system. The 'normal' family is different from the 'pathological' one, not because it is defined by an absence of problems, but because it succeeds in coping with unexpected events by creating alternative functioning models.

The roles played by the family members are conclusive in this respect. Their tasks are strongly linked to the timing – a kind of social calendar marking the socially expected behaviours for the single family life phases. A social clock is introjected, which will adjust the individual behaviour in relation to the different ages and periods of life.[53] We are confronted with a three-dimensional phenomenon in relation to which the individual and the family life cycle are considered in a wider social context, because cultural and temporal aspects have stressed the importance of peculiar periods and characterized them as prominent life cycle phases.

The transition to parenthood and that to adolescence of children are among the most relevant life cycle phases. The transition to parenthood is crucial not only for the family but also for the couple's life cycle. When a new member joins the family, a different history begins to develop, as the nature of the partner union is denoted.[54] Here the developmental tasks are making room for the child through a change in the couple system, and the parental role-taking that is strictly connected to the change in partner relationship. A new generation calls for a new definition of the family bounds within a broadened context, and the partners' task is 'climbing up a generation' in order to take care of the previous one.[44] The couple is defined by a constant recreation of different balances, and the adjustment of rules and roles to new functioning needs is crucial.[55,56]

Adolescence is also a crisis factor in the family life cycle, and it inevitably entails rebuilding. Minuchin[57] described this phase as one of transition, with important changes brought about by the adolescent moving towards and playing a new role in the outside world. The redefinition of the boundaries between the subsystems is necessary both for the adolescent to move away in order to be more independent and responsible, and for a more mature parent–adolescent relationship.

The presence of 'symptoms' in adolescence may be seen to be the result of a family dysfunction, and the therapeutic treatment aims to modify the system by marking out new boundaries in the family organization.

Haley[48,58] considered the adolescence crisis as a struggle for preserving the hierarchical status quo within the family. Being part of a relational 'perverse triangle',[58] the adolescent may be seen as a mediator of the parents' relationship. When he or she goes away, the marital balance, so far centred around him,

has to be changed. The adolescent may inadequately react to this, showing difficulties or even failing to move away. In this case, his or her behaviour will 'take shelter' in the family conflict, and once again the system will be cohesive and goal oriented through the symptom. Families with such problems in this life cycle phase are stuck with an old child representation that no longer fits the present.[59] They keep the child under an unsuitable control, with stiff rules and strict dependence relationships.

Otherwise, they may promote the assumption of adult behaviour too early in the child. In such a case, Minuchin described the parental child as a real substitute for the parents, overwhelmed by duties, responsibilities, expected competence and excessive autonomy for his or her age, and whose developmental needs have misled him or her.

Families with adolescents should indeed mark out qualitatively different boundaries from those of families with small children. Total control is no longer suitable, and the boundaries should be more flexible.[59]

Olson et al developed the circumflex model[55] for the study of normal family functioning, and described more flexible boundaries for the family in this phase as a precondition for the adolescent's unbinding, whereas the family with small children should be characterized by a stronger emotional proximity. Therefore, the developmental tasks in the adolescence phase necessitate flexible boundaries and rules because the changes required put every single member under stress. The changes in the parent–child relationship are interfaced with changes in the couple relationship and in both of the parents.

All the different generations are confronted with the task of proceeding towards a better differentiation and individuation, and to this final aim they must be able to adjust to the kind of tie that keeps them together.

The study of family gives us crucial elements for the general framing of headache disorders. Analysis of family relationships, the weight of headache on them and the phase of the family's life cycle are important to know for diagnostic and therapeutic implications. A systematic evaluation of the family addresses part of the therapeutic intervention (e.g. psycho-pedagogic suggestions, through to indications for family therapy).

## Acknowledgements

The section on conceptualization of pain and illness is written with a contribution from Dr Tiziana Franceschini, Child Psychologist, University 'La Sapienza', Rome. A special thank you to Gianpaolo Nicolais for his contribution to the translation of this chapter.

## References

1. Piaget J, Inhelder B, *Memory and Intelligence.* New York: Basic Books, 1973.
2. Piaget J, Piaget's theory. In: Mussen PH, ed., *Carmichael's Manual of Child Psychology* 3rd edn. New York: Wiley, 1970.
3. Peterson L, Coping by children undergoing stressful medical procedures: Some conceptual, methodological and therapeutic issues. *J Consult Clin Psychol* 1989; **57**: 380–7.
4. Rudolph KD, Denning MD, Weisz JR, Determinants and consequences of children's coping in the medical setting: Conceptualization, review and critique. *Psychol Bull* 1995; **118**: 328–57.
5. Gaffney A, Dunne EA, Developmental aspects of children's definition of pain. *Pain* 1986; **26**: 105–17.
6. Brewster AB, Chronically ill children's concepts of their illness. *Pediatrics* 1982; **69**: 355–62.
7. Campbell JD, Illness is a point of view: the development of children's concepts of illness. *Child Dev* 1975; **46**: 92–100.
8. Ross DM, Ross SA, Childhood pain: the school-aged child's viewpoint. *Pain* 1984; **20**: 179–91.
9. Gaffney A, Dunne EA, Children's understanding of the causality of pain. *Pain* 1987; **29**: 91–4.
10. Crow CS, Children's pain perspectives inventory (CPPI): developmental assessment *Pain* 1997; **72**: 33–4.
11. Willis D, Elliott C, Jay S, Psychological effects of physical illness and its concomitants. In: *Handbook for the Practice of Pediatric Psychology.* New York: Wiley, 1982.
12. Varni JW, *Clinical Behavioral Pediatrics: An interdisciplinary biobehavioral approach.* New York: Pergamon Press, 1983.
13. Brewester AB, Chronically ill hospitalised children's concept of their illness. *Pediatrics* 1982; **69**: 355–62.
14. Maddux JE, Roberts MC, Sledden EA, Wright L, Developmental issues in child health psychology. *Am Psychol* 1986; **41**: 25–34.
15. Harbeck C, Peterson L, Elephants dancing in my head: A developmental approach to children's concept of specific pain. *Child Dev* 1992; **63**: 138–49.
16. Hurley A, Whelan EG, Cognitive development and children perception of pain. *Pediatr Nurs* 1988; **14**: 21–9.
17. Kager VA, Arndt EK, Kenny TJ, Psychosomatic problems of children.
18. Spirito A, Stark LJ, Tyc VL, Stressors and coping strategies described during hospitalization by chronically ill children. *J Clin Child Psychol* 1994; **23**: 314–22.
19. Gardner R, The guilt reactions of parents of children with severe physical diseases. *Am J Psychiatry* 1969; **126**: 636.
20. Bibace R, Walsh ME, Children's conceptions of illness. In: Bibace R, Walsh ME, eds, *Children's Conceptions of Health, Illness and Bodily Functions.* San Francisco: Jossey-Bass, 1981: 48.
21. Lazarus RS, Folkman S, *Stress, Appraisal and*

*Coping.* New York: Springer, 1984.

22. Varni JW, Pediatric pain: a decade biobehavioral perspective. *Behav Therap* 1995; **18**: 65–70.

23. Band EB, Weisz F, How to feel better when it feels bad: Children's perspectives on coping with everyday stress. *Dev Psychol* 1988; **24**: 247–53.

24. Curry SL, Russ SW, Identifying coping strategies in children. *J Clin Child Psychol* 1985; **14**: 61–9.

25. Folkman S, Lazarus RS, The relationship between coping and emotion: Implications for theory and research. *Soc Sci Med* 1988; **26**: 309–17.

26. Weisz JR, McCabe M, Denning MD, Primary and secondary control among children undergoing medical procedures: Adjustment as a function of coping style. *J Consult Clin Psychol* 1994; **62**: 324–32.

27. Roth S, Cohen LJ, Approach, avoidance and coping with stress. *Am Psychol* 1986; **41**(7): 813–19.

28. Band EB, Children's coping with diabetes: Understanding the role of cognitive development. *J Pediatr Psychol* 1990; **15**: 27–41.

29. Altshuler JL, Ruble DN, Developmental changes in children's awareness of strategies for coping with uncontrollable stress. *Child Dev* 1989; **60**: 1337–49.

30. Weisz JR, Development of control-related beliefs, goals and styles in childhood and adolescence: A clinical perspective. In: Rodin J, Schooler C, Schaie K, eds, *Self-directedness: Cause and effects throughout the life course.* Erlbaum: Hillsdale, NJ, 1990: 103–45.

31. Comas BE, Coping with stress during childhood and adolescence. *Pyschol Bull* 1987; **101**: 393–403.

32. Peterson L, Toler SM, An information seeking disposition in child surgery patients. *Health Psychol* 1986; **4**: 343–59.

33. Garrison WT, The conceptual utility of the temperament construct in understanding coping with pediatric conditions. In: La Greca AM, Siegel LJ, Wallander JL, Walker CE, eds, *Stress and Coping in Child Health.* New York: Guilford Press, 1992: 72–84.

34. Ciccone DS, Grzesiak RC, Cognitive dimensions of chronic pain. *Soc Sci Med* 1984; **19**: 1339–45.

35. Holm JE, Hiroyd KA, Hursey KG, Penzien MS, Penzien DB, The role of stress in recurrent tension headache. *Headache* 1986; **26**: 160–7.

36. Freud A, The concept of developmental lines. *Psychoanal Study Child* 1963; **18**: 245–65.

37. Klein M, On the development of mental functioning. *Int J Psychoanal* 1958; **39**: 84–90.

38. Holmes J, *John Bowlby and Attachment Theory.* London: Routledge, 1993.

39. Bowlby J, *A Secure Base.* London: Routledge, 1988.

40. Main M, Solomon J, Discovery of an insecure, disorganized/disoriented attachment pattern: procedures, findings and implications for the classification of behaviour. In: Yogman M, Brazelton TB, eds, *Affective Development in Infancy.* Ablex: Norwood, 1986: 95–124.

41. Ainsworth MDS, Blehar M, Waters E, Wall S, *Patterns of Attachment: Assessed in strange situation and at home.* Erlbaum: Hillsdale, NJ, 1978.

42. Main M, Kaplan N, Cassidy J, Security in infancy, childhood and adulthood: a move to the level of representation. In: Bretherton I, Waters E, eds, *Growing Points in Attachment: Theory and research.* Monographs of the Society of Research in Child Developmental Serial, 209. Chicago: University of Chicago Press, 1985 (p. 50).

43. Breunlin DC, Oscillations theory and family development. In: Falicov CJ, ed., *Family Transitions: Continuity and Change over the Life Cycle.* New York: Guilford Press, 1988 (pp. 133–55).

44. McGoldrick M, Heiman H, Carter E, The changing family life cycle: A perspective on normalcy. In: Walsh F, ed., *Normal Family Processes,* 2nd edn. New York: Guilford Press, 1993.

45. Duvall E, *Marriage and Family Development.* Philadelphia: Lippincott, 1977.

46. Hill R, Social theory and family development. In: Cuisenier J, ed., *The Family Life Cycle in European Societies.* Paris: Mouton, 1977 (pp. 31–9).

47. Wynne L, An epigenetic model of family

process. In: Falicov C, ed., *Family Transitions: Continuity and change over the life cycle.* New York: Guilford Press, 1988.

48. Haley J, *Leaving Home. The Therapy of Disturbed Young People.* New York: McGraw Hill, 1980.

49. Malagoli Togliatti M, Tafà M, De Gregorio F, Il contributo dei terapeuti della famiglia attraverso l'analisi delle pubblicazioni dei soci della Società Italiana di Psicologia e Psicoterapia Relazionale. In: Malagoli Togliatti M, ed., *Psicologia della Famiglia. Tendenze e sviluppi.* Milano: Franco Angeli, 1996.

50. Bowen M, *Dalla famiglia all'individuo.* Roma: Astrolabio, 1979.

51. Bowlby J, *The Making and Breaking of Affectional Bods.* London: Tavistock, 1979.

52. Boszormenyi-Nagy I, Spark G, *Invisible Loyalties: Reciprocity in intergenerational family therapy.* New York: Harper & Row, 1973.

53. Scabini E, *Psicologia sociale della famiglia.* Torino: Bollati Boringhieri, 1995.

54. Tafà M, Malagoli Togliatti M, Rivelli MC, La coppia e la transizione alla genitorialità. *Rassegna di Psicologia* 2000; **17**(1): 95–125.

55. Olson D, Russell C, Sprenkle D, Circumflex model of marital and family systems: VI. Theoretical update. *Fam Process* 1985; **22**: 69–84.

56. Olson D, Family stress and coping: A multisystem perspective. In: Cusinato M, ed., *Research on Family Resources and Need Across the World.* Milano: Edizioni Universitarie di Lettere Economia Diritto, LED, 1996 (pp. 73–105).

57. Minuchin S, *Families and Family Therapy.* Cambridge, MA: Harvard University Press, 1976.

58. Haley J, *Uncommon Therapy.* New York: WW Norton, 1973.

59. McGoldrick M, Carter E, The family life cycle. In: Walsh F, ed., *Normal Family Processes.* New York: Guilford Press, 1982 (pp. 259–96).

# 35

## What does it mean to treat headache in children and adolescents? Dealing with patients; dealing with families; dealing with teachers.

*Çiçek Wöber-Bingöl*

The management of headache in children and adolescents requires not only knowledge about and experience of the principles of diagnosis and treatment, but also a certain style of dealing with all the people involved, including the patient and his or her parents as well as others in the patient's environment, particularly teachers. Knowing the expectations of the patients and parents is extremely important. Lewis et al[1] asked 100 children suffering from headache for more than 3 months what they wanted to receive from their clinic visit. The choices included identification of cause, medication for pain, explanations, laboratory tests, radiographs or computed tomography (CT), physical examinations, pain relief, eye examinations, talking to others with headaches and reassurance. Of these ten choices, three were consistently ranked as the most important: to find the cause, to get pain relief and to receive reassurance that they did not have a brain tumour. In our own department, we asked the parents about their expectations and we received similar results. The vast majority of parents wanted information and reassurance, followed by adequate treatment, whereas only a small group expected examinations such as computed tomography or magnetic resonance imaging (MRI) (unpub-

lished data). This chapter highlights some essential aspects of dealing with patients, parents and teachers, covering diagnostic procedures as well as therapeutic management, it also provides the text of leaflets that have been distributed by me to parents and teachers for several years.

## Diagnosis of headache

The principles of the diagnostic procedure in headache in children and adolescents are described earlier. From the point of view of the patients and their parents, it is essential to explain the diagnostic steps and to clarify that a careful history and clinical examination in patients presenting with headache are prerequisites for further diagnostic and therapeutic management.

The history must include the family history, the patient's previous history and headache history, as well as questions about the social environment. Usually, an adolescent is able to give a detailed description of the headache and answers all questions adequately.[2] Taking the history in a child requires more time and patience, but asking the questions in a proper way means that we can get many headache details from the child him- or herself. Describing the headache quality seems to be most difficult for children and questions about the onset of the headache history, as well as the duration and frequency of headaches, are answered more reliably by the parents.[2] In small children who are unable to express themselves adequately, restlessness and irritability may be the only signs of head pain. In addition, it is essential to ask for factors that precipitate, exacerbate or alleviate the headache. According to a study by Lewis et al,[1] tension and pressure, bright lights, noise and missed meals are the most important triggers in children with recurrent or chronic idiopathic headache, and this finding agrees with our own experience. Furthermore, it is important to explore the patient's psychosocial environment.[3]

The clinical examination includes a general as well as a neurological examination. The child should be informed that the examination will not be painful. The parents will usually watch the examination closely and, therefore, the findings should be discussed in detail immediately after the examination.

After taking the history and doing the clinical examination, further steps must be discussed with the parents and the patient. In patients with (suspected) idiopathic headache, additional examinations are not routinely required. It is essential to explain that the cause of idiopathic headache cannot be detected by additional examinations and that such examinations are performed only to exclude an organic disease. In cases with severe or frequent headache attacks or episodes, it may be difficult to convince the parents, the patients and sometimes even other doctors that there is no underlying organic disease. In such cases it will be necessary to perform cranial MRI, CT or other examinations, even if the history and the clinical examination do not provide any evidence of an underlying organic disease, to reassure the parents and the patient. In children with headache after physical exercise, a cardiological examination may be useful. A child with exhausting attacks of migraine with aura, accompanied by visual field defects, sensory symptoms, disturbances of speech as well as nausea and vomiting, may be fearful of a further attack and the parents may be afraid of a life-threatening disease. In such situations, the physician must be calm and try to get the parents' confidence. Reassuring the patient and the parents requires not only good arguments, but also a doctor who is convinced of these arguments from the bottom of her or his heart.

In patients with (suspected) symptomatic headache, it is easier to explain the cause of the headache and specific additional examinations must be arranged. Frequent causes of symptomatic headache include common cold, tonsillitis, sinusitis, other infections and sometimes uncorrected vision disorders. None of these disorders causes much fear among patients and parents. It may be a little bit different, however, if a child has a severe headache after falling and hurting his or her head. In such cases, a cranial fracture and an intracranial bleed or other lesions must be excluded quickly by radiographs of the skull or cranial CT scans. In rare cases, headache may be the presenting symptom of an intracranial tumour, which requires very careful handling. The child and his or her family are fearful and frightened, and they do not know what is going to happen. In this situation, it is essential to speak very clear and simply, and to explain the situation with great patience.

Dealing with headache in young patients and explaining the necessary steps to the parents, we should never forget that the important person is the child or adolescent. The doctor must speak to the young patient explaining diagnostic and therapeutic steps, in order to gain the patient's confidence.

# Treatment of headache

In cases with symptomatic headache, information must be provided about whether or not a causal therapy is possible, e.g. antibiotics in acute sinusitis or spectacles in uncorrected vision disorders. Sometimes the response to a causal therapy may also be important for establishing the definite diagnosis (e.g. tension-type headache vs headache resulting from an uncorrected vision disorder).

For treating migraine and tension-type headache in children and adolescents, a broad spectrum of therapeutic measures has been recommended, but only a few have been examined in controlled trials. Considering this lack of information, it is not practicable to rely exclusively on the findings of controlled clinical trials, although it is necessary to include further treatment options.[4] However, there should be at least some scientific evidence that such treatment is efficacious and well tolerated, and the possible benefit of the treatment must clearly outweigh potential risks. Dogmatic principles such as restricted views of the aetiology and pathogenesis of the headache ('food allergy', 'hypotension', 'sinusitis', 'psychosomatic disease'), as well as monocausal therapies (restrictive diets, medication for raising the blood pressure, antibiotics for 'treating' sinusitis) and therapeutic nihilism ('you must live with your headache'), must be rejected strongly.[5]

Considering the expectations of the patients and parents, the first therapeutic step is there-fore to provide sufficient information about the headache and – in patients with migraine or tension-type headache – to explain why there is no evidence for any underlying serious disease. The second step is to provide a specific therapeutic concept. The parents must be informed about pharmacological and non-pharmacological treatment options for acute therapy as well as prophylaxis, and about the major advantages and disadvantages of these therapies.

In acute migraine attacks, children with short attacks may experience meaningful relief from pain and associated symptoms by resting in a darkened, quiet room and falling asleep for a few hours (or less). Another group of children with short attacks that may not require pharmacotherapy are those who vomit within less than 1 or 2 hours of the onset of the attack and who experience complete or significant pain relief immediately thereafter. All other patients require additional pharmacological therapy (see the start of this chapter). Several factors must be considered to achieve successful treatment: (1) the diagnosis must be correct; (2) the medication must be given as early as possible; (3) the dose administered must be sufficient; (4) parents (and patient) must be informed about the maximum doses per day and per month, as well as (5) about the effect and possible adverse effects of the drug; (6) the patient should not experience (additional) discomfort caused by the administration of the drug; (7) a drug should not be administered against the wishes of the patient or parents; (8) in coexisting migraine and tension-type headache, patient and parents should be instructed to differentiate the two headache types and to treat migraine attacks only; and (9) the patient (and parents) must be instructed to deal with the medication carefully and responsibly in order to avoid the development of analgesic-induced headache from uncritical use of analgesics.[4]

Besides adequate acute therapy, all migraine patients and their parents should be advised about strategies in everyday life that may help to reduce the frequency of migraine attacks. The first step is to identify trigger factors such as stress in the family or at school. The relevance of dietary triggers such as chocolate, cheese, citrus fruits, nuts, coloured sweets, processed meat ('hot-dog headache'), etc. is generally overestimated in my opinion. Prescribing a strict diet may not only be harmful to the child's health, but also cause an additional restriction to his or her quality of life.

The second step in non-pharmacological migraine prophylaxis is providing information to the patient and parents about a certain lifestyle, including sufficient sleep, a morning free of stress, regular meals, sufficient breaks while studying and sufficient physical exercise. Children and adolescents experiencing headache associated with physical exercise should be trained to pay attention to adequate drinking. In children and adolescents with frequent migraine attacks at the first visit, i.e. more than two or three attacks per month lasting for more than 6–12 hours, the patient (and/or parents) should be asked to keep a headache diary for 4 weeks. A prophylactic therapy should not be started at the first visit, because in my experience many patients show at least some degree of improvement at the second visit. In patients with persistent frequent attacks, prophylactic therapy should be initiated, with discussion with the patient and parents of the advantages and disadvantages of non-pharmacological measures and pharmacotherapy.

To cope with an acute episode of tension-type headache, any kind of distraction or relaxation exercises may be useful. Analgesics should be avoided in episodic tension-type headache and are contraindicated in chronic tension-type headache. If an analgesic is administered, the patient and the parents must be advised to treat only a more severe, but not every, episode of tension-type headache.

In the prophylaxis, many of the recommendations discussed for migraine therapy can also be applied in tension-type headache. In particular, this is true for avoidance of precipitating or exacerbating factors and provision of a certain lifestyle.

In patients with refractory headaches, a re-evaluation of the diagnosis, taking into consideration organic as well as psychosocial, psychological and psychiatric factors, is necessary.

## Headache at school

If a child or adolescent complains of headache at school, the teacher is also confronted with the problem and it is extremely important to provide sufficient information for teachers about how to deal with headache in an individual patient. If a pupil gets a severe headache, the teacher often calls the parents to take their child home. However, in children diagnosed as having migraine, for example, it is much more useful to instruct the teacher on how to deal with the headache at school, e.g. to allow the patient to lie down for a while or to take an analgesic. Apart from this, teachers may also contribute in evaluating precipitating factors of idiopathic headache by observing the child's behaviour at school or by recognizing a learning disability. Problems and stress at school are commonly put forward as predisposing or trigger factors of headache and have been investigated most comprehensively by Larsson[6] and Carlsson.[7] According to these studies, young headache patients are more often afflicted by stress in their everyday life; they spend more time on their homework, have difficulty relaxing, and are more often tired after school than headache-free controls. Therefore, it is extremely important to discuss with the patient and the parents, how to plan the time after school and to explain the importance of relaxing after school and having sufficient breaks including physical exercise when doing the homework. If a learning disability is suspected, it should be evaluated by appropriate psychological tests and, if necessary, treated with a specific training program. In the author's clinical experience successful therapy of a learning disability is often associated with an improvement of headache. Similarly, behavioural problems at school must be discussed with the teacher and if necessary psychological testing should be arranged in order to evaluate possible causes of the behavioural disturbance and to plan specific treatment.

Children and adolescents missing many days of school, must be examined very, very carefully. After exclusion of an organic disease, comprehensive psychological work-up is mandatory, since the actual cause of missing school may not be headache, but school phobia as part of social phobia. If this problem is not recognised, the child or adolescent will receive prophylactic headache medication, the medication will not be effective, further examinations regarding organic disorders will be performed, other therapies will be tried, and the parents will change from one doctor to the next resulting in "doctor shopping". As a consequences of such misdirected management the underlying problem, i.e. school phobia and social phobia respectively,

may further deteriorate. Many parents will neither recognize nor accept the severity of the actual problem, arguing that it is impossible for the child to go to school having such severe and frequent headaches. Therefore, the observations of the teacher are extremely important. The teacher must persuade the parents to present the child or adolescents to a specialist for comprehensive neuropsychiatric and psychological evaluation and adequate therapy. The treatment of school phobia requires inpatient therapy. The first step is to gain the patient's and parents' confidence, the second step is to explain that not headache, but school phobia is the actual problem. Accepting this fact is the prerequisite for further successful therapy including special training programs for attending school.

## Conclusion

In children and adolescents with headaches, it is extremely important to provide information about diagnostic and therapeutic steps and reassurance in order to gain the patients' and the parents' confidence. In addition, it may be necessary to cooperate with the patients' teachers about possible precipitating factors of idiopathic headache, as well as individual management of acute headache at school.

## When children have headache: information for parents and teachers

### What is headache?

Headache is a pain anywhere in the head, which may occur without an underlying disease or be associated with an organic disorder.

## Headaches unassociated with an organic disease

The two major types of headaches unassociated with an organic disease are migraine and tension-type headache.

### Migraine
- A child suffering from an acute migraine attack usually stops playing or studying, looks 'sick', wants to lie down, and may wish to sleep.
- The headache is usually severe, localized on one or both sides of the forehead, and may be made worse by physical activity.
- The child may also be nauseated or vomit and may dislike light or loud noise. Sometimes, he or she may have difficulties thinking or speaking. Occasionally he or she may experience visual disturbances. Rarely, tingling feelings or weakness may occur on one side of the body.
- The headache usually lasts a few hours, whereas neurological symptoms should subside within an hour.

### Tension-type headache
- This is the second major type of headache not associated with organic disease.
- It is less severe than migraine.
- It is not associated with nausea, vomiting, difficulties in thinking or speaking, or visual disturbances.

## What are the causes of migraine and tension-type headache?

- The exact cause of migraine as well as tension-type headache is still unknown, although there are various factors that may trigger these headaches.
- Some of these trigger factors are:
  - alteration of sleep–wake cycle
  - missing or delaying a meal
  - stress at school
  - familial problems
  - chronic anxiety.
- Foods such as ripened cheese, chocolate or nuts may trigger a migraine attack. However, not all of the foods trigger headaches in all migraine sufferers all of the time.
- Weather changes are often thought to cause migraine, but these should not exclude the other possible trigger factors that are treatable and changeable.

## Headaches associated with an organic disease

### Frequent causes
- Common cold, angina, sinusitis
- Flu and any other infection
- Head or neck injury
- Uncorrected vision disorders.

### Life-threatening causes
These diseases are rare and require immediate admission to a hospital:
- Meningitis, encephalitis
- Cerebral haemorrhage (e.g. after head injury)
- Brain tumour.

## How to recognize headache in young children

- Restlessness and irritability may be the only signs of head pain in young children who are unable to express themselves adequately, but this may also be true in older children.

## When to worry about headache

### Acute headaches

If they are associated with any of the following symptoms:

- Fever and/or stiff neck
- Drowsiness or lethargy
- Neurological symptoms such as weakness of an arm or leg, difficulty in walking, visual disturbance, or speech disorder, when symptoms last more than 1 hour
- Severe vomiting
- First epileptic seizure
- Sudden onset like an explosion.

### Recurrent or chronic headaches

- If frequency and/or intensity of headache increases
- If the headache pattern changes
- If associated neurological symptoms last longer than usual or if new neurological symptoms (including personality changes) develop
- If epileptic seizures occur
- If pain killers do not work anymore.

## What to do

### In acute headaches

- If headache is associated with any of the symptoms mentioned above, call a doctor immediately.
- If none of these symptoms is present:
  - encourage the child to relax in a quiet and darkened room
  - observe the child.
- If the headache has not subsided on the following day, or if any of the above symptoms occur, call a doctor.

### In recurrent or chronic headaches

- Every child with recurrent or chronic headaches should be seen by a doctor.
- Chronic progressive headaches require further investigations as soon as possible.
- Chronic non-progressive headaches are usually the result of migraine or tension-type headache.
- To find out whether headache is caused by an organic disorder or not the doctor will:
  - take a careful history
  - perform a clinical examination
  - decide whether further investigations are necessary.
- Usually, these investigations are not painful.
- Sometimes a venepuncture may be required.
- In young children, it may be necessary to give a sedative before some special investigations.

### In migraine or tension-type headache

- It is important to find out what the headache triggers are.
- Preventing such triggers is the first step to reduce the frequency of headaches.
- The second step is to elucidate possible psychological factors, such as learning difficulties or family friction.
- An important element is to produce a certain lifestyle with a regular change of learning and leisure, regular meals and regular sleeping hours, as well as a warm interest on the part of the parents in their child's emotions.
- Pain killers may be necessary in acute migraine attacks, but should be avoided in tension-type headache. In any case, ask your doctor and do not give more than five per month on average.
- If the child has frequent headache attacks, prophylactic treatment may be required, e.g. special psychological therapies such as

relaxation training, training of learning disabilities or certain medications given over a period of several months.

## Special remarks about headache, school and studying

- The pressure to be successful in general, as well as pressure at school in particular, may trigger headaches. Causes of this pressure may be:
  - extreme achievement orientation and excessive ambition of the child him- or herself or
  - learning disabilities, difficulties in reading, spelling or mathematics, or difficulties in concentration.
- However, reduced concentration or hyperactivity may be the only expression of headache when the child cannot or does not verbalize the symptom.
- Observations of school performance are essential in children recurrently complaining of headache.
- Teachers may notice a disturbance before the parents do.

## Concluding remarks

- Diagnosing childhood headache as soon as possible ensures that an organic cause of headache is not overlooked and represents the prerequisite for a specific treatment.
- If a child has migraine or tension-type headache, the child, the parents and the teachers can learn to control and cope better with the headaches. Psychological and medical strategies will provide support.

## Acknowledgement

The author is grateful to Dr Marcia Wilkinson (London, UK), Professor Dr WD Gerber (Kiel, Germany) and Dr V Pfaffenrath (Munich, Germany) for providing their experience and comments in establishing the 'Information for parents and teachers'.

## References

1. Lewis DW, Middlebrook MT, Mehallick L, Rauch TM, Deline C, Thomas EF, Pediatric headaches: What do the children want? *Headache* 1996; **36**: 224–30.
2. Wöber-Bingöl Ç, Wöber Ch, Karwautz A et al, Diagnosis of headache in childhood and adolescence: a study in 437 patients. *Cephalalgia* 1995; **15**: 13–21.
3. Karwautz A, Wöber C, Lang T et al, Psychosocial factors in children and adolescents with migraine and tension-type headache: A controlled study and review of the literature. *Cephalalgia* 1999; **19**: 32–43.
4. Wöber Ch, Wöber-Bingöl Ç, Clinical management of young patients presenting with headache. *Funct Neurol* 2000; **15**(suppl): 89–105.
5. Hermann C, Kim M, Blanchard EB, Behavioral and prophylactic pharmacological intervention studies of pediatric migraine: an exploratory meta-analysis. *Pain* 1995; **60**: 239–55.
6. Carlsson J, Larsson B, Mark A, Psychosocial functioning in school children with recurrent headaches. *Headache* 1996; **36**: 77–82.
7. Larsson B, Carlsson J, A school-based, nurse-adminstered relaxation training for children with chronic tension-type headache. *J Pediatr Psychol* 1996; **21**: 603–14.

# 36

# Pain experience in children
*Federica Galli, Tiziana Franceschini and Vincenzo Guidetti*

Clinical pain can never be seen as primarily a biologic phenomenon or as only a psychologic event, nor can pain be divorced from the social context

(McGrath, 1989)[1]

The experience of pain is universal. Attempts to relieve and comprehend the nature of and the reasons for pain concerns many fields, from religion to medicine, from ethnology and anthropology to psychology, philosophy, etc. The etymology of the word 'pain' contains the Greek term *poinè* (suffering) and the Latin *poena* (punishment), deriving from a common Indo-European matrix meaning 'to pay' (e.g. having a pain as punishment or accepting pain to redeem the sin is a central aspect of Christianity).

Pain is always surrounded by a composite matrix of biological psychological and social interactions. Perhaps, the complex embedding of these factors is the raison d'être for the difficulties in finding a general definition of the concept of pain.

Franklin[2] defined pain as an emotion caused by any cognitive or physical stimulation. This concept of pain emphasized the experience of unpleasantness or displeasure, without including as a criterion any associated tissue damage or noxious physical stimulation.

By the mid-twentieth century, a 'specific' theory of pain postulated the presence of specific receptors, and pain was explained in terms of stimulation of pain receptors.[3] Sanders[4] defined pain as a cluster of gross motor (complaints of pain, crying, grimacing, distorted walk), cognitive (thoughts, feelings, images) and physiological responses (neurological events). Fordyce[5] recognized four elements of a pain episode: nociception, pain perception, suffering and pain behaviour.

Merskey[6] offered a definition of pain, including both unpleasant subjective experience and physical stimulation. The Task Force on Taxonomy of the International Association of Pain defined pain as 'an unpleasant sensory and emotional experience associated with actual or potential tissue damage, or described in terms of such damage'.[7]

Similar to Merskey, Owen[8] stated that an infant has an unpleasant subjective experience when (1) there is evidence of tissue damage and (2) the infant responds with signs of distress, such as crying, increased heart rate, or facial expression consistent with distress or other signs.

In line with his idea of pain, Owen[8] defined headache as a 'borderline case' of the concept of pain: children with headache express signs of distress through verbal reports or behavioural indices, from which it is even possible to infer the presence of a tissue damage, not evident by itself. In addition, the role of age-related differences in understanding and expressing pain remains unaccounted for.

Factors such as cognitive maturation, language development, pain memories, perceiving coping ability, self-regulation capabilities, cultural, and familial and individual attributions contribute individually and together to the pain experience and the development of chronic pain.[9]

The weight of each factor in modulating pain experience and expression is unknown. We apply adult categories in the understanding and analysis of children's pain. The characteristics of infants' pain can only be deduced by adults on the basis of non-verbal clues. The younger the child, the more emphasis lies on symptoms inferred by adults from behavioural and physiological signs of distress.[10]

## Synopsis of developmental characteristics of children's pain

Biological maturation influences the perception and response to pain. This assumption outlines the role of age-related physiological features in the modulation of pain, but also the expression of pain does change with age. Sensation of pain differs from cognition of pain, e.g. several factors (age, previous pain experiences, coping style, skills or answers from family or social setting) are implicated in communicating pain. 'The development of a communication system ... would appear to require not only the ability to transcend concrete stimulus–response linkages, but also the

presence of an intentional, observing self and the belief in the existence of other self-conscious individuals'.[11] The process is related to the development of anatomical and physiological pathways. Cognitive operations imply that sensory information undergoes attentional modulation and elaboration by associative areas. Prefrontal cortex and limbic area maturity plays a critical role in determining the developmental process from sensation to cognition of pain in children.[11]

The systemic principle of 'totality'[12] may help us to explain the consequences of the developmental patterns. The outcome of the number of individual age-related factors is different by the simple sum of each factor. The outcome of the relationship of the factors within a system (such as the pain system) is not simply a 'heap' of the involved elements, depending on the related process.

Bearing in mind this view, we should consider the child as not being a 'little adult'. This also means that many individual factors run together to affect the expression and modulation of pain, always resulting in different outcomes. To start by considering the child as a whole of his or her development, taking into account neurobiological and psychological maturational processes, familial and social environmental factors, is crucial to avoid a limiting and unilateral approach to the disease. Taking all these factors into account has critical importance in the assessment process and for the choice of the better drug or non-drug treatment.

The central nervous system is the most multifaceted and fascinating structure in the body and the related processes show at least the same complexity. A developmental perspective involves physiological and psychological factors related to the modulation and expression of pain in a bidirectional way. 'Pain perceptions result from complex neural interactions that also reflect the impact of psychologic and environmental factors'.[11]

However, little is known about the relative weight and reciprocal modulation of physiological and environmental factors. The historical nature–nurture controversy is strictly brought in, even though the current view has a strong transformation. In contemporary neurobiology, the focus is not related to the questions 'Is nature or nurture the major contributor to the biological processes?', but to the questions 'To what degree is this biological process determined by genetic and developmental factors? To what degree is it environmentally or socially determined? To what degree is it determined by a toxic or infectious agent?'.[13]

Kandel[14] outlined that 'The mind will be to the biology of the twenty-first century what the gene has been to the biology of the twentieth century'. The current perspective goes well beyond the mind–body dualism, opening up the need for an integrated framing (nature *and* nurture), from analysis of the basic processes.

The emotions should be considered as a fundamental component of the pain experience.[15] On the 'nature side' the tissue trauma (pain) activates both spinothalamic pathways that convey to the somatosensory cortex and spinoreticular pathways that lead to the limbic areas through noradrenergic projections.[15] The link with the 'nurture side' is related to the adaptation and survival reasons of emotional phenomena associated with pain. The limbic system is present in all mammals. The activation of limbic structure involved in attention processes – fear or panic – leads to the 'fight or flight' responses. The child's expression of pain and the related emotions

activate the care-giving environment in defensive terms. The role of the environment in shaping the characteristics of the subsequent responses to the pain cues is critical, even though we should always take into account the biological and physiological bases of grafting.

It is crucial to stress that the early pain experiences can not only affect the future patterns of management pain of that child, but may also play a critical role in shaping the pain system in biological terms.[16]

Traditionally, lack of complete myelination has been proposed as an index of immaturity in the neonatal nervous system and used frequently to support the argument that neonates and infants are not capable of pain perception.[1,17–19]

The adults' inference for recognizing children's pain can explain the discordance of research about non-verbal infants' pain. Beliefs about infants' non-perception of pain after tissue damage had been supported by studies that found a total lack of response by newborns to pin-prick or electrical stimulation.[20] Often, clinicians administered little or no anaesthetic to infants for procedures such as endotracheal intubation[21] or circumcision.[22]

There is increasing evidence that pain experiences during infancy lead to changes in the structure and function of the pain system (e.g. lower pain threshold in pre-term neonates after exposure to painful stimuli).[16] Studies on neonatal circumcision pain showed higher pain-related behaviours in later routine immunization.[23] Direct empirical investigations showed a great deal of objective and subjective distress associated with pain in infants.[24] Pain is associated with levels of catecholamines, glucagons, insulin, endogenous corticosteroids and biochemical markers for protein catabolism.[25] In neonates, the catecholamine responses to surgery are more acute than in adults: the responses are very rapid and these increased peak concentrations, and reinstatement of baseline levels.[26] Cortisol responses in neonates are greater than in adults and return rapidly to baseline within 24 h.[26]

The short-term risk of the misconception that neonates do not feel or have low sensitivity to pain, and do not have a memory for pain, may lead to inadequate and/or infrequent analgesic medication,[27] under-medication and limited treatment.[28] To date, the long-term consequences on the modulation of the child's development and responses to pain are unknown.

Children can recall pain experiences, understand the nature of pain and associate pain with particular feelings; children's understanding of pain can, however, show some conceptual deficiencies, which correlate with their level of cognitive development (see later).[29]

Recent, better-controlled data unequivocally demonstrate that neonates do feel pain: anatomical, functional and neurochemical systems are sufficiently well developed at birth to permit pain perception and memory.[15,16,18,19] In line with the ethological view,[30] Izard and Dougherty[31] claimed that competence for pain perception and expression must be present at birth, because the expression of distress in response to tissue damage is adaptive and helpful to survival. Newborn infants have the anatomical and functional components necessary for appreciation of painful stimuli:[19] further development of the pain pathways during infancy and childhood involves the enhancement of these sensory modalities and intracortical connections with the limbic system and the affective and associative areas located in the frontal cortex, parietal cortex and the insula.[19]

In relation to the memory of pain in children, only a few studies have been carried out in children compared with adults.[32] Moreover, most studies have been realized in relation to the external provision of painful stimuli (inoculation, lumbar puncture, dental restoration, etc.) and related contexts, principally to obtain information about children's abilities to provide testimony in legal situations, and not assessing children's memory of the pain itself.[33] Sensation and cognition or representation of pain are different (but not unrelated) levels of analysis, modulated by several factors as cited above. It is important to bear in mind that not having a clear cognition and capacity to recall pain does not mean that pain does not influence later pain experience. Earlier experiences of pain may give rise to indelible traces on a biological basis, and subsequent memory may be influenced by them. In addition, memory of pain has been involved in the establishment of chronic pain syndromes.[34]

Currently, the prevailing theory on the brain–behaviour relationship stresses the plasticity of the brain and the force of psychological and social experiences in modulating its structures and functions.[35] Pain perception depends on complex neural interactions activated by tissue damage and modulated by ascending and descending gating systems, in relation to environmental and psychological factors.[36] This general description of pain's activation and modulation gives rise to several questions on the mechanisms involved in the process (e.g. which mechanism explains the placebo effect?).

'Studies on learning in simple animals provided the first evidence that experience produces sustained changes in the effectiveness of neural connections by altering gene expression'.[12] Rats exposed to repetitive neonatal pain showed decreased pain threshold during development. However, the difference was not maintained during adulthood, even though the long-term effects had been noted in relation to stress-related behaviours (more freezing, running, jumping than the control sample).[37] Drawing conclusions by direct analogy between animal and human development is at best approximate, even though there are hypotheses that neonatal intensive painful care, occurring at a time of rapid cortical maturation, may lead to crucial changes in the neural architecture and may be retained in the memory, with consequences on the structuring of the pain system and subsequent pain-related experiences.[38,39] The central nervous system may be altered by nociceptive experiences; repeated exposure to painful stressors may redirect the growth of neural pathways and result in a nociceptual neural architecture that renders the individual 'pain vulnerable' or 'pain resilient'.[40]

The specific role of environmental factors in the refinement of these sensory modalities, and of intracortical connections with the limbic system, the affective and associative areas, is not well known. Recently, more attention has been given to the interconnectivity of physiological factors (such as the status of the autonomic nervous system, threshold of sensory receptors, synaptic connections, activation of the hypothalamic–pituitary–adrenal axis, locus ceruleus, noradrenaline [norepinephrine] production, etc.) and psychological factors (cognitive maturation, language development, memory, coping abilities, and cultural, familial and individual attributions about pain) in pain modulation and chronic progression.[8] Consideration of all these variables may help to explain why the same tissue damage may lead to different pain experiences in both

adults and children,[41] even though finding the relative weight of each factor in modulating pain experience, length and expression is the real challenge of modern-day research.

The interactions between child and maternal factors stress the complexity of pain modulation and behaviour in infancy. In early infancy, individually based reactivity level (temperament is the related index) better predicts behaviour. In late infancy, pain behaviour is more strongly related to the patterns of maternal responsivity to pain cues over time and immediate maternal behaviour during pain.[42] This shows the function of environmental factors in modulating physiological response to pain, and the importance of analysing and considering the role of individual differences.

Pain's complex neurophysiology is the result of mediator molecules or other stimuli acting on nociceptors, which evoke subsequent responses within many neural circuits: several neurotransmitters act within these diverse multilevel circuits. Each class of mediator occurs centrally in pain pathways, as a primary neurotransmitter or as a modulator of underlying synaptic transmission. The density of these neurotransmitters increases gradually during gestation, with marked increases around the perinatal period and changes until the puberty.

## Expression of pain in children

The differentiation between sensitivity to pain and expression of pain represents an anchor point to consider in research and clinical practice. The smaller the child, the more the possibilities of expressing distress by age-related ways, other than adult ones. The expression of pain changes with age, showing behavioural age-related features. The most striking difference between the adult and infant response to pain is the non-verbal nature of the infant repertoire. Infants and young children primarily respond with physical withdrawal from the stimulus, large body movements and crying. Children and adolescents are less likely to cry. They are more likely to describe their distress verbally. On an age-related background, only a context-related analysis may give us data to decode pain-related behaviours in children.

Over time, the expression of pain from an innate and adaptive response to environmental dangers may assume symbolic meanings, becoming a way of expressing emotional states, to achieve the proximity of caregivers and to obtain 'secondary gains'. Knowledge about developmental processes involved in the modulation of children's pain is of critical interest for practitioners, to tailor the assessment and management of clinical conditions (Table 36.1).

Hurley and Whelan[43] have found an evolution of children's perspectives on pain (on the meaning, cause and value of pain), according to Piaget's four stages of cognitive development.

Crow[44] designed the Children's Pain Perspectives Inventory (CPPI) to assess children's concepts about definition, cause, description and value of pain, with questions such as: 'How do you feel when you have pain?', 'What does cause pain?', 'What makes you

---

**0–3 months**
- No apparent understanding of pain
- Memory for pain likely but not conclusively demonstrated
- Responses are perceptually dominated

**3–6 months**
- Pain response of infancy supplemented by anger response of toddlers

**6–18 months**
- Children develop clear fear of painful situations
- Words are common to express pain
- Localization of some pain

**Up to 6 years**
- Prelogical thinking characterized by concrete thinking and egocentrism, and transductive logic

**7–10 years**
- Concrete operational thinking characterized by child being able to distinguish self from the environment
- Use of behavioural coping strategies

**>11 years**
- Formal logic thinking, characterized by abstract thinking and introspection
- Increased use of mental or cognitive processes
- Coping strategies

**Table 36.1**
*Developmental sequence of understanding pain.[1]*

feel better when you have pain?', 'Is there more than one kind of pain?' In a sample of children aged between 5 and 13 years with orthopaedic problems, Crow[44] found a highly significant correlation between children's pain perspectives measured by the CPPI and Piaget's stages of cognitive development measured with the Cartoon Conservation Scale (CCS). The children's verbal responses were consistent with cognitive developmental progression from preoperational to concrete operations through formal operations. Children at the 'preoperational' level did not comprehend the questions or responded inappropriately, with answers that were global, circular or magic. During the 'concrete' operational stage children's responses provided concrete rules or transgressions of some rules associated with pain; at the same time some responses began to reflect the notion of internalization of the causal processes or mechanisms of pain. Children at the higher cognitive level ('formal' operational stage) demonstrated the onset of the notion of pain causation and the role of the body as a possible agent in causing pain. Children with the most mature understanding of pain described both psychological and physiological processes in pain causation.

Gaffney and Dune[45] found that half of their sample of children aged 5–14 years mentioned, as causes of pain, explanations involving one or more elements of transgression or self-causality. This kind of explanation in younger children is coherent with their finalistic thinking and the sense of imminent justice. 'Transgression' explanations persist also in older children where they coexist with more objective causes, indicating a progression from single to multiple causation.[45]

At the opposite end of the scale, neither Ross and Ross[24] nor Schultz[46] reported significant developmental patterns in children's understanding of pain.

The difficulty in studying the development of children's response to painful events, and the consequent discrepant results of research, may depend on the biases in the systematic evaluation of the distress:[29] older children manifest qualitatively different types of distress behaviour, which are not always included in observational measures.[47] Older children exhibit greater muscular rigidity and verbal expression of pain, whereas younger children manifest anxiety through vocal protest and skeletal activity.[48]

When pain has been experienced, children present a wide range of behavioural expressions from vocalizations to non-verbal body actions.[9] Facial expressions may offer insights of pain in infants. There is an empirical distinction between the expression of pain in infants and that in adults: in the first half hour of life, facial expression in response to the heel lance consisted of brows down and together, eyes tightly closed and the mouth angular, whereas adults in pain situations have open eyes and mouth corners stretched downwards and outwards.[49]

The expression of pain through body movements changes according to neuromuscular development. McGraw[50] analysed the reactions to a noxious stimulation (a pin prick) in infants from birth to age 4 years. Until the age of 10 days, the neonates do not respond at all or respond with diffuse body movements. The reaction increased in intensity during the first month and declined during the second. Between 6 months and 1 year of age, the infants exhibited purposeful withdrawal of the stimulated limb, often preceded by visual fixation on the point of stimulation. By the age of a year, infants touched the area of stimulation after the stimulus was withdrawn. Further development was characterized by anticipatory response designed to protect the infant from the pin prick.

Infants also express pain by crying. The pain cry is unlike a hungry or angry cry, because it is characterized by a sudden onset of loud crying without preliminary moaning, an initial long cry and an extended period of breathholding in expiration.[51]

Wasz-Hockert et al[52] claimed that pain cry is dysphonated or hyperphonated, and it is likely to have any melody other than rising–falling and to last longer. Murray[53] summarized the literature about children's crying, concluding that qualitative properties do not allow differentiation between pain cries and other cries. The crying intensity may allow discrimination, increasing with the increased amount of discomfort experienced by the infant and with increasing infant motivation to send a message to the listener.

Crying is also a social signal. It recalls the caregivers' presence, strengthening the attachment system.[54] The infants' crying may be influenced by the answers from the social context, supporting the link between pain and attachment system.

The infants' cardiac activity showed a developmental pattern in response to age-related stressful events. For 5-month-old infants, the heart rate decreases in the presence of height, whereas at 9 months of age the heart rate shows an increase in the presence of strangers, similar to adults in stressful or painful events.[55]

Craig et al[56] investigated developmental changes in pain expression of healthy infants receiving routine immunization injections during the first 2 years of life. The categories

of expressive behaviour observed are vocal actions (crying, pain vocal, pain–fear verbal), non-vocal–face (distorted face, eye orientation, eye opened–closed), non-vocal–torso (rigid, withdrawing), non-vocal–limbs (protect/touch, kick/thrash). Craig et al[56] reported that younger children vocalized more, expressed rigidity primarily after the injection and did not orient towards the injection area at all. The older children cried for a shorter span of time, vocalized less than the younger children after the injection, used language primarily before the injection, watched the nurse and their mothers, and viewed the injection, protected and/or touched the injection area after needle penetration.

Ross and Ross[24] studied the children's verbal report on painful experiences. The authors designed a semi-structured interview to study the children's knowledge and understanding of pain, their ability to describe pain, specific pain experiences, use of coping strategies and maladaptive pain in hospitalized children aged between 5 and 12 years. Data showed the absence of a developmental trend, which the authors explained with the lack of opportunities of intentional training or incidental learning about physical pain in the children's socialization process. This hypothesis was confirmed by the parents' interviews, in which most of the parents stated that they discourage the discussion of pain experiences with their children.

Ross and Ross[24] found that most pain definitions were one-dimensional (see below), with the children's description of pain being of a general discomfort or focused on specific pain events. The children had no understanding of the warning and diagnostic values of pain; they could not think of anything good about pain.

The pain experiences were attributed to clearly *related* and *immediate* causes, such as accidents, environmental factors, illness or surgery. There was no evidence of the children's conception of the pain as a punishment, differing from other research on illness causality,[57] which found a sense of imminent justice in children's definition of pain. The children were able to communicate effectively about their pain and provided excellent descriptions and information about their pain experiences.

Ross and Ross[58] stressed that three procedural components that have fostered the possibility of obtaining such information from the children: the type of questions used, the child's perception of his or her role and capabilities, and the psychological climate of the interview setting. Most of the children mentioned that headache was the type of pain that they frequently encountered. There was relatively low use of self-initiated coping strategies, with a prevalence for distraction and physical procedures. About 40% of the sample reported at least one instance of using pain for secondary gains, mainly in the form of increased parental and peer attention, and avoidance of school and athletic training activities.

Gaffney and Dunne,[59] studying a sample of Irish schoolchildren aged 5–14 years, found that the acquisition of a concept of pain follows a developmental sequence consonant with Piaget's theory of cognitive development (see also Chapter 34).

The responses of younger children in the pre-operational stage of cognitive development tended to be perceptually dominated and very concrete: pain is 'a thing', something located in the body or an unpleasant physical property. In this stage, the understanding of the relationship between pain and illness and the value of pain as a warning system are lacking.

Progressive age levels showed a shift from perceptual to conceptual functioning, manifested in increasing abstraction, more generalized views and a developing awareness of the psychological/emotional concomitants of pain. Children in the 'concrete operational' stage can use analogies to describe pain, which result in more vivid qualitative descriptions; there was a developmental awareness of the psychological concomitants of pain in the context of its ability to affect the mood of the suffer.

At the 'formal operation' stage, older children and adolescents are capable of introspection: they defined pain as a feeling or a sensation, and used abstract definitions, which included a reference to both physical and psychological dimensions of pain. Older children had a more active view of the pain, as something that has to be coped with or dealt with.[59]

## Conclusion

Several points remain uncovered in the contemporary comprehension of pain mechanisms and modulating factors. The lack of a general and commonly recognized definition is a probable corollary to the complexity of this matter.

On the other hand, knowledge about the mechanisms related to pain's perception and modulation is crucial for specialists dealing with patients who cope with painful disorders. Somatic pain has always had psychological consequences, because psychological distress may manifest itself in somatic ways. Head pain may be framed on this general background, even though the existence of distinct patterns of interaction between biological and psychological variables should be better analysed.

The social and environmental context within which pain occurs gives us crucial information about environmental contingencies and social modelling which may shape the expression of pain. Physical symptoms may be related to attention and interest by a parent, to obtain 'secondary gain', etc. Antecedents and consequences of recurrent headache have been considered to have a crucial role in determining the outcome (increasingly chronic nature) of headache.[60] Only a multilevel approach gives us the possibility of a complete framing of child pain.

Knowledge about the biological and physiological components of pain is not enough for complete understanding of a pain's dimensions.

Learning has been implicated in the development and maintenance of some somatic disorders:[61] the importance of health beliefs and practices of family members and the presence of family models for the patient's illness should always be examined when dealing with pain disorders. Developmental cognitive patterns of codifying the reality (e.g. understanding illness and therapeutic interventions) should be kept in our mind when taking care of young patients, for both for diagnostic and therapeutic planning of clinical interventions.

# References

1. McGrath PJ, Developmental and psychological factors in children's pain. *Pediatr Clin North Am* 1989; **36**: 823–36.
2. Franklin B, *A Dissertation on Liberty and Necessity*. New York: The Facsimile Text Society, New York, 1930.
3. Wolff HG, Wolf S, *Pain*. Springfield, IL: Thomas, 1958.
4. Sanders SH, A trimodal behavioral conceptualization of clinical pain. *Percep Motor Skills* 1979; **48**: 551–5.
5. Fordyce WE, Pain and suffering: A reappraisal. *Am Psychol* 1988; **43**: 276–83.
6. Merskey H, On the development of pain. *Headache* 1970; **10**: 116–23.
7. Merskey H, Classification of chronic pain: descriptions of chronic pain syndromes. 1986; *Pain* (suppl 3): 51.
8. Owens ME, Pain in infancy: conceptual and methodological issues. *Pain* 1984; **20**: 213–30.
9. Zeltzer L, Bursch B, Walco G, Pain responsiveness and chronic pain: a psychobiological perspective. *Dev Behav Pediatr* 1997; **18**: 413–22.
10. Owens ME, Pain in infancy: conceptual and methodological issues. *Pain* 1984; **20**: 213–30.
11. Sifford LA, Psychiatric assessment of the child with pain. *Child Adolesc Psychiatr Clin North Am* 1997; **6**: 745–81.
12. Watzlawick P, Beavin JH, Jackson DD, *Pragmatics of Human Communication. A study of interactional patterns, pathologies, and paradoxes*. New York: WW Norton & Co, 1967.
13. Kandel ER, A new intellectual framework for psychiatry. *Am J Psychiatry* 1998; **155**: 457–69.
14. Kandel ER, Biology and the future of psychoanalysis: a new intellectual framework for psychiatry revisited. *Am J Psychiatry* 1999; **156**: 505–24.
15. Chapmann CR, Limbic processes and affective dimension of pain. In: Carli G, Zimmermann M, eds, *Progress in Brain Research*. Amsterdam: Elsevier Science, 1996: p. 110.
16. Anand KS, Grunau R, Oberlander TF, Developmental character and long-term consequences of pain in infants and children. *Child Adolesc Psychiatr Clin North Am* 1997; **6**: 703–23.
17. Tilnet F, Rosett J, The value of brain lipoids as an index of brain development. *Bull Neurol Inst NY* 1931; **1**: 28–37.
18. Fletcher AB, Pain in neonate. *N Engl J Med* 1988; **317**: 1347–8.
19. Anand KJS, Carr DB, The neuroanatomy, neurophysiology and neurochemistry of pain, stress and analgesia in newborns and children. *Pediatr Clin North Am* 1989; **36**: 795–822.
20. Canestrini S, *Uber das sinnesleben des neugeborenen*. Monogr Gesamtgab Neurol Psychiat.

Berlin: Springer, 1913: 5, 1a.

21. Craig KD, Ontogenetic and cultural influences on the experience of pain in man. In: Kosterlitz HW, Terenius LY, eds, *Pain and Society*. Weinheim: Verlag Chemie, 1980: 37–52.

22. Kirya C, Werthmann MW, Neonatal circumcision and penile dorsal nerve block: a painless procedure. *J Pediatr* 1978; **96**: 998–1000.

23. Taddio A, Katz J, Ilersich AL, Effect of neonatal circumcision on pain response during subsequent routine vaccination. *Lancet* 1997; **349**: 599–603.

24. Ross DM, Ross SA, Childhood pain: The school-aged child's viewpoint. *Pain* 1984; **20**: 179–91.

25. Anand KJS, Sippell WG, Aynsley-Green A, Randomized trial of fentanyl anaesthesia in preterm babies undergoing surgery: effects on stress response. *Lancet* 1987; **i**: 243–8.

26. Anand KJS, Neonatal responses to anaesthesia and surgery. *Clin Perinatol* 1990; **17**: 207–14.

27. Eland JM, Anderson JE, The experience of pain in children. In: Jacox AK, ed., *Pain: A source book for nurses and other health professionals*. Boston: Little Brown, 1977.

28. Thompson KL, Varni JW, A developmental–cognitive–biobehavioral approach to pediatric pain assessment. *Pain* 1986; **25**: 283–96.

29. Rudolph KD, Denning, MD, Weisz JR, Determinants and consequences of children's coping in the medical setting: Conceptualization, review and critique. *Psychol Bull* 1995; **118**: 328–57.

30. Charlesworth WR, An ethological approach to research on facial expressions. In: Izard CE, ed., *Measuring Emotions in Infants and Children*. Cambridge: Cambridge University Press, 1982: 317–34.

31. Izard CE, Dougherty LM, Two complementary systems for measuring facial expressions in infants and children. In: Izard CE, ed., *Measuring Emotions in Infants and Children*. Cambridge: Cambridge University Press, 1982: 97–126.

32. Zonneveld LNL, McGrath PJ, Reid GJ, Sorbi MJ, Accuracy of children's pain memories. *Pain* 1997; **71**: 297–302.

33. Ornstein PA, Manning EL, Archer Pelphrey K, Children's memory for pain. *Dev Behav Pediatr* 1999; **20**: 262–77.

34. Flor H, Birbaumer N, Acquisition of chronic pain: Physiological mechanisms. *Am Pain Soc* 1994; **32**: 119–27.

35. Cicchetti D, Cannon TD, Neurodevelopmental processes in the ontogenesis and epigenesis of psychopathology. *Dev Psychopathol* 1999; **11**: 375–93.

36. Melzack R, Wall PD, *The Challenge of Pain*. New York: Penguin, 1982.

37. Anand KJS, Thrivikraman KV, Engelmann M, Sü Y, Plotsky PM, Adult rat behavior and stress responses following pain in neonatal period. *Pediatr Res* 1995; **37**: 57A.

38. Anand KJS, Grunau RE, Oberlander TF, Developmental character and long-term consequences of pain in infants and children. *Child Adolesc Psychiatr Clin North Am* **6**: 703–24.

39. Grunau RE, Children's judgments about pain at age 8–10 years: do extremely low birthweight (≤1000g) children differ from full birthweight peers? *J Child Psychol Psychiatry* 1998; **4**: 587–94.

40. Barr RG, Boyce WT, Zeltzer LK, The stress-illness association in children: A perspective from the biobehavioral interface. In: Haggerty RJ, Sherrod LR, Garmezy N, Rutter M, eds, *Stress, Risk and Resilience in Children and Adolescents: Processes, mechanisms and interventions*. Cambridge: Cambridge University Press, 1994: 182–224.

41. McGrath P, *Pain in Children*. New York: Guilford, 1990.

42. Sweet SD, McGrath PJ, Symons D, The role of child reactivity and parenting context in infant pain response. *Pain* 1999; **80**: 655–61.

43. Hurley A, Whelan EG, Cognitive development and children's perception of pain. *Pediatr Nurs* 1988; **14**: 21–9.

44. Crow CS, Children's pain perspectives inventory (CPPI): developmental assessment. *Pain* 1997; **72**: 33–40.

45. Gaffney A, Dunne EA, Children's understanding of the causality of pain. *Pain* 1987; **29**: 91–4.

46. Schultz NV, How children perceive pain. *Nurs Outlook* 1971; **19**: 670–3.

47. LeBaron S, Zeltzer L, Assessment of acute pain and anxiety in children and adolescents by self-reports, observer reports and a behavioral checklist. *J Consult Clin Psychol* 1984; **52**: 729–38.

48. Katz ER, Kellerman J, Siegel SE, Behavioral distress in children with cancer undergoing medical procedures: Developmental considerations. *J Consult Clin Psychol* 1980; **48**: 356–65.

49. Izard CE, Huebner RR, Risser D, McGinnes GC, Dougherty LM, The young infant's ability to produce discrete emotion expressions. *Devel Psychol* 1980; **16**: 132–40.

50. McGraw MB, *The Neuromuscular Maturation of the Human Infant*. New York: Hafner, 1945.

51. Wolff PH, The natural history of crying and other vocalizations in early infancy. In: Foss B, ed., *Determinants of Infant Behavior*. London: Methuen & Co., 1969: 81–115.

52. Wasz-Hockert O, Lind J, Vuorenkoski V, Partenen T, Valanne E, The infant cry: a spectrografic and auditory analysis, Clinics in Developmental Medicine. London: Spastics International Medical Publications, 1968.

53. Murray AD, Infant crying as an elicitor of parental behavior: an examination of two models. *Psychol Bull* 1979; **86**: 191–215.

54. Kagan J, *Psychological Research on the Human Infant: An evaluative summary*. New York: William T Grant Foundation, 1982.

55. Campoe JJ, Emde J, Gaensbauer T, Henderson C, Cardiac and behavioral interrelationships in the reactions of infants to strangers. *Dev Psychol* 1975; **11**: 589–601.

56. Craig KD, McMahon RJ, Morison JD, Zaskow L, Developmental changes in infant pain expression during immunization injections. *Soc Sci Med* 1984; **19**: 1331–7.

57. Kister MC, Patterson CJ, Children's conceptions of the causes of illness: understanding of contagion and the use of immanent justice. *Child Dev* 1980; **51**: 839–46.

58. Ross DM, Ross SA, The importance of type of question, psychological climate, and subject set in interviewing children about pain. *Pain* 1984; **19**: 71–9.

59. Gaffney A, Dunne EA, Developmental aspects of children's definition of pain. *Pain* 1986; **26**: 105–17.

60. Martin PR, *Psychological Management of Chronic Headaches*. New York: The Guilford Press, 1993.

61. Garralda ME, Somatisation in children. *J Child Psychol Psychiatry* 1996; **1**: 13–33.

# XII

## Organization of services for children and adolescents with headaches

# 37

## Childhood and adolescence headache centres

*Vincenzo Guidetti, Federica Galli*

The aim of this chapter is to give practical suggestions for the implementation of a headache centre for children and adolescents, analysing the decision-taking steps in the management of headache.

Headaches vary in severity from moderate to severe and prolonged disability, in a diagnostic range from a minor symptom to serious underlying disease. The wide range of physical and psychological factors in co-morbid headache emphasizes the importance of tailoring both the diagnostic process and the treatment according to the peculiarities of the single case, and of not limiting the clinical intervention to routine practice, but addressing further examinations according to the whole patient history (detailed anamnesis *and* general and neurological examinations). This allows a reduction in the economic costs of services related to unnecessary examinations.

The impact of headache crises on economics has been analysed in adults,[1–7] but not in children and adolescents. There is little in the literature even on the organization and models of headache centres, in either adults or most of all children or adolescents.[8,9]

The organizational structure of headache centres needs to take account of the national health care systems across the various countries. The headache centre may be affiliated to hospital or medical schools, or be independent (freestanding clinics). The former is more diffuse and, historically, the original type. Institutional affiliations can facilitate benefits to patients from a range of services offered by the institution, even though freestanding clinics can also provide a wide range of diagnostic services. Headache centres may offer outpatient and inpatient treatment units, with specialized sections, some of which may be dedicated to young patients.[10]

The quality of care and quality assurance, outcomes and the satisfaction of patients are areas of investigation that need further studies in order to implement quality systems for headache centres.[11]

Our aim is to give general guidelines about the organization of a headache centre for children and adolescents, even though much will depend on the resources of any centre. We promote a multidisciplinary approach from diagnosis to treatment of headache, encouraging networking of health care resources. Headache centres may offer opportunities for training experience and education and research, as well as care of patients.

Referral to this third level, a specialized centre, may not be immediate for headache patients, and sometimes it does not happen at all. In spite of the high prevalence rates of headache, the estimates for consultation rates in adults are about 30%,[12,13] with self-treatment interventions by over-the-counter medications being prevalent. However, a study on adult migraineurs who were referred to a headache specialist showed that the patients were more satisfied with the care and improvement in headache frequency, duration and intensity than those referred to primary care physicians.[14] More headache specialists than primary care physicians asked patients to take prophylactic medication and keep headache diaries and educated them in avoidance of trigger factors, spending more time with the patients.

A study on childhood migraine showed that the most important factors linked to the consultation rates were aura symptoms and high frequency of attacks, with more missed school days than among those children who had not consulted a doctor for migraine.[15]

The referral of children and adolescents to a third-level headache centre assumes particular importance when considering how many factors may be related to headache, factors that may be missed because attention has been focused only on headache symptoms. Education of the patient about correct drug intake is crucial at the developmental ages, and also with regard to such help as how to recognize and avoid triggering factors.

Treatment choices should be guided not only by diagnosis, but also by a general framing of headache attacks, with regard to the impact on the daily activities of patients.

Planning of therapy should be influenced by a complete and specific analysis of the impact of headaches on the patient's daily life, and not only because of the use of a diagnostic label. This implies two parallel diagnostic methods (medical and psychological), which converge on therapy planning. Only biopsychosocial or holistic framing of headaches can assure complete understanding of the disease and its consequences on daily life, predisposing to the most adequate treatment.

The conjunction of drug treatment with psychological/behavioural suggestions may be useful in improving the course of the headache and preventing chronic evolution. An important challenge is to understand whether or not the onset of migraine precedes or follows the occurrence of other problems (e.g. psychopathology or impaired functional status).

## Timing of diagnosis

The treatment of headache patients start with a complete anamnesis (see Chapter 5), as well as neurological and objective examinations (Fig. 37.1). Further steps address the presence of neurological signs and symptoms.

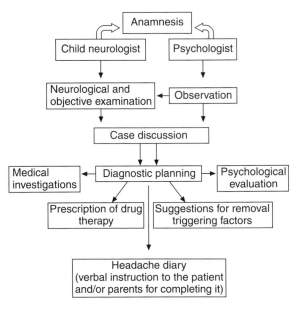

**Figure 37.1**
*First examination.*

The familial recurrence of a number of pathologies (e.g. allergy, hypertension, tumour, epilepsy, stroke, thrombocytosis) opens itself to occasional examinations.

We promote multidisciplinary work from the first meeting to the planning of therapy and follow-ups. A child neurologist should be involved in this first meeting, together with a clinical psychologist, for the observation of non-verbal language and focus on elements by the past and present history, from which hypotheses can be built for verification. The presence of the psychologist at the neurological visit may add important diagnostic elements. The mother–child interaction, the level of autonomy, inhibition or opposition of the child to the visit, and the adequacy of the behavioural patterns for the age strengthen the diagnostic framing. Multidisciplinary work

needs adequate training to define and learn protocols of diagnosis and treatment.

At this point, sufficient elements should be present to address further diagnostic steps. Neurological signs and symptoms, 'secondary' clinical features of headache, familial history for some pathologies (e.g. hypertension, hypercholesterolaemia, epilepsy) guide towards testing for organic causal diseases by specific investigations.

But which medical examinations? The limitations of this chapter do not allow inclusion of detailed indications (see Chapter 35), but just some general suggestions (Fig. 37.2).

The contribution of electroencephalographic (EEG) examination in the diagnosis of chronic headache in children appears to be limited.[16,17] However, EEG study must be performed when there is suspicion of headache as

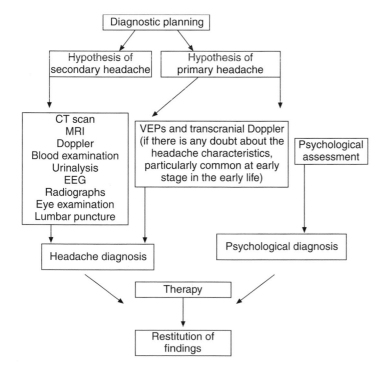

**Figure 37.2**
*Diagnostic planning for medical and psychological assessment. CT, computed tomography; MRI, magnetic resonance imaging; VEP, visual evoked potentials.*

a 'bridge' symptom in epilepsy,[18–21] in cases of post-traumatic headache, and when there is evidence of meningitis or encephalitis, metabolic disorders or intoxication, or headache associated with cognitive deficits and behavioural disorders.[22] The EEG cannot exclude intracranial lesions.

Neuroimaging studies (computed tomography [CT] and magnetic resonance imaging [MRI]) should be required only in patients with abnormal neurological findings, atypical headache pattern and/or change of pre-existing characteristics of head pain.[23–26]

Blood examinations are useful when infectious or metabolic causes are suspected, or in the case of unclear untreatable headache.[22,27]

A lumbar puncture is indicated when there is evidence of subarachnoid haemorrhage, meningitis, encephalitis, brain abscess, septic sinus thrombosis, cerebral vasculitis, meningiosis carcinomatosa, lymphomatosis, leukaemia or pseudotumour cerebri.[22]

Medical and psychological diagnoses have different timing (Fig. 37.3). The psychological evaluation requires more time (if not limited to structured screening) and different tools according to the case's characteristics (see Chapter 6). It may be difficult to organize the process of psychological assessment independently of medical controls, depending on the different organization of each centre, even if it may be useful to separate the psychological assessment by time.

The psychological evaluation should particularly be recommended when the patient's history shows evidence of elements such as the tendency to somatization,[28–30] previous or actual psychiatric disorders or symptoms[28–31] (see Chapter 14), or important life changes or specific stress (e.g. separation of parents, recent bereavement, school prob-

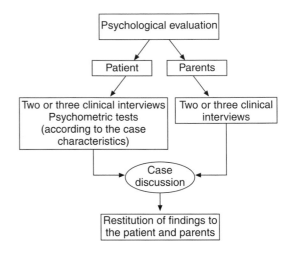

**Figure 37.3**
*Planning the psychological assessment.*

lems). However, more subtle, disabling situations may become visible only within a diagnostic process.

We suggest taking no more than a month to 6 weeks to complete the diagnostic process. In the mean time, the medical examinations will be ready and the complete framing of 'that headache in that patient' will be available.

## Timing of therapy planning

The planning of therapy depends on the whole framing of a single situation. In general, after the first visit, we should have sufficient elements, even if it is only at the end of the whole diagnostic process that we have sound evidence to implement therapy (Fig. 37.4). The therapeutic intervention may begin at the first meeting, with behavioural and life-style suggestions for significant improvement in the quality of life, acting on trigger factors for headache crises (e.g. suggestions for improved

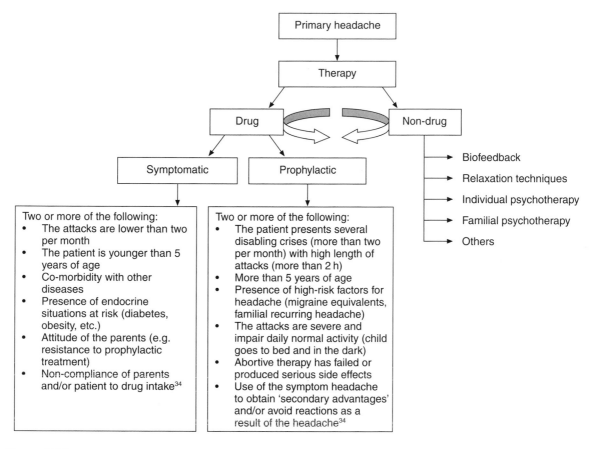

**Figure 37.4**
*Therapy planning.*

sleep hygiene[32] or diet, limits to time spent playing videogames or watching TV, reduction in pressure for school achievement and adequate physical exercise).

The prescription for symptomatic drug therapy may also be done during the first visit, even though it is sometimes better to wait for the second examination until the elements of both the diagnostic process and the clinical situation before prescribing prophylactic therapy. In fact, it is a common experience to record a spontaneous reduction in headache frequency after the first visit, an aspect from which diagnostic and therapeutic directions can be drawn. However, specific cases (e.g. severe disabling headache or previous, but unsuccessful, attempts with prophylactic therapy) may suggest that preventive therapy be planned at the first visit. At the second visit, we will have data from the medical examinations and the headache diary[33] to provide better framing of the clinical situation.

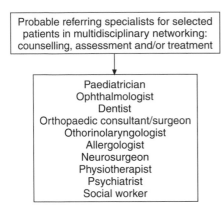

**Figure 37.5**
*Specialists for counselling, assessment and/or intervention on specific cases.*

Co-morbid diseases, suspicions about the involvement of various factors that influence head pain, may suggest referral to other specialists for counselling, assessment and/or interventions at different levels (Fig. 37.5). Other pathologies, whether or not related to headache, may be highlighted during the diagnostic process, requiring occasional referrals. Often, the same specialists receive our referrals for all our headache patients.

## Emergency unit inside headache centres?

The presence of an emergency department inside a headache centre is uncommon. The type of response to headache patients presenting as urgent situations depends on the organization of the different centres. Usually, as for adults,[8] therapy planning provides the indications for treatment of acute attacks at home. However, answers for patients and their families who need help to cope with an acute attack should always be given (also by phone), pro-

viding details about emergency departments or preferential ways of accessing the centre. Indirect evaluation of these cases may be difficult, considering the worrisome impact of certain headache symptoms or the disabling severity of some attacks.

In spite of the high prevalence of headache in children or adolescents, the percentage of visits to the paediatric emergency department resulting from headache is low (1.3%),[35] and similar to those in adults (1.3–2.5%).[36,37] No serious conditions, which present with headache as the chief complaint, appear to be common in the paediatric emergency departments.[35,38,39] Most of the headaches seen at the emergency departments seem to be secondary to concurrent illnesses (mainly upper respiratory tract infections) and minor head trauma, even if the proportion of cases with primary headache is lower (10–38%)[35,38,39] in children and adolescents than in adults (23–55%).[37,40] However, we do know that night onset of headache, projectile vomiting, lack of triggering or relieving factors, headache with changed characteristics, fixed unilateral localization of head pain, delay of growth, as well as clear objective, neurological abnormalities (papilloedema, ataxia, hemiparesis and/or abnormal eye movements) warrant neuroradiological examination to exclude the existence of brain tumours or intracranial haemorrhages.[39,41,42]

## Final comment

Headache is so common that there may be a tendency by both parents and physicians to assume an attitude of 'self-cure' or to have the idea that it is a minor and short-lived problem. However, headache may be the symptom of deeper difficulties, a way of communicating discomfort, which needs immediate recognition and treatment. This means not only the exclusion of the secondary nature of headache or simply giving a drug, but also understanding which are the triggers of headache and what 'that headache' signifies in the life of 'that patient' and his or her family.

It is clear that multilevel framing of the problem allows work in this direction, helping to find the roots of the problem and offering the patient diverse appropriate solutions, which can be integrated with the drug treatment.

# References

1. Caro JJ, Caro G, Getsios D, Raggio G, Burrows M, Black L, The migraine ACE model: evaluating the impact on time lost and medical resource use. *Cephalalgia* 2000; **40:** 282–91.

2. Michel P, Dartigues JF, Dune G et al, Incremental absenteeism due to headaches in migraine: results from the Mig-Access French national cohort. *Cephalalgia* 1999; **19:** 503–10.

3. Leonardi M, Musicco M, Nappi G, Headache as a major public health problem: current status. *Cephalalgia* 1998; **18**(suppl 21): 66–9.

4. Schwartz BS, Stewart WF, Lipton RB, Lost workdays and decreased work effectiveness associated with headache in the workplace. *J Occup Environ Med* 1997; **39:** 320–7.

5. Lipton RB, Stewart WF, von Korff M, Burden of migraine: societal costs and therapeutic opportunities. *Neurology* 1997; **48**(suppl 3): S4–9.

6. Blau JN, MacGragor EA, Migraine consultations: a triangle of viewpoints. *Headache* 1995; **35:** 104–6.

7. de Lissovay G, Lazarus SS, The economic cost of migraine. Present state of knowledge. *Neurology* 1994; **44**(suppl 4): S56–62.

8. Clifford Rose F, Lipton RB, Headache clinics. In: Olesen J, Tfelt-Hansen P, Welch KMA, eds, *The Headaches*. New York: Raven Press, 1993.

9. Nappi G, Micieli G, Cavallini A et al, Business management of headache centers. *Cephalalgia* 1998; **18**(suppl 21): 76–9.

10. Sicuteri F, Boccuni U, Pietrini U, The headache clinic: a nocipathy unit. *Panminerva Medica* 1982; **24:** 37–40.

11. Ferrari A, Baraghini GF, Sternieri E, Cavazzuti L, Roli L, Quality assurance system using ISO 9000 series standards to improve the effectiveness and efficacy of the Headache Center. *Funct Neurol* 2000; **15**(suppl 3): 230–6.

12. Lipton RB, Steward WF, Migraine in the United States: a review of epidemiology and health care use. *Neurology* 1993; **43**(suppl 3): 6–10.

13. *Migraine Management Guidelines.* Surrey: Synergy Medical Education, 1993.

14. Hu XH, O'Donnell F, Kunkel RS, Gerard G, Markson LE, Berger ML, Survey of migraineurs referred to headache specialists: care, satisfaction and outcomes. *Neurology* 2000; **55:** 141–3.

15. Metsähonkala L, Sillanpää M, Tuominen J, Use of health care services in childhood migraine. *Headache* 1996; **36:** 423–8.

16. Kramer U, Nevo Y, Neufeld MY, Harel S, The value of EEG in children and adolescents with chronic headaches. *Brain Dev* 1994; **16:** 304–8.

17. De Carlo L, Cavaliere B, Arnaldi C, Faggioli R, Soriani S, Scarpa P, EEG in children and adolescents with chronic headaches. *Eur J Pediatr* 1999; **158:** 247–8.

18. Brinciotti M, Di Sabato ML, Matricardi M, Guidetti V, Electroclinical features in children and adolescents with epilepsy and/or migraine, and occipital epileptiform EEG abnormalities. *Clin Electroencephalogr* 2000; **31:** 76–82.

19. Puca F, de Tommaso M, Clinical neurophysiology in childhood headache. *Cephalalgia* 1999; **19:** 137–46.

20. De Carlo L, Cavaliere B, Arnaldi C, Faggioli R, Soriani S, Scarpa P, EEG evaluation in children and adolescents with chronic headaches. *Eur J Pediatr* 1999; **158:** 247–8.

21. Ramelli GP, Sturzenegger M, Donati F, Karbowski K, EEG findings during basilar migraine attacks in children. *Electroen-*

*cephalogr Clin Neurophysiol* 1998; **107**: 374–8.

22. Wöber C, Wöber-Bingöl Ç, Clinical management of young headache patients. *Funct Neurol* 2000; **15**(suppl 3): 89–105.

23. Maytal J, Bienkowski RS, Patel M, Eviatar L, The value of brain imaging in children with headaches. *Pediatrics* 1995; **96**: 413–16.

24. Wöber-Bingöl Ç, Wöber C, Prayer D et al, Magnetic resonance for recurrent headache in childhood and adolescence. *Headache* 1996; **36**: 83–90.

25. Lewis DW, Dorbad D, The utility of neuroimaging in the evaluation of children with migraine or chronic daily headache who have normal neurological examinations. *Headache* 2000; **40**: 629–32.

26. Lahat E, Barr J, Barzilai A, Cohen H, Berkovitch M, Visual evoked potentials in the diagnosis of headache before 5 years of age. *Eur J Pediatr* 1999; **158**: 892–5.

27. van der Wouden JC, van der Pas P, Bruijnzeels MA, Brienen JA, van Suijlekom-Smit LWA, Headache in children in Dutch general practice. *Cephalalgia* 1999; **19**: 147–50.

28. Garralda ME, Somatisation in children. *J Child Psychol Psychiatry* 1996; **1**: 13–33.

29. Garralda ME, Practitioner review: Assessment and management of somatization in childhood and adolescence: A practical perspective. *J Child Psychol Psychiatry* 1999; **40**: 1159–67.

30. Egger HL, Angold A, Costello EJ, Headaches and psychopathology in children and adolescents. *J Am Acad Child Adolesc Psychiatry* 1998; **37**: 951–8.

31. Guidetti V, Galli F, Fabrizi P et al, Headache and psychiatric comorbidity: clinical aspects and outcome in an 8-year follow-up study. *Cephalalgia* 1998; **7**: 455–62.

32. Bruni O, Galli F, Guidetti V, Sleep hygiene and migraine in children and adolescents. *Cephalalgia* 1999; **19**(suppl 25): 57–9.

33. Metsähonkala L, Sillanpää M, Tuominen J, Headache diary in the diagnosis of childhood migraine. *Headache* 1997; **37**: 240–4.

34. Guidetti V, Galli F, Drug guidelines for juvenile headache treatment. *Semin Headache Manage* 1997; **2**: 7–8.

35. Burton LJ, Quinn B, Pratt-Cheney JL, Pourani M, Headache etiology in pediatric emergency department. *Pediatr Emerg Care* 1997; **13**: 1–4.20.

36. Dickmen RL, Masten T, The management of nontraumatic headache in a university hospital emergency room. *Headache* 1979; **19**: 391–6.

37. Dhopesh V, Anwar R, Herring C, A retrospective assessment of emergency department patients with complaint of headache. *Headache* 1979; **18**: 37–42.

38. Kan L, Nagelberg J, Maytal J, Headaches in a pediatric emergency department: etiology, imaging, and treatment. *Headache* 2000; **40**: 25–9.

39. Lewis DW, Qureshi F, Acute headache in children and adolescents presenting to the Emergency Department. *Headache* 2000; **40**: 200–3.

40. Letch MJ, Non-traumatic headache in the emergency department. *Ann Emerg Med* 1980; **9**: 404–9.

41. Battistella PA, Naccarella C, Soriani S, Perilongo G, Headache and brain tumors: different features versus primary forms in juvenile patients. *Headache Q* 1998; **9**: 245–8.

42. Guidetti V, Fabrizi P, Galli F, De Cesare C, Unilateral headache in early and late childhood. *Int J Neurol Sci* 1999; **20**: S56–9.

# Appendix

A. Proposal for a brief clinical record
- ❏ M
- ❏ F
- ❏ Age _____
- ❏ Age of onset _____
- ❏ First-degree relative with identical attacks

<table>
<tr>
<td>

**DURATION**

- ❏ <30 min
- ❏ >30 min
- ❏ <4 h
- ❏ >4 h
- ❏ >8 h
- ❏ 24 h
- ❏ >24 h

</td>
<td>

**NUMBER of ATTACKS**
(days/month-year)

- ❏ <15/month
- ❏ <15/month
- ❏ <180/year
- ❏ <180/year

(per day)
- ❏ 1
- ❏ 2–4
- ❏ 5–8

</td>
<td>

**QUALITY of PAIN**

- ❏ pulsating
- ❏ pressing
- ❏ tightening
- ❏ pressing–tightening

**LOCATION**

- ❏ unilateral _____

- ❏ bilateral _____

</td>
</tr>
<tr>
<td>

**INTENSITY**
- ❏ mild
- ❏ moderate
- ❏ severe
- • aggravation by routine physical activities
  - ❏ Yes
  - ❏ No

</td>
<td colspan="2">

**AURA SYMPTOMS**
- ❏ visual aura
- ❏ sensorial aura
- ❏ motor aura
- ❏ speech aura
- ❏ less typical aura

</td>
</tr>
<tr>
<td>

**ACCOMPANYING SYMPTOMS**
- ❏ nausea
- ❏ vomiting
- ❏ phonophobia
- ❏ photophobia
- ❏ anorexia
- ❏ conjunctival injection
- ❏ lacrimation
- ❏ nasal congestion
- ❏ forehead and facial sweating
- ❏ miosis
- ❏ ptosis
- ❏ eyelid oedema
- ❏ vertigo

</td>
<td colspan="2">

**LOCATION**
- ❏ unilateral
- ❏ bilateral

**DEVELOPMENT and DURATION**

- ❏ <60 min
- ❏ >60 min

*IHS code*

</td>
</tr>
</table>

❏ **B. PROPOSAL FOR A COMPLETE CLINICAL RECORD (on the basis of the protocol by the Italian Group for the Study of Headache-Sinpi)**

## FAMILY ANAMNESIS

Primary headache (>5/year)          NO _____ YES _____
Mother _____ Father _____ Brothers and/or Sisters _____
Collaterals on mother's side _____ Collaterals on father's side _____
Diagnosis of headache (family) _____
Other pathologies in the family _____

## PERSONAL ANAMNESIS

Perinatal suffering          NO _____ YES _____
Type _____
Menarche          NO _____ YES _____          at age _____
Premenstrual syndrome          NO _____ YES _____

## REMOTE PATHOLOGICAL ANAMNESIS

Benign paroxysmal vertigo          NO _____ YES _____
Other _____
Seizures:          NO _____ YES _____ Diagnosis _____
Other _____
Head trauma          NO _____ Yes _____ 2 or more weeks before the beginning of headache _____
Concomitant or within 2 weeks from the beginning of headache _____
After the beginning _____
Head trauma:
light _____ with loss of consciousness <15 min _____ with loss of consciousness >15 min
with focal neurological signs _____ with fractures _____
Allergic disturbances:          NO _____ YES _____
Which _____
Othorhinolaryngological disturbances:          NO _____ YES _____
Which _____
Dental disturbances:          NO _____ YES _____
Which _____
Visual disturbances:          NO _____ YES _____
Which _____
Other _____
**Anamnesis registered by:** the patient _____ the father _____ the mother _____
the child + one of the parents _____ others _____

**Attacks of one type** _____ **of more than one type** _____

**Characteristics of attacks:**

NB if there are two types of attacks specify in A the characteristics of the prevalent one and in B the other.

Age at start (years, months)

A _____ B _____

Duration of headache

A _____ B _____

Total number of attacks at visiting time (if more than 10 write >10)

A _____ B _____

Frequency of attacks in the last 6 months: <1 per month = 1; from 1 to 3 per month = 2; 1 per week = 3; <15 per month = 4; >15 per month = 6.

A _____ B _____

Duration of headache:

months/year

A _____ B _____

days/month

A _____ B _____

Intensity of pain: slight = 1; medium (reduces activities) = 2; severe (interruption of activities) = 3.

A _____ B _____

Average duration of attack: <5 min = 1; 5–30 min = 2; 30 min–2 h = 3; 2–6 h = 4; 6–12 h = 5; 12–48 h = 6; >48 h = 7.

A _____ B _____

Periodicity of attacks: absent = 0; spring = 1; summer = 2; autumn = 3; winter = 4; more than one season = 5; school time = 6.

A _____ B _____

Usual days of the week: weekdays = 1; weekends = 2; both = 3; variable = 4.

A _____ B _____

usual time of head pain beginning: variable = 0; awakening = 1; morning = 2; afternoon = 3; evening = 4; night = 5.

A _____ B _____

Quality of pain: throbbing/hammering = 1; burdening/constricting = 2; 1 + 2 = 3; shooting/stinging = 4; burning/superficial = 5; other = 6.

A _____ B _____

Lateralization: bilateral = 1; unilateral = 2; alternating unilateral = 3.

A _____ B _____

Location of start: periorbital = 1; frontal = 2; temporal = 3; parietal = 4; occipital = 5; diffused = 6; facial = 7; vertex = 8.

A _____ B _____

Location of diffusion: absent = 0; periorbital = 1; frontal = 2; temporal = 3; parietal = 4; occipital = 5; diffused = 6; facial = 7; vertex = 8.

A _____ B _____

**Associated symptomatology:**

| | BEFORE | | DURING | | AFTER | |
|---|---|---|---|---|---|---|
| Photophobia | A _____ | B _____ | A _____ | B _____ | A _____ | B _____ |
| Conjunctival hyperaemia | A _____ | B _____ | A _____ | B _____ | A _____ | B _____ |
| Visual fogging | A _____ | B _____ | A _____ | B _____ | A _____ | B _____ |
| Reduction of visual field | A _____ | B _____ | A _____ | B _____ | A _____ | B _____ |
| Phosphenes | A _____ | B _____ | A _____ | B _____ | A _____ | B _____ |
| Scintillating scotomata | A _____ | B _____ | A _____ | B _____ | A _____ | B _____ |
| Negative scotomata | A _____ | B _____ | A _____ | B _____ | A _____ | B _____ |
| Amblyopia | A _____ | B _____ | A _____ | B _____ | A _____ | B _____ |
| Fortification spectra | A _____ | B _____ | A _____ | B _____ | A _____ | B _____ |
| Disperceptions | A _____ | B _____ | A _____ | B _____ | A _____ | B _____ |
| Ptosis | A _____ | B _____ | A _____ | B _____ | A _____ | B _____ |
| Pallor | A _____ | B _____ | A _____ | B _____ | A _____ | B _____ |
| Blush | A _____ | B _____ | A _____ | B _____ | A _____ | B _____ |
| Feeling of heat/cold | A _____ | B _____ | A _____ | B _____ | A _____ | B _____ |
| Sweating | A _____ | B _____ | A _____ | B _____ | A _____ | B _____ |
| Rhinorrhoea | A _____ | B _____ | A _____ | B _____ | A _____ | B _____ |
| Sensation of closed nose | A _____ | B _____ | A _____ | B _____ | A _____ | B _____ |
| Lacrimation | A _____ | B _____ | A _____ | B _____ | A _____ | B _____ |
| Nausea | A _____ | B _____ | A _____ | B _____ | A _____ | B _____ |
| Vomiting | A _____ | B _____ | A _____ | B _____ | A _____ | B _____ |
| Abdominal pain | A _____ | B _____ | A _____ | B _____ | A _____ | B _____ |
| Fever | A _____ | B _____ | A _____ | B _____ | A _____ | B _____ |
| Changing moods | A _____ | B _____ | A _____ | B _____ | A _____ | B _____ |
| Crying | A _____ | B _____ | A _____ | B _____ | A _____ | B _____ |
| Insomnia | A _____ | B _____ | A _____ | B _____ | A _____ | B _____ |
| Hypersomnia | A _____ | B _____ | A _____ | B _____ | A _____ | B _____ |
| Irritability | A _____ | B _____ | A _____ | B _____ | A _____ | B _____ |
| Exhaustion | A _____ | B _____ | A _____ | B _____ | A _____ | B _____ |
| Phonophobia | A _____ | B _____ | A _____ | B _____ | A _____ | B _____ |
| Acuphenis | A _____ | B _____ | A _____ | B _____ | A _____ | B _____ |
| Vertigo | A _____ | B _____ | A _____ | B _____ | A _____ | B _____ |
| Lipothymia/syncope | A _____ | B _____ | A _____ | B _____ | A _____ | B _____ |
| Tachycardia | A _____ | B _____ | A _____ | B _____ | A _____ | B _____ |
| Dysarthria | A _____ | B _____ | A _____ | B _____ | A _____ | B _____ |
| Ataxia | A _____ | B _____ | A _____ | B _____ | A _____ | B _____ |
| Verbal expression deficit | A _____ | B _____ | A _____ | B _____ | A _____ | B _____ |
| Sensitive deficit | A _____ | B _____ | A _____ | B _____ | A _____ | B _____ |
| Motor deficit | A _____ | B _____ | A _____ | B _____ | A _____ | B _____ |
| Loss of consciousness | A _____ | B _____ | A _____ | B _____ | A _____ | B _____ |
| Sensorium blackout | A _____ | B _____ | A _____ | B _____ | A _____ | B _____ |

Triggering factors: absent = 0; emotional stress = 1; physical stress = 2; food = 3; menstruation = 4; other factors = 5.

A _____ B _____

Which _____

Relieving factors: absent = 0; rest or sleep = 1; eating = 2; others = 3.

A _____ B _____

Which _____

Worsening factors: absent = 0; physical stress = 1; cough = 2; changing position of the head = 3; getting up from bed = 4; others = 5.

A _____ B _____

Which _____

**Clinical tests and instrumental investigations:**

Objective examination:          normal _____ altered _____

Neurological examination:          normal _____ altered _____

Laboratory examinations:          not carried out _____ normal _____ altered _____

Head radiographs:          not carried out _____ normal _____ altered _____

Intercritical EEG:          not carried out _____ in the limits _____

altered in an unspecific way _____

altered in a specific way _____

Critical EEG:          not carried out _____ in the limits _____

altered in an unspecific way _____

altered in a specific way _____

Intercritical transcranial Doppler:          not carried out _____ normal _____ altered _____

Critical transcranial Doppler:          not carried out _____ normal _____ altered _____

CT scan:          not carried out _____ normal _____ altered _____

NMR:          not carried out _____ normal _____ altered _____

**Drugs** (acute attacks therapy)          NO _____ YES _____

Which _____

**Drugs** (prophylactic therapy)          NO _____ YES _____

Which _____

## PRESENT DIAGNOSIS:

A _____ B _____

(for the diagnosis look at enclosure 2)

**Number of school absences:**

in the present school year: days of absence/school days:

_____/_____

in the last school year: days of absence/school days:

_____/_____

Interruption of school attendance for headache:

YES _____ NO _____

# Index

Page references for illustrations are in italics, and italics followed by t for tables